STATUS OF KETAMINE IN ANESTHESIOLOGY

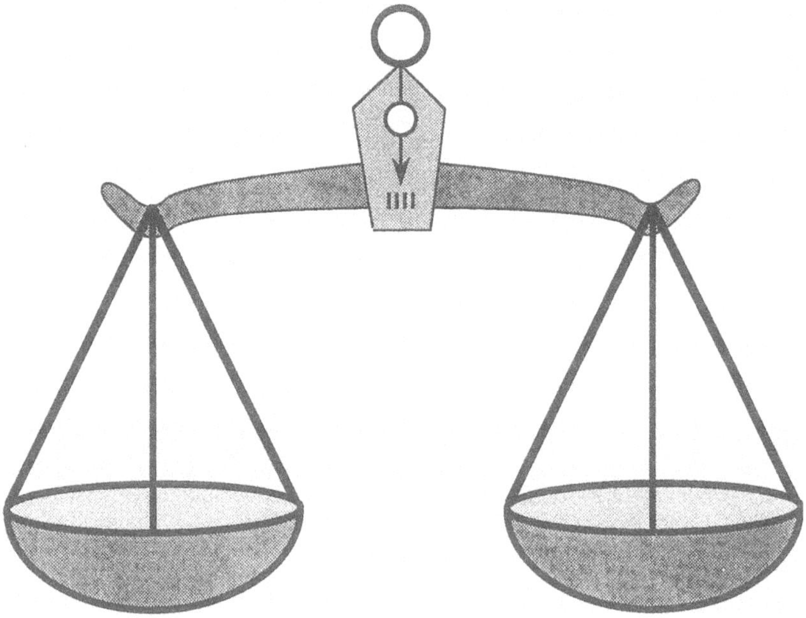

EDWARD F. DOMINO, EDITOR

Intenational Standard Book Number-13 978-0916182-31-1
Original ISBN 978-0916182-07-6
Library of Congress Catalog Card Number 89-92147

This book may be purchased through online websites, bookstores,
or directly from the publisher,
NPP Books, 15 Sunset Road, Arlington, MA 02474, U.S.A.

Nppbooks.com

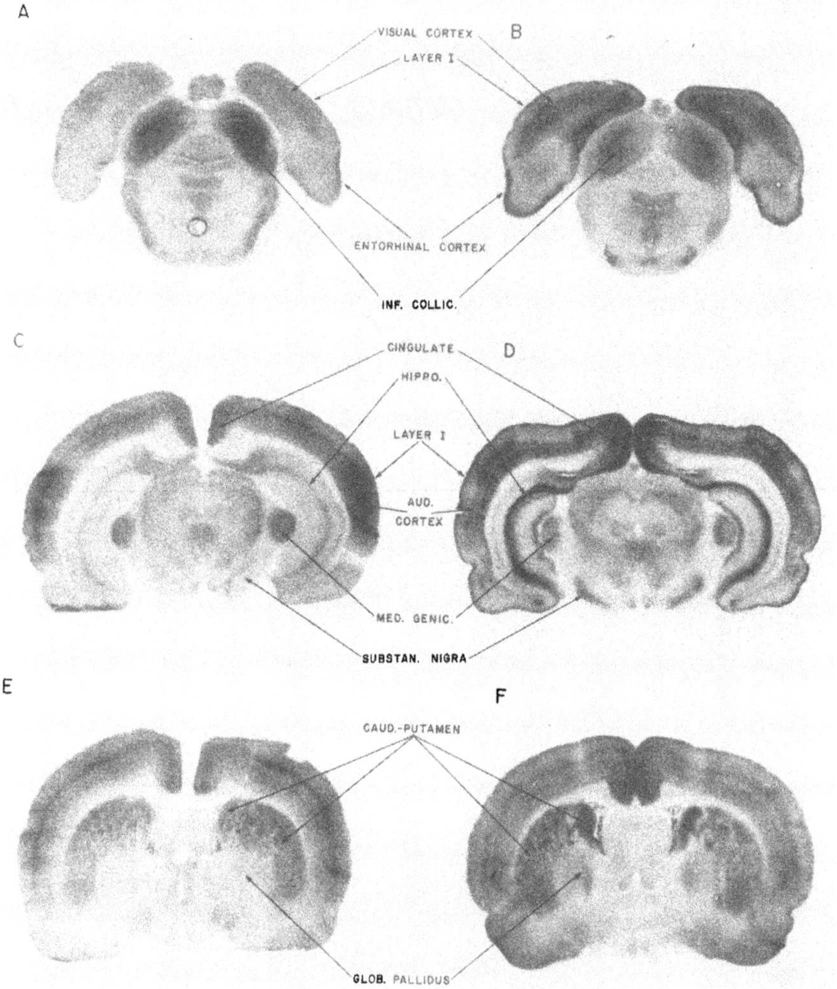

ACKNOWLEDGEMENT

The colored photograph on the front cover and the figure above are of autoradiographs of brain sections from control (left) and 30 mg/kg i.v. ketamine treated (right) rats. They are reproduced with permission of the authors, journal editor and publisher (Crosby, G., Crane, A.M. and Sokoloff, L.: Local changes in cerebral glucose utilization during ketamine anesthesia. Anesthesiol. 56:437-443, 1982.) Colorizing from the black and white original was kindly performed by A.B. Young, University of Michigan, Ann Arbor, MI 48104-1687. The editor gratefully acknowledges their cooperation.

Participants of the 25th Anniversary Symposium

Status of Ketamine in Anesthesiology
The University of Michigan, Ann Arbor, MI
June 19-21, 1989

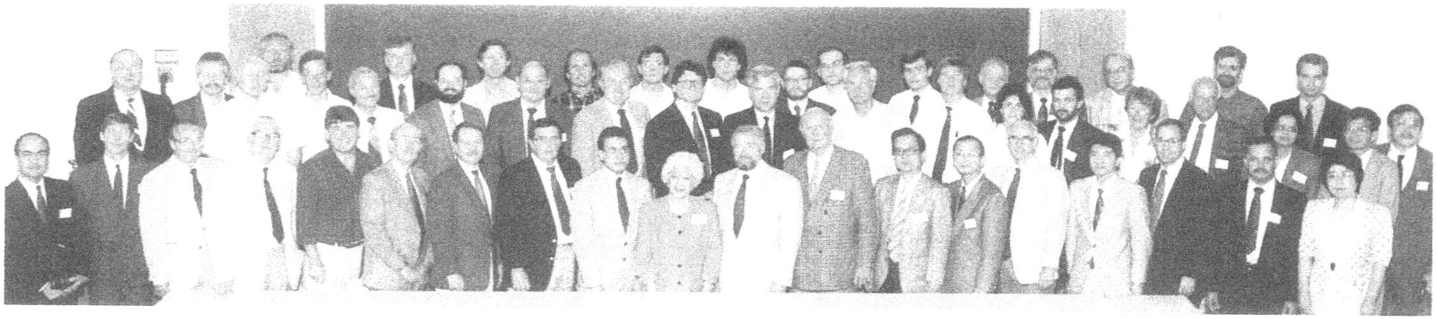

Row one (L-R): O.E. El-Khateeb, O. Brandicourt, E.K. Zsigmond, J.W. Dundee, A.J. Trevor, M.S. Albin, D.C. Sawyer, D.J. Smith, R.F. Ghaly, L.R. Reyes de Castro, H. Kreuscher, G. Corssen, H. Suzuki, J. Tatsuno, A. Doenicke, M. Irifune, S.M. Shulman, K. Ramabadran, W. Hanaoka

Row two (L-R): W.D. Winters, H.W. Gervais, W.L. Way, L. Tokics, N.E. Johnson, L. Domino, E.F. Domino, T.H. Stanley, W. Tolksdorf, D. Quade, B. Gebhardt, R. Klose, F.W. Marcoux, B. Calvo, J.L. Pedraz, G. Schulte-Steinberg, O. Schulte-Steinberg, U. Mahisekar, C. Lee, K. Hanaoka

Row three (L-R): J.P. Jantzen, L.B. Jones, A. Maurset, D.D. Rigamonti, J. Church, U.B. Hoppe, H.A. Adams, M.D. Kelland, K. Eyrich, E. Pfenninger, J. Idvall, H. Suttman, P. Migaly

Status of Ketamine in Anesthesiology

Proceedings of the 25th Anniversary of Ketamine Symposium held at the University of Michigan in Ann Arbor, MI June 19-21, 1989

Sponsors

The Symposium was sponsored by the Departments of Anesthesiology and Pharmacology of the University of Michigan Medical School and the University of Michigan School of Dentistry. The Symposium supporters included: Merck, Sharp & Dohme Research Laboratories, NPP Books, Parke Davis, Division of Warner Lambert, Morris Plains, NJ, Parke-Davis and Co., Berlin, Federal Republic of Germany, Pfizer Central Research, Groton, CT, Roche Laboratories, Hoffmann-LaRoche, Inc., Nutley, NJ, University of Michigan Department of Anesthesiology, University of Michigan Department of Pharmacology, University of Michigan Office of Vice President for Research, The Upjohn Company, Warner Lambert/Parke Davis Pharmaceutical Research Division, Ann Arbor, MI, Warner-Lambert International Operations, Morris Plains, NJ.

Facilities

The facilities of the University of Michigan School of Dentistry provided an ideal setting for presentations, discussion and exchange of ideas among all of the participants. The entire scientific program was video taped and is available on standard ½ inch VHS cassettes. Arrangements can be made for their purchase from the University of Michigan by contacting the editor.

The facilities of the University of Michigan League were utilized for the reception, poster session and banquet. The color collages on the two following pages represent selected photographs of some of these events.

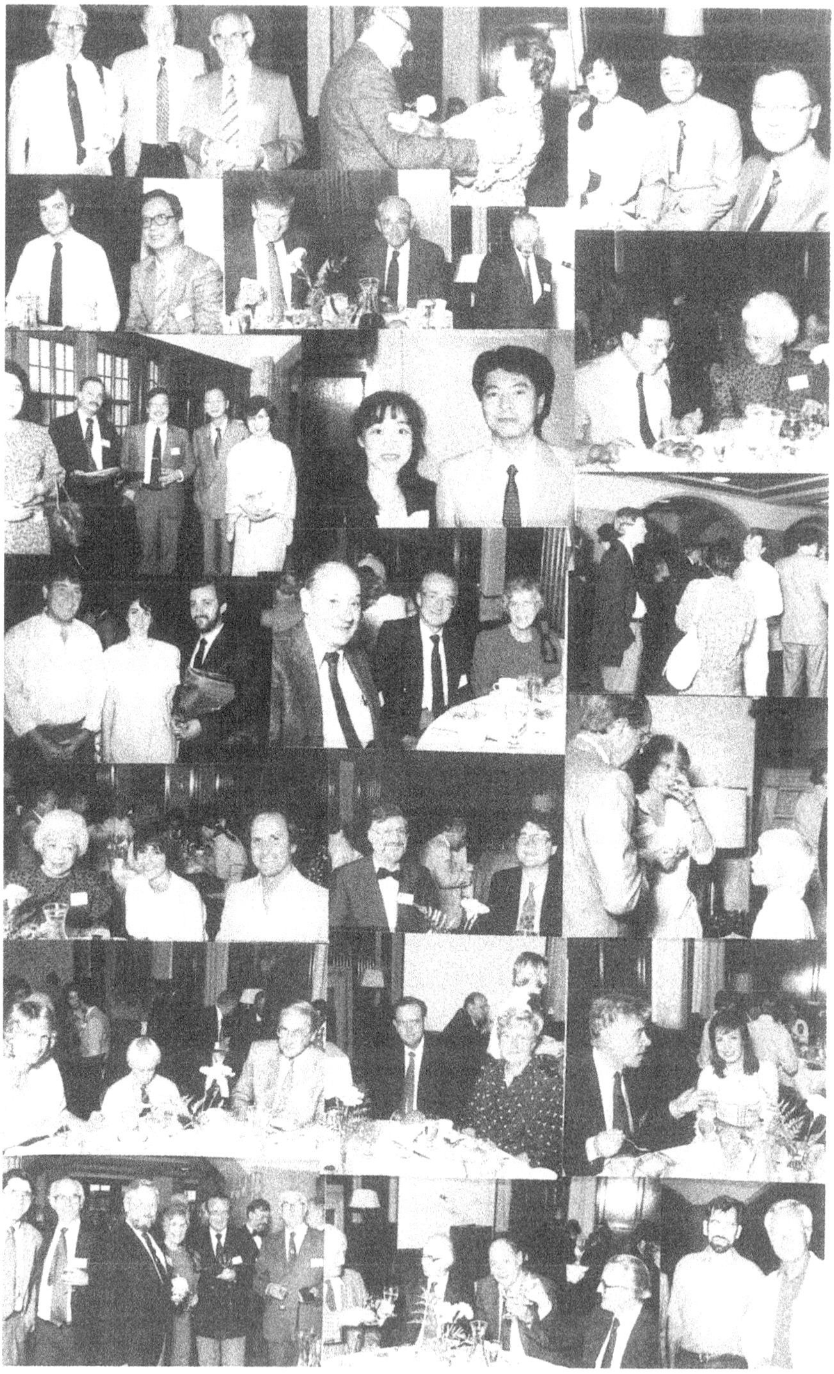

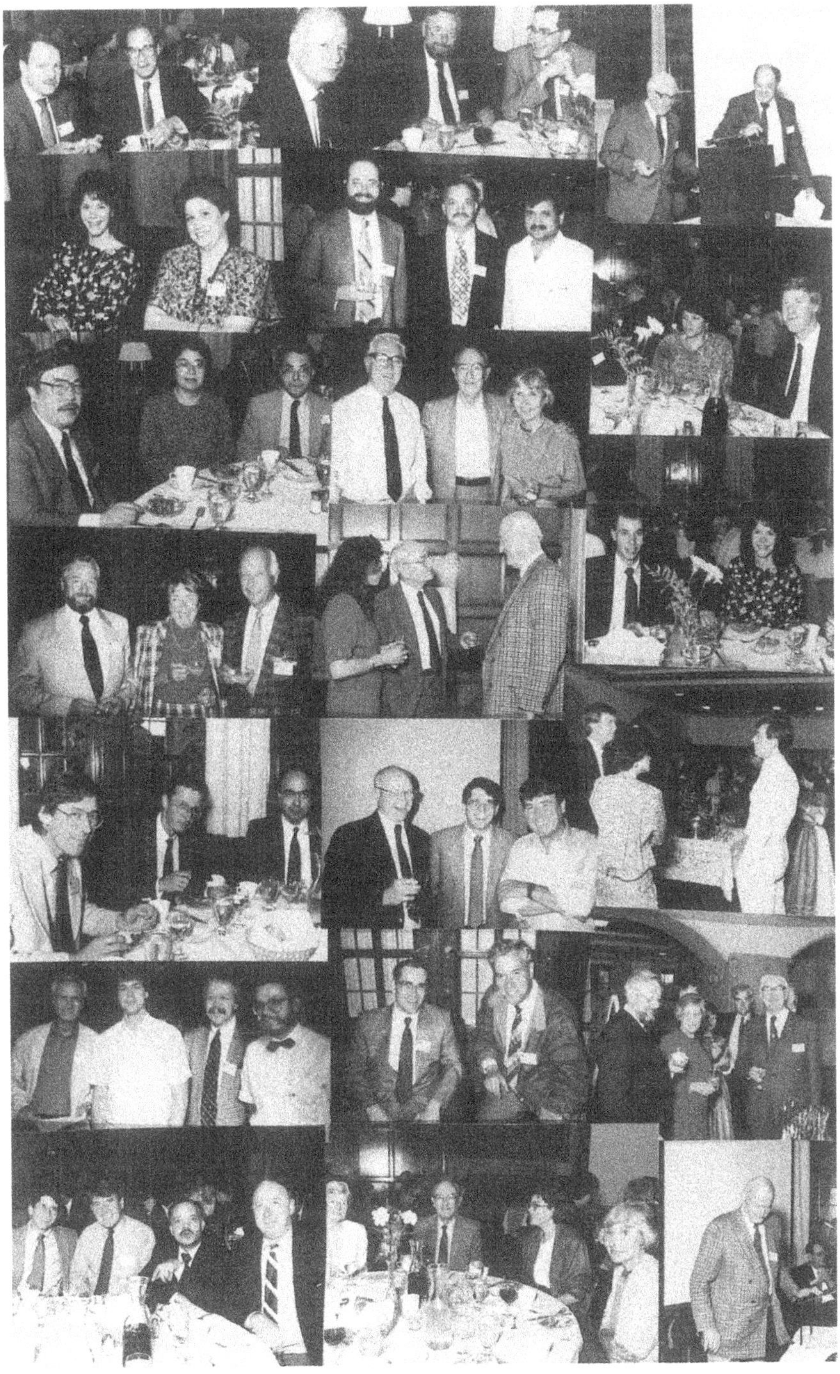

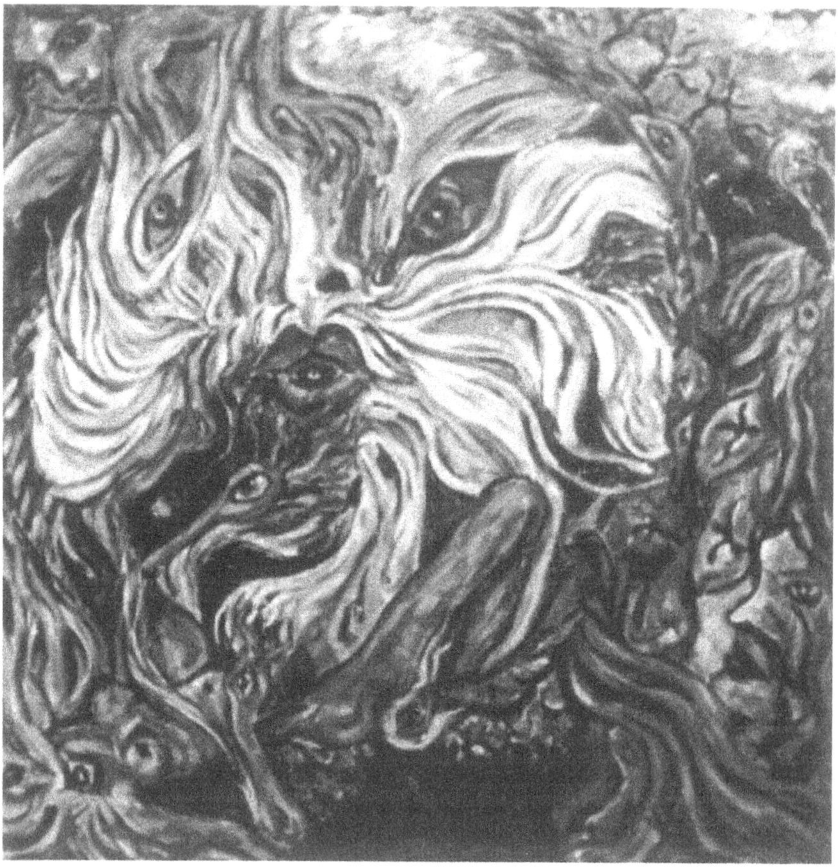

Sixteen years ago a patient was given ketamine anesthesia as part of a study conducted by Dr. Elemer Zsigmond. When the patient recovered she was asked what kind of "dreams" she experienced. At the time she was not able to fully express in words her experience under ketamine anesthesia. But it did inspire her to do a painting of her "dream." It was a "heavy experience, but a beautiful one" to her. (Courtesy of Dr. Zsigmond.)

Preface

The chapters in this book represent almost all of the presentations at the Twenty-Fifth Anniversary of Ketamine Symposium held in Ann Arbor, June 19-21, 1989 at the University of Michigan. About 82 U.S. and international scientists gave oral and poster presentations covering various aspects of this Symposium. All participants were asked to present their findings in a critical manner regarding the pros and cons of ketamine use in anesthesiology today. Clearly, ketamine is not the ideal anesthetic anesthesiologists dream will become a reality, nor is it the nightmare that many believe, at least in the United States. There is a place for ketamine in anesthesiology. The purpose of the twenty fifth anniversary ketamine symposium was to define what that place is today.

Seven sessions were held including: I. Historical and Present Perspectives; II. Biotransformation and Pharmacology; III. Analgesic Actions; IV. Pharmacokinetics; V. Clinical Applications; VI. Problems and Modern Uses; VII. New Basic Science Developments: NMDA Antagonist Actions and Neuroprotective Effects. These form the basis for the organization of this book.

The editor would like to thank Mrs. Ellen Howard and numerous students for their efforts in helping to ready this book for publication.

January 2, 1990

Edward F. Domino
Department of Pharmacology
University of Michigan
Ann Arbor, Michigan
48109-0626
U.S.A.

Notice

The authors and publisher have taken great care in an attempt to provide all information regarding dosage, side effects, indications, etc. of ketamine and other drugs described in this book to the best of their abilities. Errors may occur that have been overlooked. As a result, it is extremely important that any person planning to administer ketamine should obtain detailed instructions from persons experienced with its use as well as consulting appropriate package insert information, etc. The information contained in this book should be used merely as a guideline to supplement first hand knowledge and experience with the use of ketamine and other drugs. Although ketamine has a large therapeutic index compared to other anesthetic agents, when given alone it has significant and serious side effects that require the attention of one experienced with anesthetic and airway management.

Participants

H.A. Adams, M.D.
Department of Anesthesiology and Intensive Care
University Hospital Giessen
Klinikstr. 29
D-6300 Giessen, F.R. Germany

M.S. Albin, M.D.
Department of Anesthesiology
The University of Texas Health Science Center at San Antonio
7703 Floyd Curl Drive
San Antonio, TX 78284-7838

P.A. Boxer, Ph.D.
Warner Lambert/Parke Davis
Pharmaceutical Research Division
2800 Plymouth Road
Ann Arbor, MI 48105

P. Brandicourt, M.D.
Parke-Davis
11 Ave Dubonnet
92407 Courbevoie
Paris, Cedex, France

B. Calvo, Ph.D.
Department of Pharmacy
Faculty of Pharmacy
University of Salamanca
Salamanca, Spain

D.W. Choi, M.D., Ph.D.
Department of Neurology
Stanford University Medical School
Stanford, CA 94305

J. Church, M.D., Ph.D.
Departments of Physiology and Anesthesiology
University of British Columbia
2146 Health Sciences Mall
Vancouver, B.C., Canada V6T 1W5

G. Corssen, M.D.
The Pain Control Center of Arizona
13200 N. 103rd Avenue
Suite 10
Sun City, AZ 85351

L. Coughenour, B.S.
Warner Lambert/Parke Davis
Pharmaceutical Research Division
2800 Plymouth Road
Ann Arbor, MI 48105

A. Doenicke, M.D.
Institute of Anesthesiology of the University of Munich
Pettenkoferstr. 8A
D-8000 Munich 2, F.R. Germany

E.F. Domino, M.D.
Department of Pharmacology
M6414 Medical Science Bldg. I
University of Michigan
Ann Arbor, MI 48109-0626

L. E. Domino, M.D.
Department of Psychiatry
University of Alabama at Birmingham
Birmingham, AL 35294

J.W. Dundee, O.B.E., M.D., Ph.D.
The Oaks
24 Old Coach Road
Belfast BT9 5PR, Northern Ireland

O.E. El-Khateeb, M.D.
Anesthesia and ICU Department
Jahra Hospital
P.O. Box 40206
Jahra 01753, Kuwait

K. Eyrich, M.D.
Departments of Anesthesiology and Operative Intensive Care Medicine
The Steglitz Medical Center of the Free University of Berlin
Hindenburgdamm 30
D-1000 Berlin 45, F.R. Germany

I. Feller, M.D.
Department of Surgery
University Hospital 1B401
The University of Michigan
Ann Arbor, MI 48109-0033

J. Finch, M.D.
Department of Anesthesiology
University Hospital 1G323
The University of Michigan
Ann Arbor, MI 48109-0048

A.S. Freeman, Ph.D.
Center for Cell Biology
Sinai Hospital of Detroit
6767 W. Outer Drive
Detroit, MI 48235-2899

B. Gebhardt, M.D.
Medical Affairs Department
Parke-Davis and Company
Postfach 5620
7800 Freiburg, F.R. Germany

H.W. Gervais, M.D.
Department of Anesthesiology
Johannes Gutenberg University
Langenbeckstr. 1
D-6500 Mainz 1, F.R. Germany

R.F. Ghaly, M.D.
Department of Anesthesiology and Critical Care
Cook County Hospital
1835 W. Harrison St.
Chicago, IL 60612-9985

B. Giordani, Ph.D.
University of Michigan Medical Center
Med-Inn, Rm. 480
1500 E. Medical Center Dr.
Ann Arbor, MI 48109-0804

D.J. Gole, Ph.D.
Mediventure
655 Phoenix
Ann Arbor, MI 48104

G. Griffin, D.V.M., M.S.
Warner Lambert/Parke Davis Pharmaceutical Research Division
2800 Plymouth Road
Ann Arbor, MI 48105

K. Hanaoka, M.D., Ph.D.
Department of Anesthesiology
Tokyo University Branch Hospital
3-28-6 Mejirodai
Bunkyo-ku
Tokyo 112, Japan

U.B. Hoppe, M.D.
Department of Anesthesiology and Intensive Care Medicine
BG Unfallklinik
Ludwig Guttmannstrasse 13
6700 Ludwigshafen 25, F.R. Germany

H. I'Awson, Ph.D.
Reproductive Sciences Program
University of Michigan
300 N. Ingalls
Ann Arbor, MI 48109-0404

J. Idvall, M.D.
Department of Anesthesiology
Malmo General Hospital
S-214 01 Malmo, Sweden

M. Irifune, D.D.S.
Department of Pharmacology
Faculty of Medicine
Kagoshima University
Kagoshima 890, Japan

J.P. Jantzen, M.D., Ph.D., DEAA
Clinic for Anesthesiology
Johannes Gutenberg University
Langenbeckstrasse 1
D-6500 Mainz, F.R. Germany

N.E. Johnson, M.D., M.P.H.
Department of Emergency Medicine
Loma Linda University Medical Center
11234 Anderson St.
Loma Linda, CA 92350

L.B. Jones
Anaquest
2005 West Beltline Highway
Madison, WI 53713

M.D. Kelland, Ph.D.
Center for Cell Biology
Sinai Research Institute
6767 W. Outer Drive
Detroit, MI 48235

R. Klose, M.D.
Department of Anesthesiology
and Intensive Care Medicine
BG Unfallklinik
Ludwig Guttmannstrasse 13
6700 Ludwigshafen 25, F.R. Germany

H. Kreuscher, M.D.
Department of Anesthesiology
Stadt Kliniken Osnabruck
Natruper-Tor Wall 1
D4500 Osnabruck, F.R. Germany

J.V. Kyff, D.O.
Department of Anesthesiology
University Hospital 1G323
The University of Michigan
Ann Arbor, MI 48109-0048

C. Lee, M.D.
Department of Anesthesiology
School of Medicine
Harbor-UCLA Medical Center
1000 W. Carson Street
Torrance, CA 90509

P. Lipton, Ph.D.
Department of Physiology
University of Wisconsin-Madison
Medical School
225 Services Memorial Institute
Madison, WI 53706

D. Lodge, Ph.D.
Department of Physiology
The Royal Veterinary College
University of London
Royal College Street
London NW1 OTU,
United Kingdom

U. Mahisekar, M.D.
Department of Anesthesiology
The University of Illinois
College of Medicine at Chicago
1740 West Taylor Street
Chicago, IL 60612

F.W. Marcoux, Ph.D.
Department of Pharmacology
Warner Lambert/Parke Davis
Pharmaceutical Research Division
2800 Plymouth Road
Ann Arbor, MI 48105-2430

A. Maurset, M.D.
Department of Pharmacology
University of Oslo
P.O. Box 1057 Blindern
Oslo 3, Norway 0316

P. Migaly, M.D.
31600 Harlo, Apt. 3-F
Madison Heights, MI 48071

J.L. Pedraz, Ph.D.
Department of Pharmacy
Faculty of Pharmacy
University of Salamanca
Salamanca, Spain

E. Pfenninger, M.D.
University Clinic of Anesthesiology
University of Ulm
Albert Einstein Allee 11
D-7900 Ulm, F.R. Germany

S.J. Pryn, M.D.
University of Michigan Medical Center
Section of Pediatric Anesthesiology
Mott Children's Hospital
OPB Room C 4139
Ann Arbor, MI 48109-0800

D. Quade
Marketing Department
Parke-Davis and Company
Postfach 5620
7800 Freiburg, F.R. Germany

L.L. Radulovic, Ph.D.
Warner Lambert/Parke Davis
Pharmaceutical Research Division
2800 Plymouth Road
Ann Arbor, MI 48105

K. Ramabadran, Ph.D.
Department 426, AP-9A
Abbott Laboratories
Abbott Park, IL 60064

L.R. Reyes de Castro, M.D.
Division of Anesthesiology
University of Santo Tomas
Manila, The Philippines

D.D. Rigamonti, Ph.D.
Walter Reed Medical Center, Bldg. 40
WRAIR, Department of Medical Neuroscience
Washington, D.C. 20012

L. Robichaud, B.S.
Warner Lambert/Parke Davis
Pharmaceutical Research Division
2800 Plymouth Road
Ann Arbor, MI 48105

D.A. Rosen, M.D.
Department of Anesthesia, Pediatrics, and Communicable Disease
University of Michigan Medical Center
Ann Arbor, MI 48109

S.Y. Sakurai, B.S.
Neuroscience Laboratory
University of Michigan
1108 E. Huron
Ann Arbor, MI 48109-1687

D.C. Sawyer, D.V.M., Ph.D.
A-132 E. Fee Hall
College of Veterinary Medicine
Michigan State University
East Lansing, MI 48824-1316

O. Schulte Steinberg, M.D.
Dietrichweide 7
8130 Starnberg 2, F.R. Germany

T. Steinberg, M.D.
Dietrichweide 7
8130 Starnberg 2, F.R. Germany

S.M. Shulman, M.D.
Department of Anesthesiology
Columbia Presbyterian Medical Center
630 West 168th Street
New York, NY 10032

D.J. Smith, Ph.D.
Department of Anesthesiology
West Virginia University
Health Sciences Center
Morgantown, WV 26506

T.H. Stanley, M.D.
Department of Anesthesiology
University of Utah
50 North Medical Drive
Salt Lake City, UT 84132

H. Suttmann, M.D.
Institute of Anesthesiology
University of Munich
Pettenkoferstr. 8A
D-8000 Munich 2, F.R. Germany

H. Suzuki, M.D.
Department of Anesthesiology
Tokyo Women's Medical College
8-1 Kawada-cho
Shinjuku-ku
Tokyo, Japan

J. Tatsuno, M.D.
Department of Physiology II
National Defense Medical College
3-2, Namiki
Tokorozawa, Saitama
359, Japan

L. Tokics, M.D.
Department of Anesthesiology
Huddinge University Hospital
S-14186 Huddinge, Sweden

W. Tolksdorf, M.D.
Clinic for Anesthesiology
Medical Faculty
University of Technology
D-5100 Aachen, F.R. Germany

A.J. Trevor, Ph.D.
Department of Pharmacology
University of California
School of Medicine
San Francisco, CA 94143

K.J. Tuman, M.D.
Department of Anesthesiology
Rush-Presbyterian-St. Luke's Medical College
1753 West Congress Parkway
Chicago, IL 60612

W.L. Way, M.D.
Department of Anesthesiology (C-455)
University of California
School of Medicine
San Francisco, CA 94143-0648

P.F. White, M.D.
Department of Anesthesiology
Washington University School of Medicine
Box 8054
660 S. Euclid Avenue
St. Louis, MO 63110

W.D. Winters, M.D., Ph.D.
Department of Pharmacology
University of California-Davis
School of Medicine
Davis, CA 95616

T.F. Woolf, Ph.D.
Department of Drug Metabolism/Pharmacology
Warner Lambert/Parke Davis
Pharmaceutical Research Division
2800 Plymouth Road
Ann Arbor, MI 48105

E.K. Zsigmond, M.D.
Department of Anesthesiology
The University of Illinois
College of Medicine at Chicago
1740 West Taylor Street
Chicago, IL 60612

Table of Contents

Section I. Historical and Present Perspectives

Section II. Biotransformation and Pharmacology

Section VI. Problems and Modern Uses

Status of Ketamine in Anesthesiology,
edited by E.F. Domino©1990, NPP Books
P.O. Box 1491, Ann Arbor, MI 48106

Historical Aspects of Ketamine—First Clinical Experience

G. Corssen

Central Arizona Anesthesiology, Ltd.
Scottsdale, AR

The synthesis of phencyclidine (CI-395, PCP, Sernyl, Sernylan) by Maddox (1981), laboratory testing by Chen *et al.* (1959), and clinical testing by Greifenstein *et al.* (1958) and Johnstone *et al.* (1959) provided the basis for human pharmacologic studies and clinical exploration of the chloroketone analogue of PCP, CI-581, later known as ketamine (Ketalar, Ketaject). Ketamine was synthesized by Stephens (1963) and initial laboratory testing with CI-581 was conducted by McCarthy *et al.* (1965). This was followed by human pharmacologic studies carried out by Domino and Corssen and their associates (Domino *et al.*, 1965). Clinical trials were begun in 1964 and the first clinical experience in 130 patients was reported by Corssen and Domino (1966). At that time, the authors introduced the term "dissociative anesthesia" to describe the peculiar state of unconsciousness produced by ketamine in which the subject is profoundly analgesic and in a trance-like state, not appearing to be asleep or anesthetized, but rather disconnected from the surroundings. Corssen and Domino attributed the special features of this state to a dissociation between the thalamoneocortical and the limbic systems. Since visual and somatosensory impulses travel unimpaired from the periphery to the primary sènsory cortex, it appeared that the sensory isolation occurred within the brain, presumably in the association areas. The authors postulated that under the effect of ketamine the patient is unable to interpret impulses and make the appropriate response; therefore, there is no reaction to light impulses introduced into the eye nor to pain impulses that ordinarily would be evoked by surgical stimulation (Fig. 1).

In subsequent studies conducted in primates at the University of Alabama in Birmingham (Sparkes *et al.*, 1973, 1975), the effects of ketamine on visually evoked potentials recorded from the visual cortex were compared with those recorded from non-specific midbrain and

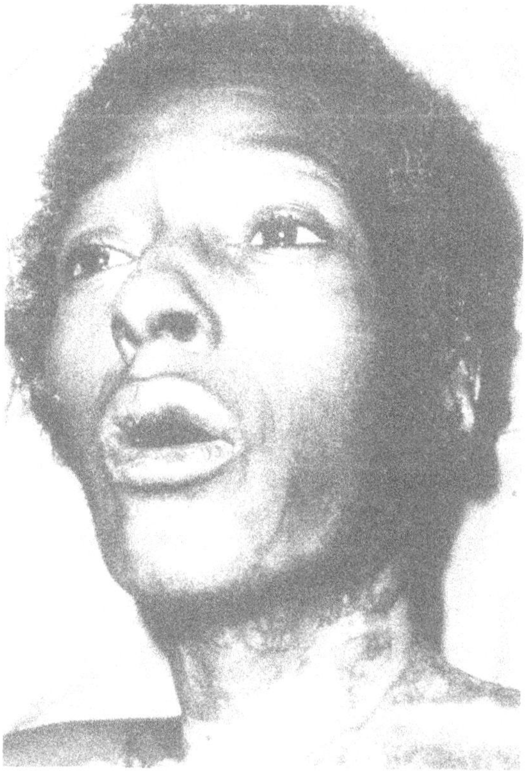

Fig. 1. Patient anesthetized with ketamine.

thalamic areas. The results indicated that the diffuse neocortical projection system is the primary site of action of ketamine. Furthermore, the results showed that the profound analgesic action of the drug probably results from the functional disorganization of nonspecific pathways in midbrain and thalamic areas.

Initial experiences with the clinical use of ketamine at the University of Michigan, and later at the University of Alabama, corroborated the observations made earlier in human volunteers; namely, that ketamine differs markedly from conventional intravenous and inhalational anesthetic agents. This difference results from its selective, dissociative action on the central nervous system which produces a unique anesthetic state characterized by profound analgesia, cardiovascular stimulation, lack of respiratory depression, maintenance of protective reflexes and amnesia.

Early during the exploratory use of ketamine in surgical patients, it became apparent that the drug was particularly suitable when the procedure involved skin, bone, and joints (Corssen *et al.*, 1968). Therefore, ketamine was successfully employed in body surface procedures such as wound debridement and skin grafting in burn therapy. Also, repetitive orotracheal intubation could be avoided in the surgical treatment of thermal injury since preservation of the laryngo-pharyngeal reflexes under ketamine anesthesia facilitated the maintenance of an unobstructed airway. For the same reason, positional problems often encountered during radiodiagnostic and radiotherapeutic procedures in infants and in children were largely overcome by ketamine's ability to preserve airway patency.

The sympathomimetic effects of ketamine (increases in cardiac output, pulse rate, and systolic and diastolic pressures) may be of benefit in the anesthetic management of poor risk patients. In particular, these effects may benefit patients suffering from hypovolemic shock following massive hemorrhage where transfusion cannot promptly restore the blood volume and where temporary improvement of cardiovascular function is of vital importance (Corssen *et al.*, 1974). We also found ketamine suitable as the sole anesthetic or in combination with nitrous oxide-oxygen for pain control during cardiac surgery, especially in infants and children (Corssen *et al.*, 1970).

Ketamine is an excellent bronchodilator and may be the anesthetic of choice for induction of anesthesia in the asthmatic. We have successfully administered ketamine by i.v. infusion to terminate an asthma attack after conventional methods of treatment failed (Corssen *et al.*, 1972).

When administered in subanesthetic amounts, a painless state is produced without loss of consciousness in which shortlasting ambulatory surgery and dental procedures may be performed. Being water soluble, ketamine does not irritate veins and does not cause pain on injection. When administered i.m., the drug is rapidly absorbed without local irritation or induration. During our initial human pharmacologic and clinical trials, ketamine's psychedelic properties presented a drawback, particularly in the human volunteers in whom any type of preanesthetic medication was omitted. In fact, emergence reactions of agitation, delusions, illusions, hallucinations, and delirium occurred with such frequency in the volunteers and, to a lesser degree, in surgical patients who received commonly used preanesthetic medication, that we began to have serious doubts of successfully introducing ketamine as a clinically useful anesthetic.

Other disadvantageous properties of ketamine which were of concern to us during the first months of clinical usage included its tendency to raise intracranial pressure and to produce hypertonicity, causing involuntary muscle movements and profuse salivation. Therefore, we became increasingly more aware of the need to find methods and drugs to eliminate or attenuate the ketamine-induced undesirable and potentially dangerous effects.

Efforts to reduce the adverse effects of ketamine became partially successful by including various combinations of opiates, tranquilizers and belladonna drugs in the preanesthetic medication. Droperidol appeared to be especially effective in providing preanesthetic tranquility, reducing the incidence of unpleasant dreams under ketamine anesthetic, and terminating acute psychomotor emergence reactions. A real breakthrough in effectively "taming" ketamine by minimizing the incidence and degree of emergence psychic phenomena and reducing its adverse cardiovascular and musculo-skeletal effects came with the use of diazepam and its derivatives administered before, during, or after ketamine anesthesia (Coppel *et al.*, 1973).

It appears that most of our initial skepticism and doubts regarding ketamine's role as a general anesthetic have gradually been overcome and the drug has found its place as an unusually safe, rapidly acting parenteral anesthetic. Naturally, we fully agree with M. Johnstone, as quoted by T. Boulton (1987) of Reading, United Kingdom, that ketamine is probably the most important advance in the symptomatic treatment of pain since the discovery of aspirin.

References

Boulton, T.B.: Twenty years of dissociative anesthesia with ketamine (CI-581). Its origin and present significance. Survey of Anesthesiol. 31: 62-67, 1987.

Chen, G., Ensor, C.R., Russell, D., and Bohner, B.: The pharmacology of 1-(1-phenylcyclohexyl) piperidine HCl. J. Pharm. Exp. Ther. 127: 241, 1959.

Coppel, D.L., Bovill, J.G., and Dundee, J.W.: The taming of ketamine. Anaesthesia 28: 293, 1973.

Corssen, G.: Recent developments in the anesthetic management of burned patients. J. Trauma 7: 152, 1967.

Corssen, G., Allarde, R., Brosch, F., and Arbenz, G.: Ketamine as the sole anesthetic in open heart surgery. A preliminary report. Anesth. Analg. 49: 1025, 1970.

Corssen, G. and Domino, E.F.: Dissociative anesthesia: Further pharmacologic studies and first clinical experience with the phencyclidine derivative CI-581. Anesth. Analg. 45: 29, 1966.

Corssen, G., Gutierrez, J., Reves, J.G., and Huber, F.C.: Ketamine in the anesthetic management of asthmatic patients. Anesth. Analg. 51: 588, 1972.

Corssen, G., Miyasaka, M., and Domino, E.F.: Changing concepts in pain control during surgery: Dissociative anesthesia with CI-581: A progress report. Anesth. Analg. 47: 746, 1968.

Corssen, G., Reves, J.G., and Carter, J.R.: Neuroleptanesthesia, dissociative anesthesia and hemorrhage. Int. Anesth. Clin. 12: 145, 1974.

Domino, E.F., Chodoff, P., and Corssen, G.: Pharmacologic effects of CI-581, a new dissociative anesthetic in man. Clin. Pharmacol. Ther. 6: 279, 1965.

Greifenstein, F.E., DeVault, M., Yoshitake, J., and Gajewski, J.R.: A study of 1-aryl cyclohexyl amine for anesthesia. Anesth. Analg. 37: 283, 1958.

Johnstone, M., Evans, V., and Baigel, J.R.: Sernyl (CI-395) in clinical anesthesia. Brit. J. Anaesth. 31: 433, 1959.

Maddox, V.H.: The historical development of phencyclidine. In PCP (Phencyclidine): Historical and Current Perspectives. E.F. Domino, ed., pp. 1-8, NPP Books, Ann Arbor, 1981.

McCarthy, D.A., Chen, G., Kaump, D.H., and Ensor, C.: General anesthetic and other pharmacologic properties of 2-(o-chlorophenyl)-2-methylamino cyclohexanone HCl (CI-581). J. New Drugs 5: 21, 1965.

Sparkes, D.L., Corssen, G., Aizenman, B., and Black, J.: Further studies of the neural mechanisms of ketamine-induced anesthesia in the rhesus monkey. Anesth. Analg. 54: 189, 1975.

Sparkes, D.L., Corssen, G., Sides, J., Black, J., and Kholeif, A.: Ketamine-induced anesthesia: neural mechanisms in the rhesus monkey. Anesth. Analg. 52: 288, 1973.

Status of Ketamine in Anesthesiology,
edited by E.F. Domino©1990, NPP Books
P.O. Box 1491, Ann Arbor, MI 48106

Early British Experience with Ketamine

J.W. Dundee

Department of Anaesthetics
The Queen's University of Belfast
Northern Ireland

Ketamine had a long "gestation period" by standards of the 1960's. Almost 5 yr elapsed since the description of its pharmacology by Chen (1965) and McCarthy and associates (1965) and the clinical pharmacologic studies of Domino *et al.* (1965) and its clinical launch in North America. There was a prolific spate of American publications in early 1970, reflecting studies carried out in 1968-69, some of which drew attention to side effects both during (hypertension, tachycardia and hypertonus) and after anesthesia (emergence delirium and dreams).

The present requirements for organized clinical trials in the country of use, and consideration of reports by the national drug regulatory organization—Committee on Safety of Medicines (CSM) in the UK—equivalent to Federal Drug Administration (FDA) in the USA—did not exist in Britain 30 yr ago. A pharmaceutical firm could provide data in an "investigator's manual", based on studies carried out elsewhere. This happened when ketamine was introduced in Britain late in 1969 and early 1970.

A chemically similar drug, phencyclidine (CI-395, Sernyl) also introduced by Chen and colleagues (1959), was studied by Johnstone *et al.* from the Manchester Royal Infirmary in England. Their report, published in 1959, described its effects in 67 patients. Greifenstein and De Vault (1958) described maniacal excitement following surgery under phencyclidine lasting up to 3 hr. The significance of these findings, in relation to ketamine, was not appreciated at the time.

One can say without much doubt the introduction of ketamine into Britain was a "disaster" from which the drug never recovered. Yet it was one from which many lessons have been learned. The reasons for this fiasco are reviewed. Table 1 summarizes the information available to initial British investigators. Table 2 gives the manufacturer's main indications for the use of ketamine.

The wording of Table 1 caused much concern with the early British

TABLE 1. Guidelines available for the first British use of ketamine

1. Rapidly acting nonbarbiturate general anesthesia (manufacturer's brochure).
2. Producing "dissociative anesthesia" characterized by complete analgesia with only superficial sleep (Corssen and Domino, 1966).
3. A compound with a cataleptic analgesic and anesthetic action, but without hypnotic properties.
4. Catalepsy = a characteristic akinetic state, with a loss of orthostatic reflexes, but without impairment of consciousness (Chen, 1965).

TABLE 2. Early recommended indications for the use of ketamine

1. As the sole anesthetic agent for diagnostic and surgical procedures. Although best suited for short procedures, it can be used with additional doses, in procedures requiring anesthesia for periods of 6 hr or longer.
2. For the induction of anesthesia prior to the administration of other general anesthetic agents.
3. To supplement low potency agents such as nitrous oxide.

(From the literature supplied to clinical investigators in Britain)

anesthetists. First, a recognized classification (Dundee and Wyant, 1974) divides intravenous anesthetics into rapidly acting and slower acting. Rapidly acting drugs will, in adequate doses, induce loss of consciousness in one arm-brain circulation time. When injected as a bolus at the height of forearm reactive hyperemia, this can be as short as 10-12 sec, and in normal clinical conditions is in the 30-40 sec range. Attempts to achieve this expected rapid onset by increasing dosage also increased sequelae (Knox *et al.*, 1970).

The new terms "dissociative anesthesia" and catalepsy were never fully understood by those who had little previous experience with neurolept anesthesia. While popular in continental Europe, this had not been widely used in Britain. In retrospect, one can appreciate the greater American familiarity with this technique when Pender (1971) described the effects of ketamine as resembling that of neurolept drugs, but produced by one agent. Clearly those advising the initial investigators were unaware of these transatlantic differences in practice. The difficulty of rapidly placing a woman's legs in lithotomy stirrups caused frustration and problems with which we had no previous experience.

It was (and still is) common British practice to concentrate initially on "pure" studies—no or little premedication, no supplementary drugs and a standard large patient population providing facilities for using the drug as the main agent. Clearly, the first indication listed in Table 2 pointed to its initial use as the sole (or main) agent for women having minor gynecologic operations, which was one of the specific fields of use recommended by the company. This typical short operation seldom lasted more than 5 to 6 min, which was very different from North American practice. It was not unusual to have a turnover of one such operation every 10 min in a single operating room, often with one anesthetist. With hindsight, we know we had most of the factors which contribute to an unacceptably high incidence of emergence delirium, *i.e.*, unpremedicated young women, very short operations, and no other sedation or hypnotic drugs.

The situation was made worse by the then common practice of returning patients directly to their ward (often an open "Florence Nightingale" type with 10-20 beds) without a stay in the recovery ward. While it is often stated that patients themselves are unaware of and not upset by emergence delirium, this does not apply to other patients, some of whom may be waiting for an operation. Patients having the minor operation discussed above do not normally receive (or require) postoperative sedation and one can imagine how the emergence deliriums of the other patients contributed to the chaos in the ward during these early studies.

Without being critical of the individuals involved, one realizes that medical advisors to the pharmaceutical industry have to deal with a wide spectrum of drugs. The British advisors to Parke Davis & Company, headed by Dr. John Gorringe, while being most helpful, had no previous experience with anesthetics and certainly were unaware of the differences between British and American practice. The author had worked in Philadelphia and was aware of American practice, as were two of our fellow investigators. Even this experience did not alert us to the problems which we were to experience. The Lancet of June 27, 1970, contained the report of our experience in over 450 anesthetic inductions with ketamine (Dundee *et al.*, 1970). This was a very intensive clinical trial, carried out in about three months in four hospitals. It involved adult gynecology and general surgery patients and 40 children undergoing minor surgical procedures. Our findings are best described by a direct quote from our final paragraph ". . .narcosis with ketamine is quite different from that produced by other available drugs, and the term dissociated anesthesia is very descriptive. Anesthesia is accompanied and followed by a high incidence of undesirable side effects in adults. Although these are decreased by certain forms of premedication, more work is needed to find the most suitable adjuvants and to clarify the specific indications for its use."

Looking back on the British experience with this drug, this was a temperate understatement of our problems. Some of my coworkers felt that there was no place for this drug in British anesthetic practice. Others of us appreciated its analgesic action and its possible potential in certain limited fields. It certainly was not the universal, non-hypotensive substitute for thiopental which we had expected. If only our pharmaceutical advisors had been more knowledgeable, the situation would have been quite different. Yet it was a privilege to learn so much about clinical trials in such a short time.

ACKNOWLEDGEMENTS

The author is appreciative of the help of the many stalwart colleagues in these early studies.

REFERENCES

Bovill, J.G., Clarke, R.S.J., Davis, E.A. and Dundee, J.W.: Some cardiovascular effects of ketamine. Br. J. Pharmacol. 41: 411, 1971.

Chen, G.: Evaluation of phencyclidine-type cataleptic activity. Arch. Int. Pharmacodyn. 157: 193-201, 1965.

Chen, G., Ensor, C.R., Russell, D. and Bohner, B.: The pharmacology of 1-(1-phenylcyclohexyl)piperidine HCl. J. Pharmacol. Exp. Ther. 127: 241-250, 1959.

Corssen, G. and Domino, E.F.: Dissociative anesthesia: Further pharmacologic studies and first clinical experience with the phencyclidine derivative CI-581. Anesth. Analg. 45: 29-40, 1966.

Domino, E.F., Chodoff, P. and Corssen, G.: Pharmacologic effects of CI-581, a new dissociative anesthetic in man. Clin. Pharmacol. Ther. 6: 279-290, 1965.

Dundee, J.W., Bovill, J., Knox, J.W.D., Clarke, R.S.J., Black, G.W., Love, S.H.S., Moore, J., Elliott, J., Pandit, S.K. and Coppel, D.L.: Ketamine: a preliminary report on its use as an induction agent. Lancet 1: 1370-1371, 1970.

Dundee, J.W. and Wyant, G.M.: Intravenous Anaesthesia, Churchill Livingstone, Edinburgh and London, 1974.

Greifenstein, F.E. and De Vault, M.: A study of a 1-arylcyclohexylamine for anesthesia. Anesth. Analg. Cur. Res. 37: 283-294, 1958.

Johnstone, M., Evans, V. and Baigel, S.: Sernyl (CI-395) in clinical anaesthesia. Br. J. Anaesth. 31: 433-439, 1959.

Knox, J.W.D., Bovill, J.G., Clarke, R.S.J. and Dundee, J.W.: Clinical studies of induction agents. XXXVI: Ketamine. Br. J. Anaesth. 42: 875-885, 1970.

McCarthy, D.A., Chen, G., Kaump, D.H. and Ensor, C.: General anesthetic and other pharmacological properties of 2-(o-chlorophenyl)-2-methylaminocyclohexanone HCl (CI-581). J. New Drugs 5: 21-33, 1965.

Pender, J.W.: Dissociative anesthesia. J. Amer. Med. Ass. 215: 1126-1130, 1971.

Status of Ketamine in Anesthesiology,
edited by E.F. Domino©1990, NPP Books
P.O. Box 1491, Ann Arbor, MI 48106

The Taming of Ketamine

J.W. Dundee

Department of Anaesthetics
The Queen's University of Belfast
Northern Ireland

The early British experience with ketamine has been described as disasterous (Dundee, 1990), with an unexpectedly high incidence of emergence delirium and hypertension. The first large British study, involving more than 450 administrations, although highlighting the problems encountered, concluded "Ketamine has certain actions not possessed by other agents, and these should guarantee it a place in anesthesia . . . Although these (undesirable side effects) are decreased by certain forms of premedication, more work is needed to find the most suitable adjuvants and to clarify the specific indications for its use." (Dundee *et al.*, 1970)

This paper describes these early studies, which were aimed at minimizing the side effects of the drug, while retaining its desirable properties. Some of these attempts involved the use of adjuvant drugs while others looked at the types of procedures and patients for which the drug would be more suitable. The title "The Taming of Ketamine" is taken from a paper by Coppel *et al.* (1973) which describes studies carried out to retain the best and minimize the worst effects of this unique drug.

Unpleasant Sequelae

Table 1 lists the most common sequelae encountered with ketamine anesthesia (Bovill and Dundee, 1972). The severity of these have been shown to depend on a number of factors such as individual predisposition, the nature and duration of the operation and the (supposed) circumstances of awakening. The emergence delirium does not upset the patients, but does upset their attendants and other patients. By contrast unpleasant dreams do upset the patients but not their attendants, who are unaware of them. Early fears of "flashback" incidents, whereby patients can relive the dreams after several days, have been exaggerated.

Early in the use of ketamine, we demonstrated (Knox *et al.*, 1970) that dosage is a factor influencing the occurrence of unpleasant dreams

TABLE 1. Main problems associated with the use of ketamine

Intraoperative	*Postoperative*
Hypertonus	Emergence delirium
Hypertension	Unpleasant dreams
	Emetic sequelae

and emergence delirium. With a constant patient population and operations (women having short gynecologic operations) the incidence increased with dosage (Table 2). Contrary to a widely expressed view, the condition of patients on leaving the operating room was not found to be a factor (Table 3).

The early British studies were carried out in adult women. It was difficult to get a comparable group of men and women having a similar short operation to compare the incidence (there being no male equivalent to minor gynecologic operations). The data in Table 4 were obtained from patients having longer but otherwise comparable operations. This shows that the tendency of women to have both emergence delirium and unpleasant dreams (Coppel *et al.*, 1973; Lilburn *et al.*, 1978) is greater than with men.

Studies described to date show that the two factors predisposing to a high incidence of emergence sequelae were short operations in young women and the administration of large doses of ketamine. Table 4 shows that in this susceptible group of patients orthodox premedication clearly

TABLE 2. The percentage of sequelae are related to the dose of ketamine

	<2 mg kg^{-1}	*2-3 mg kg^{-1}*	*3+ mg kg^{-1}*
Dreams	23	33	38
Delirium	19	12	27

(Knox *et al.*, 1970)

TABLE 3. Percentage incidence of emergence delirium following 2 mg/kg ketamine in patients who were awake or asleep on leaving the operating room

Condition arrival in recovery ward	*N*	*Emergence upset*		
		Mild	*Severe*	*Total*
Awake	70	18	16	34
Asleep	55	14	22	36

modifies the incidence and severity of complications. However, this may be achieved at the cost of delayed recovery.

Even with major operations lasting 1 1/2 hr, the importance of premedication cannot be underestimated. The patients listed in Table 5 had ketamine as the main anesthetic, yet in the absence of an opioid, one quarter were unhappy about the anesthesia. The data in Tables 4 and 5 are drawn from different patient populations, yet they show similar results.

Protection by benzodiazepines

The early use of ketamine coincided with the increasing use of oral benzodiazepines as premedication and the availability of parenteral preparations of flunitrazepam and lorazepam, in addition to diazepam. There are many studies on this topic. Table 6 summarizes some of these, while Table 7 shows the benefit of giving a small dose near the end of the

TABLE 4. Effect of sex, nature and duration of the operation, and premedication on the percent incidence of unpleasant sequelae from ketamine

	Emergence Delirium	*Unpleasant Dreams*
Men	6	6
Women	24	14
Atropine premedication		
Minor operations	34	40
Major operations	20	10
Opioid premedication		
Minor operations	11	26
Major operations	5	0
Droperidol premedication		
Minor operations	5	36
Major operations	6	15

TABLE 5. Percent incidence of unpleasant sequelae and acceptability of anesthesia in patients undergoing body surface operations, related to premedication

	Atropine 0.6 mg	*P 20 mg H 0.4 mg*	*D 5 mg F 0.1 mg*
Mean duration of operation (min)	64 (23-90)	85 (31-180)	80 (38-150)
Severe emergence delirium	75	0	0
Unpleasant dreams	50	0	75
Acceptable to patient	75	90	95

(P = papaveretum; H = hyoscine; D = droperidol; F = fentanyl)

TABLE 6. Percent of sequelae associated with i.m. benzodiazepine premedication

	Prolonged emergence sequelae	*Unpleasant dreams*
0.9% NaCl	40	30
Diazepam 15 mg	25	32
Flunitrazepam 1.5 mg	22	2
Lorazepam 4 mg	4	4

TABLE 7. Percent incidence of troublesome sequelae, and patients dissatisfied with anesthesia. The patients were unpremedicated women having short minor gynecological operations under ketamine-nitrous oxide anesthesia. Supplements were given at the end of the operation.

Additional drug given i.v.	*Nil*	*Droperidol 5 mg*	*Diazepam 5 mg*
Emergence upset	34	5	65
Unpleasant dreams	40	40	15
Patients dissatisfied with anesthesia	52	40	15

operation. Both of these sets of data were obtained from "high risk" patients, *i.e.*, women having short (5-10 min) minor gynecologic operations. The data show clearly the benefit of a longer acting benzodiazepine such as lorazepam and for many this has become the method of choice for preventing unpleasant sequelae after ketamine.

Droperidol. This drug provided benefits similar to diazepam but some patients were unhappy about their condition on awakening. They felt disorientated or "dissociated" and, since lorazepam is more effective, it is probably preferred to droperidol. When given i.v., the relatively long duration of action of droperidol should be remembered.

In summary, the following factors affect the severity of ketamine emergence sequelae:

Doses of ketamine (2 + mg kg^{-1})
Nature and duration of operation
Preanesthetic medication (more frequent with "light premedication")
Sex of patient (women more susceptible than men)
Use of concurrent drugs

The circumstances of awakening, whether in a busy operating room, the quieter surroundings of the recovery room, or the ward, do not appear to be as important a factor as once thought. Preoperative briefing may reduce the incidence, but this has not been adequately researched. Sequelae become less frequent and severe on repeated use, as during the treatment of burns.

Reduction of Hypertension

Early in the clinical use of ketamine, Bovill *et al.* (1971) demonstrated that, with a constant dose of 2 mg kg^{-1}, the rate of administration did not influence the cardiovascular response to ketamine. Neither was there less hypertension when the equivalent dose (10 mg kg^{-1}) was given i.m.

A wide variety of drugs have been studied to reduce this ketamine induced hypertension. These include hexamethonium, adrenoreceptor blockers, droperidol, labetalol, promethazine, procaine amide, and phentolamine. Since most of these drugs were without effect in reducing hypertension and tachycardia, this work is not described in detail. Furthermore, with proper selection of cases, we no longer consider tachycardia and/or hypertension a major clinical problem except when the drug is given by continuous infusion (Coppel and Dundee, 1989). It is sufficient to say that best results were obtained from pretreatment with the adrenoreceptor blocker, labetalol. The best overall effect was produced by following ketamine with a low concentration of halothane and avoiding pancuronium with its known chronotropic effects.

Summary

Careful selection of patients, operations, and correct premedication can be used successfully to mitigate the unpleasant sequelae from ketamine, while retaining its desirable properties.

References

Bovill, J.G., Coppel, D.L., Dundee, J.W. and Moore, J.: Current status of ketamine anaesthesia. Lancet i: 1285-1288, 1971.

Bovill, J.G. and Dundee, J.W.: Attempts to control the cardiostimulatory effect of ketamine in man. Anaesthesia 27: 309-312, 1972.

Coppel, D.L., Bovill, J.G. and Dundee, J.W.: The taming of ketamine. Anaesthesia 28: 293-296, 1973.

Coppel, D.L. and Dundee, J.W.: Present position of ketamine infusions. A study of 100 cases and a comparison with propofol. In Status of Ketamine in Anesthesiology, E.F. Domino, ed., this volume, NPP Books, Ann Arbor, 1990.

Dundee, J.W.: Early British experience with ketamine. In Status of Ketamine in Anesthesiology, E.F. Domino, ed., this volume, NPP Books, Ann Arbor, 1990.

Dundee, J.W., Bovill, J.G., Knox, J.W.D., Clarke, R.S.J., Black, G.W., Love, S.H.S., Moore, J., Elliott, J., Pandit, S.K. and Coppel, D.L.: Ketamine: a preliminary report on its use as an induction agent. Lancet i: 1370-1371, 1970.

Knox, J.W.D., Bovill, J.G., Clarke, R.S.J. and Dundee, J.W.: Clinical studies of induction agents. XXXVI: Ketamine. Br. J. Anaesth. 42: 875-885, 1970.

Lilburn, J.K., Dundee, J.W., Nair, S.G., Fee, J.P.H. and Johnston, H.M.L.: Ketamine sequelae-evaluation of the ability of various premedicants to attenuate its psychic actions. Anaesthesia 33: 307-311, 1978.

Status of Ketamine in Anesthesiology,
edited by E.F. Domino©1990, NPP Books
P.O. Box 1491, Ann Arbor, MI 48106

Ketamine and Postanesthetic Emergence Reactions

M.S. Albin, L. Bunegin, and C. Garcia

Neuroanesthesia Laboratory and Service
Department of Anesthesiology
University of Texas Health Science Center
San Antonio, TX

The ability of anesthetic agents to produce unusual psychogenic and neurobehavioral responses can be exemplified by the description of Sir Humphrey Davy (1800) concerning inhalation of nitrous oxide when he reported that self-inhalation was "—attended by a highly pleasurable thrilling, particularly in the chest and extremities. The objects around me became dazzling and my hearing more acute. Towards the last inspiration, the thrilling increased, the sense of muscular power became greater and at last an irresistible propensity to action was indulged in—." Similarly, it has been noted that psychogenic reactions have occurred from the use of virtually all anesthetic agents and adjuvants with incidence rates as high as 30% (Smaessert *et al.*, 1960; Albin and Dresner 1970). The phenomenon of postanesthetic excitation has been described following the use of nitrous oxide, thiopental, halothane, cyclopropane, thiamylal, hexobarbital, ether, methohexital, vinyl ether, ethylene, tribromethanol, chloroform, phencyclidine (PCP), ketamine, propanidid, phenoperidine-droperidol and enflurane (Albin and Dresner 1970; White *et al.*, 1982). Postanesthetic emergence responses have been characterized by restlessness, disorientation, crying, moaning, screaming, irrational verbalization, hallucinations, and vivid, terrifying or pleasant dreams.

The problem of postanesthetic emergence reactions (PER) has been one of the most undesirable side effects associated with ketamine. Early studies with ketamine involving 12,283 procedures in 10,861 patients indicated an overall PER rate of 13.3% (Parke Davis, 1969, see Table 1). An analysis of the factors influencing manifestations of PER with ketamine in the study noted above revealed that the PER appeared to be higher in the female and more frequent between 15 and 60 years of age in short procedures where ketamine was the sole anesthetic, in patients

TABLE 1. Incidence rates for select adverse reactions in 12,183 procedures (10,861 patients) participating in 88 studies with CI-581 (with and without those considered non-drug-attributable)

	Incidence Rates			
Adverse Reaction	*Including those considered non-drug-attributable*		*Excluding those considered non-drug-attributable*	
	Number	*Percent*	*Number*	*Percent*
Dreams (pleasant)	837	6.81	679	5.53
Dreams (unpleasant)	207	1.69	199	1.62
Hallucinations	210	1.71	152	1.24
Psychic abnormality	74	0.60	62	0.50
Confusion w/wo vocalization	367	2.99	327	2.66
Moaning, groaning or crying	193	1.57	184	1.50

having a good physical status or being a good operative risk, when the preoperative medication was judged to be unsatisfactory or when no premedication was given, and in the patient with preoperative anxieties (Albin and Dresner 1970; White *et al.*, 1982).

Conversely, attenuation of PER has been noted to occur when ketamine was used with inhalation agents, when the patient was prepared psychologically, with reduction of the total dose of ketamine (mg/kg/min), with the use of pharmacological agents such as narcotics, barbiturates, butyrophenones and benzodiazepines, and with the employment of the S(+) optical isomer (White *et al.*, 1982; White *et al.*, 1985). It has been noted that attempts to limit afferent input as a factor that might exacerbate PER have not been successful.

The use of a continuous infusion technique has allowed for a substantial decrease in the amount of ketamine used with subsequent decrease in PER (Oduntan and Gool 1970; Albin and Figallo 1976; White *et al.*, 1982; White, 1983). This technique has allowed for better titration of anesthesia-analgesia, a reduced total dose, and promoted rapid awakening with minimal psychic discomfort. Low i.v. dosing of ketamine, ranging from 0.025 to 0.036 mg/kg/min, with excellent anesthesia control is possible using this method (Albin and Figallo, 1976).

In reality, PER can be considered as a type of toxic organic brain syndrome (Henry and Mann, 1965) which involves impairment of orientation, memory, intellectual functions, and lability of affect. The associated reactions are determined by the pharmacological response-specificity interplaying upon the mosaic of inherent personality patterns, current emotional conflicts and the environmental substrate. Unfortunately, when Phase III ketamine studies were developed prior to submission to the FDA for approval, the categorization and evaluation of the neurobehavioral responses were not subjected to ongoing analysis using the available psychometric and psychiatric testing techniques. This might have led to an earlier recognition of the factors determining the psychogenic adverse reactions and the development of studies oriented to recognizing causative factors and, hence, possible solutions. Along a similar note, the terminology often used by the anesthesiologist to describe the psychogenic responses to ketamine PER has often been vague, confusing and contradictory. What would be of great utility is a phenomenological evaluation of the descriptions of the PER, utilizing the methodologies found in psychopharmacology (Albin *et al.*, 1972). Using this approach, we may be able to truly define the existence of states described as "sensory deprivation", "hallucinations", pseudohallucinations", "delirium", etc., (Sedman, 1966; Albin *et al.*, 1972). The phenomenological confusion that exists because of the improper categorization of symptoms with physiological correlates can best be noted where ketamine PER is often equated with the response(s) manifested by exposure to LSD. In Table 2, we

TABLE 2. Comparison of LSD and ketamine hydrochloride

Parameter	*LSD*	*Ketamine*
Chemical structure	Lysergic acid diethylamide	2-(Orthochlorophenyl)-2-methylamino-cyclohexanone
EEG response	Low voltage, fast activity	High voltage, slow activity (*theta* waves)
Anesthesia	None	Profound
Analgesia	Questionable	Intense
Food intake	Inhibited	Stimulated
Amnesia	Rare	Common
Tolerance	Common	Rare
Dreams and behavior	Difficult to repress pharmacologically	Easy to attenuate pharmacologically
	Dream states abstract divorced from reality	Dream states abstract often related to stimulation of environment
	Heightened color sense	
	Flashback phenomena very common	Flashback extremely rare if occurring at all

can note the significant differences between these two psychopharmacological agents.

Attempts to "tame" ketamine in terms of decreasing the incidence of PER has involved the use of pharmacological agents, either for premedication or in combination with ketamine intraoperatively or postoperatively. Reports have noted attenuation of PER when ketamine was used with inhalational agents, hypnotics, and narcotics. Butyrophenones, such as droperidol, have been employed with mixed results, and the consensus appears to show that this drug may enhance the occurrence of unpleasant dreams (Bovill *et al.*, 1971; Morgan *et al.*, 1971) and prolong the disorientation during recovery from anesthesia (Knox *et al.*, 1970; Bovill *et al.*, 1971; Sadove *et al.*, 1971; Erbguth *et al.*, 1972). As a drying agent, atropine has been shown to increase unpleasant dreams. Glycopyrrolate has been suggested as a preferred antisialogogue since it passes the blood brain barrier with difficulty.

The introduction of the benzodiazepines (Kothary and Zsigmond, 1977; Mattila *et al.*, 1979; Domino *et al.*, 1982; Langrehr *et al.*, 1984) has made an important difference in attenuating PER. Diazepam was the first drug in this class to be used successfully. Similarly, lorazepam (Fragen and Caldwell, 1976; Houlton and Downing, 1978; Dundee *et al.*, 1979; Barclay *et al.*, 1980) and flunitrazepam have also been of utility in decreasing these emergence responses. The most current benzodiazepine in use, midazolam, is shorter acting, water soluble, and does not appear to prolong recovery (White *et al.*, 1982; Cartwright and Pingel, 1984; Martinez-Aguirre and Sansano, 1986). Besides their effects in reducing PER, these benzodiazepines can modify the cardiovascular stimulating properties of ketamine, probably by attenuating catecholamine release.

Another approach to the problem of PER following ketamine relates to the use of centrally active cholinesterase inhibitors, such as physostigmine and tetrahydroaminoacridine (THA), to antagonize the CNS effects of ketamine. Similarly, the nondepolarizing muscle relaxant antagonist, 4-aminopyridine, has also been employed in attenuating PER. The results with physostigmine (Balmer and Wyte, 1977; Drummond *et al.*, 1979; Toro-Matos *et al.*, 1980) have been equivocal, with some studies indicating efficacy and others showing no effects in attenuating PER. The drug, 4-aminopyridine, has been noted to accelerate recovery from ketamine and ketamine-diazepam anesthesia in both the rhesus monkey and man (Agoston *et al.*, 1980; Martinez-Aguirre, 1982; Martinez-Aguirre, 1980).

THA (1,2,3,4-tetrahydro-5-aminoacridine, Tacrine), is a cholinesterase inhibitor, a mild neuromuscular blocker, and a respiratory stimulant (Hunter, 1965). It inhibits the uptake of norepinephrine, dopamine and 5-hydroxytryptamine (Drukarch *et al.*, 1988). Structurally, it is also similar to the K^+ channel blocker, 4-aminopyridine (Osterreider, 1987; Rogawski, 1987). THA has been shown to reverse the psychosis due to the synthetic anticholinergic, Ditran (Gershon and Olaria, 1960; Bell *et al.*, 1964), and was shown to be a partial antagonist to morphine (Shaw and Bentley, 1949; Shaw and Bentley, 1953). THA also has attenuated symptoms of physical dependence seen after morphine withdrawal (Stone *et al.*, 1961; Albin *et al.*, 1975a). The reversal of ketamine anesthesia and PER in animals and man (Albin *et al.*, 1974; Albin *et al.*, 1975b,c) has been reported with THA and includes the reversal of PCP anesthesia and PER in animals (Albin *et al.*, 1974; Maayani *et al.*, 1973; Maayani *et al.*, 1974). It also has been noted that THA has had no effects on anesthesia sleep time or PER after thiamylal (Albin *et al.*, 1974) while it has been efficacious in attenuating the acute central anticholinergic syndrome in man (Summers *et al.*, 1980). Among its other CNS effects, THA has recently been reported to modify the delirium seen in senile dementia, Alzheimer type (Summers *et al.*, 1986). Memory enhancement in mice (Fitten *et al.*, 1987) has also been described using this interesting chemical moiety. The potent PCP analogue, TCP, has been shown to be inhibited by THA in its ability to bind to the dissociative anesthesia receptor site (Young *et al.*, 1987). THA has been shown to have an excitatory action on hippocampal pyramidal neurons (Stevens and Cotman, 1987) and also blocked N-methyl-D-aspartate (NMDA) induced cytotoxicity in cultured murine neurons (Davenport, to be published). Recent work has indicated that the distribution of PCP and NMDA binding sites appear to be identical (Maragos *et al.*, 1986). These PCP and NMDA receptors appear to be coupled and probably inversely related (Comptom *et al.*, 1987; Tamminga *et al.*, 1987). Thus, in many ways, the THA effects may be due to interactions with the PCP-NMDA receptor complex.

With our present knowledge, the optimal use of ketamine to minimize PER would involve the adequate psychological preparation of the patient, the use of a continuous infusion low dose technique of ketamine delivery, the choice of the S(+) optical isomer, and the employment of a short acting, water soluble benzodiazepine like midazolam. Of interest would be further evaluation of compounds similar to THA, not only because of their effects on PER, but in helping to explain the complex interactions relating to receptor binding sites and neuroprotective responses.

References

Agoston, S., Salt, P.J., Erdmann, W., *et al.*: Antagonism of ketamine—diazepam anaesthesia by 4-aminopyridine in human volunteers. Br. J. Anaesth. 52: 367-370, 1980.

Albin, M.S. and Dresner, A.J.: Emergence reactions associated with the administration of ketamine hydrochloride. Arc. Med. 1: 179-203, 1970.

Albin, M.S., Dresner, A.J., Paolino, A.F., *et al.*: Long term personality evaluation in patients subjected to ketamine hydrochloride and other anesthetic agents. In Advances in Anaesthesiology and Resuscitation, ed. by J. Hoder, R. Jedlicka and J. Pokorny, pp. 627-662, Avicenum, Prague, 1972.

Albin, M.S., Bunegin, L., Massopust, L.C. Jr., and Jannetta, P.J.: Ketamine-induced post-anesthetic delerium attenuated by tetrahydroaminoacridine. Exp. Neurol. 44: 126-129, 1974.

Albin, M.S., Orr, M.D., Bunegin, L., *et al.*: Tetrahydroaminoacridine antagonism to narcotic addiction. Exp. Neurol. 46: 644-688, 1975a.

Albin, M.S., Bunegin, L., Jannetta, P.J., *et al.*: Tetrahydroaminoacridine (THA). I. Effect on postanesthetic emergence responses and anesthesia sleep-time after ketamine, phencyclidine and thiamylal in animals. In Recent Progress in Anesthesiology and Resuscitation, ed. by A. Arias, pp. 143-146, Excerpta Medica, Amsterdam, 1975b.

Albin, M.S., Aguirre, E.M., and Albin, R.L.: Tetrahydroaminoacridine (THA). II. Modification of postanesthetic emergence responses and anesthesia sleep-time after ketamine hydrochloride (KH) in the human. In Recent Progress in Anesthesiology and Resuscitation, ed. by A. Arias, pp. 147-149, Excerpta Medica, Amsterdam, 1975c.

Albin, M.S. and Figallo, E.: The use of an intravenous ketamine hydrochloride drip technique for fractured hip repair in the geriatric patient. Proc. VI World Cong. Anesthesiology, Mexico City, April 24-30, pp. 277-279, 1976.

Balmer, H.G.R. and Wyte, S.R.: Antagonism of ketamine by physostigmine. Br. J. Anaesth. 49: 510-512, 1977.

Barclay, A., Houlton, P.C. and Downing, J.W.: Total intravenous anaesthesia-A technique using flunitrazepam, ketamine, muscle relaxants and controlled ventilation of the lung. Anaesthesia 35: 287-290, 1980.

Bell, C., Gershon, S., Carroll, B., *et al.*: Behavioral antagonism to a new psychotomimetic-JB-329. Arch. Int. Pharmacodyn. 147: 9-24, 1964.

Bovill, J.G., Dundee, J.W., Coppel, L., *et al.*: Current status of ketamine anaesthesia. Lancet 1: 1285-1288, 1971.

Cartwright, P.D. and Pingel, S.M.: Midazolam and diazepam in ketamine anaesthesia. Anaesthesia 39: 439-442, 1984.

Comptom, R.P., Contreras, P.C., O'Donohue, T.L., *et al.*: The N-methyl-D-aspartate antagonist, 2-amino-7-phosphonoheptanoate, produces phenycyclidine like behavioral effects in rats. Eur. J. Pharmacol. 136: 133-134, 1987.

Davy, H.: Researches, Chemical and Philosophical: Chiefly Concerning Nitrous Oxide, or Dephlogisticated Nitrous Air and Its Respiration, J. Johnson, London, 1800.

Domino, E.F., Zsigmond, E.K., Domino, L.E., Domino, K.E., Kothary, S.P. and Domino, S.E.: Plasma levels of ketamine and two of its metabolites in surgical patients using a gas chromatography/mass fragmentography assay. Anesth. Analg. 61: 87-92, 1982.

Drukarch, B., Leysen, J.E., and Stoof, J.C.: Further analysis of the neuropharmacological profile of 9-amino-1,2,3,4-tetrahydroacridine (THA), an alleged drug for the treatment of Alzheimer's disease. Life Sci. 42: 1011-1017, 1988.

Drummond, J.D., Brebner, J., Galloon, S., *et al.*: A randomized evaluation of the reversal of ketamine by physostigmine. Can. Anaesth. Soc. J. 26: 288-295, 1979.

Dundee, J.W., McGowan, A.W., Lilburn, J.K. *et al.*: Comparison of the actions of diazepam and lorazepam. Br. J. Anaesth. 51: 439-445, 1979.

Erbguth, P.H., Reiman, B. and Klein, R.L.: The influence of chlorpromazine, diazepam and droperidol on emergence from ketamine. Anesth. Analg. 51: 693-700, 1972.

Fitten, L.J., Flood, J.F., Baxter, C.F., *et al.*: Long term oral administration of memory-enhancing doses of tacrine in mice: a study of potential toxicity and side effects. J. Gerontol. 42: 681-685, 1987.

Fragen, R.J. and Caldwell, N.: Lorazepam premedication-lack of recall and relief of anxiety. Anesth. Analg. 55: 792-796, 1976.

Gershon, S. and Olaria J.: JB-329-a new psychotomimetric, its antagonism by tetrahydroaminoacridine and its comparison with LSD, mescaline and sernyl. J. Neuropsychiatry 1: 283-288, 1960.

Henry, W.D. and Mann, A.M.: Diagnosis and treatment of delirium. Canad. Med. Assoc. J. 93: 1156-1166, 1965.

Houlton, P.J.C. and Downing, J.W.: General anaesthesia with intravenous flunitrazepam, continuous ketamine infusion and muscle relaxant. S. Afr. Med. J. 54: 1048-1049, 1978.

Hunter, H.R.: Tetrahydroaminoacridine in anaesthesia. Brit. J. Anaesth. 37: 505-513, 1965.

Knox, J.W.D., Bovill, J.G., Clarke, R.S.J., *et al.*: Clinical studies of induction agents-ketamine. Br. J. Anaesth. 42: 875-885, 1970.

Kothary, S.P. and Zsigmond, E.K.: A double-blind study of the effective antihallucinatory doses of diazepam prior to ketamine anesthesia. Clin. Pharmacol. Thes. 21: 108-109, 1977.

Langrehr, D., Agoston, S. and Sia, R.: Ataranalgesia. A review. Acta Anaesthesiol. Belg. 35: 165-187, 1984.

Maayani, S. Weinstein, H. and Cohen, S.: Acetylcholine-like molecular arrangement in psychotomimetic anticholinergic drugs. Proc. Natl. Acad. Sci., USA 70: 3103-3106, 1973.

Maayani, S., Weinstein, H., Ben-Zue, N., *et al.*: Anticholinesterase activity and antagonistic activity to acetylcholine. Biochem. Pharmacol. 23: 1263-1281, 1974.

Maragos, W.F., Chu, D.C.M., Greenamyre, J.T., *et al.*: High correlation between the localization of [3^H] TCP binding and NMDA receptors. Eur. J. Pharmacol. 123: 173-174, 1986.

Martinez-Aguirre, E.: Antagonism of 4-aminopyridine to ketamine-diazepam anesthesia in children. Acta Anaestheiol. Belg. 31: 289-291, 1980.

Martinez-Aguirre, E.: Antagonism of ketamine by 4-aminopyridine and physostigmine (letter). Br. J. Anaesth. 54: 110, 1982.

Martinez-Aguirre, E, and Sansano, C.: Comparison of midazolam (RO 21-3981) and diazepam as complement of ketamine-air anesthesia in children. Acta Anesthesiol. Belg. 37: 15-22, 1986.

Mattila, M.A.K., Larni, H.M., Nummi, S.E., *et al.*: Effect of diazepam on emergence from ketamine anaesthesia: A double-blind study, Anaesthesist 28: 20-23, 1979.

Morgan, M., Loh, L. and Singer, L.: Ketamine as the sole anesthetic agent for minor surgical procedures. Anaesthesia 26: 158-165, 1971.

Oduntan, S.A. and Gool, R.Y.: Clinical trial of ketamine (CI-581). Can. Anaesth. Soc. J. 17:411-416, 1970.

Osterreider, W.: 9-Amino-1,2,3,4-tetrahydroacridine (THA) is a potent blocker of cardiac potassium channels. Brit. J. Pharmacol. 92: 521-525, 1987.

Parke-Davis: Medical Summary, Ketalar, CI-581: A short acting anesthetic, Parke-Davis and Co., Ann Arbor, 1969.

Rogawski, M.A.: Tetrahydroaminoacridine blocks voltage-dependent ion channels in hippocampal neurons. Eur. J. Pharmacol. 142: 169-172, 1987.

Sadove, M.S., Shulman, M., Hatano, S., *et al.*: Analgesic effects of ketamine administered in subdissociative doses. Anesth. Analg. 50: 452-457, 1971.

Sedman, G.: A phenomenological study of pseudohallucinations and related experiences. Acta Psychiat. Scand. 42: 35-70, 1966.

Shaw, F.H. and Bentley, G.A.: Some aspects of the pharmacology of morphine, with special reference to its antagonism by 5-amino-acridine and other chemically related compounds. Med. J. Australia 2: 868-874, 1949.

Shaw, F.H. and Bentley, G.A.: Pharmacology of some new anticholinesterases. Australia J. Exp. Biol. Med. Sci. 31: 573-577, 1953.

Smaessert, A., Schekr, C.A. and Artusio, Jr., J.F.: Observations in the immediate postanesthesia period. II. Mode of recovery. Brit. J. Anaesth. 32: 181-185, 1960.

Stevens, D.R. and Cotman, C.W.: Excitatory actions of tetrahydro-9-aminoacridine on hippocampal pyramidal neurons. Neurosci. Lett. 79: 301-305, 1987.

Stone, V., Moon, W. and Shaw, F.H.: Treatment of intractable pain with morphine and tetrahydroaminoacridine. Brit. Med. J. 1: 471-473, 1961.

Summers, W.K., Kaufman, K.R., Altman, F., Jr., *et al.*: THA-A review of the literature and its use in treatment of five overdose patients. Clin. Tox. 16: 269-281, 1980.

Summers, W.K., Majovski, L.V., Marsh, G.M., *et al.*: Oral tetrahydroaminoacridine in long-term treatment of senile dementia, Alzheimer type. New Eng. J. Med. 315: 1241-1245, 1986.

Tamminga, C.A., Tanimoto, K., Kuo, S., *et al.*: PCP-induced alterations in cerebral glucose utilization in rat brain: Blockade by metaphit, a PCP-receptor-acylating agent. Synapse 1: 497-504, 1987.

Toro-Matos, A., Rendon-Platas, A.M., Avila-Valdez, E., *et al.*: Physostigmine antagonizes ketamine. Anesth. Analg. 59: 764-767, 1980.

White, P.F., Way, W.L. and Trevor, A.J.: Ketamine—Its pharmacology and therapeutic uses. Anesthesiol. 56: 119-136, 1982.

White, P.F.: Use of continuous infusion versus intermittent bolus administration of fentanyl or ketamine during outpatient anesthesia. Anesthesiol. 59: 294-300, 1983.

White, P.F., Schuttler, J., Shafer, A., Stanski, D.R., Horai, Y., and Trevor, A.J.: Comparative pharmacology of the ketamine isomers. Studies in volunteers. Br. J. Anaesth. 57: 197-203, 1985.

Young, A.B., Albin, R.L., Albin, M.S., *et al.*: 1,2,3,4-tetrahydro-9-aminoacridine and other acridine derivatives are displacers of specifically found [^{3}H]-N-(1-[2-thienyl]cyclohexyl) -3,4-piperidine. Soc. Neurosci. Abstracts 13: 1553, 1987.

Status of Ketamine in Anesthesiology,
edited by E.F. Domino©1990, NPP Books
P.O. Box 1491, Ann Arbor, MI 48106

Clinical Pharmacology of Ketamine

E.K. Zsigmond and E.F. Domino

Departments of Anesthesiology and Pharmacology
University of Michigan Medical School
Ann Arbor, MI

INTRODUCTION

The data presented in this chapter are reproduced from a scientific exhibit presented at the 53rd Congress, International Anesthesia Research Society, Hollywood, FL, March 11-15, 1979 and articles by Zsigmond and Domino (1980a,b). Although this research has been published in abstract form, much of it is relatively unavailable or inaccessible to currently interested persons. Hence, it was decided that there would be scientific merit to reproduce much of the pertinent clinical pharmacological studies which had been performed by the authors with the assistance of many co-workers. This research is presented in a slightly modified version and is reproduced with permission of the publishers. It represents research carried out on human normal and patient volunteers who gave written, informed consent as approved by the Institutional Committee to Review Investigations at the University of Michigan and the State Prison of Southern Michigan at the former Parke Davis research facilities at Jackson, MI.

RESULTS

Clinical Pharmacologic Studies of Ketamine Alone

The initial animal studies by Chen *et al.* (1966) indicated that ketamine had a potential as an anesthetic in humans. Subsequently, Domino *et al.* (1965) reported on the clinical pharmacology of ketamine in human volunteers.

Central nervous system effects

The effects of ketamine on the scalp electroencephalogram (EEG) of humans are unique (Domino *et al.*, 1965; Corssen *et al.*, 1969). In Fig. 1 is illustrated a typical example of a subject who received 1 mg/kg of ketamine as in i.v. infusion over 1 min.

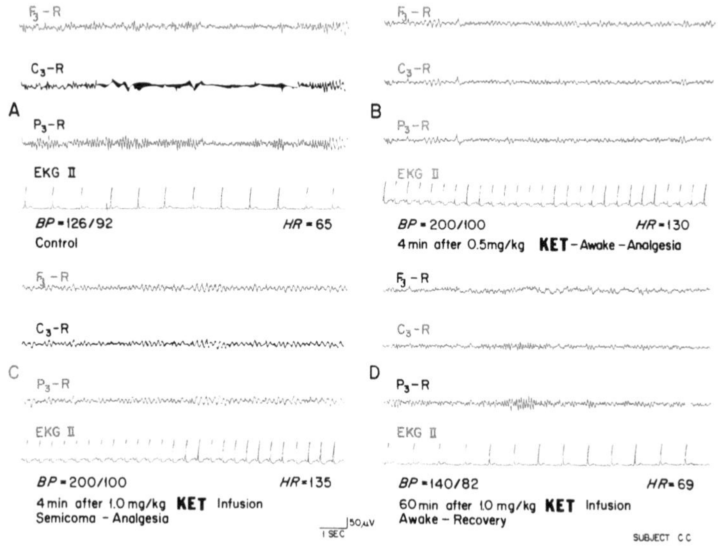

Fig. 1. EEG effects of a continuous infusion of ketamine in man.

Prior to the administration of ketamine, the arterial blood pressure was 126/92 mm Hg with a heart rate of 65/min. In panel A is shown a typical EEG with the eyes closed. Scalp recordings were taken from frontal (F3), central (C3), and parietal (P3) areas to both ears as reference using the 10-20 International System. Lead II of the EKG is shown. Four min after 1.0 mg/kg of ketamine the subject was awake and had analgesia to pin prick. At this time the arterial blood pressure was 200/100 mm Hg with a heart rate of 130/min. The EEG showed suppression of typical *alpha* rhythm and a low voltage fast wave pattern with occasional *theta* (6 Hz) activity (panel B). In panel C is shown the EEG tracing 4 min after 1.0 mg/kg of ketamine. At this time the subject had marked analgesia and was semicomatose. The EEG showed generalized *theta* wave activity. Panel D illustrates an EEG tracing taken 60 min after the last dose of 1.0 mg/kg of ketamine given over a 1 min period. At this time the subject was awake and showed partial recovery. The arterial blood pressure at this time was 140/82 mm Hg and the heart rate 69/min. The EEG tracing had not completely recovered. Occasional bouts of *alpha* activity were present but not as much as in the control period (compare panel A vs panel D).

The effects of 2.0 mg/kg i.v. ketamine on the visually evoked response (VER) in another subject are shown in Fig. 2. In the control period before ketamine administration, the VER was recorded to 100 light

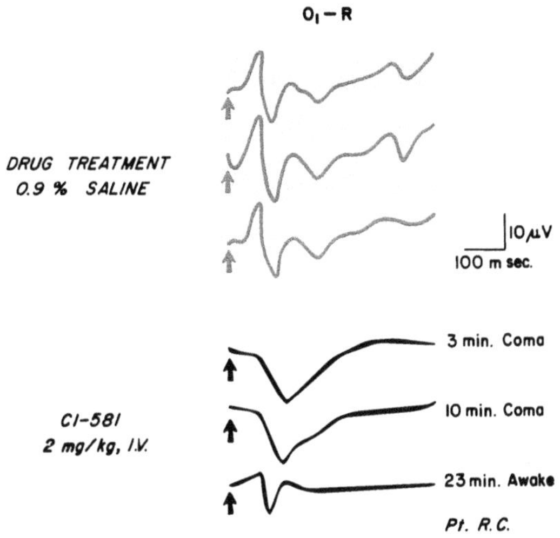

Fig. 2. Effects of ketamine on visually evoked responses.

flashes which were averaged by a computer of average transients. The recording was taken from the occipital area of the scalp (0_1) to both ears as reference (R). During an infusion of 0.9% NaC1, 3 consecutive recordings were taken at 5 min intervals. The light flash was at the arrow. One can observe a prominent visually evoked response. Ciganek's terminology is used to describe the wave forms recorded. It may be observed that a prominent wave 3 and wave 4 were present. Other waves were also seen but not as prominently. When the evoked response was repeated, some variation in the VER was noted. The subject was in deep coma 3 min after the administration of 2.0 mg/kg of ketamine i.v. At this time, the VER was markedly altered, as noted by an absent wave 3 and an exceedingly deep and broad wave 4. No other wave forms were seen. Ten min later a similar wave pattern was observed, although waves 5 and 6 were now barely detectable. Approximately 23 min after the administration of ketamine, the subject was awake and responded to simple commands. At this time, waves 3 and 4 were present which were somewhat similar to control, although still depressed.

In Fig. 3 is represented the dose response relationships of ketamine given i.v. on a mg/kg basis over a 30 sec period on the X axis vs the duration of loss of consciousness in min on the Y axis. Each solid circle represents an individual subject and the open circle the mean. The height

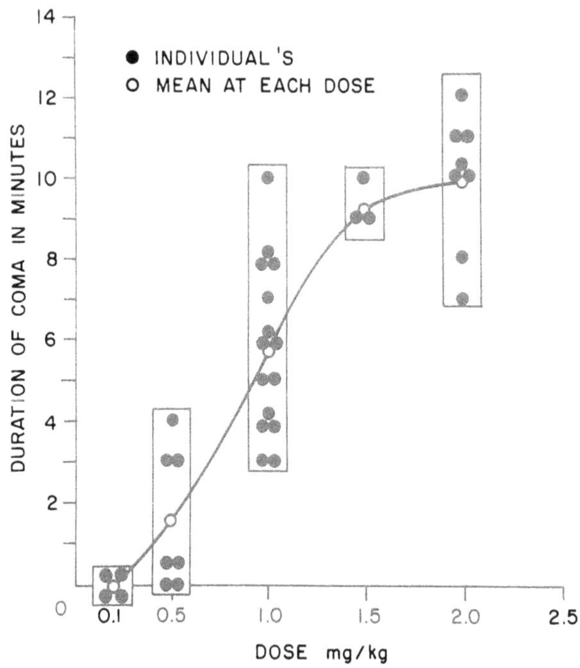

Fig. 3. Relation of i.v. ketamine dose to duration of anesthesia.

of the vertical bar represents the range of variability. It can be seen that a dose of 0.1 mg/kg ketamine induced loss of consciousness for approximately 1.5 min. There was individual variation, as noted in the figure. A dose of 1.0 mg/kg of ketamine induced a mean duration of loss of consciousness of 5.8 min. A dose of 1.5 mg/kg of ketamine induced loss of consciousness for approximately 9 min, whereas a dose of 2.0 mg/kg induced loss of consciousness for approximately 10 min. In this particular study, no preanesthetic medication was given. Under these circumstances the duration of suitable anesthesia is obviously very brief.

Cardiovascular and respiratory systems

The effects of ketamine on the arterial blood pressure and heart rate, as a function of dose, are illustrated in Fig. 4. In each case, the mean data are plotted from the same subjects whose duration of loss of consciousness is shown in Fig. 3. The mean baseline heart rate and blood pressure were obtained during the period of 0.9% NaCl infusion i.v. The change in heart rate as a function of dose was marked, with 0.1 mg/kg of ketamine inducing an increase in heart rate of only about 7 beats/min.

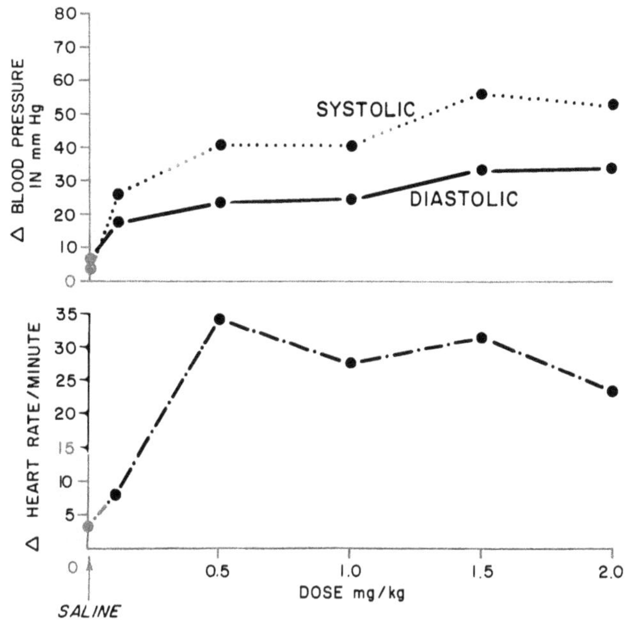

Fig. 4. Mean cardiovascular changes in relation to dose of ketamine.

However, a dose of 0.5 mg/kg of ketamine produced a mean increase in heart rate of approximately 34 beats/min. Larger doses of ketamine showed no greater change in heart rate, indicating a plateau effect. The upper portion of Fig. 4 illustrates the dose effect relationship of ketamine on the change in arterial blood pressure expressed in mm Hg. A dose effect relationship was clearly observed to a maximal dose of 1.5 to 2.0 mg/kg. Both mean systolic and diastolic blood pressure increased as a function of dose. The lower portion of Fig. 4 illustrates the mean change in heart rate from control (heart rate/min as a function of dose).

In Fig. 5 the changes in respiratory rate, blood pressure. and heart rate of one subject are plotted over an 8 min period following the administration of 1.0 mg/kg of ketamine. Obvious changes are noted.

The effects of two doses of 1.0 mg/kg of ketamine given over a 30 sec interval over time are shown in Fig. 6 in a volunteer who was observed for 50 min. The systolic and diastolic arterial blood pressure, pulse rate, relative oxyhemoglobin saturation and respiratory rate are plotted at various time intervals. In addition, the duration of loss of consciousness, as well as the presence of EEG *alpha* and *theta* waves, are shown. It can be seen that following 1.0 mg/kg of ketamine a prompt increase in arterial

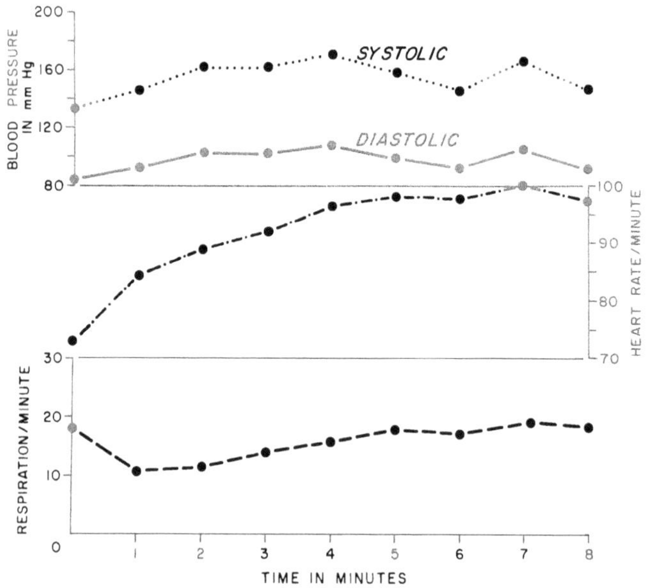

Fig. 5. Cardiorespiratory effects in a typical subject following administration of ketamine.

blood pressure and heart rate were observed. This was followed by a loss of consciousness which lasted approximately 4 min with predominant EEG *theta* waves. At this time, there was a decrease in the respiratory rate and the oximeter showed a relative decrease in 0_2 saturation. When the patient awoke approximately 5 min later, an additional dose of 1.0 mg/kg of ketamine produced a further rise in arterial blood pressure and a marked decrease in relative 0_2 saturation. Respiratory rate was not further decreased. Over the next 30 min the patient gradually recovered so that approximately 25 to 30 min later the *alpha* rhythm in the EEG was partially restored and the patient awake. However, the increase in systolic pressure had not returned to normal. The ear oximeter readings of relative 0_2 saturation and the respiratory rate were normal at this time.

Effects of diazepam ketamine combination

The human pharmacology and plasma pharmacokinetics of ketamine and diazepam-ketamine were compared in 8 volunteers in a double blind random crossover design.

Subjects:	Drug-free, adult, male volunteers
Drugs:	Placebo 0.9% NaC1 (P)-ketamine 2.2 mg/kg (K)

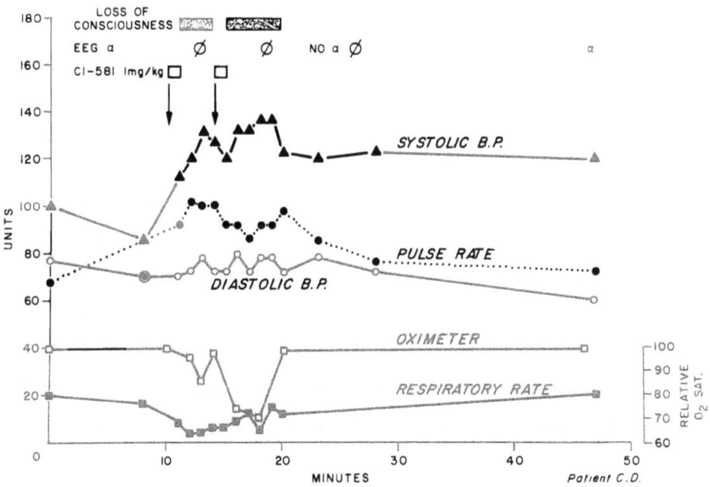

Fig. 6. Effects of ketamine anesthesia on vital signs in a typical volunteer.

Diazepam 0.3 mg/kg (D)-ketamine 2.2 mg/kg (K)

Route of administration: I.V.

Timing: − 15 min baseline measurements
− 10 min P or D given over 5 min
− 0 min ketamine infused over 30 sec

Assay for ketamine: Gas chromatography-mass fragmentography

Monitoring: EEG: 4 channels (F_3, C_1, P_1, 0_1 to both ears as reference) power frequency computer analyses. EKG: Lead II. B.P.: Strain gauge via radial or brachial arterial catheter #18 g, chest plethysmography, phonocardiography, table tilt to 75°, pupil diameter by stroboscopic photography, tape recording of verbal responses

Central nervous system

A total of 8 volunteers were given ketamine (2.2 mg/kg) and either placebo or diazepam (0.3 mg/kg) 10 min prior to ketamine anesthesia. Both 0.9% NaCl-ketamine (PK) and diazepam-ketamine (DK) caused loss of consciousness as well as alterations in the scalp EEG. The control (C) period was from -15 to -10 min. The scalp EEG activity was recorded on magnetic tape and analyzed for power frequency spectra by an IBM

1800 computer. The mean voltage²/min for each of the major frequencies is plotted in Figs. 7-10 under C, PK and DK conditions. The EEG tracings for *alpha* waves (10 Hz), *beta* waves (15 Hz), *delta* waves (4 Hz), and *theta* waves (6 Hz) are shown for the control period. Mean EEG wave amplitude is in $\mu V^2 \pm$ S.E.

Ketamine reduced *alpha* wave activity in the EEG which was not antagonized by diazepam. After PK and DK, a similar reduction in mean

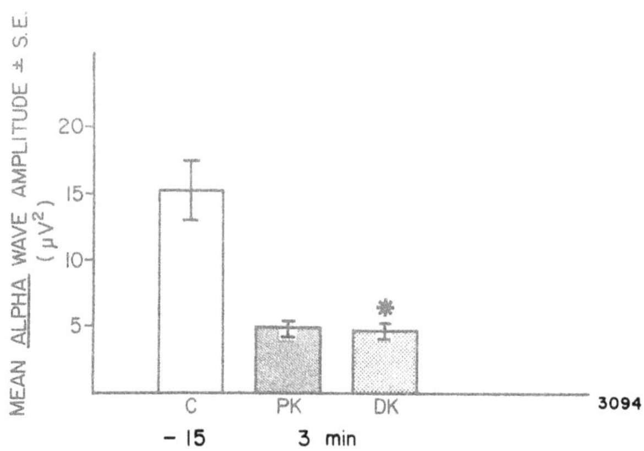

Fig. 7. Placebo-ketamine and diazepam-ketamine induced reduction of *alpha* waves (10 Hz) in the EEG.

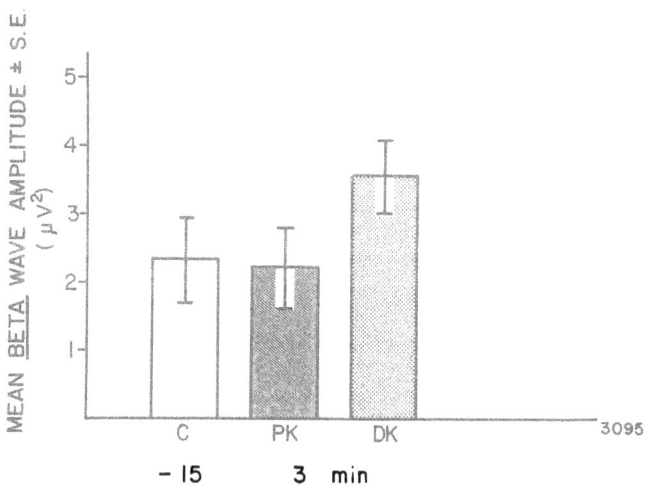

Fig. 8. Lack of effect of placebo-ketamine in altering *beta* waves (15 Hz) in the EEG.

alpha wave amplitude was observed. As illustrated in Fig. 8, ketamine did not alter *beta* activity in the EEG. Three min after DK, there is a slight increase in mean *beta* wave amplitude, but this is not statistically different from control (P <0.1). As illustrated in Fig. 9, ketamine induced *delta* wave activity in the EEG. The mean *delta* wave amplitude was significantly increased following PK compared to the control period. DK increased mean *delta* wave amplitude similar to that of PK. As illustrated in

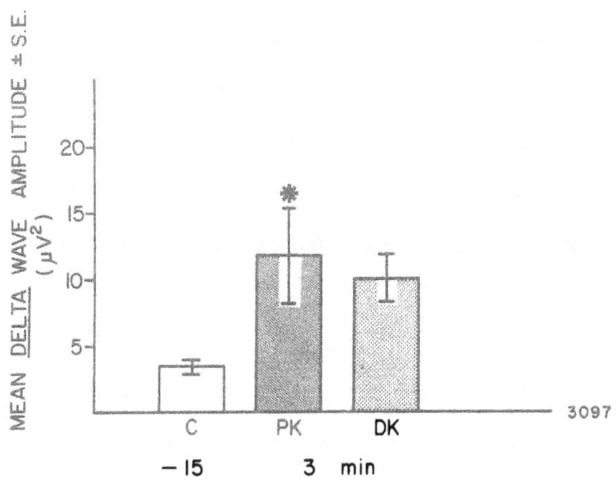

Fig. 9. Placebo-ketamine and diazepam-ketamine induction of *delta* waves (4 Hz) in the EEG.

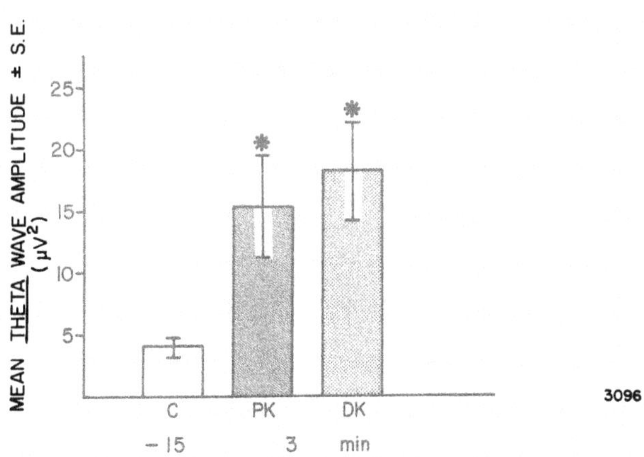

Fig. 10. Placebo-ketamine and diazepam-ketamine induction of *theta* waves (6 Hz) in the EEG.

Fig. 10, ketamine induced a profound increase in mean *theta* wave amplitude under PK and DK conditions.

Diazepam pretreatment significantly prolonged ketamine induced loss of consciousness. As illustrated in Fig. 11, the time to return of the ability to follow simple commands and to verbalize coherently increased from a mean duration of 15 to 22, and 16 to 25 min, respectively.

Cardiovascular system

The effects of PK and DK on mean maximum and mean minimum arterial blood pressure in normal volunteers are shown in Fig. 12.

Diazepam pretreatment significantly reduced the hypertensive effects of ketamine. Maximum arterial blood pressure was reduced much more than minimum arterial blood pressure.

The effects of PK and DK on mean cardiac rate (HR) and respiratory rate (RR) in normal volunteers is illustrated in Fig. 13. In this particular study there were no significant changes in heart or respiratory rate following premedication with diazepam as compared to the 0.9% NaCl placebo.

As illustrated in Fig. 14, there was a significant reduction in the cardiac ejection fraction in normal volunteers receiving diazepam as compared to placebo prior to the administration of ketamine.

Respiratory system

Ketamine alone caused a significant decrease in arterial PaO_2, an increase in arterial $PaCO_2$ and a slight but statistically significant decrease in mean arterial pH (see Figs. 15-17).

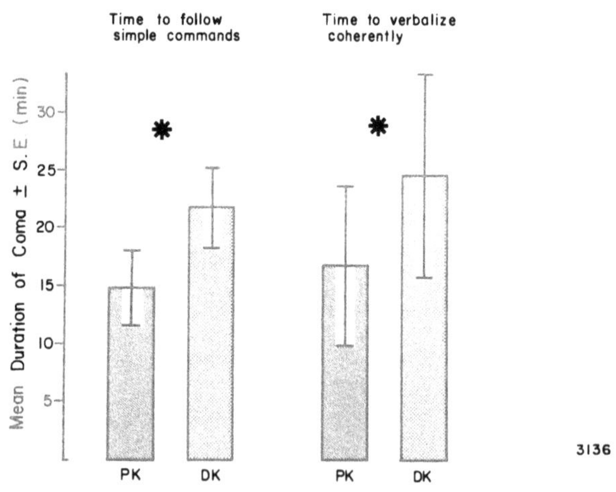

Fig. 11. Diazepam prolongation of ketamine induced loss of consciousness.

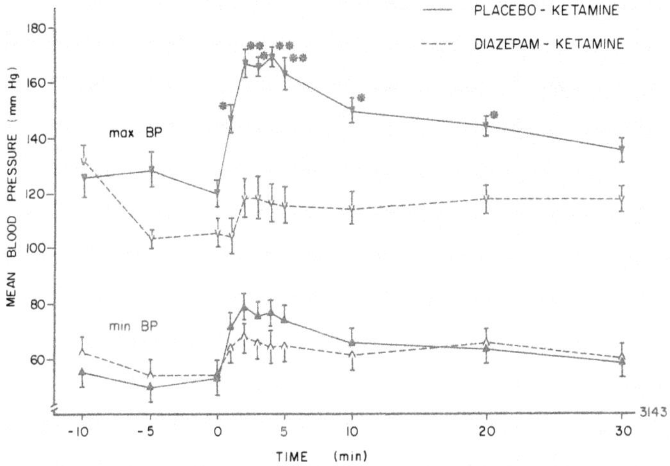

Fig. 12. Effects of placebo-ketamine and diazepam-ketamine on mean maximum and minimum radial arterial blood pressure in normal human volunteers.

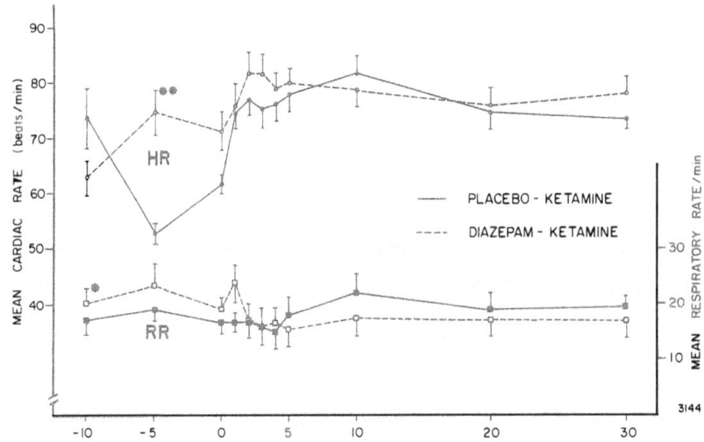

Fig. 13. Effects of placebo-ketamine and diazepam-ketamine on mean cardiac rate and respiratory rate in normal human volunteers.

Diazepam premedications enhanced the depressant effects of ketamine on the respiratory system. It should be noted that in this study in volunteers respiration was not assisted and was in the absence of surgical stimuli. It is obvious that these changes could be readily overcome with simple ventilatory support and, hence, are not clinically significant.

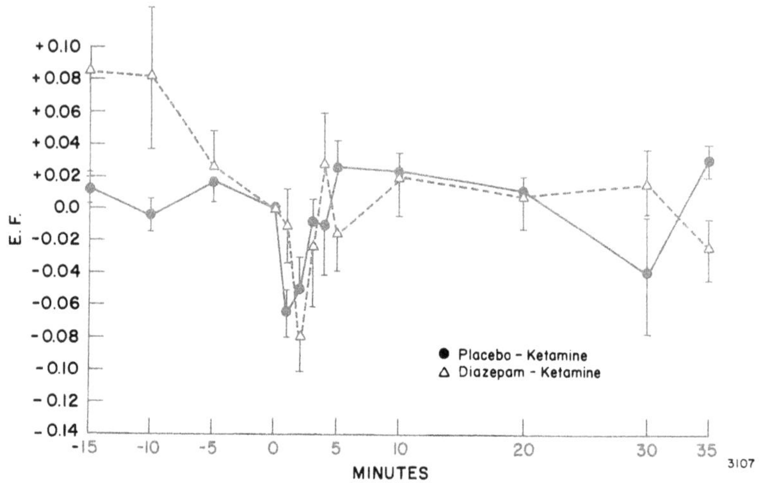

Fig. 14. Change in cardiac ejection fraction in volunteers receiving placebo-ketamine or diazepam-ketamine.

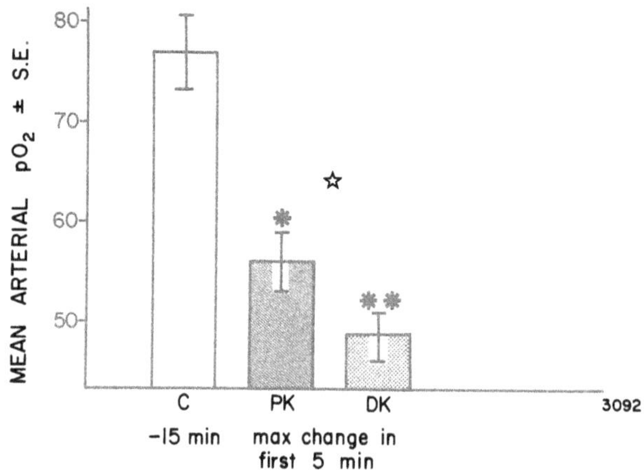

Fig. 15. Diazepam enhancement of ketamine induced PaO_2 decrease (maximum change in first 5 min).

Pharmacokinetics

The plasma levels of ketamine, ketamine metabolite I, and artifactual extraction induced ketamine metabolite II were determined by a gas chromatographic-mass fragmentographic assay (GV-MG) (Lau and Domino, 1977). The mean plasma levels of ketamine and its metabolites are plotted over a 30 min period in Fig. 18.

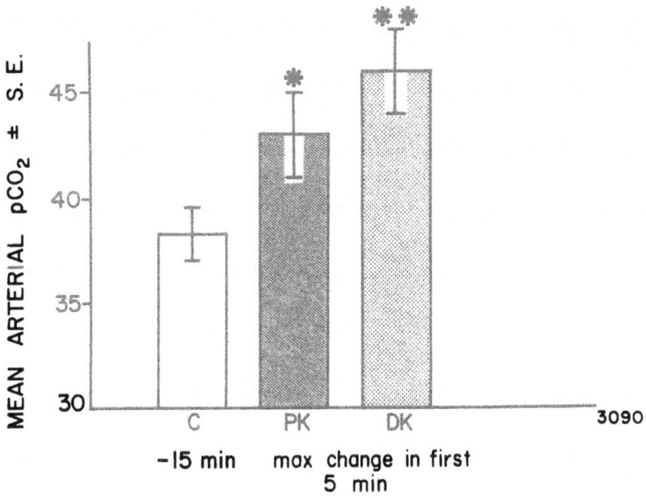

Fig. 16. Diazepam enhancement of ketamine induced increase in $PaCO_2$ (maximum change in first 5 min).

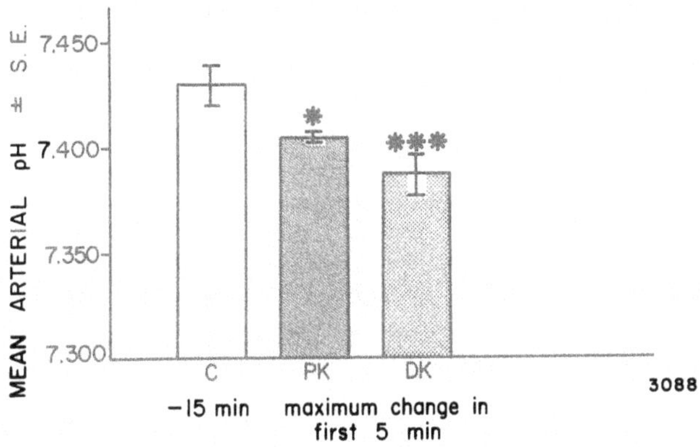

Fig. 17. Diazepam enhancement of ketamine induced reduction in arterial pH (maximum change in first 5 min).

Diazepam significantly elevated the levels of ketamine. Although its two metabolites tended to be elevated as well, the latter changes were not statistically significant. In Figs. 19 and 20 the plasma levels of ketamine and its two metabolites are shown to illustrate individual variability. It can be seen in both subjects that ketamine disappeared very rapidly from the plasma. At about 10 to 15 min after ketamine administration, the plasma

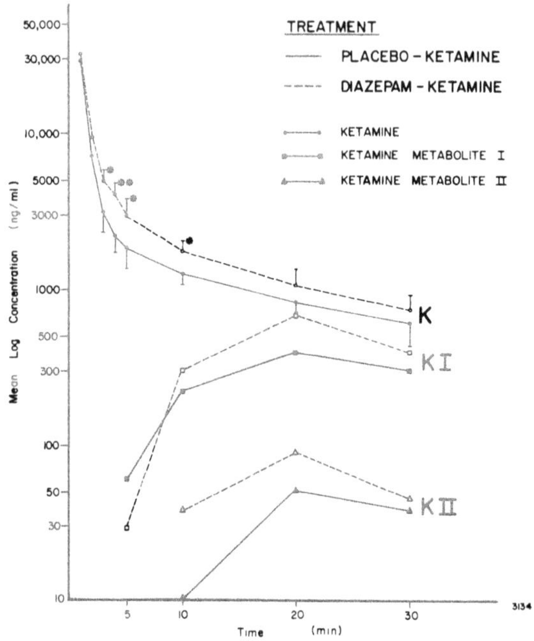

Fig. 18. Mean levels of ketamine, ketamine metabolite I and artifactual extraction induced ketamine metabolite II in normal human volunteers (GC-MF Assay).

levels were approximately 1000 ng/ml. This apparently represents the minimal anesthetic level of ketamine. Ketamine metabolite I appears more rapidly in the plasma than the artifactual ketamine metabolite II following ketamine administration. In subject #6 (Fig. 19) ketamine metabolite II was evident. In contrast, in subject #7 (Fig. 20) ketamine metabolite II was detected about 30 min following ketamine anesthesia. The levels of ketamine metabolite I are easily detectable approximately 5 to 10 min after ketamine administration. The delayed appearance of these two metabolites at the time of recovery from anesthesia suggests that ketamine biotransformation is not a significant factor in its short duration of anesthesia. It is apparent from all three figures (Figs. 18-20) that ketamine very rapidly disappears from the plasma compartment. Although the plasma disappearance of ketamine is fairly complex, a two compartment open model can be used to describe its pharmacokinetics. The mean plasma ketamine half lives ± S.E. are as follows:

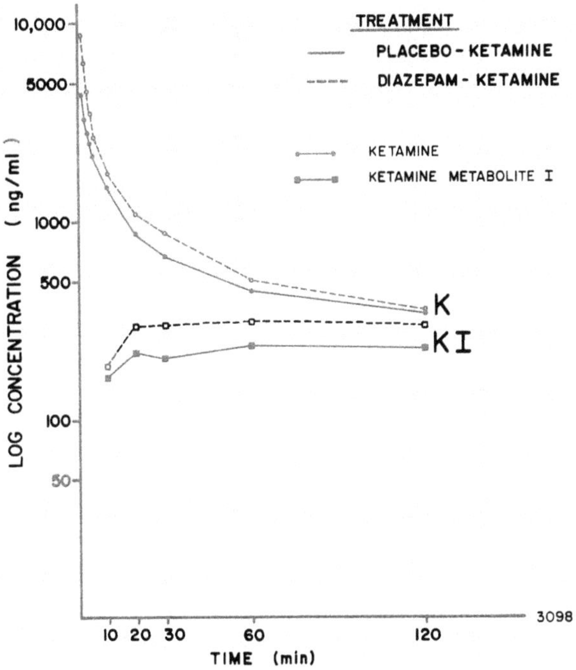

Fig. 19. Levels of ketamine and ketamine metabolite I in a normal human volunteer (subject #6—GC-MF assay).

Alpha *phase* *(min)*	**Beta** *Phase* *(hr)*	*P Value* ($\alpha + \beta$)
PK 7.15 ± 4.56	2.19 ± 0.64	—
DK 7.11 ± 2.44	2.38 ± 0.60	NS

These results were not statistically significant using each subject as his own control under PK and DK conditions.

Table tilt response

In Figs. 21 and 22 are illustrated the effects of PK and DK on table tilt of 75°. No significant differences between PK and DK conditions were noted.

Hepatic function

As illustrated in Fig. 23, there was no effect of PK and DK on plasma SGOT, taken at 0, 2 and 24 hr postanesthesia. Likewise, there was no effect on plasma SGPT (see Fig. 24).

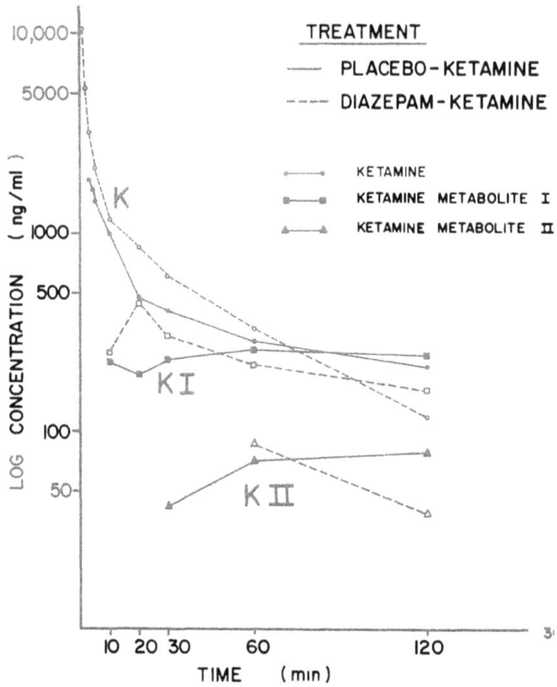

Fig. 20. Levels of ketamine, ketamine metabolite I and artifactual ketamine metabolite II in a normal human volunteer (subject #7—GC-MF assay).

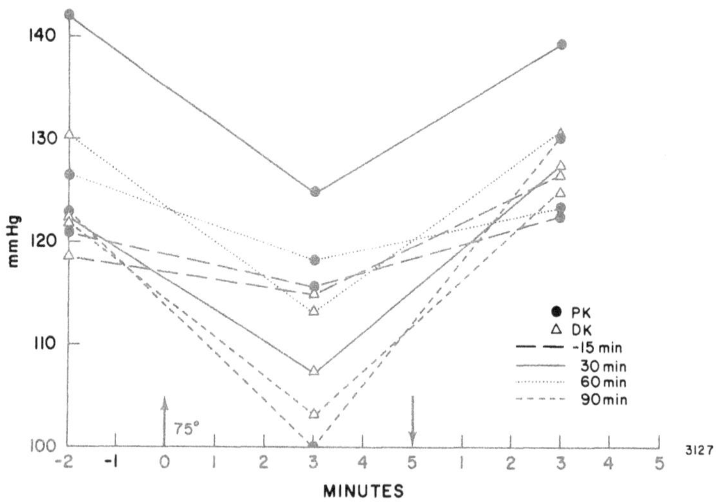

Fig. 21. Maximum direct arterial pressure in volunteers after placebo-ketamine (PK) and diazepam-ketamine (DK) changes following table tilt.

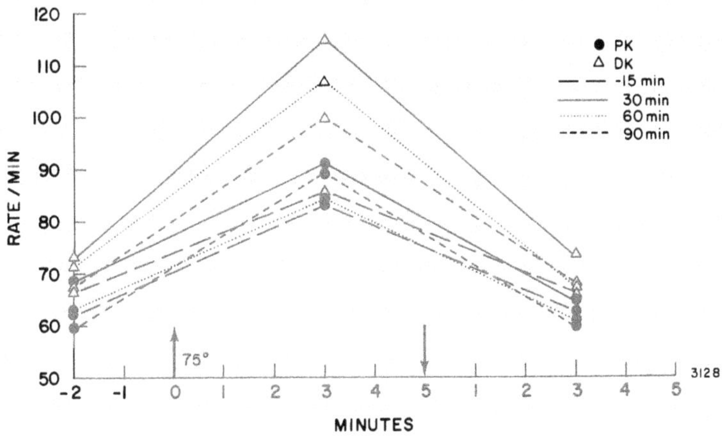

Fig. 22. Cardiac rate in volunteers after placebo-ketamine (PK) and diazepam-ketamine (DK) changes following table tilt.

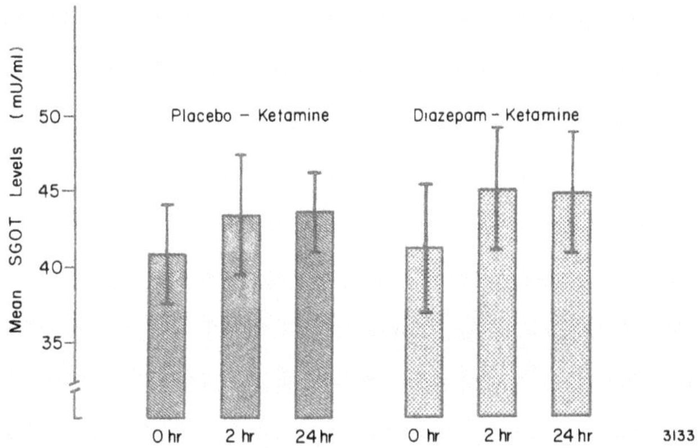

Fig. 23. Lack of effect of placebo-ketamine and diazepam-ketamine on plasma SGOT.

Plasma alkaline phosphatase was not significantly altered by ketamine anesthesia (see Fig. 25). In fact, it appeared to be reduced over time. Hepatic function, as measured by plasma cholinesterase, also was not reduced following ketamine (see Fig. 26).

Comparison of ketamine alone with thiamylal

Since its introduction by Corssen and Domino (1966) and Corssen *et al.* (1968) into clinical anesthesia, ketamine i.v. or i.m. has proven to be a

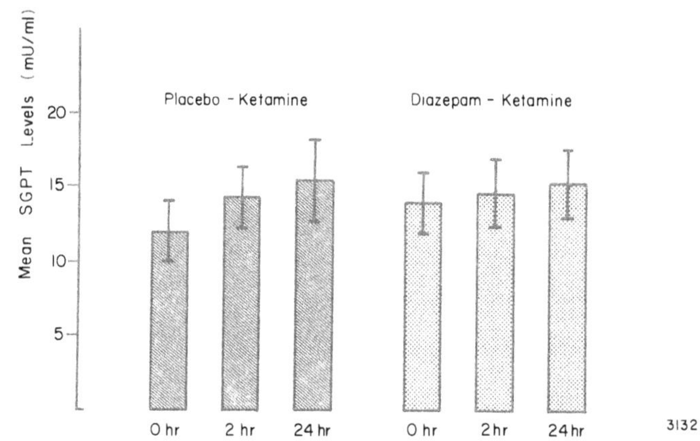

Fig. 24. Lack of effect of placebo-ketamine and diazepam-ketamine on plasma SGPT.

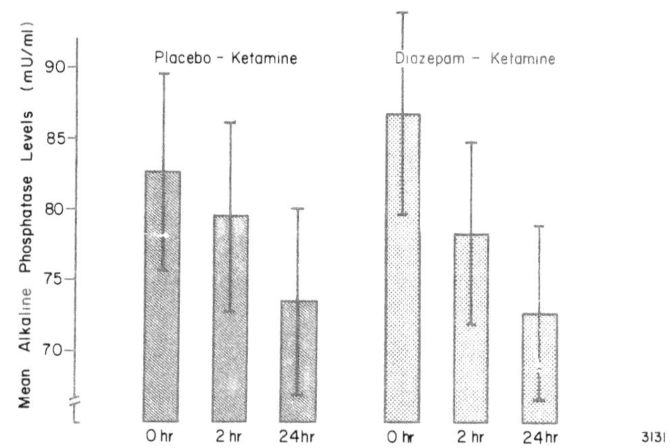

Fig. 25. Effects of placebo-ketamine and diazepam-ketamine on plasma alkaline phosphatase.

safe and effective agent for the induction of anesthesia in patients in poor cardiocirculatory state, in shock and in burn patients. Between 1966 and 1972 we became convinced of the value of ketamine compared to thiobarbiturates like thiamylal based upon clinical experience of anesthetizing thousands of patients. However, clinical impressions need to be substantiated by double blind studies. We conducted a number of these using patient volunteers. We have investigated the cardiovascular, respiratory, metabolic, catecholamine releasing and psychic effects of 2.0 mg/kg/30

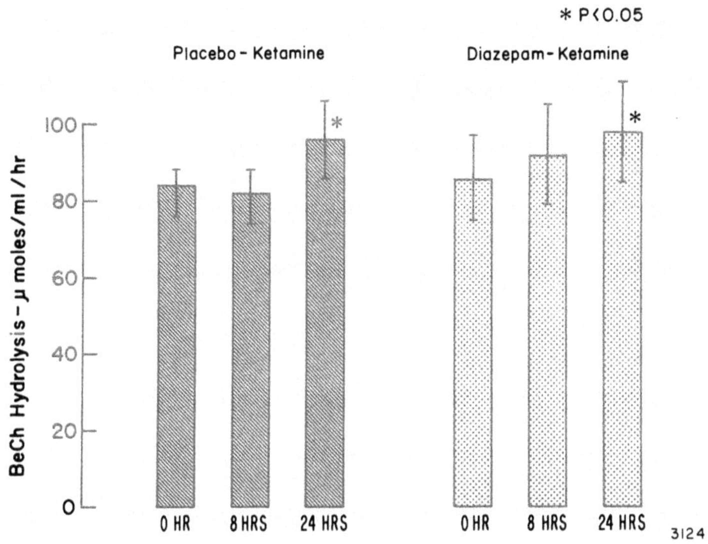

Fig. 26. Effects of placebo-ketamine and diazepam-ketamine on plasma cholinesterase activity.

sec ketamine induction in many patient volunteers since 1968. These are briefly summarized below.

We determined the cardiocirculatory effects of ketamine with respiratory assistance for the induction of anesthesia in 20 healthy volunteer gynecologic patients in good physical state ASA I-II. Details of this study have been published previously (Zsigmond *et al.*, 1972).

Cardiovascular system

As illustrated in Fig. 27, 2.0 mg/kg/30 sec i.v. ketamine ($N = 12$) caused a significant ($P < 0.01$) increase in systolic blood pressure in contrast to 5.0 mg/kg/30 sec i.v. thiamylal ($N = 8$) which caused a significant ($P < 0.05$) reduction in systolic blood pressure 5 to 20 min following its administration. Although the initial baseline blood pressures of the 2 groups vary, it is obvious that ketamine elevates and thiamylal decreases systolic blood pressure with normalization of the data.

The induction of ketamine anesthesia was followed by a significant increase in heart rate ($P < 0.05$), while no change in heart rate followed the i.v. administration of thiamylal, as illustrated in Fig. 28. Again, the initial

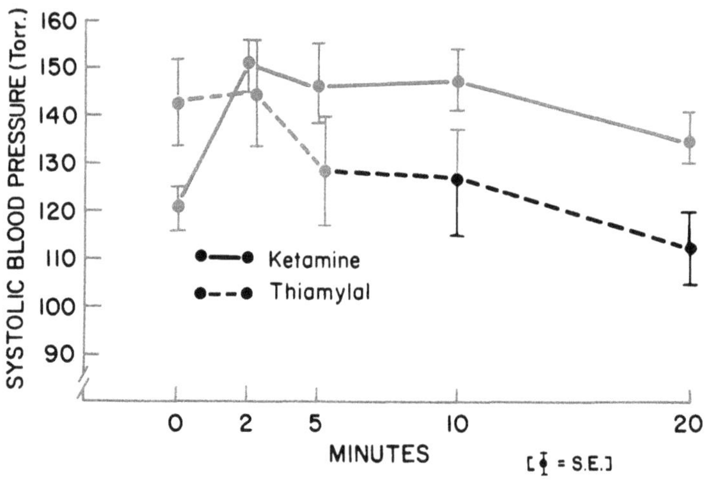

Fig. 27. Changes in systolic blood pressure after i.v.administration of ketamine and thiamylal.

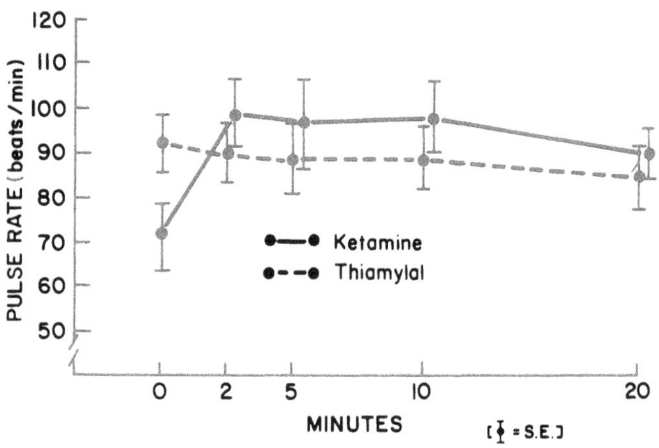

Fig. 28. Changes pulse rate after i.v.administration of ketamine or thiamylal.

mean heart rates of two groups vary, but normalization of the data further stresses the induction of a tachycardia by ketamine alone.

Plasma free norepinephrine and epinephrine levels

As illustrated in Fig. 29, i.v. ketamine caused a significant increase in venous plasma free norepinephrine concentrations peaking at 5 min ($P<0.001$) in contrast to i.v. thiamylal, which caused no significant

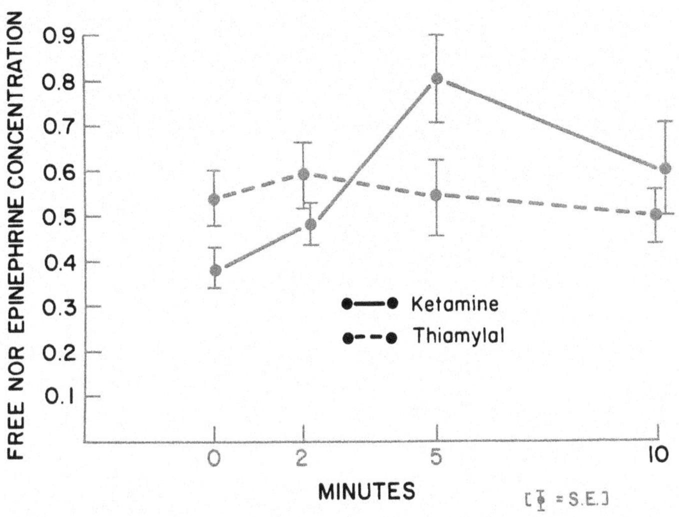

Fig. 29. Plasma free norepinephrine concentration in patients given ketamine or thiamylal for induction of anesthesia.

change in either venous plasma free norepinephrine or venous plasma free epinephrine concentrations. Epinephrine concentrations were not detectable in most of the patient volunteers receiving either ketamine or thiamylal; therefore, these results are not shown in Fig. 29.

The circulatory effects of ketamine are caused by central sympathetic stimulation since the increase in plasma free norepinephrine concentration followed the increase in both systolic and diastolic blood pressures and heart rate. Studies in the isolated perfused hemisphere of goats show that the site of action of ketamine is central and not peripheral or reflex in nature (Ivankovich *et al.*, 1974). Thiamylal i.v. not only reduced the arterial blood pressure, but also depressed the compensatory increase in heart rate and in venous plasma free norepinephrine that normally occurs in response to a decrease in blood pressure (Matsuki *et al.*, 1973). This lack of compensatory increase in central sympathetic activity following thiamylal in combination with its obligatory cardiac depressant effect (Zsigmond *et al.*, 1970; Etsten and Li, 1955) might explain the occurrence of sudden cardiac arrests which have followed the i.v. administration of rapidly acting barbiturates in critically ill patients (Dinnick, 1969), shock patients (Edwards *et al.*, 1956; Barron, 1974) and burn patients (McCaughey, 1962) who are highly dependent for the maintenance of adequate circulation on intact central sympathetic autonomic activity.

As listed in Table 1, ketamine has a number of advantages as compared to i.v. thiamylal for the induction and maintenance of anesthesia.

Ketamine alone and diazepam-ketamine combination in clinical practice

Ketamine has four basic, useful actions in clinical anesthesiology: a) anesthesia, b) a unique central cardiovascular stimulant effect and maintenance of vital reflexes, c) analgesia, and d) emergence reactions. Our research was directed towards methods of minimizing the disadvantages of ketamine while retaining its advantages. We believe that this can be accomplished through premedication with i.v. diazepam followed within 8 to 10 min by ketamine.

Ketamine central cardiovascular stimulation and its attenuation by diazepam

The central actions of ketamine to stimulate the cardiovascular system through sympathetic discharge resemble, but are not identical in mechanism of action to, the effects of lobeline or doxapram. However, respiration is depressed by ketamine. This cardiovascular action of ketamine has advantages in patients in whom the maintenance of adequate cardiovascular function and cardiac contractility are dependent on intact central sympathetic circulatory reflex regulation (Corssen *et al.*, 1970). Reduction in the basal vessel tone resulting in sudden vasodilatation, decreased venous return and decreased cardiac output induced by i.v.

TABLE 1. Comparison of ketamine and i.v. thiamylal for anesthetic induction

	Anesthetic induction agent	
Action	*1.0 mg/kg ketamine*	*5.0 mg/kg thiamylal*
Cardiac	↓	↓↓
Blood pressure	↑↑	↓
Peripheral vascular resistance	↑↑	↓
Cardiac output	↑↑	↓↓
Perfusion of vital organs	↑	↓
Central regulation of the circulation	↑↑	↓↓
Minute ventilation	↓	↓↓
Bronchial muscle tone	↓	↑
Pulmonary shunting	=	↑↑
Cerebral blood flow	↑	↓
Histamine release	=	↑

rapidly acting barbiturates may lead to simultaneous and sometimes catastrophic decrease in both cardiac contractility and peripheral vascular tone. Decreased coronary perfusion may lead to cardiac arrhythmias and/or cardiac arrest. Therefore, ketamine has definite advantages in the management of cardiac patients. This is documented in the data of Fig. 30 in which a comparison was made of the influence of diazepam and ketamine (N = 25) and thiamylal (N = 22) on the incidence of complications during induction of anesthesia in critically ill cardiac patients (Zsigmond *et al.*, 1974).

It is evident from Fig. 30 that although diazepam-ketamine (DK) caused a higher incidence of tachycardia during induction of anesthesia than i.v. thiamylal (T), the incidence of hypotension and bradycardia were markedly reduced. Hypotension and bradycardia, especially in combination, in a patient with an impaired coronary blood supply may result in sudden cardiac arrest as a result of sudden decrease in coronary perfusion pressure head. These findings further support the notion that ketamine is superior to i.v. barbiturates for the induction of anesthesia in critically ill patients (Virtue *et al.*, 1967; Corssen *et al.*, 1970; Tweed *et al.*, 1972; Chaspakis *et al.*, 1973 and Zsigmond *et al.*, 1974).

Analgesic action of ketamine

Clinical experience in critically ill, hemorrhagic shock, and burn patients first suggested that, in addition to the somatic analgesic effect of

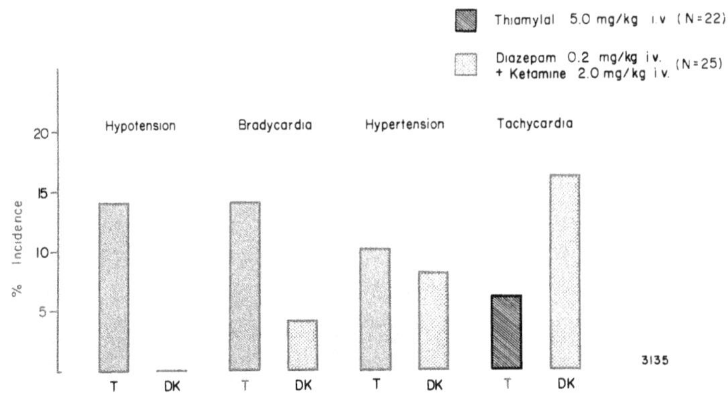

Fig. 30. Comparison of circulatory complications associated with diazepam-ketamine and thiamylal induction.

ketamine, it also has a visceral analgesic effect. Many patients who recovered from loss of consciousness to full awareness following ketamine anesthesia had prolonged analgesia and no recall of painful procedures (Virtue *et al.*, 1967; Corssen *et al.*, 1968; Tweed *et al.*, 1972; Chasapakis *et al.*, 1973; Zsigmond *et al.*, 1974). The dose requirements for analgesia are markedly lower than for anesthesia with loss of consciousness, as shown by both clinical pharmacologic studies and blood level determinations (Idvall, 1978). The analgesic effect of ketamine i.m. can be used with advantage in children or adults in whom no i.v. route is necessary for a short but painful procedure, *i.e.*, dressing or suture removal or other short, painful procedures. Intramuscular injection of 1.0-5.0 mg/kg ketamine caused no marked respiratory depression or excessive circulatory stimulation in such patients.

Ataract analgesia with diazepam-ketamine for induction of anesthesia for ASA I-II patients

The marked circulatory stimulation following the induction of anesthesia with ketamine as a sole agent forced us to consider the concomitant or prior use of agents which may alleviate the circulatory stimulation in response to 2.0 mg/kg/30 sec ketamine administration. In a former clinical pharmacological study comparing droperidol-fentanyl with diazepam-fentanyl analgesia we observed a moderation of excessive shifts in both sympathetic and parasympathetic autonomic activity during anesthesia with the i.v. administration of diazepam 0.2 to 0.3 mg/kg/4 min. Therefore, we carried out a pilot study in healthy gynecologic patient volunteers to determine whether 0.2 mg/kg diazepam may also reduce the cardiocirculatory stimulation induced by ketamine. These volunteers received no respiratory support or supplemental oxygen. Arterial blood samples were used for the determination of norepinephrine by Vendsalu's method (1960).

Circulatory effects

In this double blind study, we observed a highly significant ($P < 0.001$) reduction in the direct arterial blood pressure and heart rate ($P < 0.01$) increases following 2.0 mg/kg ketamine by pretreatment with diazepam 0.2 mg/kg, both given i.v. This can be seen by comparing the data in Figs. 31 and 32.

Diazepam, when given i.v. at least 5 min but not later than 15 min before ketamine, caused a marked reduction in increased sympathetic activity induced by ketamine, as reflected in a significant reduction in arterial plasma free norepinephrine concentrations, systolic blood pressure and

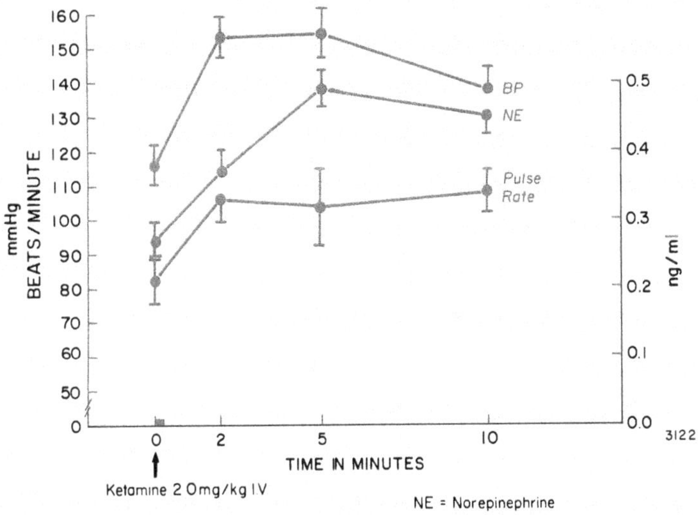

Fig. 31. Arterial plasma free norepinephrine, blood pressure and pulse rate changes in six patients given ketamine alone.

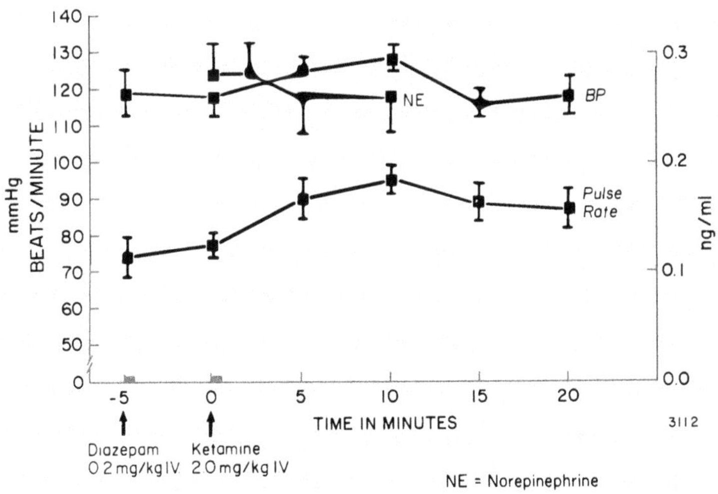

Fig. 32. Arterial plasma free norepinephrine, blood pressure, and pulse rate changes in six patients given diazepam-ketamine.

heart rate. This is illustrated again in 2 groups of 8 patients, in each of whom plasma free norepinephrine was assayed, as shown in Fig. 33.

In two other groups of healthy ASA I-II patients, each of whom underwent minor surgery but received oxygen and respiratory assistance, identical findings were obtained. As Figs. 34 and 35 show, arterial plasma free norepinephrine showed changes identical to those found in the previous study (Zsigmond *et al.*, 1974, as illustrated in Fig. 33).

Pretreatment with diazepam (0.2 mg/kg) 5 min before ketamine (2.0 mg/kg), both given i.v. to 6 patients in each group, lowered plasma free norepinephrine and epinephrine levels (Fig. 36).

Respiratory effects

In order to rule out that ketamine might have altered blood gases, primarily $PaCO_2$, which in turn might have caused central sympathetic stimulation, we carried out an additional study in ASA I-II gynecologic patients who received ketamine (2.0 mg/kg/30 sec), or diazepam (0.2 mg/kg/3 min) and 5 min later ketamine (2.0 mg/kg/30 sec) for induction of anesthesia. Chest plethysmographic recordings and arterial blood gases

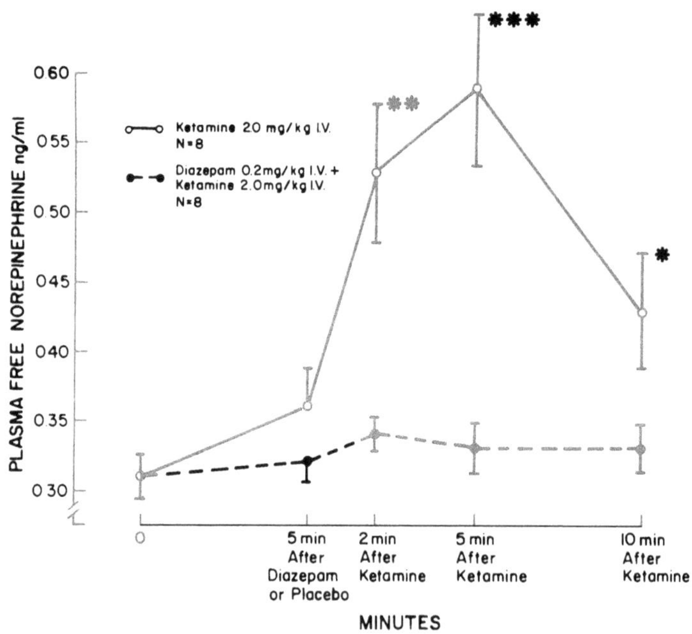

Fig. 33. Plasma free norepinephrine concentration in patients induced with ketamine or diazepam-ketamine.

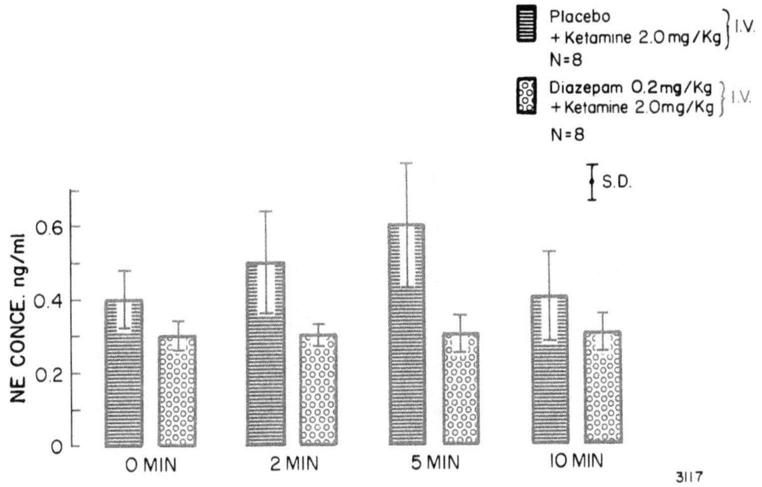

Fig. 34. Plasma free norepinephrine levels in patients following ketamine and diazepam-ketamine anesthetic induction with oxygenation.

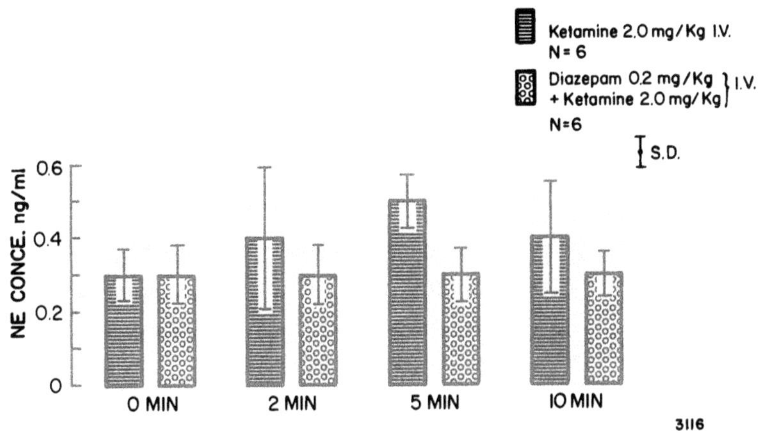

Fig. 35. Plasma free norepinephrine levels in patients following ketamine and diazepam-ketamine anesthetic induction without additional oxygenation.

showed that ketamine caused a marked respiratory depression lasting for 5 to 8 min without a significant increase ($P<0.01$) in $PaCO_2$, significant reduction ($P<0.01$) in PaO_2 and a significant reduction in respiratory rates in both groups (see Fig. 37 for blood gas data). Some volunteers became apneic for 40 to 70 sec following the i.v. administration of ketamine.

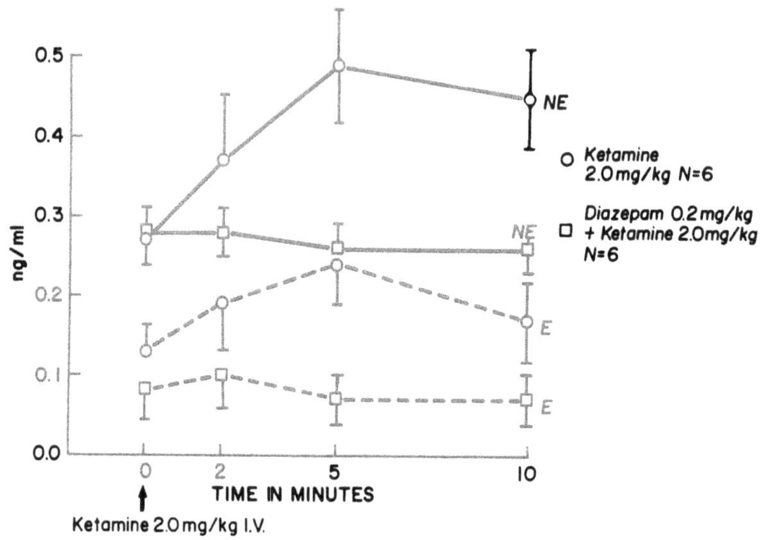

Fig. 36. Arterial plasma free epinephrine and norepinephrine concentrations in patients induced with ketamine or diazepam-ketamine.

Pretreatment with diazepam in a dose of 0.2 mg/kg caused no significant change except at 2 min ($P<0.05$), a further increase in $PaCO_2$, but no change in the PaO_2 reduction induced by ketamine. Diazepam neither counteracted nor potentiated the marked respiratory depression and apnea which occurred following the i.v. administration of ketamine in the volunteers (Fig. 37). Larger doses of diazepam (0.3 mg/kg/5 min), however, caused a potentiation of respiratory depression in volunteers who received ketamine for anesthetic induction, as illustrated previously in Figs. 15-17. This transient but potent respiratory depressant effect of ketamine must be taken into consideration when this agent is used for induction of anesthesia. The patient must receive assisted ventilation and enrichment of the inhaled atmosphere with oxygen in order to avoid hypoxemia, hypercarbia, and metabolic acidosis as consequences of respiratory depression (Zsigmond *et al.*, 1976).

The increase in norepinephrine concentration following ketamine administration without respiratory assistance was of the same magnitude as in the patients who did receive respiratory assistance and oxygen (see Figs. 34 and 35). Hence, it is not likely that the circulatory changes and increase in the arterial plasma free norepinephrine were the result of secondary circulatory changes triggered by primary respiratory depres-

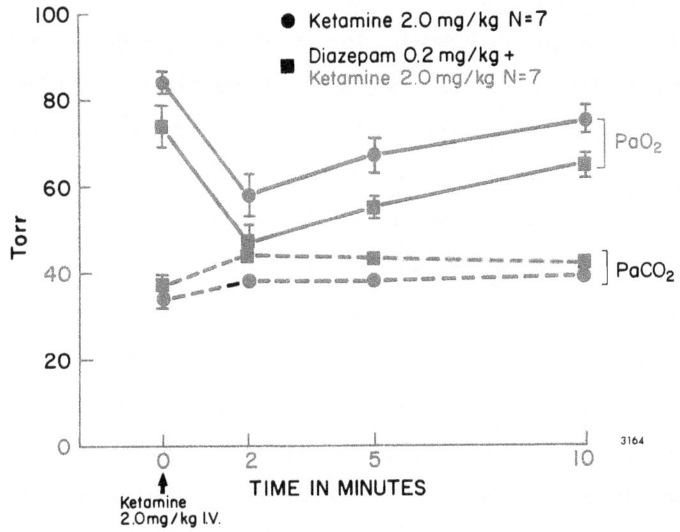

Fig. 37. Effects of ketamine and diazepam-ketamine on arterial blood gases.

sion induced by increased autonomic activity (Kothary and Zsigmond, 1975), as suggested by the work of Dowdy and Kaya (1968). They observed increased autonomic reflex activity following i.v. ketamine administration.

Airway maintenance during diazepam-ketamine

The present series of studies further corroborates the original observations of Corssen and Domino (1966) and Corssen *et al.* (1968) in that none of the patients required insertion of an artificial airway. No relaxation of the jaw muscles followed the administration of i.v. ketamine, in contrast to the marked relaxation of jaw muscles that leads to airway obstruction following the i.v. administration of rapidly acting barbiturates or other currently available anesthetic induction agents. This maintenance of jaw muscle tone following the administration of ketamine is a great advantage when anesthesia is to be given to patients in whom there is difficulty in maintaining an open airway or in whom endotracheal intubation may prove to be difficult to impossible, *e.g.*, patients with facial and airway burns. These patients may receive ketamine anesthesia safely if an increased concentration of oxygen is supplied through a face mask even without respiratory assistance, since ketamine respiratory depression is short lived. No arrhythmia or metabolic acidosis developed in any of the volunteers after ketamine induction without respiratory assistance but with oxygen inhalation. Indeed, adequate oxygenation was observed in the patients receiving ketamine anesthesia without the insertion of an oropharyngeal or nasal airway and/or any support of the jaw during the induction of anesthesia simply by increasing the inhaled oxygen concentration.

Diazepam-Ketamine Analgesia for Induction of Anesthesia in ASA III-V Physical State Patients

Plasma free norepinephrine and epinephrine and circulatory effects

After the initial studies in ASA I-II physical state patients proved that i.v. pretreatment with diazepam markedly reduced the cardiovascular stimulation induced by ketamine, we immediately began to utilize this combination for the management of anesthesia in cardiac and critically ill patients. Between 1970 and 1973 we administered anesthesia to 500-600 patients who were in ASA physical states IV-V and IVE-VE.

A controlled clinical study by Yoon *et al.* (1975) demonstrated the safety of diazepam-ketamine in 30 patients before undergoing aorto-coronary bypass. The circulatory data of this study are plotted in Fig. 38.

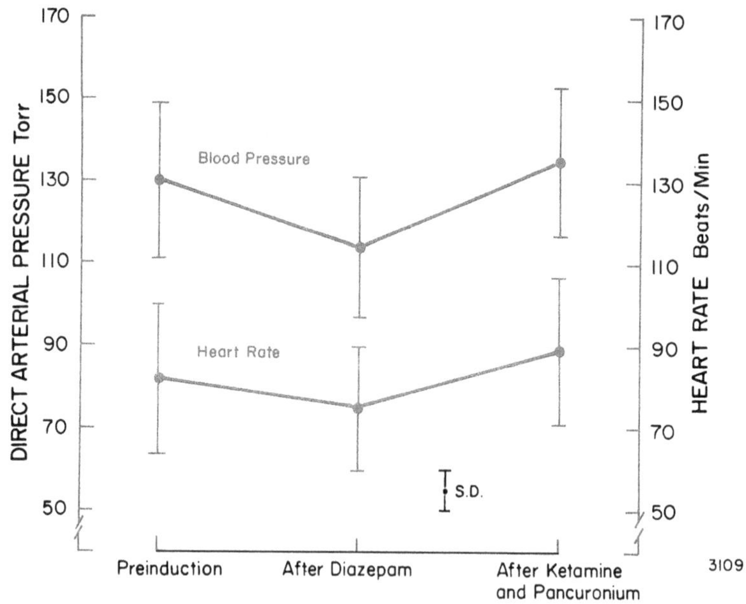

Fig. 38. Circulatory changes following diazepam-ketamine induction in 30 cardiac patients undergoing aorto-coronary bypass operations.

After the i.v. administration of diazepam, both blood pressure and heart rate were reduced. After the sequential administration of pancuronium and ketamine, a slight mean increase in both direct arterial blood pressure and heart rate occurred. However, no significant increase over the initial blood pressure and heart rate occurred following completion of the induction sequence.

In order to further objectively authenticate these observations, we set up another study in 12 cardiac patients prior to undergoing cardiac surgery under cardiopulmonary bypass for valvular reparative or coronary bypass procedures (Kumar *et al.*, 1978).

Circulatory effects

As illustrated in Figs. 39 and 40, the combination of diazepam and ketamine caused no significant increase in either systolic or diastolic arterial blood pressure directly recorded from the radial artery, in heart rate recorded from the R-R interval of the electrocardiogram and in the arterial plasma free norepinephrine and epinephrine levels.

If one compares the plasma free catecholamine levels and circulatory changes in healthy volunteers and cardiac patients, it is evident that no difference between these 2 groups was observed. Of course, in the cardiac patients respiration was always manually assisted, and an enriched oxy-

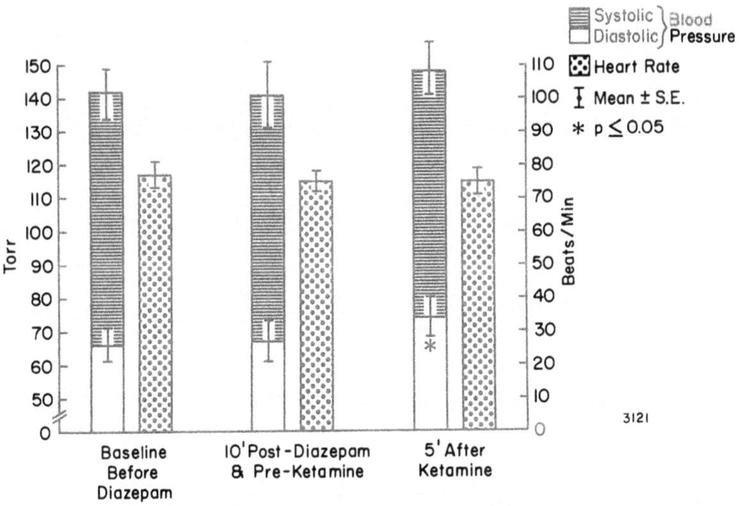

Fig. 39. Direct arterial pressure and heart rate changes during diazepam-ketamine induction in cardiac surgical patients.

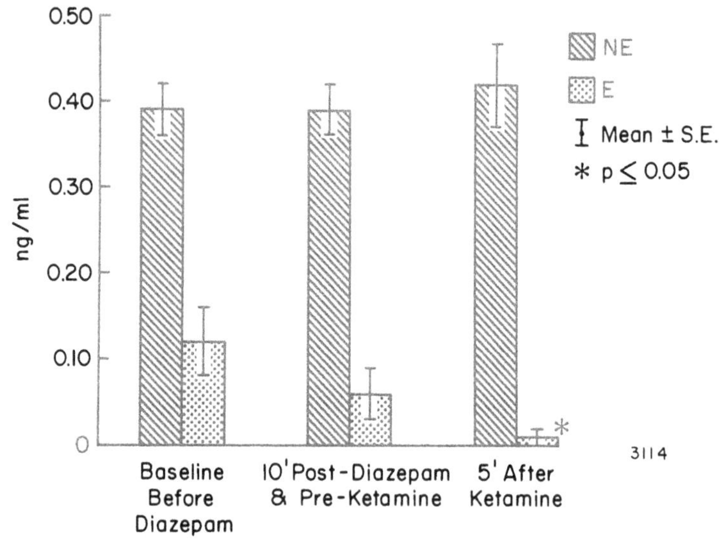

Fig. 40. Plasma free norepinephrine and epinephrine concentrations during diazepam-ketamine induction in cardiac surgical patients.

gen concentration was always used in the inhaled atmosphere in order to prevent any circulatory changes secondary to ventilatory depression and alterations in arterial blood gases or acid base balance.

Fig. 41 illustrates that although cardiac patients initially had higher arterial plasma free norepinephrine and epinephrine concentrations than normal volunteers, no greater increase in plasma free norepinephrine concentration occurred following diazepam-ketamine induction in cardiacs than in normal volunteers. A significant decrease in plasma free epinephrine concentration occurred in cardiac patients after diazepam-ketamine induction, as can be noted in Fig. 41.

Diazepam-ketamine induction for cardiac surgical patients

The circulatory sequelàe following the administration of 0.3 mg/kg/4 min diazepam—2.0 mg/kg/30 sec ketamine induction in a poor risk ASA V patient undergoing coronary bypass surgery—is shown in Fig. 42.

Note that the plasma free norepinephrine and epinephrine levels remain normal during induction of anesthesia with the diazepam and

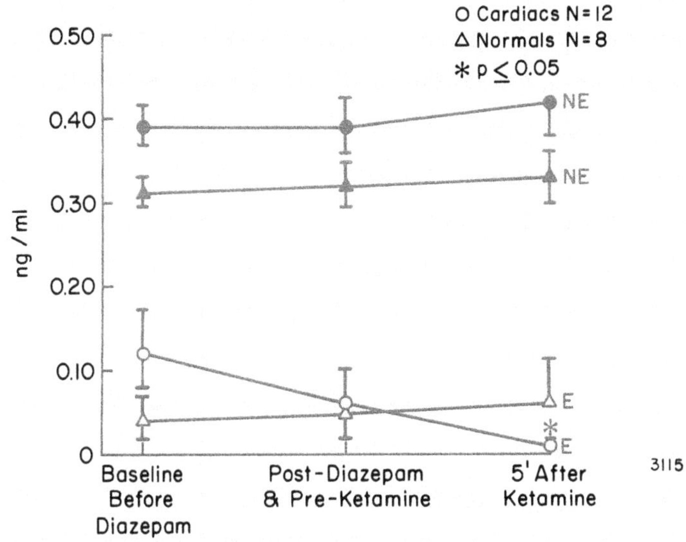

Fig. 41. Comparison of the plasma free norepinephrine and epinephrine concentrations of healthy and cardiac surgical patients during diazepam-ketamine induction.

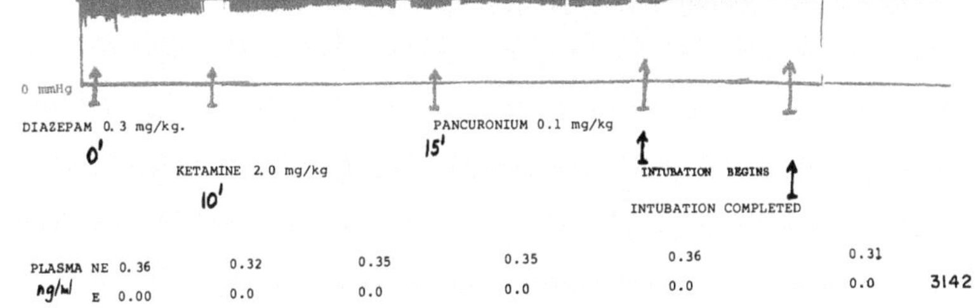

Fig. 42. Diazepam-ketamine anesthesia in a patient in physical state ASA V.

ketamine combination. No significant increase in arterial pressure (directly recorded) was observed following induction. Furthermore, the subsequent administration of pancuronium did not elicit marked cardiocirculatory stimulation on the combination of ketamine with a skeletal muscle relaxant. We must emphasize, however, that when this technique is used, respiration must be assisted. The arterial $PaCO_2$ increased from 32 to 57 Torr during intubation. The pharynx, larynx and trachea were not sprayed with a local anesthetic, resulting in a marked increase in arterial blood pressure during and following intubation, as seen in Fig. 42.

Diazepam-ketamine induction for carotid vascular surgical patients

There are advantages of diazepam-ketamine anesthetic induction in a patient in physical state IVE scheduled for a carotid artery bypass. An example is illustrated in Fig. 43. It may be noted that the administration of ketamine was followed by a moderate rise and certainly no decrease in arterial blood pressure. As is well known in this type of patient, severe hypotension, especially in response to head up tilt resulting in reduction of the already impaired cerebral blood flow, may lead to cerebral hypoxia and hemiplegia. Diazepam-ketamine anesthetic induction has a definite advantage in patients undergoing carotid vascular surgery over other induction agents, such as i.v. rapidly acting barbiturates which may cause sudden reduction in arterial blood pressure and cerebral blood flow.

Use of diazepam-ketamine in a patient with pheochromocytoma

The test of the safety of diazepam-ketamine induction was made when we had to provide emergency anesthesia for a reoperation of a patient with pheochromocytoma in an extremely bad physical state of VE.

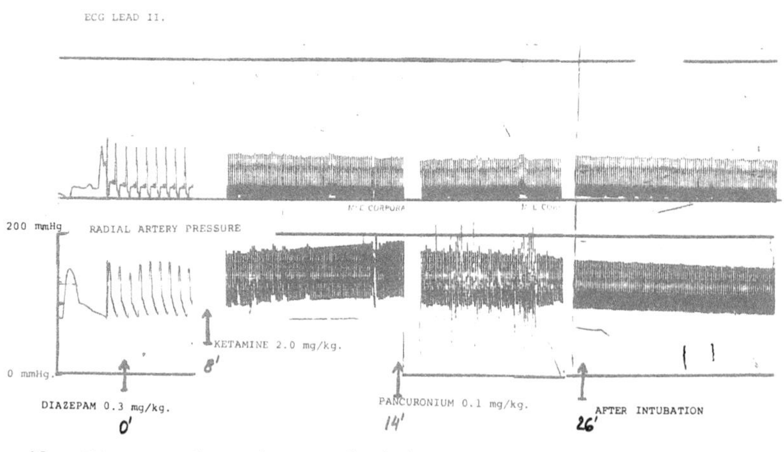

Fig. 43. Diazepam-ketamine anesthesia in a patient in physical state ASA IVE.

As illustrated in Fig. 44, the combination of diazepam-ketamine safely achieved our aim to induce anesthesia without adverse sequelae.

No hypotension, bradycardia, arrhythmias, or bronchospasm occurred in this individual. Since this initial study, we have provided safe induction of anesthesia for two additional patients with pheochromocytoma with a combination of diazepam-ketamine. These cases further corroborate our findings that circulatory changes induced by ketamine have a central origin, since no adrenomedullary stimulation occurred in these pheochromocytoma patients receiving diazepam-ketamine induction. These findings are in striking contrast to the cardiocirculatory and norepinephrine increases which follow the administration of large i.v. doses of morphine for induction of anesthesia. Zsigmond and Martinez (1974) showed a marked rise in plasma free norepinephrine levels in response to the severe hypotension following the i.v. administration of 3.0 mg/kg/10 min morphine in critically ill cardiac patients. Bradycardia followed by tachycardia, hypotension followed by hypertension in many other patients triggered cardiac arrhythmias and myocardiac infarcts during the utilization of i.v. morphine bolus (3.0 mg/kg/5 min) technique. Therefore, after an initial trial of this technique, we replaced i.v. morphine with 0.4 mg/kg/10 min diazepam followed by 2.0 mg/kg/20 sec ketamine 5 min later. Also, diazepam 0.4 mg/kg/5 min followed by fentanyl 10 g/kg/5 min or

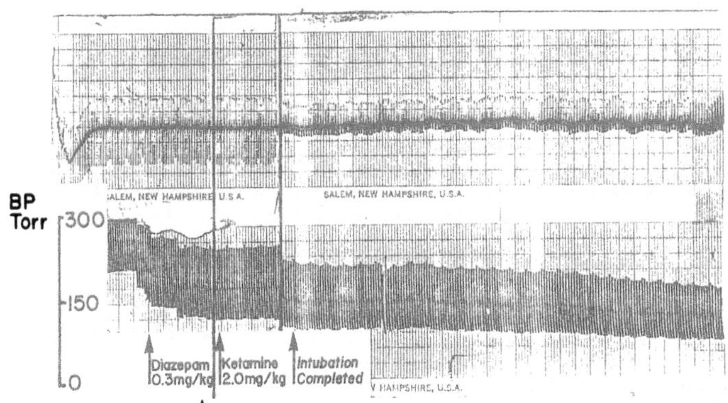

Fig. 44. Diazepam-ketamine in a patient with pheochromocytoma.

1.0 mg/kg/10 min morphine can be used for the induction of anesthesia in ASA III-V or poor risk patients (Zsigmond *et al.*, 1976).

The advantages of induction with 0.2-0.4 mg/kg diazepam followed by 1.0-2.0 mg/kg/30 sec ketamine 5 min later are: 1) lack of cardiac depression as compared to other available induction techniques, 2) the lack of depression of central sympathetic circulatory regulation, 3) probable lack of histamine release, 4) lack of increase in muscle tone and increase in metabolic oxygen demand which follows the administration of N-methylated barbiturates and of ketamine as a sole agent used for i.v. induction of anesthesia, 5) no adverse psychic sequelae to ketamine administration, 6) no organotoxicity. Therefore, this technique can be used in patients with renal and/or hepatic failure.

Psychic effects

Although these investigations showed an antagonism of the cardiocirculatory effect of ketamine by i.v. diazepam, the question whether the adverse psychic side effects are also reduced or eliminated by pretreatment with diazepam remained unsettled. Our hypothesis was that ketamine may induce the psychic adverse effects (Kothary and Zsigmond, 1975) by the same central mechanism as the circulatory stimulation. Therefore, a double blind study was conducted in a large group of healthy gynecologic patients in ASA I-II physical state. Half of the patients

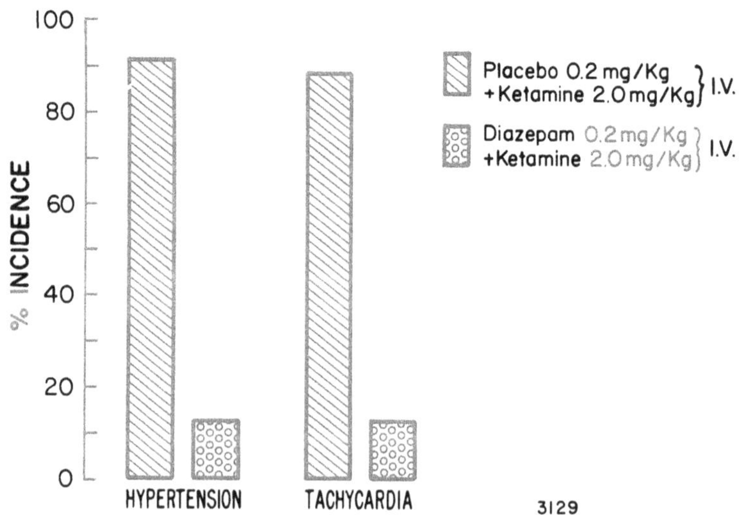

Fig. 45. Antagonism of ketamine induced circulatory changes by pretreatment with diazepam.

received 0.3 mg/kg diazepam pretreatment and half of them received placebo prior to the i.v. administration of 2.0 mg/kg/30 sec ketamine. Pretreatment with diazepam markedly reduced cardiocirculatory stimulation in those patients given i.v. ketamine in the doses shown in Fig. 45. The mean maintenance dose requirements for ketamine in patients with ASA I-II physical states is shown in Fig. 46.

Pretreatment with diazepam successfully prevented the recall of bad dreams, visual disturbances, pleasant dreams and hallucinations induced by ketamine, as illustrated in Fig. 47. We were surprised to observe such a high incidence of hallucinations using this technique with ketamine alone.

Ketamine infusion for maintenance of anesthesia

Since 1973, we have utilized diazepam 0.3 mg/kg/5 min and ketamine 2.0 mg/kg/30 sec for induction of anesthesia in several hundred patients without adverse psychic sequelae. From the study on psychic effects, it also became evident that a dose of 2.0 mg/kg/hr ketamine for maintenance of anesthesia and analgesia following 2.0 mg/kg/30 sec induction dose caused complete amnesia and analgesia for the events in the operating room. These patients received only diazepam and ketamine i.v., oxygen and an i.v. succinylcholine drip. Since ketamine caused little relaxation of skeletal muscles, we were forced to use i.v. succinylcholine drip for the maintenance of muscle relaxation in these patients. Since

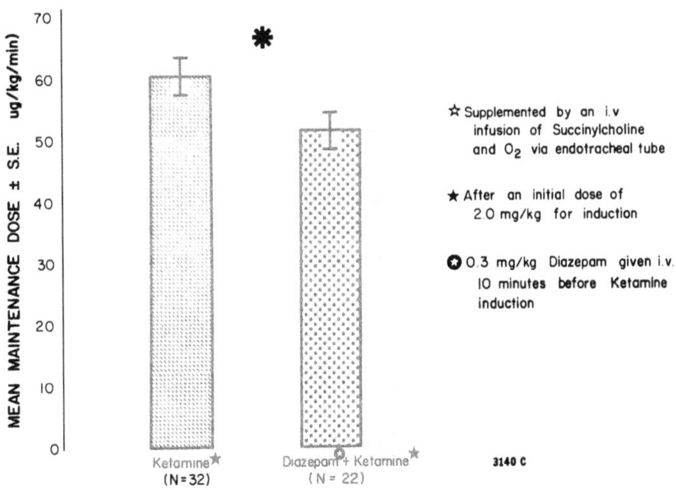

Fig. 46. Maintenance dose requirements for ketamine in patients with ASA I-II physical states.

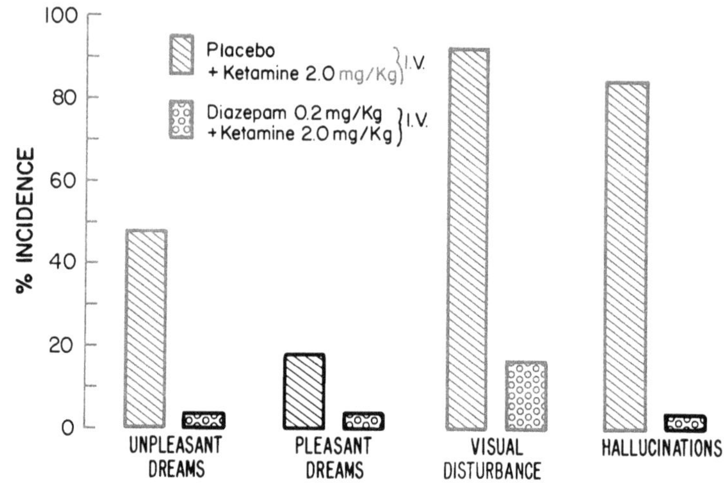

Fig. 47. Antagonism of ketamine induced psychic sequelae by pretreatment with diazepam.

these patients underwent primarily intra-abdominal procedures with no recall of pain or the events, this study also supports the contention that ketamine has both anesthetic and analgesic effects, not only for somatic but also for visceral pain. Interview of these patients in the recovery room immediately following anesthesia and 24 hr later revealed a favorable acceptance of diazepam-ketamine as compared to ketamine alone. Fig. 48 illustrates that the patients who received diazepam-ketamine were discharged from the recovery room in about the same time as those who received ketamine only.

The mean recovery room stay of both groups was the same as the mean period following inhalation anesthesia in our institution. Therefore, no marked prolongation of the recovery room stay was observed in either group of these patients, since the excitement of the patients who received placebo-ketamine was well controlled by i.v. diazepam. The use of low doses of both diazepam (0.2 mg/kg/2 min) and ketamine (1.0 mg/kg/30 sec) for the maintenance of short anesthesia, even in patients scheduled for outpatient surgery, allows early discharge from the recovery room. A dose of 0.3 mg/kg i.v. diazepam followed 10 min later by an induction dose of 1.0 mg/kg of ketamine and subsequent 1 mg/kg/hr of ketamine i.v. drip in combination with N_20-0_2 and muscle relaxants proved to be effective and safe to maintain adequate amnesia and analgesia in hundreds of surgical patients. Only 4 patients reported unpleasant recall to the administration of this combination over a 5 yr period.

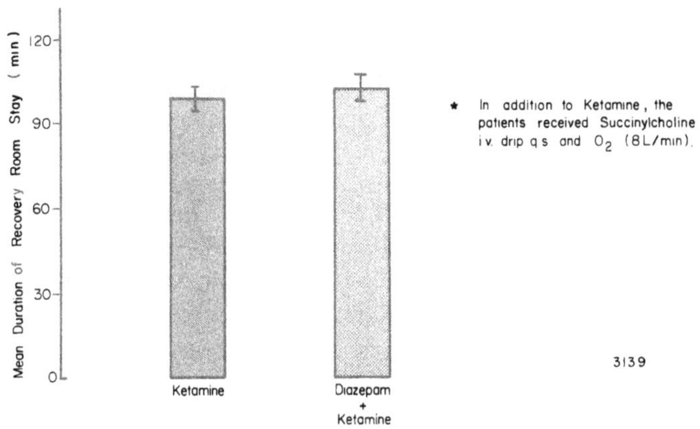

Fig. 48. Duration of recovery room stay in patients with ASA I-II physical state receiving ketamine i.v.drip.

EEG effects of ketamine i.v. drip administration

Determination of EEG recordings in the patients who received placebo-ketamine *vs* diazepam-ketamine induction followed by i.v. maintenance by ketamine showed that the EEG effects of diazepam are superimposed on the EEG effects of ketamine. No convulsions were observed even in epileptic patients who received ketamine for several hours as the sole agent.

Special studies on the safety of ketamine and diazepam-ketamine

Liver function. Special attention was paid to liver function following the administration of placebo-ketamine or diazepam-ketamine for induction and ketamine i.v. drip for the maintenance of anesthesia in all volunteer studies. We were unable to demonstrate any adverse effect on liver function in patients anesthetized with diazepam-ketamine in the 220 volunteer patients studied. This further supports the findings that ketamine did not adversely alter liver function in healthy volunteers who received it about one week apart on two occasions, as summarized in Figs. 23-26.

Other organ functions. No adverse effects of ketamine on renal function were revealed by any of the clinical follow-ups of the volunteers and/or patients. Serum creatinine and BUN remained normal following the administration of either ketamine or diazepam-ketamine combination. In a study conducted in 10 healthy gynecologic patient volunteers, it was shown that, although a reduction in plasma cholinesterase activity followed ketamine administration i.v., this was very transient and enzyme activity returned to normal after 10 min (Kothary and Zsigmond, 1978). Creatinine phosphokinase levels following induction with ketamine remained normal for the subsequent 24 hr in 8 healthy gynecologic patients who received repeated doses of ketamine for maintenance of anesthesia (Zsigmond, 1971).

Reflex circulatory regulation in response to positional changes

Since many operations require head up tilt or lateral tilt of surgical patients, it was essential to know the influence of surgical positioning on circulation during diazepam-ketamine and placebo-ketamine induction and maintenance of anesthesia. The positioning may cause changes in the ventilation and perfusion in the lung, in cerebral perfusion, and in the regulation of blood pressure and cardiac output. As illustrated in Fig. 49, the table tilt responses were not adversely affected by the use of either diazepam-ketamine or placebo-ketamine i.v. induction.

We carried out a double blind study in 18 healthy gynecologic pa-

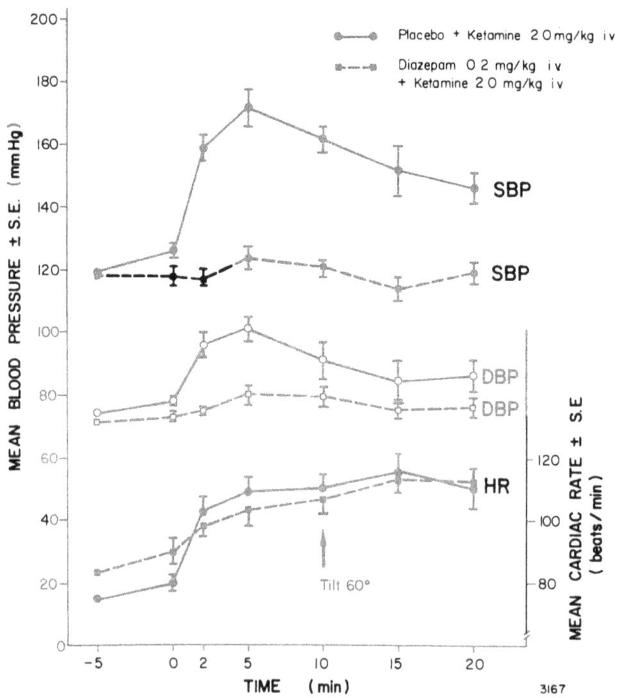

Fig. 49. Blood pressure and cardiac rate changes before and after table tilt following placebo-ketamine or diazepam-ketamine induction.

tients to determine whether patients induced with diazepam-ketamine or placebo-ketamine tolerate table tilt and gained insight into its comparison with other induction techniques (Kumar *et al.*, 1978). It is well known that i.v. barbiturates cause a marked reduction in reflex circulatory regulation in response to table tilt. The expected increase in plasma free norepinephrine following table tilt did not occur in those patients induced with ketamine or diazepam-ketamine. Norepinephrine levels, elevated at the time of table tilt, were not altered following table tilt (see Fig. 50).

These findings in healthy gynecologic patients were further confirmed in patients receiving anesthesia for induction who were positioned in the head up tilt position. Most of these patients underwent carotid bypass surgery in whom hypotension and reduction in circulatory response to table tilt might result in reduced cerebral blood flow with possible adverse or fatal sequelae. Cardiac patients who had to be induced in head up tilt because of the extreme hypoxia and pulmonary edema also tolerated well diazepam-ketamine in head up tilt in contrast to i.v. barbiturates. Thoracic surgical patients who require lateral position immediately following intubation well tolerated the tilt. No adverse sequelae were observed in this type of patient. This is in agreement with findings of Silvay *et al.* (1978) that no shunting in the lung was observed in thoracic surgical patients during thoracotomy maintained with ketamine anesthesia.

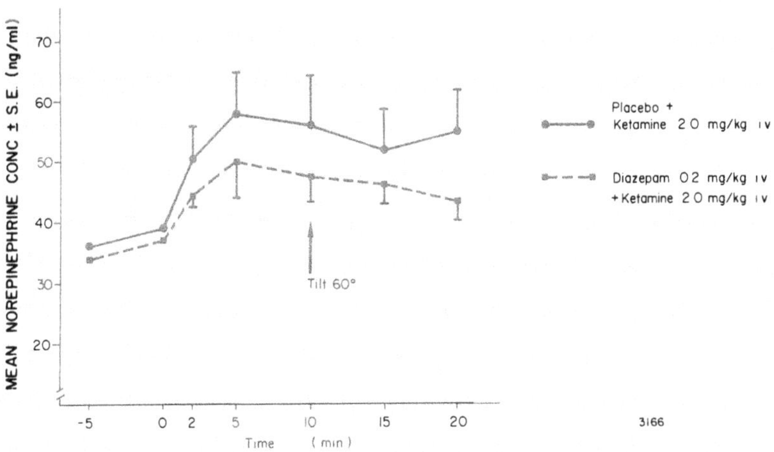

Fig. 50. Plasma free norepinephrine levels before and after table tilt following placebo-ketamine or diazepam-ketamine induction.

Interaction with Skeletal Muscle Relaxants

Effect of ketamine on the circulatory effects of pancuronium

The advantages of pancuronium for intubation and maintenance of skeletal muscle relaxation are well documented. No ganglionic block, histamine release or cardiac arrhythmias follow its administration (Zsigmond *et al.*, 1974). Therefore, this agent is widely utilized in poor risk, cardiac and burn patients for endotracheal intubation and maintenance of skeletal muscle relaxation. Pancuronium, however, causes an increase in the pulse rate, probably by an atropine like action (Saxena and Bonta, 1971). In order to determine whether this vagolytic effect in any way increased the adverse circulatory sequelae following ketamine administraiton, we studied ketamine (N = 5) and thiamylal (N = 8) in combination with pancuronium during induction of anesthesia (Zsigmond *et al.*, 1976). Contrary to our expectations, the combination of ketamine with pancuronium resulted in no greater increase in plasma free norepinephrine levels or pulse rate than ketamine alone, as illustrated in Figs. 51 and 52. Pancuronium, surprisingly, reduced significantly the increase in blood pressure and pulse rate induced by ketamine (Matsuki *et al.*, 1974).

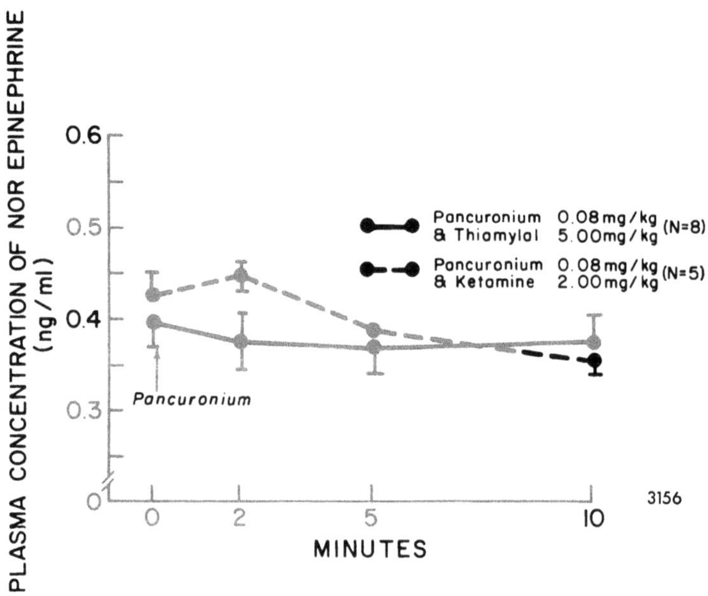

Fig. 51. Concentration of norepinephrine in patients receiving pancuronium in addition to thiamylal or ketamine.

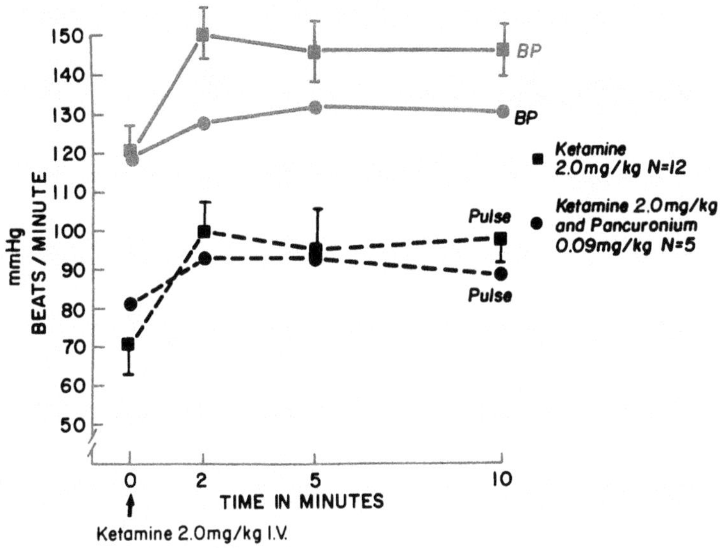

Fig. 52. Cardiovascular effects in patients receiving ketamine or ketamine-pancuronium.

Although we can offer no explanation for this antagonistic effect of pancuronium on ketamine induced cardiocirculatory effects, this combination can be used with advantage for intubation following a safe induction with diazepam-ketamine in a poor risk or cardiac patient (Kumar *et al.*, 1977).

Effect of ketamine on skeletal muscle relaxant requirements

Succinylcholine requirements were not different between patients receiving i.v. ketamine alone or diazepam-ketamine. When compared to the requirements for maintenance of relaxation during thiopental anesthesia, it appears that more succinylcholine was required for the ketamine groups (Fig. 53). Amaki *et al.* (1978) showed a markedly altered response to all skeletal muscle relaxants in the rate of blockade of the rat phrenic nerve hemidiaphragm preparation. However, Johnston *et al.* (1974) found a marked reduction only in *d*-tubocurarine and a slight reduction in succinylcholine requirements in patients anesthetized with halothane (0.95-1.05%) who received 75.0 mg/m^2 ketamine i.v. prior to these skeletal muscle relaxants. As shown in Fig. 54, the pancuronium dose requirement was less affected than the dose requirements of *d*-tubocurarine and succinylcholine. The latter study involved the interaction of many

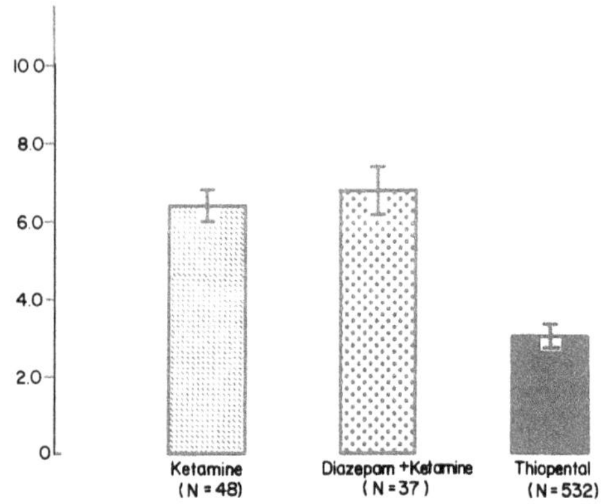

Fig. 53. Influence of ketamine and diazepam-ketamine and thiopental on succinylcholine requirements.

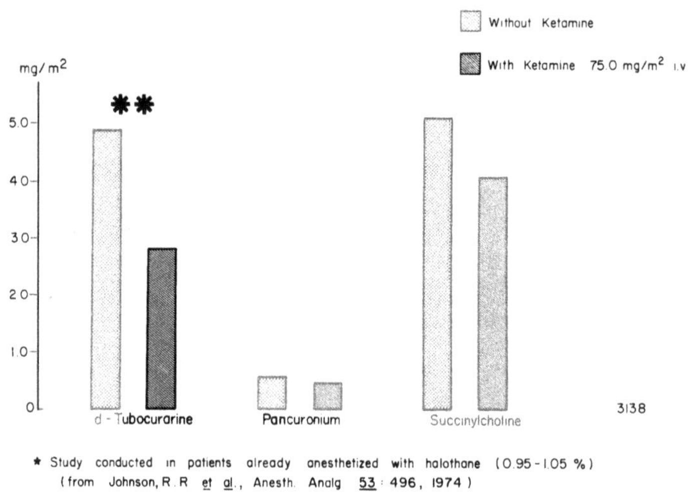

Fig. 54. The influence of ketamine on the ED_{50} of neuromuscular blocking drugs.

agents. Obviously, more research needs to be done in this area, as described in the chapter by Lee *et al.* in this volume.

Conclusions

1. Ketamine alone reduces *alpha* and increases *theta* waves in the human EEG.
2. Ketamine alters markedly the visually evoked response from scalp electrodes. It does not block visual input but alters it.

3. Ketamine produces anesthesia which is dose related and short lasting. Individual differences are noted.
4. Ketamine induces a dose related increase in the duration of loss of consciousness, respiratory depression, arterial hypertension (both systolic and diastolic), EEG slow waves, and depression of the VER. Analgesia is profound. Ketamine alone has useful anesthetic properties but also a number of disadvantages, especially hypertension, tachycardia and psychic side effects.
5. Diazepam prolongs ketamine loss of consciousness. The EEG shows superimposed patterns of both drugs.
6. Diazepam pretreatment reduces ketamine induced hypertension.
7. Diazepam enhances slightly ketamine respiratory depression.
8. Ketamine blood levels fall rapidly following 2.2 mg/kg i.v./30 sec.
9. Pharmacokinetics of ketamine (although more complex) can be described by a two compartment open model.
10. The marked cardiorespiratory effects of ketamine occur during its *alpha* phase of redistribution.
11. Diazepam elevates the plasma concentrations of ketamine.
12. The plasma concentrations of ketamine metabolite I and the extraction artifact ketamine and metabolite II are not altered by diazepam.
13. Urinary excretion of ketamine is unchanged by diazepam (not shown in a figure).
14. Ketamine induced sleeping time is prolonged by diazepam.
15. Diazepam reduces the hypertensive effects of ketamine.
16. The normal table tilt response is well maintained following both placebo-ketamine and diazepam-ketamine.
17. Emergence reactions are reduced by diazepam.
18. Liver function is not altered by ketamine.
19. Ketamine causes plasma cholinesterase inhibition, both *in vitro* and *in vivo*. However, this is transient. It is followed by a slight increase.
20. Ketamine has many advantages over thiamylal in patients whose diseases contraindicate the use of i.v. rapidly acting barbiturates. These include:
    a) Patients with congestive heart failure
    b) Hypovolemic patients owing to acute hemorrhage
    c) Patients with reduced cerebral blood flow (such as occlusive diseases
    d) Hypertensive cardiovascular disease with hypovolemia
    e) Patients in whom positional changes are required for the operation
    f) Asthmatic patients
    g) Patients with allergic diathesis

h) Patients in renal failure whose excretion of barbiturates is reduced
i) Patients in hepatic failure whose metabolism of barbiturates is reduced

21. The central stimulant effect of ketamine is advantageous in patients in whom increased central sympathetic activity prevents reduction in the perfusion of vital organs, *e.g.*, burn patients, patients in shock and patients in heart failure.
22. Both somatic and visceral analgesia can be provided by reduced doses of ketamine in an i.v. drip (1.0 mg/kg/hr after an initial 1.0 mg/kg/30 sec dose) or by 2.0-5.0 mg/kg i.m. ketamine.
23. Diazepam (0.2-0.3 mg/kg/4 min) given 8 to 10 min prior to ketamine antagonizes the marked circulatory stimulation and increase in norepinephrine and epinephrine induced by 2.0 mg/kg/30 sec ketamine induction.
24. Although the jaw muscles are well maintained during ketamine anesthesia, a transient respiratory depression occurs in the absence of surgical stimulation that is further increased by diazepam in a dose greater than 0.2 mg/kg. Oxygen administration and/or respiratory assistance are, therefore, required when ketamine is used in a rapid i.v. injection (30 sec).
25. Diazepam-ketamine induction in ASA III-V physical state patients causes minimal circulatory changes and no alterations in sympathetic activity when oxygen and respiratory assistance are provided.
26. Diazepam markedly alleviates the psychic adverse sequelae to ketamine administration.
27. Ketamine can be safely employed for maintenance of anesthesia after diazepam pretreatment or in a slow i.v. drip.
28. The EEG effects of diazepam-ketamine anesthesia represent a composite of the actions of these agents.
29. No hepatotoxicity or muscle injury is evident following ketamine or diazepam-ketamine anesthesia.
30. Ketamine or diazepam-ketamine anesthesia allows adequate circulatory regulation in head up or lateral tilt surgical positioning.
31. No increase in muscle relaxant requirements is observed by ketamine alone compared to diazepam-ketamine anesthesia.

Advantages of Diazepam-Ketamine in Anesthetic Practice

Clinical Pharmacology	*Clinical Practice*
High therapeutic index	Safe in poor risk patients
Rapid redistribution	Amenable to i.v. continuous infusion
Adequate metabolism	Low cumulation potential
No sustained cardiocirculatory effects	Consider using in cardiac patients
No apparent histamine release	Allergic response is rare
No alteration of table tilt response	Positional changes are not hazardous
Stimulates central nervous system sympathetic activity	Sudden cardiovascular collapse is unlikely
Stimulates reflexes	Circulatory stimulant effect, if desired
No organ toxicity	No hazard to patient
Abuse potential present	Patient or occupational hazards negligible with restricted access to drug

References

Amaki, Y., Nagashima, H., Radnay, P.A., and Foldes, F.F.: Ketamine interaction with neuromuscular blocking agents in the phrenic nerve hemidiaphragm preparation of the rat. Anesth. Analg. 57: 238-243, 1978.

Barron, D.N.: The disadvantages of the barbiturates as induction agents, in Recent papers in anesthesiology and resuscitation. Arias, Llaurado, Nalda-Felipe and Lunn, eds., Exp. Med. Int. Cong. 347: 79-80, 1974. Proc. IV European Congress of Anesthesiology, Madrid, Spain, Sept. 5-11, 1974.

Chasapakis, G., Kekis, N., Sakkalis, C., and Kolios, D.: Use of ketamine and pancuronium for anesthesia for patients in hemorrhagic shock. Anesth. Analg. 52: 282-287, 1973.

Chen, G., Ensor, C.R., and Bohner, B.: The neuropharmacology of 2-(o-chlorophenyl)-2-methylaminocyclohexanone hydrochloride. J. Pharmacol. Exp. Ther. 152: 332-339, 1966.

Corssen, G., Allarde, R., Brosch, F., and Arbenz, G.: Ketamine as the sole agent in open heart surgery. A preliminary report. Anesth. Analg. 49: 1025-1031, 1970.

Corssen, G. and Domino, E.F.: Dissociative anesthesia: Further pharmacologic studies and first clinical experience with a phencyclidine derivative CI-581. Anesth. Analg. 45: 29-40, 1966.

Corssen, G., Domino, E.F., and Bree, R.L.: Electroencephalographic effects of ketamine anesthesia in children. Anesth. Analg. Curr. Res. 48: 141-147, 1969.

Corssen, G., Miyasaka, M., and Domino, E.F.: Changing concepts in pain control during surgery: Dissociative anesthesia. A progress report. Anesth. Analg. 47: 746-758, 1968.

Dinnick, P.O.: Deaths associated with anesthesia: Observations on 600 cases. Anaesth. 19: 536-556, 1969.

Domino, E.F., Chodoff, P., and Corssen, G.: Pharmacologic effects of CI-581, a new dissociative anesthetic in man. Clin. Pharmacol. Exp. Ther. 6: 279-291, 1965.

Dowdy, E.G. and Kaya, K.: Studies on the mechanism of cardiovascular responses to CI-581. Anaesth. 29: 931-943, 1968.

Edwards, G., Morton, H.J.V., Pask, E.A., and Wyliz, W.D.: Deaths associated with anesthesia: A report of 1000 cases. Anaesth. 11: 194-200, 1956.

Etsten, B. and Li, T.H.: Hemodynamic changes during thiopental anesthesia in humans: Cardiac output, stroke volume, total peripheral resistance and intrathoracic blood volume. J. Clin. Invest. 34: 500-510, 1955.

Idvall, J.: Hemodynamic and respiratory effects of ketamine in relation to plasma levels. Excerp. Med. Int. Cong. Ser. 542: 443, 1978. Proc. V. European Congress of Anesthesiology, Sept. 4-9, 1978, Paris, France.

Ivankovich, A.D., Miletich, D.J., Reimann, C., Albrecht, R.F., and Zahed, B.: Cardiovascular effects of centrally administered ketamine in goats. Anesth. Analg. 53: 924-931, 1974.

Johnston, R.R., Miller, R.D., and Way, W.L.: The interaction of ketamine with *d*-tubocurarine, pancuronium and succinylcholine in man. Anesth. Analg. 53: 496-501, 1974.

Kothary, S.P. and Zsigmond, E.K.: Prevention of ketamine induced psychic sequelae by diazepam. Clin. Pharmacol. Ther. 17: 238, 1975.

Kothary, S.P. and Zsigmond, E.K.: The effect of ketamine on human plasma cholinesterase *in vitro* and *in vivo*. Excerp. Med. Int. Cong. Ser. 452: 241, 1978. Proc. V. European Congress of Anesthesiology, Paris, France, Sept. 4-9, 1978.

Kumar, S.M., Kothary, S.P., and Zsigmond, E.K.: Plasma free norepinephrine and epinephrine concentrations following diazepam-ketamine induction in patients undergoing cardiac surgery. Abstract #505. Abstracts of papers presented at the 1977 Annual Meeting, Amer. Soc. Anesth., New Orleans, La., Oct. 17-20, 1977.

Kumar, S.M., Kothary, S.P., and Zsigmond, E.K.: Plasma free norepinephrine and epinephrine concentrations following diazepam-ketamine induction in patients undergoing cardiac surgery. Acta anesth. scand. 22: 593-600, 1978.

Lau, S.S. and Domino, E.F.: Gas chromatography-mass spectrometry assay for ketamine and its metabolites in plasma. Biomed. Mass. Spec. 4: 317-321, 1977.

Matsuki, A., Kothary, S.P., and Zsigmond, E.K.: Lack of compensatory increase in plasma free norepinephrine during hypotension induced by intravenous thiamylal anesthesia. Der Anesthetist 22: 289-291, 1973.

Matsuki, A., Zsigmond, E.K., Kelsch,R.C., and Kothary, S.P.: The effect of pancuronium bromide on plasma norepinephrine concentrations during ketamine induction. Canad. Anesth. Soc. J. 21: 315-320, 1974.

McCaughey, T.: Hazards of anesthesia for the burned child. Canad. Anaesth. Soc. J. 9: 220-223, 1962.

Sadove, M.S., Shulman, M., Hatano, S., and Ingold, N.: Analgesic effects of ketamine administered in subdissociative doses. Anesth. Analg. 50: 452-457, 1971.

Saxena,P.R. and Bonta, I.L.: Specific blockade of the cardiac muscarinic receptors by pancuronium bromide. Arch. int. Pharmacodyn. 189: 410, 1971.

Silvay, G., Weinrich, A., Lumb, P., and Shiung, H.: Continuous ketamine for one lung anesthesia as an alternative to halothane. Excerp. Med. Int. Cong. Ser. 452: 140-141, 1978. Proc. V. European Congress of Anesthesiology, Paris, France, Sept. 4-9, 1978.

Tweed, W.A., Minnick, M., and Mymin, D.: Circulatory response to ketamine anesthesia. Anaesth. 37: 613-617, 1972.

Vendsalu, A.: Studies on adrenaline and noradrenaline in human plasma. Acta physiol. scand. 48: Suppl. 173, pp. 23-32, 1960.

Virtue, R.W., Alanis, J.M., Mori, M., LaFargue, R.T., Vogel, J.H.K., and Metcalf, D.R.: An anesthetic agent 2-ortho chlorophenyl-2-methylaminocyclohexanone HCl (CI-581). Anesth. 28: 823-833, 1967.

Wilson, E., Nicols, R., and McCoy, N.: Dissociative anesthesia with CI-581 in burned children. Anesth. Analg. 46: 719-723, 1967.

Yoon, M., Zsigmond, E.K., and Kothary, S.P.: A new anesthetic technique: Ataract analgesia with diazepam-ketamine-pancuronium in cardiac patients. Comm. in Anesth. 5: 10, 1975.

Zsigmond, E.K.: Malignant hyperthermia with subsequent uneventful general anesthesia. Comment case history. Anesth. Analg. 50: 1104-1112, 1971.

Zsigmond, E.K. and Domino, E.F.: Ketamine-clinical pharmacology, pharmacokinetics and current clinical uses. Anesthesiol. Rev. 7: 13-33, 1980.

Zsigmond, E.K. and Domino, E.F.: Clinical pharmacology and current uses of ketamine. In Trends in Intravenous Anesthesia, J.A. Aldrete and T.H. Stanley (eds) pp. 283-330, Symposia Specialists, Inc. Miami, FL, 1980.

Zsigmond, E.K. and Kelsch, R.C.: Elevated plasma norepinephrine concentrations during ketamine anesthesia. Clin. Pharmacol. Ther. 24: 149, 1973.

Zsigmond, E.K., Kelsch, R.C., Kothary, S.P., and Vadnay, L.: Plasma norepinephrine concentrations during anesthetic induction with ketamine. Rev. Brasil. Anesth. 22: 443-451, 1972.

Zsigmond, E.K. and Kothary, S.P.: Double blind evaluation of the circulatory response to 60° table tilt with diazepam-ketamine anesthesia. Excerp. Med. Int. Cong. Ser. 452: 58, 1978. Proc. V. European Congress of Anesthesiology, Paris, France, Sept. 4-9, 1978.

Zsigmond, E.K., Kothary, S.P., Matsuki, A., and Kelsch, R.C.: Diazepam for prevention of the rise in plasma catecholamines caused by ketamine. Clin. Pharmacol. Ther. 15: 223-224, 1974.

Zsigmond, E.K., Kothary, S.P., Matsuki, A., and Martinez, O.: Ataract analgesic mixtures: Diazepam-ketamine, in Recent papers in anesthesiology and resuscitation. Arias, Llaurado, Nalda-Felipe and Lunn, eds., Exp. Med. Int. Cong. 347: 136-138, 1974. Proc. IV European Congress of Anesthesiology, Madrid, Spain, Sept. 5-11, 1974.

Zsigmond, E.K. and Martinez, O.A.: Plasma epinephrine and norepinephrine levels during induction of morphine anesthesia in cardiac-surgical patients. Rev. Brasil. Anesth. 24: 220-225, 1974.

Zsigmond, E.K., Matsuki, A., Kothary, S.P., and Jallad, M.: Arterial hypoxemia caused by intravenous ketamine. Anesth. Analg. 55: 311-314, 1975.

Zsigmond, E.K., Matsuki, A., Kothary, S.P., and Kelsch, R.C.: The effect of pancuronium on plasma norepinephrine and cortisol concentrations during thiamylal induction. Canad. Anesth. Soc. J. 21: 147-152, 1974.

Zsigmond, E.K., Shively, J.G., and Flynn, K.: Respiratory and circulatory effects of diazepam in man. Clin. Pharmacol. Ther. 11: 299, 1970.

Zsigmond, E.K., Yoon, M., and Kothary, S.P.: A new anesthetic technique: Ataract analgesia with diazepam-ketamine-pancuronium in cardiac surgical patients. Excerp. Med. Int. Cong. Ser. 387: (#267) 127, 1976. Proc. VI World Cong. of Anesthesiology, Mexico City, April 24-30, 1976.

Status of Ketamine in Anesthesiology,
edited by E.F. Domino©1990, NPP Books
P.O. Box 1491, Ann Arbor, MI 48106

Clinical Pharmacologic Basis for Benzodiazepine-Ketamine Anesthesia in Patients with Coronary Occlusion

E.K. Zsigmond, S.M. Kumar, S.M. Raza, and M. Yoon

Department of Anesthesiology
University of Illinois
Chicago, IL
and
University of Michigan
Ann Arbor, MI

Introduction

Fortunately, the introduction of neuroleptanalgesia coincided with the growth of cardiac surgery. The combination of droperidol with fentanyl has been well tolerated by cardiac patients who have a good ejection fraction and a successful outcome of valvular surgery or Vineberg-procedure. However, some patients developed hypotension and bradycardia during induction, especially if they were given rapidly acting i.v. barbiturates to speed up the induction of anesthesia. It was found that diazepam caused little reduction in the ejection fraction in cardiac patients. Diazepam use brought a major improvement in the management of patients for cardioversion (Dundee and Keilty, 1969; Dalen *et al.*, 1969; Ikram and Rubin, 1971; Ikram *et al.*, 1973). We began to use diazepam as an induction agent in place of thiopental in cardiac surgical patients. In this way, three major side effects of thiopental, namely, cardiac depression, depression of central autonomic responses to decreases in peripheral vascular resistance, and histamine release were circumvented (Matsuki *et al.*, 1973). Diazepam also reduced the dose requirements of droperidol and, in some patients, obviated its use.

The introduction of ketamine was another major improvement in the management of critically ill cardiac patients who had marked hypotension and loss of normal adrenergic response to stress because ketamine caused an increase in blood pressure, heart rate, and cardiac output as a result of sympathetic stimulation (Virtue *et al.*, 1967; Tweed *et al.*, 1972; Chasapakis *et al.*, 1973). Indeed, ketamine was used as a sole anesthetic agent for patients undergoing open heart surgery (Corssen *et al.*, 1970). The severe hypertension and tachycardia induced by ketamine, however, markedly restricted its use for cardiac patients who had severe coronary occlusion limiting the myocardial oxygen supply. Such patients could not tolerate an increase in the rate-pressure product. Zsigmond and associates (Corssen *et al.*, 1972; Zsigmond *et al.*, 1974) showed that an increase in plasma free norepinephrine, but not in epinephrine, accompanied ketamine induced hypertension and tachycardia in healthy young volunteers. This represented central sympathetic stimulation, as manifested in an overflow of norepinephrine from peripheral sympathetic neurons (Corssen *et al.*, 1972, Zsigmond *et al.*, 1974). Ivankovich *et al.* (1974) elicited the same sympathetic circulatory stimulation by injecting ketamine directly into the carotid arteries of the isolated cerebral hemispheres of goats in fractions of the doses that elicited hypertension when injected into peripheral veins. It became evident that central sympathetic stimulation was the site of action of circulatory stimulation induced by ketamine.

In order to obtain additional proof for this central effect of ketamine, we carried out several double blind studies on the combination of diazepam with ketamine, using 0.9% NaCl placebo controls, in 56 healthy volunteers. We proved the protective effect of diazepam in reducing ketamine induced increases in heart rate, blood pressure and, most importantly, in plasma free norepinephrine concentrations (Zsigmond *et al.*, 1972, 1973, 1974, 1980; Kothary and Zsigmond, 1975). In another double blind study in 8 prisoner volunteers who served as their own controls, diazepam, given 10 min prior to ketamine, prevented hypertension, tachycardia, and an increase in plasma free norepinephrine concentrations (Domino and Zsigmond, 1979, 1980). Finally, in 200 healthy (ASA I or II physical state) volunteer gynecological patients who received ketamine for both induction and maintenance, ketamine induced circulatory stimulation and hallucinations were prevented by the administration of diazepam 10 min prior to ketamine (Kothary and Zsigmond, 1975, 1977). The time interval between the two drug administrations ought not to be less than 8, preferably 10, and not more than 40 min to achieve the full protection by diazepam.

Based on these multiple scientific studies, we anticipated that this combination may be safely employed for induction of anesthesia in cardiac surgical patients. However, information obtained in healthy volunteers may not be directly transposed to cardiac patients, especially to those with a poor cardiac ejection fraction. Therefore, several controlled studies were undertaken to evaluate the effectiveness and safety of diazepam-ketamine sequential administration in patients scheduled for cardiac surgery. The use of a placebo would not have been ethical, based on the already known adverse effects of ketamine when administered without benzodiazepine pretreatment. After midazolam, a water soluble congener of diazepam, became available we also investigated whether midazolam is as safe and effective as diazepam in preventing the adverse side effects of ketamine.

Materials and Methods

Pilot study

Patients (N = 30), scheduled for coronary bypass surgery with cardiac ejection fractions 0.35 were selected without further randomization (Zsigmond *et al.*, 1976). The patients received hydroxyzine (1.5 mg/kg) and meperidine (1.5 mg/kg) as preanesthetic medication. Anesthesia was induced by the i.v. administration of 0.3 mg/kg diazepam followed 10 min later by 2.0 mg/kg of ketamine. Direct arterial pressure from the radial or, preferably, brachial artery (BP), heart rate by EKG lead V5 or the lead with the tallest R wave (HR), and pulmonary artery pressure (PAP) were continually recorded. Although diazepam caused a reduction in both systolic and diastolic BP and HR, the subsequent administration of ketamine restored these hemodynamic variables to baseline levels. Tracheal intubation caused no hemodynamic changes.

Controlled studies with diazepam-ketamine sequence

Patients scheduled to undergo cardiac surgery (N = 12) were studied. Eight patients underwent valvular replacement and 4 direct aortocoronary bypass operations. Their mean age was 53 yr (29-65), mean weight 67 kg (40-95), and mean height 166 cm (150-182). All patients had an ASA physical status classification of III and IV. The patients received no propranolol for 2 weeks prior to surgery.

After preanesthetic medication with 0.15 mg/kg diazepam p.o. and 0.15 mg/kg morphine sulfate i.m., given 1 hr prior to induction, anesthesia was induced with 0.3 mg/kg diazepam followed 10 min later by 2.0 mg/kg ketamine. Afterwards, 0.1 mg/kg pancuronium was given to facilitate tracheal intubation. During this period, preoxygenation and assisted ventilation were given to avoid hypoxemia, possibly induced by ketamine (Zsigmond *et al.*, 1976a). Ventilation was assisted during the study in order to maintain $PaCO_2$ between 35-45 mm Hg and $Pa0_2$ 95 mm Hg.

Arterial blood samples for blood gas analysis and determination of plasma free norepinephrine and epinephrine concentrations were drawn prior to induction, 10 min after diazepam, 5 min after ketamine, 5 min after pancuronium, and 2.5 and 10 min after intubation. A Radiometer Copenhagen blood gas analyzer was used for blood gas analysis. Catecholamine determinations were via the Vendsalu's method (1960), modified by Kelsch *et al.* (1971). Continuous recordings of intra arterial blood pressure from the radial or brachial artery, EEG lead V5, or the lead with the tallest R wave were made via a strain gauge. Student's t-tests for paired data were used for statistical analyses. A P value of <0.05 was considered significant. The values in the text are means ± S.E.

Results

Mean systolic BP values were not significantly altered by diazepam or by subsequent ketamine administration, although the diastolic pressure

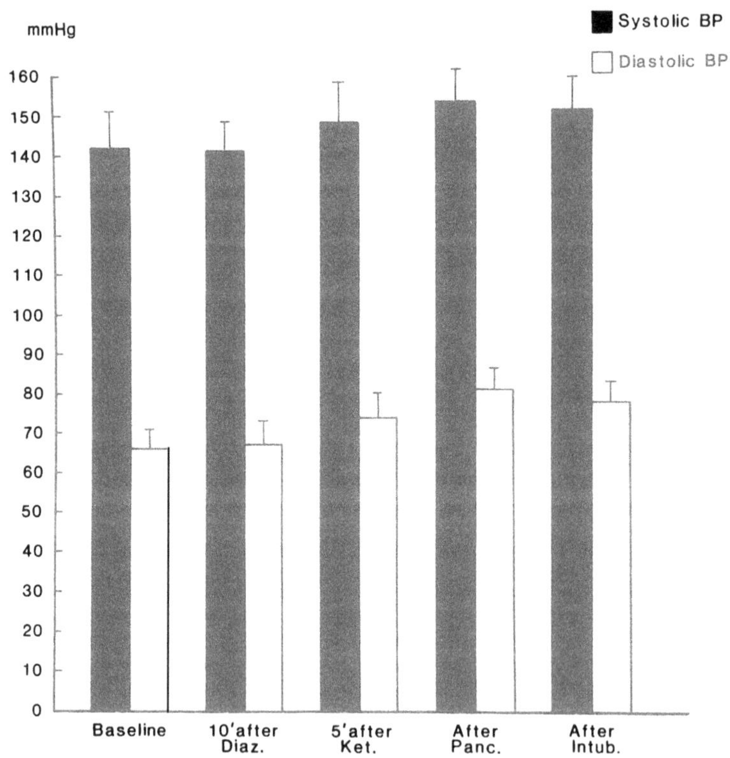

Fig. 1. Blood pressure is maintained within normal limits after diazepam-ketamine or pancuronium and intubation.

increased after ketamine (12%). Neither systolic nor diastolic pressure readings were altered by pancuronium. No significant increase in arterial pressure was seen after intubation (Fig. 1).

HR was not significantly altered following diazepam and after its combination with ketamine as compared to baseline. However, a significant increase (P <0.001) in HR was observed following pancuronium administration. Tracheal intubation resulted in no changes in HR (Fig 2).

Plasma free norepinephrine and epinephrine concentrations were not altered by diazepam *per se* nor by subsequent ketamine administration (Fig. 3 and 4). However, mean plasma epinephrine concentration decreased following ketamine. No further changes in norepinephrine and epinephrine concentration were observed after pancuronium. The pre and postintubation norepinephrine and epinephrine concentrations did not differ significantly. The mean PaO_2 and $PaCO_2$ were maintained within the normal range. No arrythmia or ST-segment changes were observed throughout the study period. No bronchospasm, hypersecretions,

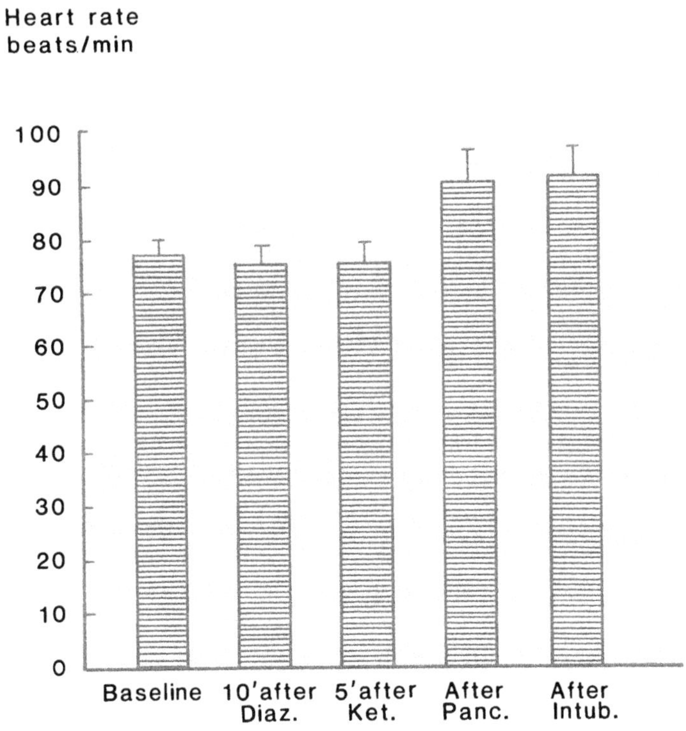

Fig. 2. Heart rate is maintained within normal limits after diazepam-ketamine; pancuronium caused an increase. *P <0.001.

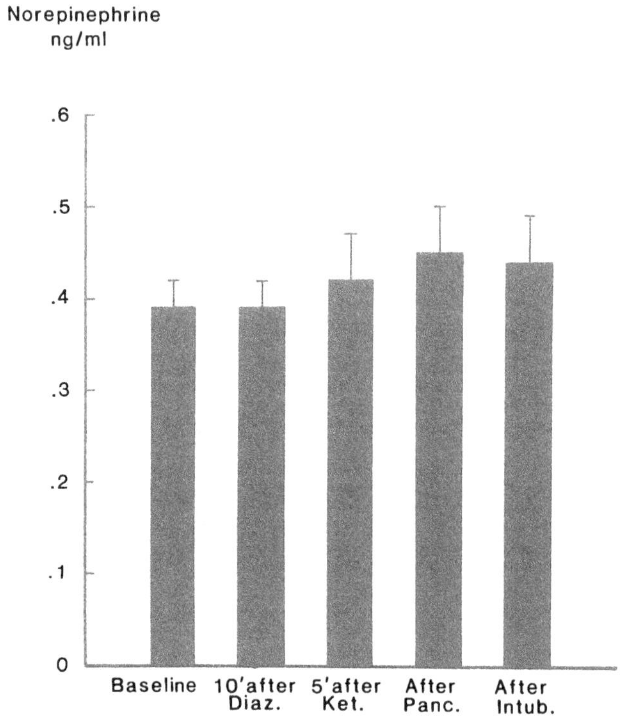

Fig. 3. Plasma norepinephrine is not altered by diazepam-ketamine-pancuronium and intubation.

awareness, or hallucinations were observed perioperatively in any of the patients.

Controlled studies with midazolam-ketamine sequence

Patients (N = 15) for elective coronary artery bypass surgery, with a mean age of 60 yr (46-71), a mean weight of 81 kg (66-102), BSA = 1.94 m^2 (1.74-2.22) were studied. After morphine (0.15 mg/kg i.m.) and diazepam (0.15 mg/kg p.o.) preanesthetic medication, the patients were induced with 0.12 mg/kg of midazolam and 10 min later with 1.0 mg/kg of ketamine. Direct arterial BP was recorded with a strain gauge via the radial artery, pulmonary artery pressure by a Swan-Ganz catheter and heart rate by the V_5 or the lead with the tallest R wave of the EKG. Cardiac output was determined by a thermodilution cardiac output injector computer in triplicate. Oxygen saturation was continuously measured by an oximeter and maintained at greater than 95% saturation. Exhaled CO_2 level was maintained between 35-45 mm Hg. ST segments were

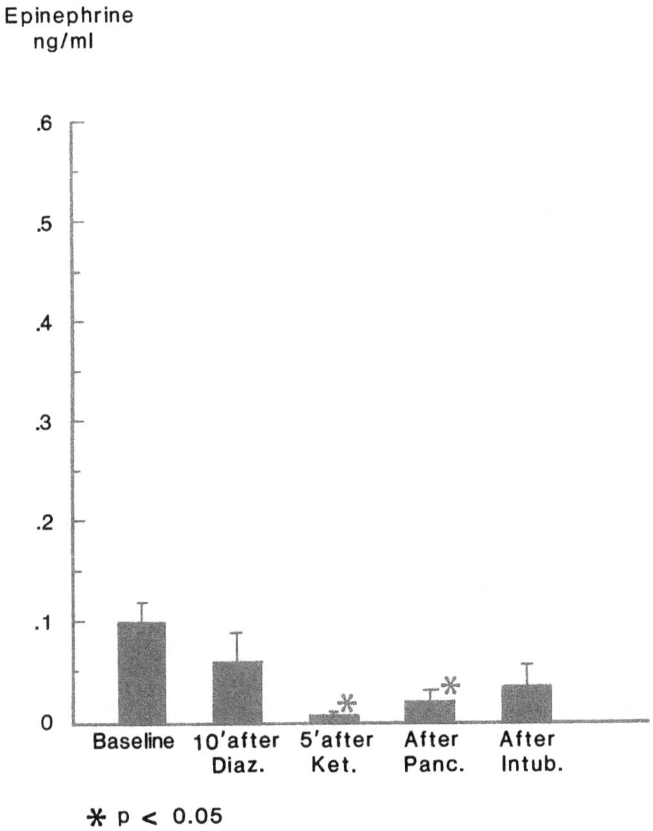

Fig. 4. Plasma epinephrine is not significantly altered by diazepam-ketamine.

observed for analysis by visual observation. Paired t-test was used to determine statistical significance. $P < 0.05$ was considered statistically significant.

Results

HR was not significantly altered by either midazolam or a midazolam-ketamine combination (Fig. 5). Systolic BP decreased significantly after midazolam and its combination with ketamine ($P < 0.01$). Neither systolic nor diastolic pulmonary/artery pressures were altered after midazolam or midazolam-ketamine (Fig. 5).

Cardiac output and cardiac index, stroke volume and stroke volume indexes were not changed by midazolam or a midazolam-ketamine com-

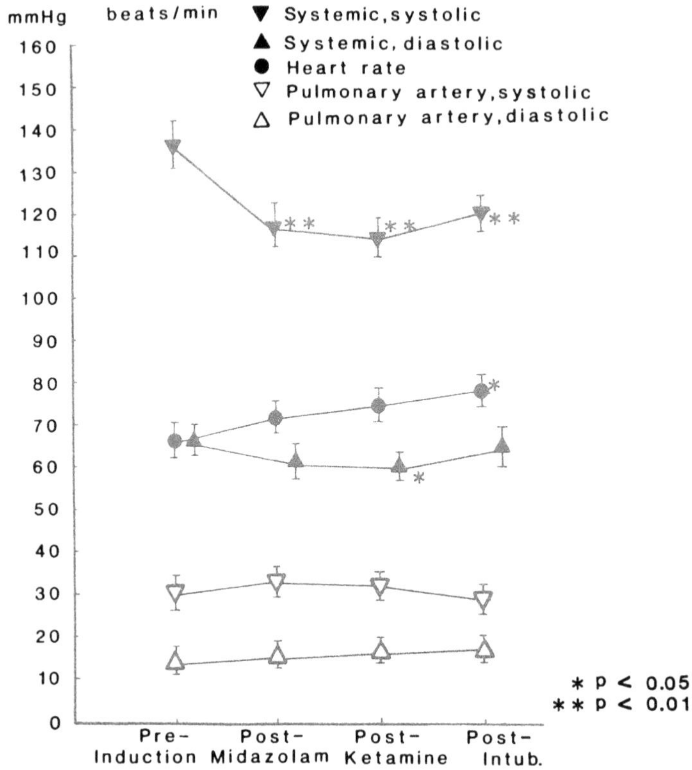

Fig. 5. Marked reduction in systemic systolic arterial pressure after midazolam alone and ketamine combination with midazolam but no change in pulmonary arterial pressure and HR even with intubation.

bination (Fig. 6). Although systemic vascular resistance was reduced by midazolam, and further by a midazolam-ketamine sequence, pulmonary vascular resistance was not altered (Fig. 7). Left ventricular stroke work indexes were reduced by midazolam (P <0.05), and further by a midazolam-ketamine sequence (P <0.01; Fig. 8).

Discussion

Ketamine as a sole anesthetic agent was found to be useful and safe in certain cardiac patients (Corssen *et al.*, 1970) and especially in pediatric cardiac surgery (Radnay *et al.*, 1974) because of its unique properties as an anesthetic agent. Ketamine provides rapid loss of consciousness, predictable dose dependent amnesia, analgesia for both

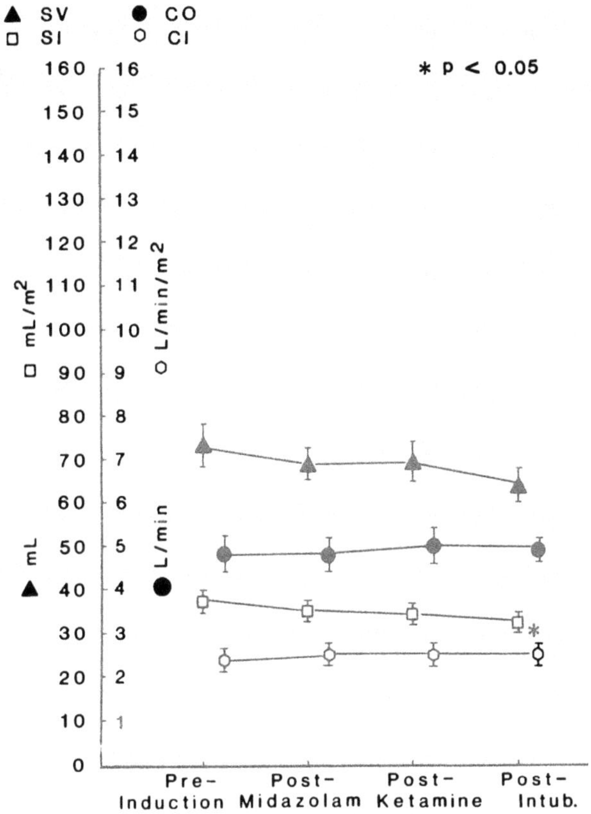

Fig. 6. Cardiac index output, stroke volume, and stroke volume index not changed by midazolam-ketamine.

somatic and visceral pain, sympathetic central stimulation in a dose dependent manner, and lacks the three major side effects of rapid acting i.v. barbiturates, *i.e.*, cardiac depression, loss of sympathetic autonomic response to stressors, and histamine release. Above all, ketamine has a therapeutic index unsurpassed by any currently used i.v. anesthetic. Nonetheless, cardiac patients with reduced myocardial oxygen supply caused by coronary stenosis and with certain anatomical defects should not receive the conventional 2.0 mg/kg ketamine i.v. dose because of the marked increase in heart rate, blood pressure, and central sympathetic stimulation leading to enhanced blood levels of norepinephrine. The influence of the three major stressors in cardiac patients during anesthesia/surgery (induction, tracheal intubation, and sternotomy) may be enhanced

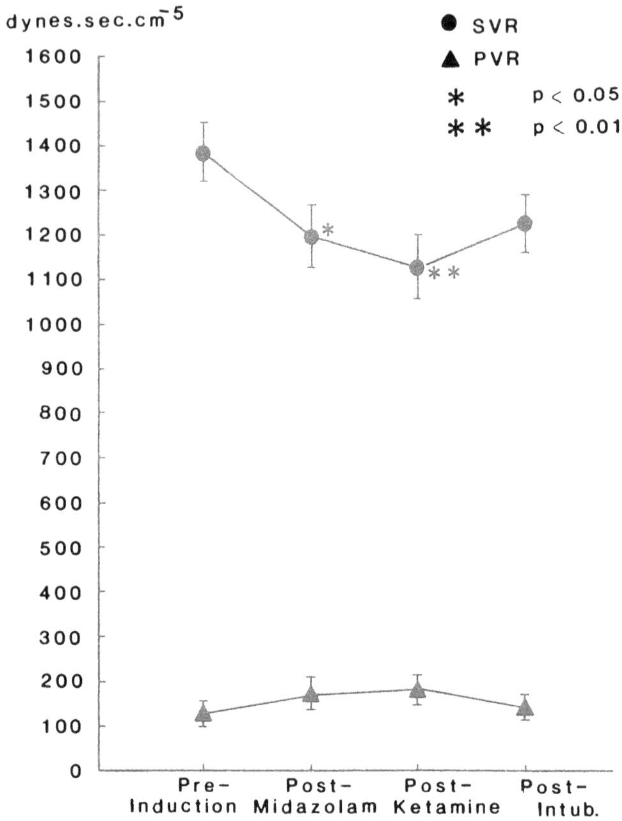

Fig. 7. Systemic but not pulmonary vascular resistance is reduced by midazolam-ketamine.

by ketamine alone. Since 1965 we have successfully utilized diazepam to prevent the excessive central sympathetic stimulation induced by these three stressors. Based on this favorable moderating effect of diazepam on excessive autonomic activity, we achieved an attenuation of ketamine induced sympathetic stimulation (Zsigmond *et al.*, 1972, 1974) in healthy volunteer gynecological patients. Moreover, diazepam (0.3 mg/kg i.v.) markedly alleviated or eliminated the tachycardia, hypertension, and increase in plasma free norepinephrine levels during ketamine anesthesia, both in healthy young volunteers (Zsigmond *et al.*, 1972, 1974, 1980) and cardiac patients (Kumar *et al.*, 1978a), while diazepam *per se* caused no adverse hemodynamic effects (Dundee, 1969; Raza *et al.*, 1987). Diazepam caused a decrease in resting sympathetic activity and a resulting

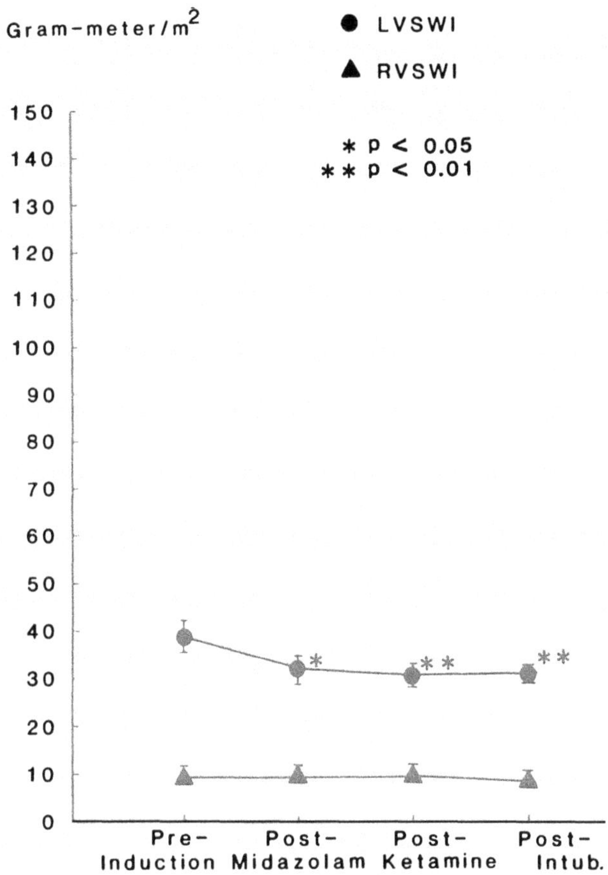

Fig. 8. Left but not right ventricular stroke work index is reduced by midazolam-ketamine.

significant decrease in plasma free epinephrine concentration (Zsigmond, 1983).

As described in detail in another chapter in this volume, we first investigated the influence of graded doses of diazepam (from 0.1 mg/kg to 0.3 mg/kg i.v.) at least 10 min prior to the i.v. administration of 2.0 mg/kg of ketamine. A marked protective effect from both the excessive sympathetic stimulation and from the emergence delirium induced by ketamine was found when volunteers were pretreated with diazepam instead of a placebo (Kothary and Zsigmond, 1975, 1976). Plasma free norepinephrine levels remained within the normal range in the diazepam pretreated group in all of our clinical pharmacologic studies in contrast to the placebo pretreated patients (Zsigmond *et al.*, 1972, 1973, 1974, 1978; Kothary and Zsigmond, 1977). Furthermore, in a double blind crossover study in 8 healthy prisoner volunteers, we reconfirmed the earlier findings that diazepam prevented the excessive sympathetic overactivity induced by placebo-ketamine and the corresponding increase in plasma free norepinephrine concentration (Domino and Zsigmond, 1980; Zsigmond and Domino, 1979). Although diazepam increased slightly ketamine blood levels, respiratory depression and enhanced the decrease in ejection fraction caused by ketamine, it also prolonged the duration of amnesia significantly, a clinically useful effect. The decrease in cardiac ejection fraction was so minimal and short lasting that it did not prevent its use in cardiac patients with even a markedly reduced ejection fraction (Silvay, 1983; Morray, 1984; Radnay, 1974). Preferably, in these patients lower pretreatment doses of diazepam or ketamine alone should be used.

Based on the foregoing clinical pharmacological studies, we carried out studies and observed remarkable hemodynamic stability with a diazepam-ketamine induction sequence (Zsigmond *et al.*, 1976b). A further controlled study in cardiac patients confirmed the results observed in healthy volunteers that diazepam prevents the hypertension, tachycardia, and increase in plasma free norepinephrine induced by ketamine (Kumar *et al.*, 1987a). The muscle relaxant, pancuronium, used for tracheal intubation, caused no alterations in hemodynamics and plasma free norepinephrine concentrations in the cardiac patients just like in the healthy volunteers (Matsuki *et al.*, 1974; Kumar *et al.*, 1978b). In healthy volunteers, pancuronium given before or simultaneously with ketamine minimized the ketamine induced circulatory changes (Matsuki *et al.*, 1974). A well controlled study confirmed the lack of pancuronium induced adverse hemodynamic changes in cardiac patients (Kumar *et al.*, 1978b). Moreover, the sequential administration of diazepam-ketamine-pancuronium allowed intubation of the trachea without adverse circulatory effects that are commonly observed with other anesthetic techniques/agents, both i.v. combinations and inhalational induction agents (Zsigmond *et al.*, 1980, 1988).

In the past few years, midazolam has gradually replaced diazepam as a sleep inducing agent in patients undergoing cardiac surgery because it has a higher potency, shorter half life and a lower incidence of thrombophlebitis associated with its use. In several well designed studies, midazolam proved to be a safe i.v. sedative or sleep inducing agent in cardiac patients (Fragen *et al.*, 1979; Reves *et al.*, 1979; Samuelson *et al.*, 1981;

Morel *et al.*, 1981; DeCastro *et al.*, 1981). In a previous study, we observed no adverse hemodynamic changes after i.v. midazolam (0.2 mg/kg) in 30 cardiac patients scheduled for cardiac surgery (Raza *et al.*, 1987a,b). Midazolam significantly reduced systemic systolic blood pressure and systemic vascular resistance, diastolic blood pressure, and left ventricular stroke work index. No other hemodynamic changes were observed. The reduction in systolic and diastolic blood pressure combined with a reduction in systemic vascular resistance with unaltered heart rate caused a reduction in cardiac work. The left ventricular stroke work index was reduced. Therefore, midazolam may safely replace diazepam in our previously described safe induction sequence with diazepam-ketamine-pancuronium. Our results from the recent study summarized here confirm the safety of midazolam-ketamine-pancuronium induction sequence in patients undergoing aortocoronary bypass surgery.

Summary

The results of several studies reported in this review clearly indicate that both diazepam-ketamine-pancuronium and midazolam-ketamine-pancuronium induction sequences are safe in cardiac surgical patients. The hemodynamic changes induced by the benzodiazepines *per se* are rather favorable. Both benzodiazepines counteracted the ketamine induced central sympathetic stimulation, if they were given at least 10 min prior to ketamine administration. Pancuronium used as a skeletal muscle relaxant caused no adverse hemodynamic effects nor altered the hemodynamic changes induced by the benzodiazepine-ketamine combination. No adverse circulatory sequelae were observed during or following tracheal intubation. Either of these combinations afforded protection against the adverse effects of tracheal intubation, as also evidenced by the lack of alteration in plasma catecholamine concentrations. Therefore, either of these techniques could provide effective and safe anesthetic induction for patients undergoing aortocoronary bypass surgery. This series of studies summarized from previously reported clinical pharmacologic investigations clearly establishes that the sequential administration of diazepam-ketamine-pancuronium causes no adverse hemodynamic or endocrine changes in patients undergoing anesthesia for cardiac surgery.

Conclusions

1. The sequential administration of diazepam and ketamine provided a safe and effective induction of anesthesia for cardiac surgical patients.

2. Diazepam-ketamine induction sequence provided a safe and effective anesthetic induction even for the cardiac patient with a low ejection fraction. Plasma free norepinephrine and epinephrine levels remained within the normal range during induction and tracheal intubation, two of the most stressful events.

3. Although midazolam per se reduced systolic BP, SVR and LVSWI, other hemodynamic variables were not altered. Ketamine potentiated some of the hemodynamic changes induced by midazolam but caused no adverse hemodynamic changes *per se*. Midazolam is as effective as diazepam in preventing the adverse hemodynamic changes induced by ketamine in patients with coronary occlusions.

Acknowledgement

The authors would like to acknowledge the technical assistance of L. Vadnay, S.P. Kothary, E. Barabas, and S. Clarke.

References

Chasapakis, G., Kekis, N., Sakkalis, C., and Kolios, I.: Use of ketamine and pancuronium for anesthesia for patients in hemorrhagic shock. Anesth. Analg. 52: 282-287, 1973.

Corssen, G., Allarde, R., Brosch, F., and Arbenz, G.: Ketamine as the sole anesthetic in open heart surgery: A preliminary report. Anesth. Analg. 49: 1025-1031, 1970.

Corssen, G. Cutierrez, J., and Reves, J.G.: Ketamine in the anesthetic management of asthmatic patients. Anesth. Analg. 51: 588-591, 1972.

Dalen, J.E., Evans, G.L., Banas, J.S., Jr., Brooks, H.L., Paraskos, J.A., and Dexter, L.: The hemodynamic and respiratory effects of diazepam (Valium). Anesthesiol. 30: 259, 1969.

DeCastro, P.J., Andrieu, S., Dubois, A., and Van Heuneghem, L.: Etude du midazolam comme inducteur, correcteur et potentialisateur d'une anesthsie analgesique a base d'alfentanil. Arzneim-Forsch/Drug Res. 31: 2251-2254, 1981.

Domino, E.F. and Zsigmond, E.K.: Pharmacokinetics of ketamine in man in relation to its circulatory effects. In Ketamine and the Cardiovascular System, D. Langrehr, ed., pp. 20-29, Excerpta Medica, Amsterdam-Geneva-Princeton, 1980.

Dundee, J.W. and Keilty, S.R.: Diazepam. In Newer Intravenous Anesthetics, R.S. Clarke, ed., International Anesthesia Clinic Series 7: 109, Little, Brown & Co., Boston, 1969.

Fragen, R.J., Meyers, S.N., Barresi, V., and Caldwell, N.J.: Hemodynamic effects of midazolam in cardiac patients. Anesthesiol. 51: S103, 1979.

Ikram, H. and Rubin, A.P.: Anaesthesia for cardioversion. Brit. Med. J. 4: 626, 1971.

Ikram, H., Rubin, A.P., and Jewkes, R.F.: Effect of diazepam on myocardial blood flow of patients with and without coronary artery disease. Brit. Heart J. 35: 626-630, 1973.

Ivankovich, A.D., Miletich, D.J., Reimann, C., Albrecht, R.F., and Zahed, B.: Cardiovascular effects of centrally administered ketamine in goats. Anesth. Analg. 53: 924-931, 1974.

Kelsch, R.C., Light, G.S., Luciano, J.R., and Oliver, W.J.: The effects of prednisone on plasma norepinephrine concentration and renin activity in salt depleted men. J. Lab. Clin. Med. 77: 267-277, 1971.

Kothary, S.P. and Zsigmond, E.K.: Prevention of ketamine induced psychic sequelae by diazepam. Clin. Pharmacol. Ther. 17: 238, 1975.

Kothary, S.P., Zsigmond, E.K., and Matsuki, A.: Antagonism of the ketamine induced rise in plasma free norepinephrine, blood pressure and pulse rate by intravenous diazepam. Clin. Pharmacol. Ther. 17: 238, 1975.

Kothary, S.P. and Zsigmond, E.K.: A double blind study of the effective anti-hallucinatory doses of diazepam prior to ketamine anesthesia. Clin. Pharmcol. Ther. 21: 108-109, 1976.

Kumar, S.M., Kothary, S.P., and Zsigmond, E.K.: Plasma free norepinephrine and epinephrine concentrations following diazepam-ketamine induction in patients undergoing cardiac surgery. Acta Anaesthesiol. Scand. 22: 593-600, 1978a.

Kumar, S.M., Kothary, S.P., and Zsigmond, E.K.: The effect of pancuronium on plasma free-norepinephrine and epinephrine in adult cardiac surgical patients. Acta Anesth. Scand. 22: 423-429, 1978b.

Matsuki, A., Kothary, S.P., and Zsigmond, E.K.: Lack of compensatory increase in plasma free-norepinephrine during hypotension induced by intravenous thiamylal anesthesia. Anaesthesist 22: 289-291, 1973.

Matsuki, A., Zsigmond, E.K., Kothary, S.P., and Kelsch, R.C.: The effect of pancuronium bromide on plasma norepinephrine and cortisol concentrations during thiamylal induction. Can. Anaesth. Soc. J. 21: 147-152, 1974.

Morray, J.P., Lynn, A.M., Stamm, S.S., *et al.*: Hemodynamic effects of ketamine in children with congenital heart disease. Anesth. Analg. 63: 895-899, 1984.

Morel, D., Forster, A., and Gardaz, J.P.: Comparative hemodynamic and respiratory effects of midazolam and flunitrazepam as induction agents in cardiac surgery. Arzneim-Forsch/Drug Res. 31: 2264-2265, 1981.

Radnay, P.A., Arai, T., and Nagashima, H.: Ketamine-gallamine anesthesia for great vessel operations in infants. Anesth. Analg. 53: 365-369, 1974.

Raza, S.M.A., Zsigmond, E.K., Neto, O.A., and Barabas, E.: Diazepam causes no adverse cardiocirculatory effects in cardiac patients. Clin. Ther. 9: 629-634, 1987a.

Raza, S.M.A., Zsigmond, E.K., and Barabas, E.: Midazolam causes no adverse hemodynamic effects in cardiac patients. Clin. Ther. 10: 40-43, 1987b.

Reves, J.G., Kissin, I., and Fournier, S.: Negative inotropic effects of midazolam. Anesthesiol. 60: 517-518, 1984.

Samuelson, P.N., Reves, J.G., Smith, L.R., and Kouchoukos, N.T.: Midazolam versus diazepam: Different effects on systemic vascular resistance. Arzneim-Forsch/Drug Res. 31: 2268-2269, 1981.

Silvay, G.: Ketamine. Mt. Sinai J. Med. 50: 300-304, 1983.

Tweed, W.A., Minuck, M., and Mymin, D.: Circulatory responses to ketamine anesthesia. Anesthesiol. 37: 613-619, 1972.

Vendsalu, A.: Studies on adrenaline and noradrenaline in human plasma. Acta Physiol. Scand. 48: Suppl. 173, pp. 23-32, 1960.

Virtue, R.W., Alanis, J.M., Mori, M., La Fargue, R.T., Vogel, J.H.K., and Metcalf, D.R.: An anesthetic agent: 2-orthochlorophenyl, 2-methylamino-cyclohexanone HCl (CI-581). Anesthesiol. 28: 823-833, 1967.

Zsigmond, E.K.: Catecholamines and Anesthesia. In Endocrinology and Anesthesia, T. Oyama and R. Hunter, eds., pp. 225-264, Elsevier Biomedical Press, Amsterdam, 1983.

Zsigmond, E.K., Barabas, E., and Korenaga, G.M.: Esmolol attenuates tachycardia caused by tracheal intubation: A double blind study. Int. J. Clin. Pharmacol. Ther. Toxicol. 26: 225-231, 1988.

Zsigmond, E.K. and Domino, E.F.: Clinical pharmacology, pharmacokinetics and clinical uses of ketamine. Scientific Exhibit at the 54th Annual Congress of the International Anesthesia Research Society, Hollywood, FL, March 11-15, 1979.

Zsigmond, E.K., Kelsch, R.C., and Kothary, S.P.: Plasma free norepinephrine concentration during induction with ketamine. Rev. Bras. Anesth. 22: 443-451, 1972.

Zsigmond, E.K., Kothary, S.P., Kumar, S.M., and Kelsch, R.C.: Counteraction of circulatory side effects of ketamine by pretreatment with diazepam. Clin. Ther. 3: 28-32, 1980.

Zsigmond, E.K., Kothary, S.P., Martinez, O.A., and Kelsch, R.O.: Diazepam for prevention of the rise in plasma catecholamines caused by ketamine. Clin. Pharmacol. Ther. 15: 223, 1974.

Zsigmond, E.K., Matsuki, A., Kothary, S.P., *et al.*: Arterial hypoxemia caused by intravenous ketamine. Anesth. Analg. 55: 311-314, 1976a.

Zsigmond, E.K., Yoon, M., and Kothary, S.P.: A new anesthetic technique: Ataract-analgesia with diazepam-ketamine-pancuronium in cardiac surgical patients. Abst. VI World Congress of Anesthesiology, Mexico City, April 24-30, 1976. Excerpta Medical Int. Cong. Series No. 387: 267, 1976b.

Status of Ketamine in Anesthesiology,
edited by E.F. Domino©1990, NPP Books
P.O. Box 1491, Ann Arbor, MI 48106

Biotransformation of Ketamine

A.J. Trevor

Department of Pharmacology
University of California School of Medicine
San Francisco, CA

INTRODUCTION

Despite the large number of investigations on the metabolism and biodisposition of ketamine [(R,S)-2-o-chlorophenyl-2-methylamino-cyclohexanone], the overall metabolic fate of the drug is still not completely understood. Early studies by Chang, Glazko and their colleagues (Chang *et al.*, 1965; Chang and Glazko, 1974) led to the identification of N-desmethylketamine (norketamine, metabolite I) as a urinary metabolite in the primate, together with an unusual unsaturated cyclohex-5-en-1-one structure (5,6-dehydronorketamine, metabolite II), shown in Fig. 1.

These 2 compounds were considered to be the primary metabolites of ketamine by most investigators who utilized the original GC analytical methods for biodisposition studies, including our own research group (Cohen *et al.*, 1973; Marietta *et al.*, 1976; Ryder *et al.*, 1978). However, only a few attempts were made to quantitate the biotransformation of ketamine *in vivo* through "balance" studies of the metabolites excreted. In humans administered tritium-labelled ketamine, over 90% of the radioactivity was recovered in the urine over 5 days (Chang *et al.*, 1970), but only 20% of the dose could be accounted for in terms of the parent drug, norketamine and 5,6-dehydronorketamine (Wieber *et al.*, 1975). Thus, in humans, and possibly other species, a major fraction of a dose of ketamine appeared to be converted to metabolites whose chemical structures (and pharmacologic activities) remained to be established. A possible explanation was the formation of hydroxylated metabolites of ketamine (Chang and Glazko, 1974; Lau and Domino, 1977), which could represent a significant fraction of a dose of the drug.

Alicyclic ring hydroxylation of ketamine

The identification of hydroxylated metabolites formed during ketamine metabolism has been aided by the introduction of newer analytical

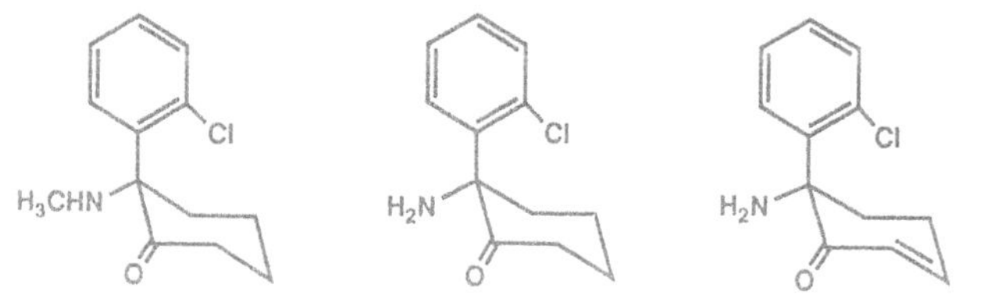

Ketamine — Norketamine (Metabolite I) — 5,6-dehydronorketamine (Metabolite II)

Fig. 1. Ketamine, the N-dealkylated metabolite (norketamine), and the urinary "metabolite" 5,6-dehydronorketamine.

methods designed to prevent the degradation of labile metabolites (Adams *et al.*, 1981; Leung and Baillie, 1986; Woolf and Adams, 1987). These include a nonselective extraction procedure to avoid base catalyzed dehydration, an initial reverse phase HPLC separative procedure, and the derivatization of metabolites with PFP or TFA to prevent thermal degradation during subsequent GLC separative procedures. The adequate resolution and identification of ketamine metabolites (often present at low concentrations in biological fluids) was accomplished by the use of capillary GLC high resolution mass spectrometry instrumentation. Confirmation of the structures of several hydroxylated metabolites derived from ketamine was achieved by their chemical synthesis (Woolf *et al.*, 1984; Leung and Baillie, 1986).

In experiments with rodent and human liver microsomes *in vitro* (Adams *et al.*, 1981; Woolf and Adams, 1987), the hydroxylation of ketamine was found to be restricted to the cyclohexanone ring system, in which carbons 4,5 and 6 were sites of metabolic attack (Fig. 2).

No evidence was found for the formation of phenolic metabolites of ketamine. The predominant member of this family of hydroxynorketamine isomers was identified as the 6-hydroxy compound. Thus,

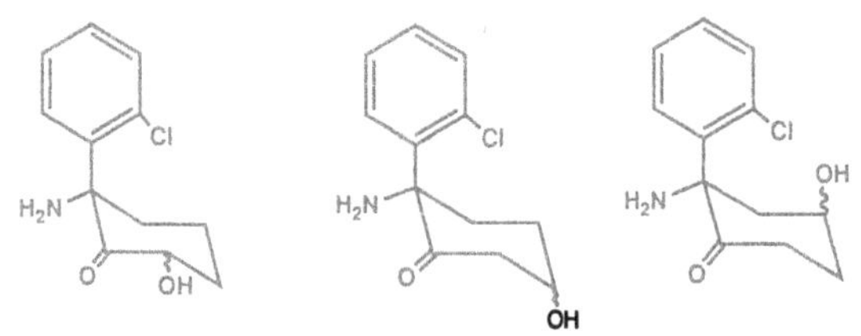

6-OH-norketamine — 5-OH-norketamine — 4-OH-norketamine

Fig. 2. Identified hydroxylated metabolites of norketamine.

the liver microsomal enzymes involved in biotransformation demonstrate partial regioselectivity in terms of the alicyclic ring hydroxylation of ketamine. Hydroxylation of the cyclohexanone ring of ketamine generates a second chiral center in the molecule, and therefore, the possibility exists for the generation of diastereomeric forms of the hydroxylated metabolites. The syntheses of the (Z)- and (E)- diastereomers of 6-hydroxyketamine (Woolf *et al.*, 1984) and of (Z)-6-hydroxynorketamine (Leung and Baillie, 1986) have confirmed that in the rat, rabbit, and human liver microsomes the (Z)- or cis-diastereomer of 6-hydroxynorketamine is formed exclusively (Woolf and Adams, 1987). Thus, the liver microsomal oxidation of carbon 6 in the cyclohexanone ring of norketamine is stereospecific.

Hydroxylation at the carbon 5 position of the ketamine molecule appears to be species dependent, in that 2 different isomeric forms of 5-hydroxynorketamine (different GLC retention times) were identified from rat versus rabbit microsomal incubates of ketamine, whereas both isomers were formed during incubation with human liver microsomes (Woolf and Adams, 1987). The relative configurations of these isomers, or of the 4-hydroxyketamine species formed in microsomal incubates, have not been determined. Pathways of metabolism of ketamine in human liver also include alicyclic ring hydroxylation of the parent molecule, leading to formation of 4- and 6-hydroxyketamine.

The major routes of biotransformation of ketamine in rodent and human microsomes *in vitro* are shown in Fig. 3. It should be emphasized that in such studies the hydroxylated metabolites are formed at much lower concentrations than norketamine, thus, the oxidation reactions involved appear to be quantitatively of less significance than the N-dealkylation of ketamine. The extent to which hydroxylation reactions involving norketamine or the parent drug occur *in vivo* is not known.

Initial studies indicated that following the N-demethylation of ketamine, dehydrogenation of the cyclohexanone ring resulted in the formation of 5,6-dehydronorketamine, a compound present in the urine of many species, including humans (Chang and Glazko, 1974). This "metabolite" could not be detected using the modified analytical procedures, which suggested that 5,6-dehydronorketamine may have been formed from 5- and/or 6-hydroxylated metabolites of norketamine, as an artifact of analytical procedures (Chang and Glazko, 1972; Lai *et al.*, 1985). Stability studies with (Z)- and (E)-6-hydroxylated ketamine failed to provide evidence for the formation of the dehydrogenation product, leading to the conclusion that the most likely sources of 5,6-dehydronorketamine

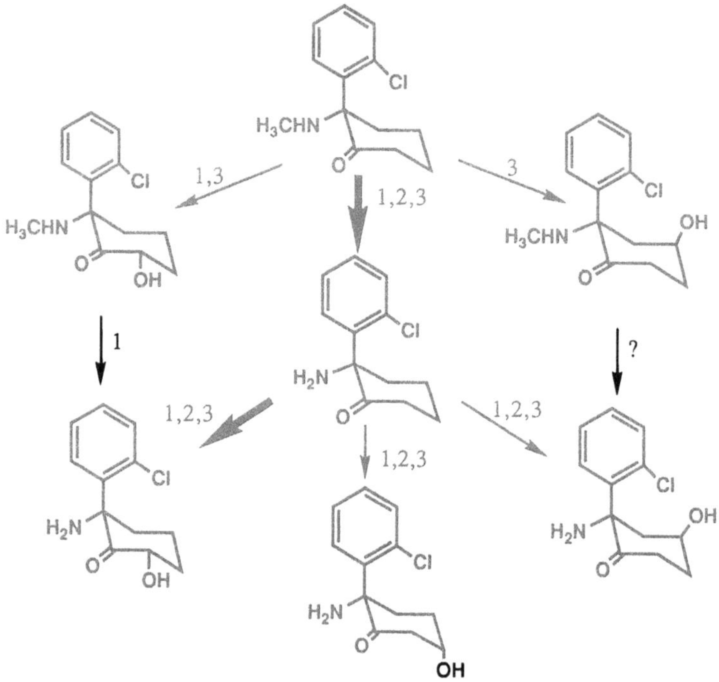

Fig. 3. Major biotransformation pathways of ketamine; 1 = Rat, 2 = Rabbit, 3 = Human.

are the 5-hydroxylated metabolites, which undergo dehydration under acidic or basic conditions (Woolf and Adams, 1987).

Enantioselectivity in ketamine metabolism

Due to the chiral center at carbon 2 of the cyclohexanone ring, ketamine exists as 2 enantiomeric structures. Almost all of the published studies on the metabolic fate of ketamine have considered the drug as a racemic mixture of its (R)- and (S)-enantiomers. Since the individual enantiomers of ketamine exhibit differences in their pharmacological effects, the biodisposition and metabolism of the optical isomers are of some interest. One approach to the investigation of the biotransformation of the ketamine enantiomers involves the preparation of "pseudoracemic" mixtures of the drugs in which 1 of the 2 enantiomers is labelled with a stable isotope for subsequent GC-MS analysis. The heavy isotope label becomes a stereochemical marker for the identification and quantitation of the metabolites derived from each isomer (Baillie, 1981).

The N-dealkylation of ketamine, leading to the formation of norketamine, is a major pathway of metabolism in all species studied (Baggot and Blake, 1976; Kaka *et al.*, 1979; Pedraz *et al.*, 1986; Sams and Pizzo, 1987; Waterman and Livingston, 1978). The reaction is catalyzed by cytochrome(s) P-450, for which ketamine is a type I substrate (Horai *et al.*, 1985) and the isozymes involved are drug-inducible (Marietta *et al.*, 1976). It is assumed that ketamine N-dealkylation occurs mainly in the liver, although other tissues, including the lungs, may also be involved (Pedraz *et al.*, 1986). The reaction is enantioselective to an extent dependent upon species. This has been shown by GC-MS analysis of products obtained from the *in vitro* liver microsomal metabolism of "pseudoracemic" mixtures containing 1 or the other of the ketamine enantiomers in deuterated form (Trevor *et al.*, 1983). In the case of human liver microsomes, (S)-ketamine was N-demethylated at a rate approximately 50% faster than the (R)-enantiomer (Fig. 4). In contrast, (R)-ketamine was metabolized 2 times faster than the (S)-enantiomer by rat liver microsomes.

Alicyclic ring hydroxylation of ketamine also exhibits enantioselectivity. The formation of (Z)-6-hydroxynorketamine in rodent and human liver microsomes is primarily from the (S)-ketamine enantiomer. The metabolite thus has the structure (R)- 5-hydroxy-(S)-norketamine. In contrast, the formation of 6-hydroxyketamine in human liver microsomes is

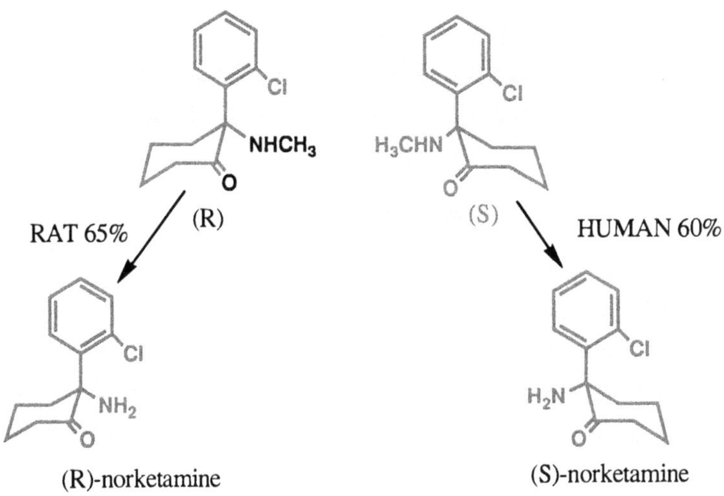

Fig. 4. N-demethylation of ketamine is enantioselective and species dependent.

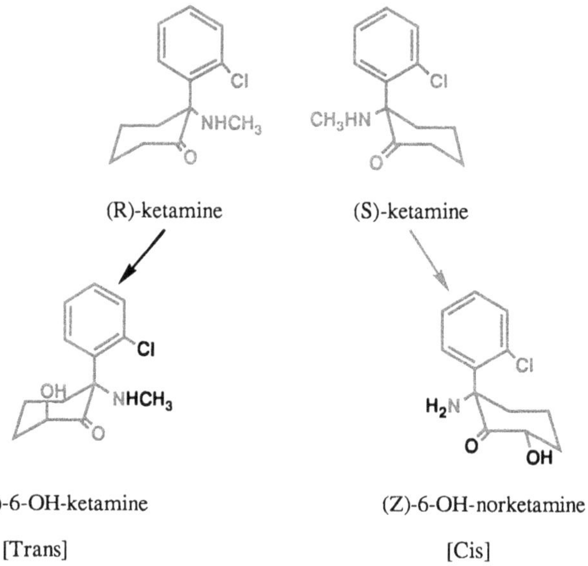

Fig. 5. Enantioselectivity in alicyclic ring hydroxylation.

largely from the (R)-enantiomer of the drug, and the metabolite has the (E)-trans-configuration (Fig. 5).

Summary

In vitro studies, using rodent and human liver microsomal preparations, have revealed that the biotransformation of ketamine is complex and characterized by stereoselectivity, certain aspects of which are species dependent. Substrate stereoselectivity occurs in terms of differences in the rates of N-dealkylation of the ketamine enantiomers, and regioselectivity occurs in the hydroxylation of the alicyclic ring. This leads to the introduction of a second chiral center in the molecule. Diastereoisomerism occurs in the formation of 6-hydroxylated metabolites of ketamine and norketamine. Unfortunately, such stereochemical characterization of N-dealkylation of ketamine and of cyclohexanone ring oxidation remains largely of academic interest since most of the metabolites formed occur at very low concentrations and no information exists suggesting that they are of pharmacologic or toxicologic importance.

References

Adams, J.D., Baillie, T.A., Trevor, A.J., and Castagnoli, N., Jr.: Studies on the biotransformation of ketamine. Biomed. Mass Spectrom. 8: 527-538, 1981.

Baggot, J.D. and Blake, J.W.: Disposition kinetics of ketamine in the domestic cat. Arch. Int. Pharmacodyn. 220: 115-124, 1976.

Baillie, T.A.: The use of stable isotopes in pharmacology research. Pharmacol. Rev. 33: 81-132, 1981.

Chang, T., Dill, W.A., and Glazko, A.J.: Metabolic disposition of 2-(o-chlorophenyl)-2-methylaminocyclohexanone.HCl (CI-581) in laboratory animals and man. Fed. Proc. 24: 268, 1965.

Chang, T. and Glazko, A.J.: A gas chromatographic assay for ketamine in human plasma. Anesthesiol. 36: 401-404, 1972.

Chang, T. and Glazko, A.J.: Biotransformation and biodisposition of ketamine. Int. Anesth. Clinics 12: 157-177, 1974.

Chang, T., Savory, A., Albin, M., Boulet, R., and Glazko, A.J.: Metabolic disposition of tritium-labelled ketamine ("Ketalar" (I-581)) in normal human subjects. Clin. Res. 18: 497, 1970.

Cohen, M.L., Chan, S.-L., Way, W.L., and Trevor, A.J.: Distribution in the brain and metabolism of ketamine in the rat after intravenous administration. Anesthesiol. 39: 370-376, 1973.

Horai, Y., White, P.F., and Trevor, A.J.: The effect of etomidate on rabbit liver microsomal drug metabolism *in vitro*. Drug Metab. Dispos. 13: 364-367, 1985.

Kaka, J.S., Klavano, P.A., and Hayton, W.L.: Pharmacokinetics of ketamine in the horse. Am. J. Vet. Res. 40: 978-981, 1979.

Lai, L., Hong, S.-C., and Davisson, J.N.: Ketamine metabolism: Identification and synthesis of a deaminated product. J. Pharm. Sci. 74: 486-488, 1985.

Lau, S.S. and Domino, E.F.: Gas chromatography-mass spectrometry assay for ketamine and its metabolites in plasma. Biomed. Mass Spectrom. 4: 317-321, 1977.

Leung, L.Y. and Baillie, T.A.: Comparative pharmacology in the rat of ketamine and its two principal metabolites, norketamine and (Z)-6-hydroxynorketamine. J. Med. Chem. 29: 2396-2399, 1986.

Marietta, M.P., White, P.F., Pudwill, C.R., Way, W.L., and Trevor, A.J.: Biodisposition of ketamine in the rat: self-induction of metabolism. J. Pharmacol. Exp. Ther. 196: 536-544, 1976.

Pedraz, J.L., Lanao, J.M., Hdez, J.M., and Dominguez-Gil, A.: The biotransformation kinetics of ketamine *in vitro* in rabbit liver and lung microsome fractions. Eur. J. Drug Metab. Dispos. 11: 9-16, 1986.

Ryder, S., Way, W.L., and Trevor, A.J.: Comparative pharmacology of the optical isomers of ketamine in mice. Eur. J. Pharmacol. 49: 15-23, 1978.

Sams, R. and Pizzo, P.: Detection and identification of ketamine and its metabolites in horse urine. J. Anal. Toxicol. 11: 58-62, 1987.

Trevor, A.J., Woolf, T.F., Baillie, T.A., Adams, J.D., and Castagnoli, N.: Stereoselective metabolism of ketamine enantiomers. In Phencyclidine and Related Arylcyclohexylamines: Present and Future Applications, ed. by J.M. Kamenka, E.F. Domino and P. Geneste, pp. 279-289, NPP Books, Ann Arbor, MI 1983.

Waterman, A. and Livingston, A.: Studies on the distribution and metabolism of ketamine in sheep. J. Vet. Pharmacol. Therap. 1: 141-147, 1978.

Wieber, J., Gugler, J.H., Hengstmann, J.H., and Dengler, H.J.: Pharmacokinetics of ketamine in man. Anaesthetist 24: 260-263, 1975.

Woolf, T.F. and Adams, J.D.: Biotransformation of ketamine, (Z)-6-hydroxyketamine, and (E)-6-hydroxyketamine by rat, rabbit, and human liver microsomal preparations. Xenobiotica 17: 839-847, 1987.

Woolf, T.F., Trevor, A.J., Baillie, T.A. and Castagnoli, N. Jr.: Synthesis of (Z)- and (E)-6-hydroxyketamine. J. Org. Chem. 49: 3305-3310, 1984.

Status of Ketamine in Anesthesiology,
edited by E.F. Domino©1990, NPP Books
P.O. Box 1491, Ann Arbor, MI 48106

Pharmacology of the Ketamine Enantiomorphs

W.L. Way, A.J. Trevor and P.F. White*

Departments of Anesthesia and Pharmacology
University of California
San Francisco, CA
and
*Department of Anesthesiology**
Washington University School of Medicine
St. Louis, MO

In a 1965 paper, Domino *et al.* stated that "the remarkable analgesic and anesthetic properties of phencyclidine have stimulated a search for derivatives that would offer the same benefits with fewer psychotomimetic effects." It was further suggested in this same paper that CI-581 (ketamine) was able to produce immobilization and/or general anesthesia in a variety of animals in a broad range of doses and perhaps represented a compound which, although less potent than phencyclidine, might allow the production of a more controllable and acceptable anesthetic state. Domino and his colleagues also felt that since there were fairly significant sympathomimetic properties and a cerebral "dissociative action," a new term was needed to designate such drugs. The suggestion was made that drugs of this type be called "dissociative anesthetics". The term "dissociative anesthesia" is interesting in that it seemed to originate from studies based on electroencephalographic effects of ketamine. These studies showed a depression of thalamoneocortical systems, while simultaneously there was seen activation in the limbic system which was termed a "functional dissociation" between the two systems. However, Winters *et al.* (1972) interpreted the electroencephalographic effects of ketamine in a somewhat different fashion, attributing these effects to a functional disorganization due to subliminal seizure activity in both the thalamus and limbic systems. The question of the proper term used to designate the type of anesthesia produced by ketamine is probably less important than the fact that over the intervening years ketamine has been utilized millions of times for the production of a satisfactory anesthetic state, useful in a variety of surgical procedures. It is not surprising that this distinct anesthetic state was a stimulus to the many basic and clinical investigations that have been carried out over the ensuing years.

Most studies have used the clinically available form of ketamine, a racemic mixture (RK) containing equal amounts of the two ketamine enantiomers. These enantiomers had been resolved by 1965, but when we embarked on our work in the early 1970s, no pharmacologic studies specific to the enantiomers had been reported in the literature. An examination of the pharmacology of ketamine isomers seemed warranted since many drugs, including the opioids, autonomic nervous system drugs, etc., have been demonstrated to show different pharmacologic effects depending on which enantiomer was selected (Casey, 1970; Fig. 1).

The animal studies reported here were carried out utilizing a supply of drugs given us by Bristol Laboratories. We had reason to believe that these were relatively pure compounds and the possibility of racemization seemed very unlikely given the fact that there is no labile functionality about the chiral center.

Our first study (Marietta *et al.*, 1977) demonstrated the increases in the duration of loss of righting reflexes following caudal vein administration to Sprague-Dawley rats of equimolar doses of ketamine and its enantiomorphs ranging from 10-40 mg/kg (Table 1).

It should be noted that significant lethality occurred following administration of the 40 mg/kg dose of both the (+) enantiomer (PK) and the RK, but not with the (−) enantiomer (MK).

It is interesting that posthypnotic stimulation, as measured by locomotor activity following i.v. administration of equimolar doses of these compounds, was not statistically different. However, in our observations, there was a suggestion that the locomotor activity of the MK was more intense than that of the PK. Thus, when we administered equihypnotic

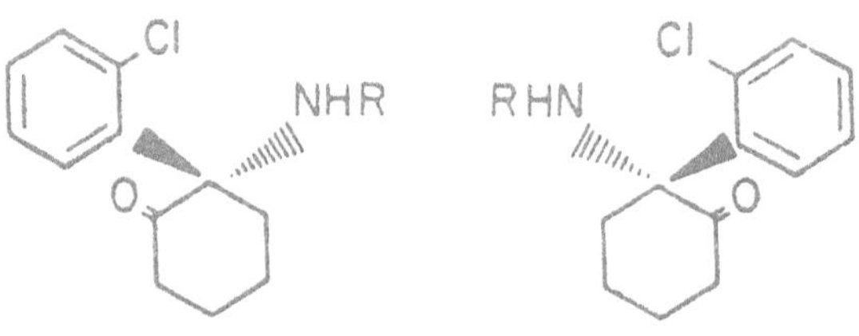

S R

Fig. 1. Ketamine and norketamine enantiomers.

TABLE 1. The duration of loss of righting reflex following i.v. administration of the ketamine enantiomers

Dosage (mg/kg)	*(-)-Ketamine (min)*	*(±)-Ketamine (min)*	*(+)-Ketamine (min)*
10	1.76 ± 0.30*	3.10 ± 0.26	4.10 ± 0.38*
20	3.84 ± 0.24*	5.80 ± 0.64	7.80 ± 0.42*
30	5.02 ± 0.20*	7.50 ± 0.55	11.90 ± 1.48*
40	8.72 ± 0.72	—	—

* P value < 0.05 by Student's unpaired t test

dosages of the PK, RK, and MK, we confirmed that the locomotor activity with the PK was significantly less intense than that with the MK.

Subsequent studies in male ICR mice (20-30 g) demonstrated that the analgesic action of ketamine was more pronounced with the PK than with the MK (Ryder *et al.*, 1978, Fig. 2).

These studies were conducted using the phenylquinone writhing test as a measure of analgesia in mice. The analgetic dose (AD_50) in these experiments was determined to be approximately 11 with the MK, approximately 6.5 with the RK, and approximately 3.7 with the PK (Table 2).

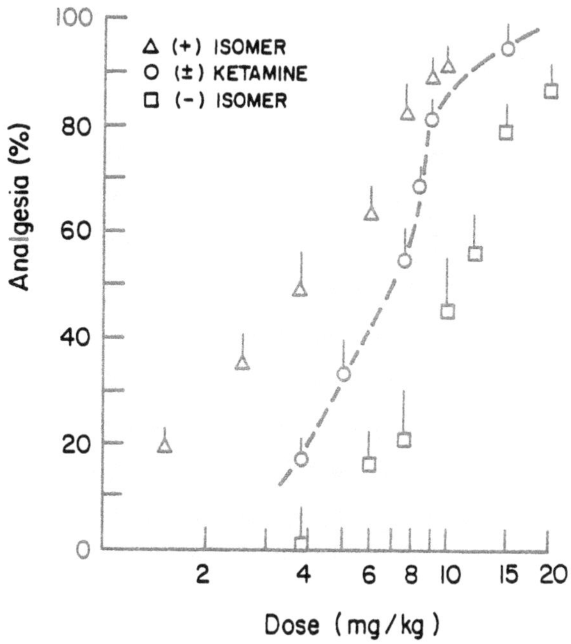

Fig. 2. Differential analgesic actions of ketamine enantiomers.

TABLE 2. (A) The median effective analgesic and hypnotic doses of (±)-ketamine and its isomers in mice[1]. (B) The potency ratios for analgesia and hypnosis of the isomers.[1]

(A) Drug	*AD_{50}[2] mg/kg s.c. (95% C.L.)*	*HD_{50}[3] mg/kg s.c. (95% C.L.)*
(−)-isomer	11 (9.2–13)	56 (46–68)
(±)-ketamine	6.5 (5.2– 8.1)	45 (41–49)
(+)-isomer	3.7 (2.6– 5.2)	38 (35–41)
(B)	Analgesia	Hypnosis
Potency ratio[4]	3.0 (2.1– 4.3)	1.5 (1.2– 1.9)

[1]The median effective doses, confidence limits and potency ratios were determined by the Litchfield-Wilcoxon test (1949).
[2]Analgesic dose necessary to inhibit writhing by 50% in the phenylquinone writhing test. Six to 7 doses and at least 9 animals per dose were used for each drug.
[3]Hypnotic dose necessary to cause the loss of righting reflex in 50% of the animals. Five doses and 10 animals per dose were used for each drug.
[4]Potency ratio is the relative potency of the (+) isomer compared to the (−) isomer.

Again, a ratio of about 3 between the PK and MK AD_50 dose was noted, but this potency difference with regard to hypnosis was not maintained, PK only being about 1.2 to 1.5 times as potent as MK when loss of righting reflex is used as a measure of hypnosis in mice. (Table 2).

In both the Marietta (1977) and Ryder (1978) studies, the observed pharmacokinetic profiles for the individual isomers of ketamine did not differ significantly from the racemic mixture, suggesting that the potency differences were not due to differences in biodisposition.

In another study in our laboratory, the behavioral effects in rats of the enantiomers were examined with regard to schedule controlled responding as a function of time, dose, and initial control rates (rate dependency) (Meliska *et al.*, 1980). This study demonstrated a qualitative as well as quantitative difference in the effects of the drugs on schedule controlled responding. PK *decreased* overall rates of responding at 30 and 60 mg/kg in contrast to MK, which *increased* rates of responding at all doses.

Based on these animal data, a protocol was designed to assess the efficacy of PK when compared to MK and RK as the sole anesthetic in man. It was formulated to allow an assessment of the relative anesthetic potencies of the ketamine enantiomers, the adequacies of anesthesia produced, the cardiovascular stimulation produced, possible correlations between plasma levels of ketamine and durations of anesthesia, and, finally, emergence behavior and side effects in the recovery room. In this study (White *et al.*, 1980), 60 healthy patients undergoing elective outpatient operations were given either the RK, the PK, or the MK in a randomized double blind fashion after informed consent had been obtained. In addition, a number of psychologic assessments were made in the recovery room by a psychologist blinded to the drug given. Samples of plasma and urine were obtained for analysis of ketamine and its major metabolites. The doses administered initially were 2 mg/kg for RK, 1 mg/kg for PK, and 3 mg/kg for MK. No other medications were used other than a dose of 0.005 mg/kg of glycopyrrolate administered 5-10 min prior to the induction of anesthesia as an antisialagogue. After induction of anesthesia with the above mentioned doses, further anesthetic was administered by titrating the dose of ketamine against the clinical signs of anesthesia. In cases where adequate surgical anesthesia could not be achieved, thiopental and nitrous oxide were employed. The total dosage of drug varied from a high total dose of 557 mg for MK to a low total dose of 143 mg for PK, but the durations of anesthesia produced were not significantly different (Table 3).

This study demonstrated differences in anesthetic potency, analgesia side effects, and anesthetic preferences among the optical enantiomers of ketamine. Since the kinetic curves and patterns of excretion of ketamine and its metabolites were similar for the three groups, we believe that this parallelism suggests that differences were due to pharmacodynamic factors (Fig. 3).

This report would not be complete without mention of two more recent studies. The first was carried out by White and his colleagues (1985) at Stanford University and was a study of 5 volunteers who received each of the drugs, *i.e.*, RK, PK, and MK, on separate occasions. Again, there appeared to be no differences pharmacokinetically. However, they did note that EEG evaluation revealed less overall slowing of EEG activity with the MK as compared to the PK and RK. This was taken as an indication that both PK and RK are better CNS depressants than

TABLE 3. Intraoperative assessment of ketamine anesthesia

	Racemate	*(+) Ketamine*	*(−) Ketamine*
Induction dose (mg/kg)	2	1	3
Total dosage			
(mg)	348±48	148±10*	557±101*
(mg/kg)	5.4	2.4	8.5
Duration of anesthesia (min)	41±8	32±4	33±7

*Isomer group that differed significantly ($P \leq 0.05$) from either the racemic group or its enantiomer

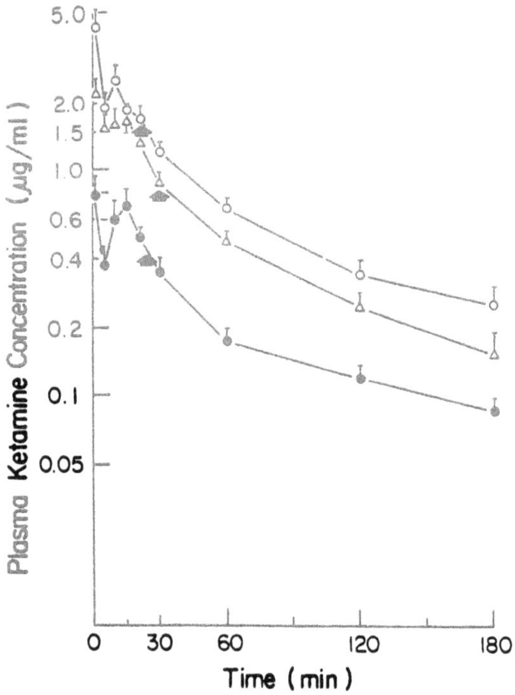

Fig. 3. Plasma levels of ketamine on a logarithmic scale as a function of time in those patients who received at most two additional bolus injections after induction with racemic ketamine, 2 mg/kg, i.v. (N = 7, △–△), (+)Ketamine, 1 mg/kg, i.v. (N = 8, ●–●), or (−)ketamine, 3 mg/kg, i.v. (N = 7, ○–○). Arrowheads indicate time of emergence from anesthesia (*i.e.*, time of purposeful response to a command). Values are means ± S.E.

than MK. They also concluded that PK was associated with more rapid recovery than the currently used racemic mixture.

A final study conducted by Schuttler *et al.* (1987) used the median frequency of the EEG power spectrum, which is meant to be a continuous noninvasive measure of the degree of central nervous system depression. This pharmacodynamic measurement was related to measured serum concentrations of drug. Essentially their observations confirmed that the MK caused less EEG slowing than did the PK or RK, *i.e.*, more CNS depression occurs with RK and PK than with MK. They again drew the conclusion that the pharmacokinetic distribution and elimination of each enantiomer are not different from the racemic compound. They felt that the pharmacodynamic interaction of the enantiomers suggests that the effect of the racemic mixture of ketamine may be primarily accounted for by classical competitive interaction (non-synergistic).

The results of the early animal work and the subsequent clinical studies would suggest that there may be merit in utilizing the PK enantiomer. However, the differences between the enantiomers and the racemic mixture are relatively small when compared to other drugs where activity of the drug may reside entirely in one or the other of the enantiomers. Pharmacologic differences have been demonstrated in these studies, but whether or not PK is a clinically superior anesthetic remains as an incompletely answered question. The original studies some 25 years ago by Domino and his colleagues (1965) certainly resulted in the start of an interesting and fascinating investigative path.

References

Casey, A.F.: Stereochemistry and biological activity. In Medicinal Chemistry (3rd ed.), ed. by A. Burger, pp 81-107, Wiley Interscience, New York, 1970.

Domino, E.F., Chodoff, P., and Corssen, G.: Pharmacologic effects of CI-581, a new dissociative anesthetic, in man. Clin. Pharmacol. Ther. 6: 279-291, 1965.

Marietta, M.P., Way, W.L., Castagnoli, N., and Trevor, A.J.: On the pharmacology of the ketamine enantiomorphs in the rat. J. Pharmacol. Exp. Ther. 202: 157-165, 1977.

Meliska, C.J., Greenberg, A.J., and Trevor, A.J.: The effects of ketamine enantiomers on schedule-controlled behavior in the rat. J. Pharmacol. Exp. Ther. 202: 198-202, 1980.

Ryder, S., Way, W.L., and Trevor, A.J.: Comparative pharmacology of the optical isomers of ketamine in mice. Eur. J. Pharmacol. 49: 15-23, 1978.

Schuttler, J., Stanski, D.R., White, P.F., Trevor, A.J., Horai, Y., Verotta, D., and Sheiner, L.B.: Pharmacodynamic modeling of the EEG effects of ketamine and its enantiomers in man. J. Pharmacokin. Biopharm. 15: 241-253, 1987.

White, P.F., Ham, J., Way, W.L., and Trevor, A.J.: Pharmacology of ketamine isomers in surgical patients. Anesthesiol. 52: 231-239, 1980.

White, P.F., Schuttler, J., Shafer, A., Stanski, D.R., Horai, Y., and Trevor, A.J.: Comparative pharmacology of the ketamine isomers. Brit. J. Anaesth. 57: 197-203, 1985.

Winters, W.D., Ferrar-Allado, T., Guzman-Flores, C., and Alvarez, M.: The cataleptic state induced by ketamine. A review of the neuropharmacology of anesthesia. Neuropharmacol. 11: 303-315, 1972.

Status of Ketamine in Anesthesiology,
edited by E.F. Domino©1990, NPP Books
P.O. Box 1491, Ann Arbor, MI 48106

Ketamine and Intracranial Pressure

E. Pfenninger and A. Reith

Albert Einstein University,
University Clinic of Anaesthesiology,
Ulm, F.R. of Germany

Introduction

Multiple injuries are almost always associated with a loss of blood, plasma, water, and electrolytes, resulting in hypovolemic shock. The combination of head injury and traumatic-hemorrhagic shock is therefore often seen in the 150,000 cases of cranial trauma occurring each year in the Federal Republic of Germany.

Ketamine has been in use for many years in the field of accident and emergency medicine, primarily for the induction and maintenance of anesthesia in patients who have suffered large blood losses (Chasapakis *et al.*, 1973; Bond and Davie, 1974; Longnecker and Sturgill, 1976). Its large scale use has been foreseen in the event of a war or major disaster.

The use of ketamine in the presence of head injury is still much debated because of reports that it leads to a rise in intracranial pressure (ICP). In an investigation carried out in 1980, Hase and Dick showed that the rise in ICP is not a constant finding. At the same time, Schalk and List in Austria (1981) proposed that an increase in ICP does not occur with low dose ketamine, or, that under the conditions of controlled ventilation and hemorrhagic shock, no increase develops when the initial ICP is within the normal range (Klose *et al.*, 1982). These findings are in agreement with those of Schwedler *et al.* (1982), who did not observe an increase in ICP after administration of ketamine to ventilated animals with normal ICP and arterial pressure levels.

Because of these different findings, the first aim of our study (using an animal model) was to look at the effect of two different doses of ketamine on ICP under emergency and hospital conditions. The second purpose of this study was to investigate the role of ketamine in injured humans with normal and increased ICP, at normotensive circulatory conditions, and during hemorrhagic shock.

Second study in ventilated patients

A second clinical investigation was undertaken on those patients who experienced an increase in ICP after the administration of ketamine (1.0 mg/kg), and who had received a nondepolorizing muscle relaxant (4.0 mg pancuronium i.v.).

Results

Animal experiments

There were no alterations in the ICP in a control group of ventilated piglets after receiving either 0.5 mg/kg or 2.0 mg/kg of ketamine. The ICP remained at the original level up to the end of the observation period (Fig. 1). Slight fluctuations of arterial blood pressure did not influence the ICP and there was no correlation between these two parameters. In normotensive animals with an elevated ICP (N-group), 0.5 mg/kg ketamine led to a negligible drop of ICP from 29 to 28.5 mm Hg at 3 and 4 min after injection. While 2.0 mg/kg ketamine lowered the ICP to 28.3 mm Hg, no increase was observed in either case. In the hypotensive group (H group) significant decreases in ICP of 3 min duration were observed. The

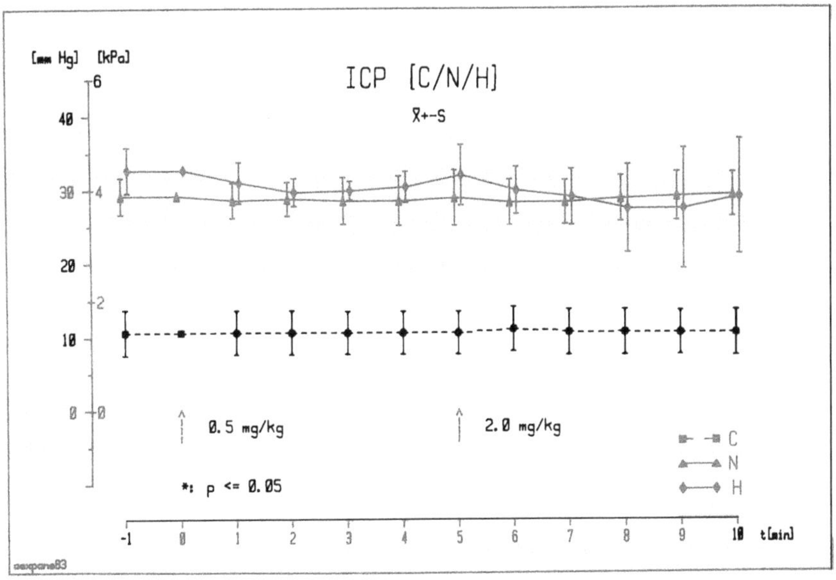

Fig. 1. Alterations in ICP in ventilated piglets after receiving 0.5 and 2.0 mg/kg ketamine (C = control group, N = normotensive blood pressure, H = hemorrhagic shock).

ICP dropped from 32.7 to 29.7 mm Hg and reached a minimum of 27.4 mm Hg after the administration of 2.0 mg/kg of ketamine. After 10 min, the ICP was still below the original level. The relationship between ICP and mean arterial pressure was reflected in a good correlation between the two parameters (r = 0.63). We must, therefore, assume that cerebral autoregulation is severely impaired during hemorrhagic shock.

In spontaneously breathing animals with normal intracranial conditions, no alterations in ICP could be observed even following 5.0 mg/kg ketamine. On the other hand, in both groups with an elevated ICP, *i.e.*, with and without hemorrhagic shock, we observed the previously reported increase in ICP. Following the higher dose of either 2.0 mg/kg or 5.0 mg/kg ketamine, the mean pretreatment ICP of 32 mm Hg rose to a peak with a mean level of 45 mm Hg (Fig. 2). Of particular interest is that none of our animals with a normal ICP died during the investigation. However, 3 out of 10 animals in the normotensive group, and 7 of the 10 animals in the hypotensive group breathing spontaneously died of apnea.

As we clearly demonstrated, 0.5 mg/kg of ketamine led to a further increase of an elevated ICP. For example, in one animal this dosage led to a rise from 30 to 60 mm Hg within a few minutes, remaining on this level over the following period of time.

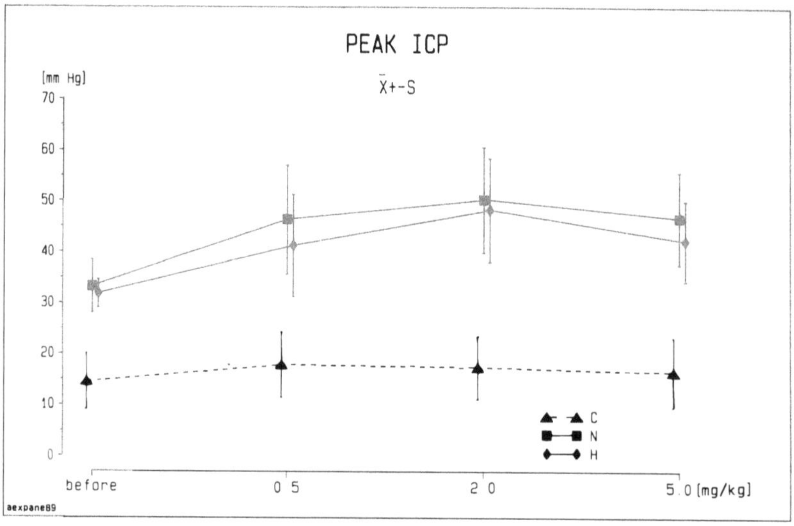

Fig. 2. Alterations in ICP in spontaneously breathing animals after receiving ketamine (C = control group, N = normotensive blood pressure, H = hemorrhagic shock).

Because the only difference in management between our two animal studies was whether ventilation was spontaneous or controlled, the arterial partial pressure of carbon dioxide levels ($PaCO_2$) was of particular interest. No changes were observed in spontaneously breathing animals, with no elevation of ICP after either 0.5 or 2.0 mg/kg of ketamine. Only with a dose of 5.0 mg/kg could a significant rise from 38 to 41 mm Hg be detected. However, an increase of such a small degree is not of clinical importance. In animals with an initially elevated ICP and normal blood pressure levels, all three doses of ketamine resulted in significant $PaCO_2$ changes. The $PaCO_2$ values rose from 37 to 44 mm Hg. In the hypotensive group, some of the piglets had potentially dangerous increases in the $PaCO_2$, particularly those animals which died from apnea. In this group the $PaCO_2$ rose from an initial value of 37 to 61 mm Hg and a significant

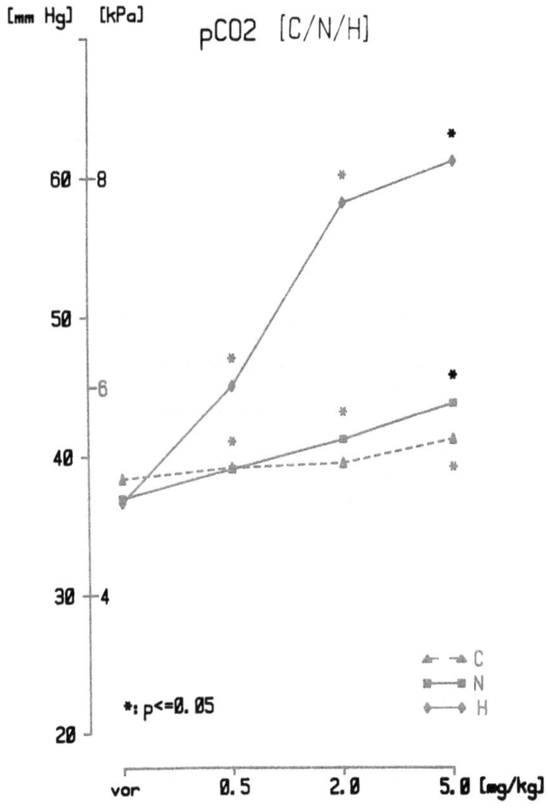

Fig. 3. $PaCO_2$ after giving 0.5 mg/kg, 2.0 mg/kg and 5.0 mg/kg ketamine.

correlation between $PaCO_2$ and ICP could be seen. In contrast, we were unable to observe any relationship between these parameters in those animals which were ventilated.

Ventilated patients

Neither 0.5 nor 1.0 mg/kg of ketamine led to an alteration of heart rate and mean arterial pressure. After the administration of 0.5 mg/kg ketamine, the ICP fell from 7 to 5 mm Hg and remained at that level until the end of the 10 min observation period. After 1.0 mg/kg ketamine, the ICP decreased from 7 to 6 mm Hg during the second minute and then rose again to 9 mm Hg (Fig. 4). None of these changes were statistically significant. It is interesting to note that the changes occurred in individual cases after the administration of 1.0 mg/kg ketamine without additional barbiturate sedation. Some of the patients had a marked decline in ICP after ketamine, whereas others had a short lasting increase. During the course of repeated measurements in the same patient, the values often varied within a wide range. Furthermore, no correlation with the baseline values could be detected.

In our second study on ventilated patients, the ICP, which was initially increased from 15 to 20 mm Hg, subsequently fell to 10 mm Hg 5

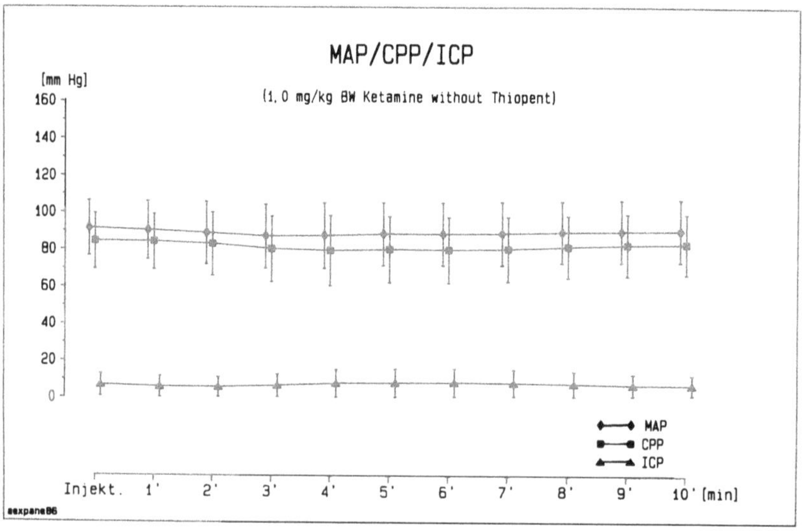

Fig. 4. Mean arterial pressure (MAP), cerebral perfusion pressure (CPP) and ICP in 10 normotensive head injury patients after receiving ketamine. Mean values and standard deviation are shown.

min after the administration of 4 mg of pancuronium (Fig. 5). The arterial pCO_2 was only slightly changed during this time (33.2 to 32.7 mm Hg).

Discussion

We have, of course, considered why our results are so different from previous reports in the literature. A review of these studies reveals that the majority of observations reporting an elevation of ICP following ketamine had been carried out on spontaneously breathing animals or patients (Gardner *et al.*, 1971; List *et al.*, 1972; Shapiro *et al.*, 1972; Takeshita *et al.*, 1972). It is interesting to note that in all the cases studied, no increase in ICP was observed during the first 3-5 min after the administration of ketamine. After this period, our ketamine induced changes were almost reversed. While some authors did not include the levels of $PaCO_2$ in their observations (Wyte *et al.*, 1972), others did not regard the changes in $PaCO_2$ which they measured as being of any clinical relevance (Gardner *et al.*, 1971; Hougaard *et al.*, 1974). Takeshita *et al.* (1972) reported a small rise in $PaCO_2$ after giving ketamine to healthy volunteers with normal ICP levels. They suggested that the increase in cerebral blood flow which they observed might be caused by the increase in CO_2 levels. Further, Shapiro

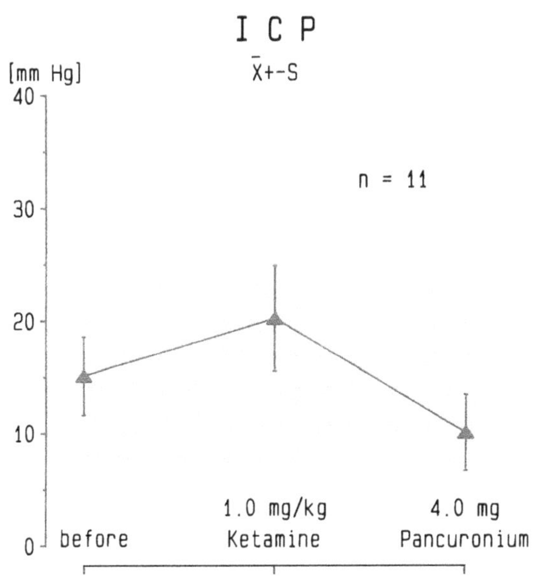

Fig. 5. ICP in 11 head injury patients with initial increasing ICP after receiving ketamine.

et al. (1972) noted that hyperventilation caused the elevated ICP seen following ketamine to revert to normal.

As a preliminary conclusion, we believe that the preexisting level of ICP is of importance for the type of $PaCO_2$ reaction following ketamine. In the presence of a normal ICP, we found no increase in $PaCO_2$. On the other hand, the combination of hypovolemic shock and increased ICP is particularly dangerous. Obviously ketamine can cause a marked increase in $PaCO_2$ and, subsequently, in ICP when given to head injury patients who are breathing spontaneously.

In some of our ventilated patients we saw an increase in ICP. A passively induced rise in ICP, as was suggested by Takeshita *et al.* (1972) and Gardner *et al.* (1971), cannot have played an important role in our patients since there was no change in arterial blood pressure. A negative inotropic effect of ketamine with subsequent venous stasis in the brain is also unlikely. As Langrehr *et al.* (1972) have shown, no cardiodepressant effects can be detected in humans up to a dose of 3 mg/kg.

Ketamine is known to cause an increase in skeletal muscle tone. Hensel *et al.* (1972) found total oxygen consumption to be 25% higher during ketamine anesthesia compared to other types of anesthesia. This excessive consumption could be normalized by injection of a non-depolarizing muscle relaxant. A general increase in muscle tone after administration of ketamine, along with increased tone of the thoracic and abdominal muscles, could lead to a rise in intrathoracic pressure. This, in turn, would impair the venous return from the head and could lead to an increased intracranial blood volume. The fact that the only difference between the animal experiments and our patients was the missing muscle relaxation favors this hypothesis.

Since patients will usually also be given a muscle relaxant with induction of anesthesia, our findings can be directly applied to the pre-hospital phase of management of cases of acute head injury. Our findings are in agreement with those of Schwedler *et al.* (1982) who did not find an increase in either ICP or in cerebral blood flow after the administration of ketamine to ventilated animals. On the other hand, when spontaneously breathing animals were examined, cerebral blood flow rose analogous to the $PaCO_2$.

We believe that the following conclusions can be drawn from our experiments:

1. Ketamine itself does not increase ICP. The decisive factor in causing an elevation in ICP is the $PaCO_2$.
2. Provided that the ICP is initially within the normal range, there

are no alterations in ICP with ketamine during spontaneous breathing. This is because changes in $PaCO_2$ are minimal, and a sufficient cranial compliance reserve is able to compensate for these minimal changes in $PaCO_2$.

3. When ICP is raised, either with or without hemorrhagic shock, ketamine can lead to a further increase via a rise in $PaCO_2$. During spontaneous breathing, the hazard of an increase in ICP exists even with low doses of ketamine.
4. In contrast, no further increase in ICP is observed during controlled ventilation, either when the ICP is normal or when it is initially raised. This is true when blood pressure is normal as well as during hemorrhagic shock.
5. Therefore, we consider ketamine, administered in a dose of 0.5 to 1.0 mg/kg, to be a suitable drug for the induction of anesthesia in polytraumatized patients with hemorrhagic shock and acute head injury. However, subsequent controlled ventilation is necessary. Of course, this does not mean that ketamine is the best drug for induction of anesthesia in patients with acute head injury *and* a normal blood pressure. For these cases, other drugs which lower ICP are available.

References

Bond, A.C. and Davie, C.K.: Ketamine and pancuronium for the shocked patient. Anaesthesia 29: 59, 1974.

Chasapakis, G., Kekis, N., and Sakkalis, C.: Use of ketamine and pancuronium for anesthesia for patients in hemorrhagic shock. Anesth. Analg. 52: 282-287, 1973.

Dawson, B., Michenfelder J.D., and Theye R.A.: Effects of ketamine on canine cerebral blood flow and metabolism: Modification by prior administration of thiopental. Anesth. Analg. 50: 443-447, 1971.

Gardner, A.E., Olson, B.E., and Lichtiger, M.: Cerebrospinal fluid pressure during dissociative anesthesia with ketamine. Anesthesiol. 35: 226-228, 1971.

Hase, U. and Dick, W.: Zum Verhalten des intrakraniellen Druckes bei Schadel-Hirn-traumatisierten Patienten nach Ketaminapplikation. In Ketamin (Ketanest) in Notfall-und Katastrophenmedizin, W. Dick, ed., pp. 77-81, Perimed, Erlangen, 1983.

Hensel, I., Braun, U., Kettler, D., Knoll, D., Martel, J., and Paschen, K.: Untersuchungen über Kreislauf und Stoffwech selveränderungen unter Ketamin-Narkose. Anaesthesist 21: 44-49, 1972.

Hougaard, K., Hansen, A., and Brodersen, P.: The effect of ketamine on regional cerebral blood flow in man. Anesthesiol. 41: 562-567, 1974.

Klose, R., Hartung, H.J, Kotsch, R., and Walz, Th.: Experimentelle Untersuchungen zur intrakraniellen Drucksteigerung durch Ketamin beim hämorrhagischen Schock. Anaesthesist 31: 33-38, 1982.

Langrehr, D., Kluge, I., and Neuhaus, R.: 5 Jahre Erfahrung mit der dissoziativen Ketamine-Anaesthesie. Anaest. Prax. 7: 5-12, 1972.

List, W.F., Crumrine, R.S., Cascorbi, H.F., and Weiss, M.H.: Increased cerebrospinal fluid pressure after ketamine. Anesthesiol. 36: 98-99, 1972.

Longnecker, D.E. and Sturgill, B.C.: Influence of anesthetic agent on survival following hemorrhage. Anesthesiol. 45, 516-521, 1976.

Pfenninger, E., Grünert, A., Bowdler, I., and Kilian, J.: The effect of ketamine on intracranial pressure during haemorrhagic shock under the conditions of both spontaneous breathing and controlled ventilation. Acta Neurochirurgica 78: 113-118, 1985.

Schalk, H.V. and List, W.F.: Liquordruckentwicklung nach Ketamin. In Ketamin (Ketanest[R]) in Notfalund Katastrophenmedizin, ed. by W. Dick, pp. 71-77 Perimed, Erlangen, 1981.

Schwedler, M., Miletich, D.J., and Albrecht, R.F.: Cerebral blood flow and metabolism following ketamine administration. Can. Anaesth. Soc. J. 29: 222-225, 1982.

Shapiro, H.M., Wyte, S.R., and Harris, A.B.: Ketamine anaesthesia in patients with intracranial pathology. Br. J. Anaest. 44: 1200-1204, 1972.

Takeshita H., Okuda, Y., and Sari, A.: The effects of ketamine on cerebral circulation and metabolism in man. Anesthesiol. 36: 69-73, 1972.

Wyte, S.R., Shapiro, H.M., Turner, P., and Harris, A.B.: Ketamine-induced intracranial hypertension. Anesthesiol. 36: 174-176, 1972.

Status of Ketamine in Anesthesiology,
edited by E.F. Domino©1990, NPP Books
P.O. Box 1491, Ann Arbor, MI 48106

Hypocapnia or Diazepam Reverses, and Midazolam or Fentanyl Attenuates Ketamine Induced Increase of Cerebral Blood Volume and/or CSF Pressure

A.A. Artru

University of Washington School of Medicine
Seattle, WA

INTRODUCTION

Ketamine generally has been reported to increase cerebrospinal fluid (CSF) pressure. For that reason, ketamine may be avoided in patients for whom an increase of CSF pressure would present a potential hazard, *i.e.*, patients with reduced intracranial compliance or a pre-existing increase of CSF pressure. The present study was designed to examine the mechanism of ketamine induced increase of CSF pressure and to determine the efficacy of treatments that might abolish or attenuate this increase of CSF pressure.

One of the issues addressed in this study was the question of whether ketamine increases cerebral blood volume (CBV) and, if so, whether ketamine induced increases of CSF pressure are accounted for by increases in CBV. Ketamine has been previously reported to increase intracranial pressure (ICP), CSF pressure, or jugular venous pressure (Evans *et al.*, 1971; Gardner *et al.*, 1971; Bock *et al.*, 1972; List *et al.*, 1972; Shapiro *et al.*, 1972; Takeshita *et al.*, 1972; Wyte *et al.*, 1972; Schulte am Esch *et al.*, 1979; Sari *et al.*, 1972). Ketamine also was previously reported to increase cerebral blood flow (CBF) (Takeshita *et al.*, 1972; Sari *et al.*, 1972; Dawson *et al.*, 1971) and to dilate isolated canine cerebral vessels (Fukuda *et al.*, 1983). Based on these studies, it has been assumed that ketamine increases ICP as a result of cerebrovasodilation (Sari *et al.*, 1972; Samuels, 1986; Campkin and Turner, 1986). However, there have been no studies that measured CBV and CSF pressure simultaneously following administration of ketamine, so this assumption remains unproven.

A second issue addressed in this study was the question of whether ketamine increases CBV indirectly, due to increased $PaCO_2$ (Schwedler *et al.*, 1982), or directly, due to its cerebral effects (Sari *et al.*, 1972; Dawson *et al.*, 1971; Fukuda *et al.*, 1983). As regards the first possibility, ketamine may increase $PaCO_2$ due to elevated CO_2 production, ventilatory depression or increase of respiratory dead space, with the increase of $PaCO_2$ causing cerebral vasodilation (Lassen, 1986). Schwedler *et al.* (1982) reported that ketamine increased CBF and ICP in awake goats when $PaCO_2$ was allowed to rise but had no effect on CBF and ICP when $PaCO_2$ was maintained at preketamine levels. It was concluded that CBF increase following ketamine resulted from increased $PaCO_2$. Alternatively, ketamine may increase CBV directly. Takeshita *et al.* (1972) reported that ketamine increased CBF and jugular venous pressure when $PaCO_2$ was allowed to rise in anesthetized patients. However, the increase in $PaCO_2$ was calculated to account for only 14% of the CBF increase, and it was concluded that CBF increase following ketamine resulted from its direct vasodilating action. Dawson *et al.* (1971) and Sari *et al.* (1972) reported that ketamine increased CBF and CSF pressure when $PaCO_2$ was maintained at preketamine levels in sedated dogs and anesthetized patients. Takeshita *et al.* (1972) and Dawson *et al.* (1971) concluded that ketamine induced increase of CBF resulted from cerebral metabolic stimulation. Unfortunately, none of these studies presented continuous, simultaneous data on CBF and CO_2. Thus, it is not certain whether CO_2 contributes in a meaningful way to the cerebral vasodilation seen with ketamine.

A third and clinically relevant issue addressed in this study was the question of whether hypocapnia, diazepam, midazolam or fentanyl reverses ketamine induced increase of CBV and/or CSF pressure. Hypocapnia has been reported to abolish or attenuate ketamine induced increase of CSF pressure when begun after ketamine is given (Wyte *et al.*, 1972; Sari *et al.*, 1972). Diazepam has been reported to abolish or attenuate ketamine induced increase of CSF pressure when begun prior to or simultaneously with ketamine (Albin *et al.*, 1978; Trop, 1978; Cabarrocas *et al.*, 1973; Thorsen and Gran, 1980; Belopavlovic and Buchthal, 1982). Ketamine was reported not to increase CSF pressure when buprenorphine (Pfenninger *et al.*, 1985) or meperidine (Gibbs, 1972) were given prior to ketamine. However, it is not known whether pretreatment with hypocapnia is as effective as posttreatment, posttreatment with diazepam is as effective as pretreatment, pretreatment with fentanyl is as effective as pretreatment with buprenorphine or meperidine, or pre- or posttreatment with midazolam is effective in abolishing or attenuating ketamine induced increase of CSF pressure. Further, it is not known whether these treatments alter the effect of ketamine on CSF pressure by antagonizing ketamine induced increase of CBV, or act independently of CBV.

METHODS

Thirty eight mongrel dogs (weight 15-21 kg) were studied. Anesthesia was induced with isoflurane (> 1.8%) and N_20 (66%) in 0_2. The trachea was intubated and ventilation was control led with a Harvard pump respirator to maintain $PaCO_2$ at 35 ± 3 mm Hg (mean ± SD) and $Pa0_2$ > 120 mm Hg. With the dog in the supine position, the right femoral artery was cannulated for arterial blood sampling for blood gas analyses and for continuous monitoring of systemic arterial blood pressure and heart rate. The right femoral vein was cannulated for fluid and drug administration, and a urinary catheter was inserted. Succinylcholine 50-120 mg/hr was infused i.v. to maintain muscle relaxation. Saline was infused i.v. at 4-6 ml/kg/hr to minimize depletion of intravascular volume. Systemic variables were monitored continuously. These included mean arterial blood pressure (MAP, determined by electronic integration), expired CO_2 (using a Beckman LB-2® medical gas analyzer) and temperature (using a nasopharyngeal thermister probe). Temperature was maintained at 37.0 ± 0.5° C by heat lamps or ice packs.

With the dog in the prone position, the head was fixed in a slightly elevated position using a stereotaxic frame. A midline scalp incision was made, and both frontalis muscles reflected laterally. Relative cerebral blood volume (CBV) was determined by measuring *gamma* emission from i.v. injected iodinated 131-I albumin (RISA). Following i.v. injection of RISA, at least 120 min were allowed for equilibration. A converging, collimated scintillation probe (NaI) was placed over the head to measure *gamma* activity. A focal length was chosen for the *gamma* detector (Picker Nuclear Magnascanner 500®) that would "view" the brain but not the muscle or skin on the opposite side of the head. Though the probe primarily measured *gamma* emission from intracerebral blood, some *gamma* emission from extracranial blood in the surrounding tissue and from background activity still contributed to the total *gamma* emission detected by the probe. During the study, the total *gamma* emission was measured and later corrected for background activity and extracranial blood. This technique for determining relative CBV was described previously (Artru, 1983; Artru, 1987).

CSF pressure was determined by placing an 18 gauge teflon catheter through a left parietal burr hole into the lateral ventricle. The burr hole was sealed and the catheter secured to the skull using a methyl methacrylate resin. Ventricular CSF pressures were recorded as mean pressures using electronic integration. The strain gauges used to measure systemic arterial pressure and intracranial CSF pressure were positioned 12 cm above heart level. The zero reference for the strain gauges was set at the level of the external auditory meatus. Following completion of the surgical preparation, wound edges were infiltrated with bupivacaine (0.75%), and the isoflurane concentration was decreased to 0.3% (end-expired value determined intermittently by gas chromatography).

Dogs then were randomly assigned to one of six groups for study. In Group I (N=7) the sequence of experimental treatments was: control, ketamine, hypocapnia and normocapnia. In Group II (N = 7) the sequence was: control, hypocapnia, ketamine and normocapnia. In Group III (N=6) the sequence was: control, ketamine and diazepam. In Group IV (N=6) the sequence was: control, diazepam and ketamine. In Group V (N=7) the sequence was either: control, ketamine and midazolam, or control, midazolam and ketamine. In Group VI (N = 5) the sequence was: control, fentanyl and ketamine. The dose of ketamine was 2.0 mg/kg, i.v., the dose of diazepam was 0.3 mg/kg, i.v., the dose of midazolam was 0.3 mg/kg, i.v., and the dose of fentanyl was 60 μg/kg, i.v. Hypocapnia was defined as $PaCO_2$ of 20-25 mm Hg, and normocapnia was defined as $PaCO_2$ of 33-37 mm Hg. The doses of ketamine, diazepam, midazolam and fentanyl were based on previously reported values for dogs (Dawson *et al.*, 1971; Albin *et al.*, 1978; Maekawa *et al.*, 1974; Artru, 1988; Artru, 1984). Each treatment was maintained for 15 min. Arterial blood gas values and heart rate were determined at each treatment. CBV, CSF pressure, expired CO_2 and MAP were determined continuously throughout all treatments. The values recorded for continuous variables were those representing maximum change associated with each treatment.

At the conclusion of the study, the dogs were sacrificed by i.v. injection of 35% KCl, a tourniquet was placed around the neck and the brain was removed via craniectomy. The *gamma* emission measured from the head after the brain was removed was taken to represent extracranial sources. CBV was calculated as the difference between total *gamma* emission and extracranial sources. The *gamma* emission measured by the collimator after it was moved away from the dog was considered to be the background portion of total extracranial *gamma* emission. The portion of *gamma* emission deriving from the extracranial circulation was taken as the difference between total extracranial sources and background activity.

Within each group cerebral and systemic values were compared between experimental conditions using repeated measures of analysis of variance. When the calculated F value exceeded the critical value for the .05 probability level, the Student-Newman-Keuls test was used to determine which differences were significant at $P < 0.05$. The coefficient of variability was used to determine the relative variability of CBV measurements at each condition.

Results

Group I: Control CSF pressure was 8.1 ± 3.4 cm H_20 (mean ± S.D., Table 1). Administration of ketamine caused an increase of CSF pressure to 14.1 ± 4.8 cm H_20, along with an increase of CBV by 12.4 ± 6.9% (Tables 2 and 3). Expired CO_2 rose by 1.5 ± 2.1 mm Hg (NS). Fifteen min after ketamine administration, hypocapnia returned CSF pressure and CBV to near control values. When hypocapnia was discontinued and normocapnia restored at 30 min after ketamine, CSF pressure increased to 10.9 ± 3.1 cm H_20 and CBV increased to 10.0 ± 4.0% above control values. There were no significant changes in $PaCO_2$ (except the desired reduction during hypocapnia), MAP or other systemic variables.

Group II: Control CSF pressure was 9.3 ± 1.8 cm H_20. Hypocapnia caused a decrease of CSF pressure to 6.6 ± 2.7 cm, along with a decrease of CBV by 6.0 ± 2.6%. Administration of ketamine during hypocapnia returned CSF pressure and CBV to near control values. Expired CO_2 rose by 0.5 ± 1.5 mm Hg (NS). When hypocapnia was discontinued and normocapnia restored at 15 min postketamine, CSF pressure increased to 17.0 ± 6.5 cm H_20 and CBV increased to 12.1 ± 7.0% above control values. Throughout these treatments there were no significant changes in $PaCO_2$ (except the desired reduction during hypocapnia), MAP or other systemic variables.

Group III: Control CSF pressure was 6.8 ± 2.7 cm H_20. Ketamine caused an increase of CSF pressure to 17.5 ± 6.4 cm H_20, along with an increase of CBV by 11.7 ± 6.6% above control. Expired CO_2 rose by 2.0 ± 2.4 cm H_20 (NS). Administration of diazepam 15 min postketamine returned CSF pressure and CBV to near control values. Neither $PaCO_2$, MAP or other systemic variables changed significantly during the experimental period.

Group IV: Control CSF pressure was 6.7 ± 2.0 cm H_20. Diazepam caused a decrease of CSF pressure to 3.2 ± 1.9 cm H_20, along with a decrease of CBV by 4.7 ± 1.9%. Administration of ketamine at 15 min

TABLE 1. Baseline cerebral and systemic values (mean ± S.D.)

	Group I (*N*=7)	*Group II* (*N*=7)	*Group III* (*N*=6)	*Group IV* (*N*=6)	*Group V* (*N*=7)	*Group VI* (*N*=5)
CSF pressure, cm H_2O	8.1 ± 3.4	9.3 ± 1.8	6.8 ± 2.7	6.7 ± 2.0	7.2 ± 2.0	6.4 ± 2.2
$PaCO_2$, mm Hg	34.8 ± 1.4	34.7 ± 1.2	34.9 ± 1.7	36.5 ± 2.5	34.4 ± 0.5	34.1 ± 1.5
PaO_2, mm Hg	149 ± 18	141 ± 20	152 ± 14	153 ± 18	151 ± 18	164 ± 11
pH	7.40 ± 0.03	7.40 ± 0.05	7.41 ± 0.03	7.38 ± 0.06	7.40 ± 0.03	7.39 ± 0.03
Bicarbonate, mEq/*l*	20.8 ± 0.7	20.9 ± 1.6	21.2 ± 1.1	20.9 ± 1.3	20.6 ± 1.3	20.1 ± 1.7
Hemoglobin, g/d*l*	12.3 ± 0.8	12.7 ± 0.5	13.4 ± 0.6	13.0 ± 0.5	12.8 ± 0.6	12.9 ± 0.5
Mean arterial pressure, mm Hg	134 ± 15	133 ± 21	130 ± 14	135 ± 11	133 ± 21	132 ± 13
Heart rate, beats/min	110 ± 16	107 ± 22	104 ± 12	104 ± 20	105 ± 23	106 ± 15
Temperature, nasopharyngeal, °C	37.3 ± 0.1	37.1 ± 0.2	37.1 ± 0.2	37.1 ± 0.2	37.0 ± 0.2	37.1 ± 0.2

TABLE 2. CSF pressure following ketamine, with and without pre- and post treatment, (cm H_2O, mean ± S.D.)

	Control	*Ketamine*	*Ketamine combined with pretreatment*	*Ketamine combined with post treatment*
Group I (hypocapnia)	8.1±3.4	14.1±4.8*	—	6.1±2.5
Group II (hypocapnia)	9.3±1.8	—	11.6±4.3	—
Group III (diazepam)	6.8±2.7	17.5±6.4*	—	7.7±3.4
Group IV (diazepam)	6.7±2.0	—	7.3±2.3	—
Group Va (midazolam)	7.0±1.4	15.0±1.4*	—	11.9±0.7#
Group Vb (midazolam)	7.3±2.3	—	12.0±4.3*	—
Group VI (fentanyl)	6.4±2.2	—	8.1±1.4#	—

* = Significantly different from control values, $P < 0.05$
# = Significantly different from both control and ketamine values, $P < 0.05$

TABLE 3. Percent change from control of cerebral blood volume following ketamine, with and without pre- and post treatment (mean±S.D.)

	Ketamine	*Ketamine combined with pretreatment*	*Ketamine combined with post treatment*	*Ketamine with reversal of pre- or post treatment*
Group I (hypocapnia)	+12.4±6.9*	—	−3.4±4.7	+10.0±4.0*
Group II (hypocapnia)	—	+4.4±7.0	—	+12.1±7.0*
Group III (diazepam)	+11.7±6.6*	—	2.2±5.7	—
Group IV (diazepam)	—	+5.5±3.0	—	—
Time, min	0–15	16–30	16–30	31–45

* = Significantly different from control values, $P < 0.05$

post diazepam returned CSF pressure and CBV to values that were not significantly different from control values. Expired CO_2 rose by 1.7 ± 2.9 mm Hg (NS). Diazepam decreased MAP to 96 ± 15 mm Hg. Ketamine returned MAP to near control values. Other systemic variables did not change significantly during the experimental period.

Group V: In dogs given ketamine prior to midazolam, control CSF pressure was 7.5 ± 2.3 cm H_20. Ketamine caused an increase of CSF pressure to 15.0 ± 1.4 cm H_20. Expired CO_2 rose by 0.9 ± 1.3 cm H_20

(NS). Following administration of midazolam 15 min postketamine, CSF pressure was 11.9 ± 0.7 cm H_20 and was increased compared to controls but decreased compared to postketamine values. Neither $PaCO_2$, MAP or other systemic variables changed significantly during the experimental period.

In dogs given midazolam prior to ketamine, control CSF pressure was 7.3 ± 2.3 cm H_20. Midazolam caused no significant change in CSF pressure. Administration of ketamine at 15 min postmidazolam increased CSF pressure to 12.0 ± 4.3 cm H_20. Expired CO_2 rose by 0.5 ± 0.4 mm Hg (NS). Midazolam decreased MAP to 120 ± 14 mm Hg. Ketamine returned MAP to near control values. Other systemic variables did not change significantly during the experimental period.

Group VI: Control CSF pressure was 6.4 ± 2.2 cm H_20. Fentanyl caused no significant change in CSF pressure. Administration of ketamine at 15 min postfentanyl increased CSF pressure to 8.1 ± 1.4, accompanied by a decrease of expired CO_2 and $PaCO_2$ by 2.3 ± 1.6 mm Hg. Fentanyl decreased MAP to 98 ± 12 mm Hg and heart rate to 63 ± 18 beats/min. MAP and heart rate remained decreased following ketamine. Other systemic variables did not change significantly during the experimental period.

The coefficient of variability for CBV measurements ranged from 3-5%. Background *gamma* activity accounted for 6-8% of measured *gamma* emission. From the determination of residual *gamma* emission following removal of the brain at the end of the study, it was calculated that 75-80% of measured *gamma* emission derived from CBV and 14-17% from the extracranial circulation.

Discussion

One aim of the present study was to determine whether ketamine increased CBV and, if so, whether ketamine induced increases of CSF pressure are accounted for by increases in CBV. The results of this study indicate that ketamine increases CBV, and that the increase in CBV is accompanied by a concomitant increase in CSF pressure. This finding is consistent with previously reported results (Takeshita *et al.*, 1972; Sari *et al.*, 1972; Dawson *et al.*, 1971). Those studies found that ketamine increased CBF in ventilated dogs sedated with nitrous oxide (Dawson *et al.*, 1971) and in anesthetized, ventilated patients (Takeshita *et al.*, 1972; Sari *et al.*, 1972). CSF pressure (Sari *et al.*, 1972; Dawson *et al.*, 1971) or jugular venous pressure (Takeshita *et al.*, 1972) increased in parallel with increase of CBF. The present finding that ketamine increased CBV also is consistent with a previous study by Fukuda *et al.* (1983) who reported that ketamine has a direct dilating effect on isolated canine middle cerebral and basilar arteries.

In contrast, others reported that ketamine causes no cerebral vasodilation and does not stimulate cerebral metabolism. Kreuscher and Grote (1967) reported that ketamine decreased CBF and cerebral metabolic rate in ventilated dogs sedated with nitrous oxide. Herrschaft and Schmidt (1973) reported that ketamine decreased CBF in anesthetized, ventilated patients. However, Kreuscher and Grote (1967) gave propanidid, 500 mg i.v., and Herrschaft and Schmidt (1973) gave propanidid, 5 mg/kg i.v., prior to ketamine. Presumably, administration of hypnotics prior to ketamine abolishes the cerebral vasodilating and metabolic stimulating properties of ketamine.

A second aim of the present study was to determine whether ketamine increases CBV indirectly, due to increased $PaCO_2$, or directly, due to its cerebral effects. The results of this study indicate that ketamine increases CBV and CSF pressure despite a lack of significant change in expired CO_2. These results argue against the proposal that ketamine produces cerebrovasodilation as a result of increased $PaCO_2$ and support the view that ketamine produces cerebrovasodilation, either by a direct dilating action on cerebrovascular smooth muscle or secondary to stimulation of cerebral metabolism. In contrast, Schwedler *et al.* (1982) reported in awake, instrumented goats that ketamine increased CBF during spontaneous ventilation when $PaCO_2$ rose from 34 ± 4 to 41 ± 7 mm Hg (mean ± SE) but did not increase CBF during mechanical ventilation when $PaCO_2$ was maintained at 30 ± 1 mm Hg. That the results of Schwedler *et al.* (1982) differ from those of Dawson *et al.* (1971), Sari *et al.* (1972) and the present study may relate either to species differences or to the fact that in the study of Schwedler *et al.* (1982) preketamine values were obtained in awake, instrumented animals. Consistent with Schwedler *et al.* (1982), Pfenninger *et al.* (1985) reported that in pigs ketamine did not increase CSF pressure during mechanical ventilation when $PaCO_2$ was maintained at normocapnia. However, Pfenninger *et al.* (1985) gave high doses of buprenorphine (mg not specified) and metomidate prior to ketamine. As discussed above, hypnotics may attenuate ketamine induced increase of CBF and CSF pressure. The cerebral action of metomidate is similar to that of thiopental (Campkin and Turner, 1986), and thiopental is reported to abolish ketamine induced increase of CBF and CSF pressure in dogs (Dawson *et al.*, 1971) and patients (Gibbs, 1972).

A third and clinically relevant aim of the present study was to determine whether hypocapnia, diazepam, midazolam or fentanyl reverses ketamine induced increase of CBV and/or CSF pressure. The results of this study indicate that the use of hypocapnia or diazepam, either pre- or postketamine, reversed the ketamine induced increase of CBV and CSF pressure. Post-treatment with midazolam and pretreatment with fentanyl attenuated but did not abolish the effects of ketamine. Pretreatment with midazolam did not abolish the increase of CSF pressure caused by ketamine. These results indicate that hypocapnia or diazepam offsets ketamine induced cerebral vasodilation so that CSF pressure does not exceed preketamine values. This finding is consistent with a previously reported case in which CSF pressure increased following administration of ketamine (Wyte *et al.*, 1972). In that report, CSF pressure decreased to preketamine values when thiopental was given and then fell to below preketamine values when hypocapnia was induced. This finding is also consistent with reports that both pretreatment or concurrent administration of diazepam abolish ketamine induced increase of CSF pressure in animals with normal or elevated (intracranial balloon) ICP (Albin *et al.*, 1978) and in patients (Thorsen and Gran, 1980). The present results also are consistent with a previous report that pretreatment with midazolam did not attenuate ketamine induced increase of CSF pressure in patients (Belopavlovic and Buchthal, 1982).

In contrast, in patients with intracranial tumors or hydrocephalus (Belopavlovic and Buchthal, 1982) or presumed intracranial pathology (patient characteristics not specified) (Trop, 1978; Cabarrocas *et al.*, 1973) pretreatment with diazepam has been reported to attenuate but not abolish ketamine induced increases of CSF pressure. These results suggest that when certain types of intracranial pathology are present, pretreatment with diazepam becomes less effective. However, because subject characteristics, intracranial conditions, use of anesthetics or other drugs and ventilatory characteristics were not specified or controlled in many of these previous studies (Albin *et al.*, 1978; Trop, 1978; Cabarrocas *et al.*, 1973; Thorsen and Gran, 1980), it is difficult to speculate further on the reasons for differences in results.

As regards the methodology of this study, it should be emphasized that in Groups I and II CBV and CSF pressure initially increased following administration of ketamine and again increased when normocapnia was restored 15 or 30 min postketamine. These results indicate that ketamine induced increase of CBV and CSF pressure last for at least 30 min. Consequently, it seems likely that the reversal of ketamine induced increase of CBV and CSF pressure seen following post treatment with hypocapnia or diazepam, and the attenuation of ketamine effect seen following post treatment with midazolam, were related to the treatments and did not occur because the effect of ketamine on CBV and CSF pressure spontaneously dissipated at 15 or 30 min. The finding that ketamine induced increase of CBV and CSF pressure lasts for at least 30 min agrees with previous reports on the duration of ketamine induced increases of CBF and CSF pressure. Dawson *et al.* (1971) reported that ketamine increased CBF for 30 min and CSF pressure for 45 min in dogs. Schulte am Esch *et al.* (1979) reported that ketamine increased CSF pressure for 40 min in patients.

In summary, the present results confirm previous assumptions that ketamine increases CSF pressure because it increases CBV. The present results indicate that ketamine can increase CBV without increasing $PaCO_2$, and are consistent with the view that ketamine increases CBV due to its cerebral effects. The findings that hypocapnia or diazepam given pre- or postketamine reverses increases of CBV and CSF pressure, and that post treatment with midazolam and pretreatment with fentanyl attenuates the effects of ketamine, suggest that these treatments may be useful adjuncts when ketamine is employed in clinical practice. For example, ketamine may be chosen for induction of anesthesia in patients who have suffered multiple traumatic injuries and whose cardiovascular stability is doubtful. Hyperventilating such patients prior to administration of ketamine may prevent CBV and CSF pressure from exceeding preketamine levels. Administration of fentanyl prior to ketamine may attenuate the effects of ketamine on CSF pressure. Should signs of increased CSF pressure appear following induction of anesthesia with ketamine, diazepam or additional hyperventilation may restore CSF pressure to preketamine values. However, it should be noted that the present studies were conducted in dogs with no known intracranial pathology. It is not known whether the cerebral responses to ketamine, hypocapnia, diazepam, midazolam or fentanyl observed here are altered when intracranial pathology is present.

REFERENCES

Albin, M.S., Gonzalez-Abola, E., Chang, J.L., Helsel, P., and Bunegin, L.: Attenuation of intracranial hypertension after ketamine by diazepam pretreatment (Vth European Congress of Anaesthesiology), pp. 213-214, Excerpta Medica, Amsterdam, 1978.

Artru, A.A.: Dose-related change in the rate of cerebrospinal fluid formation and resistance to reabsorption of cerebrospinal fluid following administration of thiopental, midazolam, and etomidate in dogs. Anesthesiol. 69: 541-546, 1988.

Artru, A.A.: Reduction of cerebrospinal fluid pressure by hypocapnia: Changes in cerebral blood volume, cerebrospinal fluid volume, and brain tissue water and electrolytes. J. Cereb. Blood Flow Metab. 7: 471-479, 1987.

Artru, A.A.: Relationship between cerebral blood volume and CSF pressure during anesthesia with halothane or enflurane in dogs. Anesthesiol. 58: 533-539, 1983.

Artru, A.A.: Relationship between cerebral blood volume and CSF pressure during anesthesia with isoflurane or fentanyl in dogs. Anesthesiol. 60: 575-579, 1984.

Belopavlovic, M. and Buchthal, A.: Modification of ketamine-induced intracranial hypertension in neurosurgical patients by pre-treatment with midazolam. Acta Anaesth. Scand. 26: 458-462, 1982.

Bock, W.J., Gobiet, W., Liesgang, J., and Grote, W.: Intracranial pressure during anaesthesia with ketamine. In Intracranial Pressure, ed. by M. Brock and H. Dietz, pp. 295-296, Springer-Verlag, Berlin, 1972.

Cabarrocas, E., Mercader, J.M., Cochs, J., and Marques, R.: Effects of ketamine in cerebral angiography. Neuroradiol. 5: 59-63, 1973.

Campkin, T.V. and Turner, J.M.: Intracranial effects of anaesthetic agents. In Neurosurgical Anaesthesia and Intensive Care, ed. by T.V. Campkin and J.M. Turner, pp. 48-72, Butterworth & Co. (Publishers) Ltd, London, 1986.

Dawson, B., Michenfelder, J.D., and Theye, R.A.: Effects of ketamine on canine cerebral blood flow and metabolism: Modification by prior administration of thiopental. Anesth. Analg. 50: 443-447, 1971.

Evans, J., Rosen, M., Weeks, R.D., and Wise, C.: Ketamine in neurosurgical procedures. Lancet I: 40-41, 1971.

Fukuda, S., Murakawa, T., Takeshita, H., and Toda, N.: Direct effects of ketamine on isolated canine cerebral and mesenteric arteries. Anesth. Analg. 62: 553-558, 1983.

Gardner, A.E., Olson, B.E., and Lichtiger, M.: Cerebrospinal fluid pressure during dissociative anesthesia with ketamine. Anesthesiol. 35: 226-228, 1971.

Gibbs, J.M.: The effect of intravenous ketamine on cerebrospinal fluid pressure. Br. J. Anaesth. 44: 1298-1301, 1972.

Herrschaft, H. and Schmidt, H.: Der Einflub von Ketamin auf die Hirndurchblutung beim Menshcen. In Ketamin, ed. by M. Gemperle, H. Kreuscher, and D. Langrehr, pp. 187-208, Springer-Verlag, Berlin, 1973.

Kreuscher, H. and Grote, J.: Die Wirkung des Phencyclidin derivates Ketamin. (CI 581) auf die Durchblutung und Sauersstoffaufnahme des Gehirns beim Hund. Anaesthesist 16: 304-308, 1967.

Lassen, N.A.: Cerebral and spinal cord blood flow. In Anesthesia and Neurosurgery, ed. by J.E. Cottrell and H. Turndorf, pp. 1-21, The C.V. Mosby Company, St. Louis, 1986.

List, W.F., Crumrine, R.S., Cascorbi, H.F., and Weiss, M.H.: Increased cerebrospinal fluid pressure after ketamine. Anesthesiol. 36: 98-99, 1972.

Maekawa, T., Sakabe, T., and Takeshita, H.: Diazepam blocks cerebral metabolic and circulatory responses to local anesthetic-induced seizures. Anesthesiol. 41: 389-391, 1974.

Pfenninger, E., Dick, W., and Ahnefeld, W.: The influence of ketamine on both normal and raised intracranial pressure of artificially ventilated animals. Eur. J. Anaesth. 2: 297-307, 1985.

Samuels, S.I.: Anesthesia for supratentorial tumor. In Anesthesia and Neurosurgery, ed. by J.E. Cottrell and H. Turndorf, pp. 115-130, The C.V. Mosby Company, St. Louis, 1986.

Sari, A., Okuda, Y., and Takeshita, H.: The effect of ketamine on cerebrospinal fluid pressure. Anesth. Analg. 51: 560-565, 1972.

Schulte am Esch, J., Pfeifer, G., Thiemig, I., and Entzian, W.: The influence of intravenous anaesthetic agents on primarily increased intracranial pressure. Acta Neurochir. 45: 15-25, 1979.

Schwedler, M., Miletich, D.J., and Albrecht, R.F.: Cerebral blood flow and metabolism following ketamine administration. Can. Anaesth. Soc. J. 29: 222-225, 1982.

Shapiro, H.M., Wyte, S.R., and Harris, A.B.: Ketamine in patients with intracranial pathology. Br. J. Anaesth. 44: 1200-1204, 1972.

Takeshita, H., Okuda, Y., and Sari, A.: The effects of ketamine on the cerebral circulation and metabolism in man. Anesthesiology 36: 69-75, 1972.

Thorsen, T. and Gran, L.: Ketamine/diazepam infusion anaesthesia with special attention to the effect on cerebrospinal fluid pressure and arterial blood pressure. Acta Anaesth. Scand. 24: 1-4, 1980.

Trop, D.: Diazepam in ketamine induced intracranial pressure increase (Vth European Congress of Anaesthesiology), pp. 221, Excerpta Medica, Amsterdam, 1978.

Wyte, S.R., Shapiro, H.M., Turner, P., and Harris, A.B.: Ketamine-induced intracranial hypertension. Anesthesiol. 36: 174-176, 1972.

Status of Ketamine in Anesthesiology,
edited by E.F. Domino©1990, NPP Books
P.O. Box 1491, Ann Arbor, MI 48106

Gas Exchange and Atelectasis During Ketamine and Halothane Anesthesia

L. Tokics

Department of Anesthesia,
Huddinge University Hospital
S-14186 Huddinge, Sweden

The impairment of arterial oxygenation during anesthesia was originally demonstrated by Campbell *et al.* (1958) to be caused by an increase of the alveolo-arterial oxygen tension difference. There are simultaneous changes in the mechanical properties of the lung with a reduction of the functional residual capacity and compliance. Although x-ray of the lungs could not disclose any structural changes, the hypothesis was proposed that microatelectasis develops during anesthesia. Experimental support for this hypothesis grew from the finding that gas exchange could be improved by inflating the lungs to high airway pressures (Bendixen *et al.*, 1963). The beneficial effect of raising the end expiratory airway pressure during anesthesia, however, has not been confirmed in subsequent investigations (Nunn *et al.*, 1965, Tokics *et al.*, 1987a).

Despite the lack of definite evidence, atelectasis continued to be regarded as a possible explanation of the alterations in lung function during anesthesia. Recently, densities in dependent lung regions in anesthetized subjects were demonstrated by computerized tomography (CT) (Brismar *et al.*, 1985), thus confirming previous suspicions.

In an experimental study, the x-ray densities have been shown to represent atelectasis (Hedenstierna *et al.*, 1989). The atelectasis develops promptly after induction of anesthesia, both during spontaneous breathing and during mechanical ventilation. In addition, its formation seems to be little influenced by the inspired gas composition (Strandberg *et al.*, 1986). These findings indicate that the cause of atelectasis formation is not gas resorption but rather a compression of the lung tissue, possibly induced by a reduction of functional reserve capacity (FRC).

Ketamine differs from most other anesthetics. Skeletal muscle tone is often maintained or even increased (Domino *et al.*, 1965). Arterial oxygenation is reported to be well maintained even in air-breathing patients (Gooding *et al.*, 1977, Rust *et al.*, 1978). A reduction of FRC occurs during spontaneous breathing with most other anesthetics (Don *et al.*, 1970, Hedenstierna *et al.*, 1985). Although this has not been investigated extensively during ketamine anesthesia, two investigations, one in children and the other in adults, support the concept that FRC is maintained with ketamine and spontaneous breathing (Shulman *et al.*, 1985, Mankikian *et al.*, 1986). These differences were the incentive to investigate the alterations in gas exchange and lung morphology with CT during ketamine anesthesia and to compare the effects of ketamine to those of halothane (Fig. 1).

METHODS

Subjects

Nineteen patients were studied awake, during anesthesia with spontaneous breathing, and during anesthesia with muscle relaxation and mechanical ventilation. Eight patients were females and 11 were males with ages ranging from 22 to 74 yr. Eight patients were given ketamine and 11 patients halothane anesthesia. All patients were scheduled for elective surgical procedures for either inguinal hernia or for cholecystolithiasis. The patients were free from cardiopulmonary diseases as judged from clinical examination and from preoperative spirometry. Informed consent was obtained in all subjects. The investigation was approved by the Ethics Committee of Huddinge Hospital.

Anesthesia

The patients received no premedication. Prior to induction, atropine (0.25-0.5 mg i.v.) was given. Ketamine anesthesia was induced by a slow (1-2 min) i.v. injection (3 mg/kg) and maintained with an i.v. infusion of 0.07-0.12 mg/kg/min. Halothane anesthesia was induced by inhalation of halothane in oxygen ($N = 6$) or by an i.v. injection of thiopental (150-500 mg) and it was maintained with halothane 0.6-1.2% inspired concentration.

During anesthesia, the inspired oxygen fraction was 0.40-0.45, and the balance nitrogen, in both groups. Before mechanical ventilation (Servo 900C Ventilator, Siemens-Elema, Sweden), the trachea was intubated. Muscular relaxation was achieved with succinylcholine and maintained with pancuronium, as indicated.

Catheterization

A triple lumen thermistor tipped catheter (Swan-Ganz 7 F, Edward's Laboratories, Santa Ana, CA) was introduced percutaneously and ad-

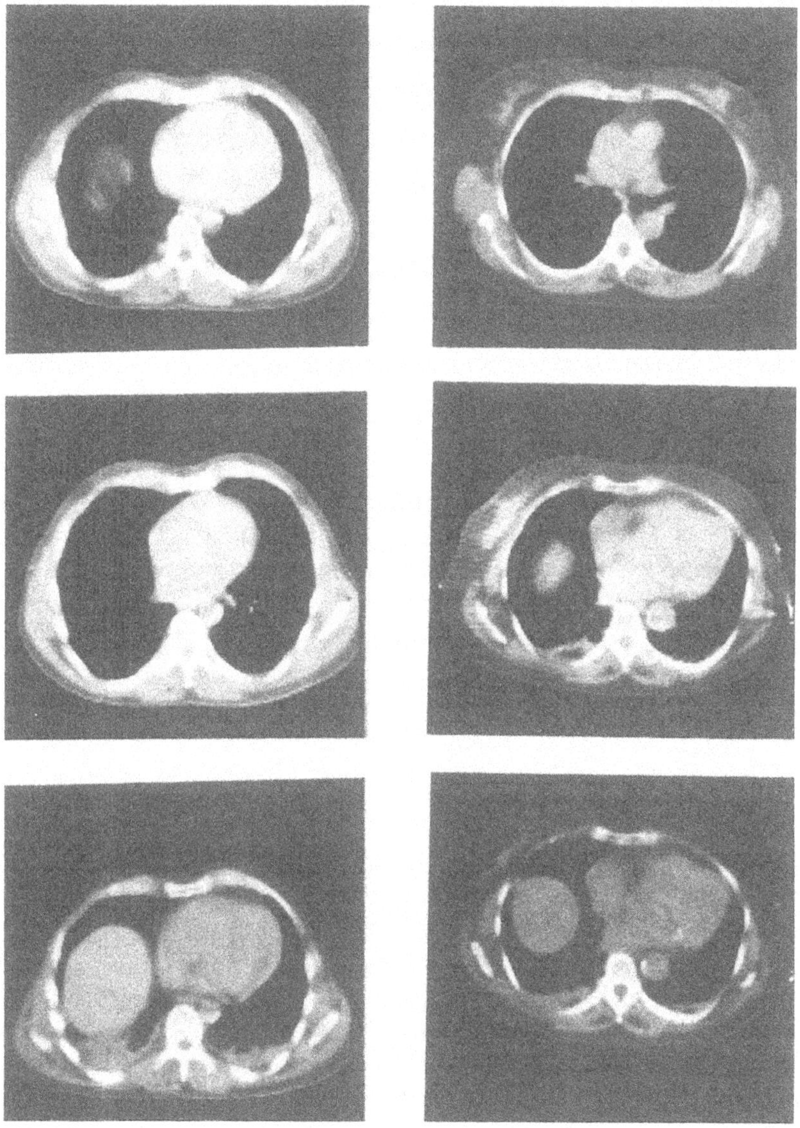

Fig. 1. CT scans from top to bottom: awake, during anesthesia and spontaneous breathing, and during mechanical ventilation. Left panel: ketamine; right panel: halothane anesthesia. Note the development of atelectasis during halothane but not during ketamine anesthesia with spontaneous breathing.

vanced to the pulmonary artery. Pulmonary vascular pressures relative to atmospheric pressure were recorded with zero reference at midthoracic level. A brachial artery was also cannulated for pressure recording and blood sampling. Additional venous catheters were inserted for infusion of inert gases and anesthetic drugs. Cardiac output was determined by thermodilution.

Ventilation-perfusion ratios

Six gases (sulphur hexafluoride, ethane, cyclopropane, enflurane, diethylether, and acetone) were dissolved in isotonic saline (0.9% NaCl) and infused into a vein at a rate of 3 ml/min. After 40 min of infusion under steady-state conditions and after arterial and mixed venous blood samples were taken and mixed, expired gas was collected for analysis by gas chromatography (Sigma 3, Perkin-Elmer). Blood gas partition coefficients were determined in each subject (Wagner *et al.*, 1974a). Arterial/mixed venous and mixed expired/mixed venous gas concentration ratios (retention and excretion, respectively) were plotted against blood gas partition coefficients. These relationships were transformed into a multicompartmental plot of blood flow and ventilation against VA/Q (Wagner *et al.*, 1974b, Evans and Wagner, 1977). Of the available information related to the distribution of the ventilation/perfusion ratios (VA/Q, see Fig. 2), we present data on shunt (Qs; perfusion of lung regions with VA/Q < 0.005), "low VA/Q regions" (Qlow; perfusion of lung regions with $0.005 <$ VA/Q < 0.1), and the log standard deviation of blood flow (QSD) and of ventilation (VSD) distributions.

Additional gas analysis

Arterial oxygen and carbon dioxide tensions (PaO_2, $PaCO_2$) were measured by standard techniques (blood-gas analyzer: ABL-2, Radiometer). Samples of inspired gas were analyzed for oxygen concentration by mass spectrometry. The alveolar-oxygen tension difference was calculated as PIO_2-$PaCO_2$/0.8-PaO_2 where PIO_2 is the inspired oxygen tension and 0.8 is an assumed respiratory gas exchange ratio.

CT of the chest

The structure and density of the lungs were studied by CT scanning. The subject lay supine on the tomograph table (Somatom 2, Siemens). A frontal scoutview covering the chest was initially obtained. CT scans in the transverse plane from a level just above the top of the diaphragm are presented. The same scan level, relative to the spine, was used during all measurements. The scan time was 5 sec, energy 115 mAs and 125 kV, slice thickness 8 mm, and window setting was ± 0/512.

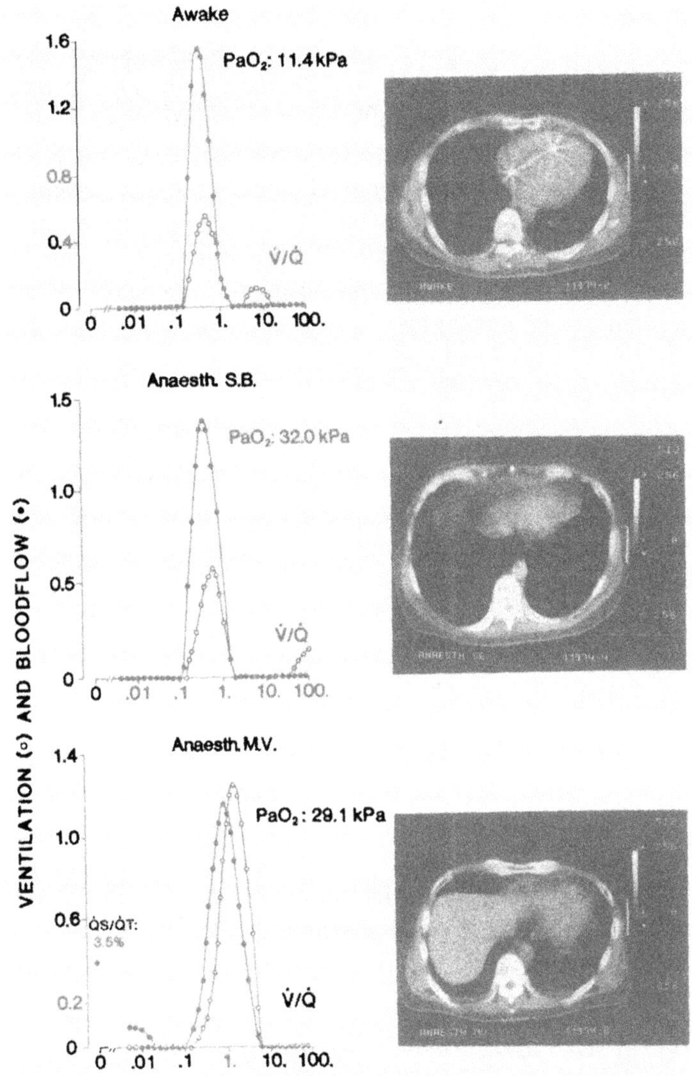

Fig. 2. CT scans and VA/Q distribution curves from the three measurements in one patient in the ketamine group. Shunt and atelectasis appear during MV. There is also a widening of the perfusion distribution in that situation.

The thoracic area on the CT scans is defined as the area contained within the inner walls of the thorax, thus including the mediastinal organs. Atelectasis was quantified by its transverse area and is presented as a fraction of the thoracic area.

Procedure

The catheters were introduced before anesthesia (ketamine N = 6, halothane N = 5), and the infusion of the inert gases was started. After at least 20 min of complete rest (40 min of infusion), recordings of central hemodynamics and gas exchange variables were made while the patient was breathing air. CT scans were obtained, and the patient was then anesthetized. After 15 min of stable anesthesia with spontaneous breathing, the measurements and CT scanning were repeated. The patients were then paralyzed and mechanically ventilated. A new set of measurements were made after 15 min of stable conditions. All recordings while both awake and under anesthesia, were made with the patient in the supine position.

Statistics

Mean values and S.E. are presented. The significance between 3 groups was tested by two way analysis of variance, and comparisons between means by Scheffe's contrast. Regression lines were compared with analysis of co-variance (Snedecor and Cochran, 1967).

RESULTS

Awake

Circulatory variables were normal in all awake patients (Table 1). The derived VA/Q distribution curves (see example in Fig. 2) were narrow in most cases with no or low shunt fractions. One patient in the ketamine and two in the halothane group had shunts amounting to more than 1% (2, 1.6 and 4.9%, respectively) which raised the alveolo-arterial oxygen tension difference in the halothane group (Table 2).

There were no abnormalities on the CT scans of the lung in the awake state.

Anesthesia with spontaneous breathing

Circulation. The circulatory reaction to anesthesia in the ketamine group was characterized by stimulation with an increase of heart rate (HR) and cardiac output (Qt) by 46% and 47%, respectively. Halothane anesthesia was accompanied by an increase of HR by 33% and a decrease of the systemic arterial pressure (SAP) by 21%. The other circulatory variables were unchanged.

Gas exchange. Gas exchange was essentially unaffected by ketamine anesthesia (Table 2). One patient developed a shunt of 4% and a blood flow to low VA/Q regions (Qlow:VA/Q_A < 0.01) of the same

TABLE 1. Circulatory variables awake and during anesthesia with spontaneous breathing (SB) and during muscular relaxation with mechanical ventilation (MV) in the ketamine (N = 6) and the halothane (N = 5) groups. HR-heart rate; SAP, PAP, PCV—mean systemic arterial, pulmonary arterial, and pulmonary venous (wedge) pressures, respectively; Qt-cardiac output. Mean ± S.E.

Ketamine	*Awake*	*Anesth, SB*	*Anesth, MV*
HR, min^{-1}	71 ± 5.7	104 ± 9.8[b]	106 ± 11.4[b]
SAP, mmHg	100 ± 3.0	117 ± 5.3	112 ± 5.3
Qt, l/min	6.2 ± 0.4	9.1 ± 0.7[c]	7.1 ± 0.6[e]
PAP, mmHg	13.5 ± 0.8	17.3 ± 1.5	15.0 ± 1.5
PCV, mmHg	7.5 ± 1.5	7.5 ± 1.5	9.8 ± 1.5
Halothane	***Awake***	***Anesth, SB***	***Anesth, MV***
HR, min^{-1}	66 ± 3.5	88 ± 7.9[a]	79 ± 4.6
SAP, mmHg	91.6 ± 5.2	72.0 ± 3.7[a]	54.8 ± 3.4[cd]
Qt, l/min	5.5 ± 0.1	5.7 ± 0.3	4.5 ± 0.4[d]
PAP, mmHg	13.4 ± 1.5	13.0 ± 1.8	12.2 ± 1.6
PCV, mmHg	6.6 ± 0.6	5.8 ± 0.3	5.8 ± 0.8

[a,b,c]Significantly different from awake, $P<0.05$, $P<0.01$, $P<0.001$, respectively.
[d,e]Significantly different from anesth, SB, $P<0.05$, $P<0.01$, respectively.

TABLE 2. Data on gas exchange awake and during anesthesia with spontaneous breathing (SB) and during muscular relaxation with mechanical ventilation (MV). Qs-shuntfraction; Qlow-fractional blood flow to lung units with VA/Q <0.01; $P_{A-a}O_2$-alveoloarterial oxygen tension difference; P_aCO_2: arterial carbon dioxide tension; ketamine (N = 6); halothane (N = 5). Mean ± S.E.

Ketamine	*Awake*	*Anesth, SB*	*Anesth, MV*
Qs, %	0.5 ± 0.4	0.9 ± 0.6	3.1 ± 0.9[bd]
Qlow, %	0.6 ± 0.6	3.0 ± 2.3	3.7 ± 1.4
QSD	0.50 ± 0.05	0.58 ± 0.14	0.95 ± 0.17[bd]
VSD	0.56 ± 0.10	0.86 ± 0.23	0.65 ± 0.07
$P_{A-a}O_2$, mmHg	11.3 ± 3.8*	31.6 ± 9.0	69.9 ± 15.0[d]
P_aCO_2, mmHg	39.1 ± 1.5	45.9 ± 1.5[b]	33.1 ± 0.8[af]
Halothane	***Awake***	***Anesth, SB***	***Anesth, MV***
Qs, %	1.5 ± 0.9	3.7 ± 0.7[a]	5.0 ± 1.2[a]
Qlow, %	0.0 ± 0.0	3.1 ± 3.1	3.5 ± 2.4
QSD	0.60 ± 0.08	0.81 ± 0.07	1.06 ± 0.17[e]
VSD	0.58 ± 0.07	1.38 ± 0.19[c]	0.71 ± 0.07[e]
$P_{A-a}O_2$, mmHg	20.3 ± 5.2*	66.6 ± 23.1	99.4 ± 24.3[e]
P_aCO_2, mmHg	40.0 ± 1.5	52.4 ± 1.6[c]	45.6 ± 1.7[bd]

[a,b,c]Significantly different from awake, $P<0.05$, $P<0.01$, $P<0.001$ respectively.
[d,e]Significantly different from anesth, SB, $P<0.05$, $P<0.01$, respectively.
*FIO_2 = 0.21 awake, 0.43 during anesthesia.

magnitude. In another patient Qlow was 14% (4% awake). The major modes of ventilation and of perfusion were narrow with log standard deviation of blood flow (QSD) and ventilation (VSD) of 0.58 and 0.76, respectively. $P_{A-a}O_2$ was only moderately increased, considering $FIO_2 = 0.43$.

Halothane anesthesia was accompanied by a development of shunt in all patients, ranging from 1.8% to 5.3%. In one patient, there was a blood flow to low VA/Q regions of 12%. The overall matching of ventilation to blood flow deteriorated in this group with an increased spread of the distributions of VA/Q ratios, as evidenced by QSD = 0.84 and VSD = 1.76. The $P_{A-a}O_2$ was 66.6 mm Hg with the same inspired oxygen concentration as during ketamine anesthesia.

CT. CT was normal in 7 of the 8 patients during ketamine anesthesia. In the same patient who also had a detectable shunt, a small atelectasis (0.6%) had developed. In the halothane group, atelectasis was found in all patients but one.

The largest area amounted to 6.2%. There was no significant correlation between the atelectatic area and the shunt fraction during spontaneous breathing in the 5 patients subjected to VA/Q studies.

Anesthesia and muscle paralysis with mechanical ventilation

Circulation. Cardiac output decreased in the ketamine group. The other circulatory variables remained unchanged, compared to the previous measurement. There was a continuous decrease of SAP and also a decrease of Qt in the halothane group.

Gas exchange. There was a deterioration of gas exchange during ketamine anesthesia and muscular paralysis. Shunt appeared in all patients except one who continued to have blood flow to low VA/Q regions, decreasing to 9% from 14% of cardiac output. Qlow, ranging from 3% to 5%, was also seen in 3 additional patients. The blood flow distribution widened to QSD = 0.95. VSD was unchanged, and $P_{A-a}O_2$ increased significantly. There were no significant changes in shunt fraction or blood flow to poorly perfused lung regions in the patients anesthetized with halothane, although the mean values of both variables increased. There was a further increase of $P_{A-a}O_2$.

CT. Atelectasis (ranging from 0.7% to 5.7%, Table 3), now appeared in the CT scans in 7 of the 8 patients in the ketamine group. There was a correlation between atelectatic area and shunt in the ketamine group ($Y = 1.04 + 1.41*X$, $r = 0.81$, $P = 0.05$, Fig. 3) and in the halothane group ($r = 0.95$, $P < 0.05$).

TABLE 3. Atelectatic area (Area, %) from the transverse CT scans given in per cent of the intrathoracic area (Th-area); SB-spontaneous breathing; MV-mechanical ventilation and muscle paralysis; ketamine (N = 8); halothane (N = 11). Mean ± S.E.

Ketamine	*Awake*	*Anesth, SB*	*Anesth, MV*
Area, %	0.0±0.0	0.1±0.1	1.9±0.7[ad]
Th-area, cm^2	348.7±16.2	362.4±17.1	342.1±15.0[e]
Halothane	***Awake***	***Anesth, SB***	***Anesth, MV***
Area, %	0.0±0.0	2.5±0.6[c]	4.1±0.7[cd]
Th-area, cm^2	339.9±10.7	332.6±10.7	328.7±11.7

Two-way analysis of variance with Scheffe's contrast.
[a,b,c]Significantly different from awake, P<0.05, P<0.01, P<0.001, respectively.
[d,e,f]Significantly different from anesth, SB, P<0.05, P<0.01, P<0.001, respectively.

Data from another 18 patients subjected to a similar investigation and anesthetized with halothane and muscular relaxation have been added in Fig. 3, making a total of 23 patients in the halothane group. Their data have been plotted together with data from the ketamine group. The regression line for halothane was $Y = 0.88 + 1.77*X$ ($r = 0.85$, $P < 0.001$). The slope and position of the two regression lines were not different.

Discussion

A high prevalence of lung collapse in dependent lung regions during halothane anesthesia has been reported in several previous studies (Brismar *et al.*, 1985, Strandberg *et al.*, 1986, Hedenstierna *et al.*, 1986, Tokics *et al.*, 1987a). The findings during ketamine anesthesia await further confirmation (Tokics *et al.*, 1987b). As evidenced by the present data, the anesthetic state, per se, is not necessarily accompanied by the development of atelectasis, even in the presence of an increased inspired fraction of oxygen. This indicates that the anesthetic regime must have some specific influence on the respiratory system for atelectasis to occur. An important factor may be changes in the chest wall mechanics. Halothane anesthesia reduces inspiratory muscle activity, with decreasing phasic activity of the intercostal muscles (Tusiewicz *et al.*, 1977) and a reduced resting tone of the diaphragm (Muller *et al.*, 1979). The end expiratory position of the diaphragm is displaced cranially (Froese and Bryan, 1974, Hedenstierna *et al.*, 1985), and there is a reduction of the cross-sectional thoracic area (Hedenstierna *et al.*, 1985). This is probably the main cause of the reduction of FRC during halothane anesthesia (Don *et al.*, 1970,

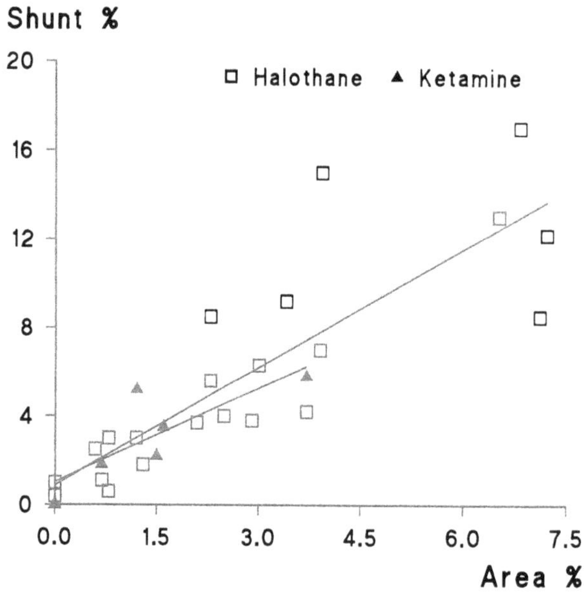

Fig. 3. Regression line of percent shunt *vs* percent transverse atelectatic area. Data from 23 patients during halothane and 6 patients during ketamine anesthesia. All patients were paralyzed and mechanically ventilated.

Hedenstierna *et al.*, 1985). During ketamine anesthesia, FRC seems to be maintained (Shulman *et al.*, 1985, Mankikian *et al.*, 1986), and the end expiratory level of the chest and the abdomen increases (Mankikian *et al.*, 1986). Although we did not measure FRC, the changes in transverse thoracic area on the CT scans are in accordance with the cited studies (Table 3) even though our measurements during spontaneous breathing could not be obtained at a true end expiratory level.

There is a vertical pressure gradient of 1 cm H_20/cm in the abdomen, whereas in the pleura the pressure gradient is much less (0.2-0.3 cm H_20/ cm, Agostoni *et al.*, 1970). In the supine subject, the difference in pressure gradients is maintained by the tension of the diaphragm. In awake, supine subjects, thoracoabdominal strapping does not produce atelectasis, in spite of a reduction of FRC of 0.5-0.7 1 (Tokics *et al.*, 1988). There is an increased transdiaphragmatic pressure during thoracoabdominal strapping (Hussain and Pardy, 1985), protecting the pleura and the lungs from the abdominal pressure gradient. When the diaphragm is relaxed, the abdominal pressure is increasingly transmitted to the thorax, reducing the volume of dependent lung regions (Roussos *et al.*, 1977). The combined effect of a lowered FRC and a reduced diaphragmatic tone may be the prerequisite for the development of atelectasis during anesthesia.

The situation during ketamine anesthesia is quite different. FRC is unchanged, and the high inspiratory air flows in early inspiration (Jaspar *et al.*, 1983, Shulman *et al.*, 1988) implies a preserved respiratory muscle function. Another protective mechanism against development of atelectasis during ketamine anesthesia could be the prolonged inspiratory duty time (Shulman *et al.*, 1988) which keeps the lungs inflated above FRC during the greater part of the breathing cycle. Muscular relaxation should abolish the differences in chest wall mechanics between these anesthetics, serving as the explanation to the development of atelectasis with ketamine during muscle paralysis.

There was a low alveolo-arterial oxygen tension difference in the ketamine group during spontaneous breathing in accordance with previous investigations (Gooding *et al.*, 1977, Rust *et al.*, 1978). During mechanical ventilation with air, Rust *et al.* (1978) reported a P_aO_2 close to the awake value. This finding seems to be at variance with the present data. However, shunt fractions in the range of 1-4% may not cause a dramatic fall in arterial oxygen tension if there is a high mixed venous oxygen content.

The gas exchange impairment, at least in the context of shunt, was related to atelectasis with both anesthetics, suggesting that atelectasis is the main cause of shunt during anesthesia (Hedenstierna *et al.*, 1986, Tokics *et al.*, 1987a). The regression lines were not different in slope. However, it cannot be concluded that these agents affect hypoxic pulmonary vasoconstriction to the same extent, even limiting the conclusion to the dosages used here, because of the confounding effects of pulmonary artery, left atrial, and alveolar pressures on the pulmonary vasoconstrictor response (Marshall, 1989). Also, the mean difference in atelectatic area between the ketamine and the halothane group (Table 3, MV) should be interpreted with caution. Lung regions with airway closure but initially not atelectatic may eventually collapse. In the halothane group, any such regions were given more time to lose their air content because lung volume is reduced during spontaneous breathing.

In conclusion, it can be stated that ketamine anesthesia with spontaneous breathing was associated with only an occasional development of atelectasis, and gas exchange was hardly affected at all. With halothane atelectasis and gas exchange impairment was a regular finding. Muscle paralysis abolished these differences. The findings suggest that changes in chest wall mechanics cause the lung collapse and, consequently, intrapulmonary shunt.

Acknowledgements

This study was supported by grants from The Swedish Society of Medicine, No 716/88.

References

Agostoni, E., D'Angelo, E., and Bonanni, M.V.: The effect of the abdomen on the vertical gradient of pleural surface pressure. Respir. Physiol. 8: 332-346, 1970.

Bendixen, H.H., Hedley-Whyte, J., and Laver, M.B.: Impaired oxygenation in surgical patients during general anesthesia with controlled ventilation: a concept of atelectasis. New Engl. J. Med. 269: 991-999, 1963.

Brismar, B., Hedenstierna, G., Lundquist, H., Strandberg, Å., Svensson, L., and Tokics, L: Pulmonary densities during anesthesia with muscular relaxation—A proposal of atelectasis. Anesthesiol. 62: 422-428, 1985.

Campbell, E.J.M., Nunn, J.F., and Peckett, B.W.: A comparison of artificial ventilation and spontaneous respiration with particular reference to ventilation-bloodflow relationships. Brit. J. Anaesth. 30: 166-175, 1958.

Domino, E.F., Chodoff, P., and Corssen, G.: Pharmacologic effects of CI-581, a new dissociative anesthetic in man. Clin. Pharmacol. Ther., 6: 279-291, 1965.

Don, H.F., Wahba, M., Cuadrado, L., and Kelkar, K.: The effects of anesthesia and 100 per cent oxygen on the functional residual capacity of the lungs. Anesthesiol. 32: 521-529, 1970.

Evans, J.W., and Wagner, P.D.: Limits of VA/Q distributions from analysis of experimental inert gas elimination. J. Appl. Physiol. 42: 889-898, 1977.

Froese, A.B., and Bryan, A.C.: Effects of anesthesia and paralysis on diaphragmatic mechanics in man. Anesthesiol. 41: 242-255, 1974.

Gooding, J.M., Dimick, A.R., Tavakoli, M., and Corssen, G.: A physiological analysis of cardiopulmonary responses to ketamine anesthesia in noncardiac patients. Anesth. Analg. 27: 205-212, 1977.

Hedenstierna, G., Löfström, B., and Lundh, R.: Thoracic gas volume and chest-abdomen dimensions during anesthesia and muscle paralysis. Anesthesiol. 55: 499-506, 1981.

Hedenstierna, G., Strandberg, Å., Brismar, B., Lundqvist, H., Svensson, L., and Tokics, L.: Functional residual capacity, thoraco-abdominal dimensions and central blood volume during general anesthesia with muscle paralysis and mechanical ventilation. Anesthesiol. 62: 247-254, 1985.

Hedenstierna, G., Strandberg, Å., Tokics, L., Lundqvist, H., and Brismar, B.: Correlation of gas exchange impairment to development of atelectasis during anaesthesia and muscle paralysis. Acta Anaesthesiol. Scand. 30: 183-191, 1986.

Hedenstierna, G., Lundquist, H., Lundh, B., Tokics, L., Strandberg, Å., Brismar, B., and Frostell, C.: Pulmonary densities during anaesthesia. An experimental study on lung morphology and gas exchange. Eur. Respir. J. 2: 528-535, 1989.

Hussain, S.N.A., and Pardy, R.L.: Inspiratory muscle function with restrictive chest wall loading during exercise in normal humans. J. Appl. Physiol. 58: 2027-2032, 1985.

Jaspar, N., Mazzarelli, M. Tessier, C., and Milic-Emili, J.: Effect of ketamine on control of breathing in cats. J. Appl. Physiol. 55: 851-859, 1983.

Mankikian, B., Cantineau, J.P., Sartene, R., Clergue, F., and Viars, P.: Ventilatory pattern and chest wall mechanics during ketamine anesthesia in humans. Anesthesiol. 65: 492-499, 1986.

Marshall, B.E.: Anesthetic influences on the pulmonary circulation. In Anesthesia and the Lung, ed. by T.H. Stanley and R.J. Sperry, pp. 69-78, Kluwer Academic Publishers, Dordrecht, The Netherlands, 1989.

Muller, N., Volgyesi, G., Becker, L., Bryan, M.H., and Bryan, A.C.: Diaphragmatic muscle tone. J. Appl. Physiol. 47: 279-284, 1979.

Nunn, J.F., Bergman, N.A., and Coleman, A.J.: Factors influencing the arterial oxygen tension during anaesthesia with artificial ventilation. Br. J. Anaesth. 37: 898-914, 1965.

Roussos, C.S., Martin, R.R., and Engel, L.A.: Diaphragmatic contraction and the gradient of alveolar expansion in the lateral posture. J. Appl. Physiol. 43: 32-38, 1977.

Rust, M., Landauer, B., and Kolb, E.: Stellenwert von Ketamin in der Notfallsituation. Anaesthesist. 27: 205-212, 1978.

Shulman, D., Beardsmore, C.S., Aronson, H.B., and Godfrey, S.: The effect of ketamine on the functional residual capacity in young children. Anesthesiol. 62: 551-556, 1985.

Shulman, D., Bar-Yishay, E., and Godfrey, S.: Drive and timing components of respiraton in young children following in induction of anaesthesia with halothane or ketamine. Can. J. Anaesth. 35: 368-374, 1988.

Snedecor, G.W., and Cochran, W.G.: Statistical Methods, Iowa State Univ. Press, Ames, IA, 1967.

Strandberg, Å., Brismar, B., Hedenstierna, G., Lundqvist, H., and Tokics, L.: Atelectasis during anaesthesia and in the postoperative period. Acta Anaesthesiol. Scand. 30: 154-158, 1986.

Tokics, L., Hedenstierna, G., Strandberg, Å., Brismar, B., and Lundqvist, H.: Lung collapse and gas exchange during general anesthesia—effects of spontaneous breathing, muscle paralysis and positive end-expiratory pressure. Anesthesiol. 66: 157-167, 1987a.

Tokics, L., Strandberg, Å., Brismar, B., Lundquist, H., and Hedenstierna, G.: Computerized tomography of the chest and gas exchange measurements during ketamine anaesthesia. Acta Anesthesiol. Scand., 31: 684-692, 1987b.

Tokics, L., Hedenstierna, G., Brismar, B., Strandberg, Å., and Lundqvist, H.: Thoracoabdominal restriction in supine men: CT and lung function measurements. J. Appl. Physiol. 64: 599-604, 1988.

Tusiewicz, K., Bryan, A.C., and Froese, A.B.: Contributions of changing rib cage—diaphragm interactions to the ventilatory depression of halothane anesthesia. Anesthesiol. 47: 327-337, 1977.

Wagner, P.D., Naumann, P.F., and Laravuso, R.B.: Simultaneous measurement of eight foreign gases in blood by gas chromatography. J. Appl. Physiol. 36: 600-605, 1974a.

Wagner, P.D., Salzman, H.A., and West, J.B.: Measurement of continuous distribution of ventilation-perfusion ratios. Theory. J. Appl. Physiol. 36: 588-599, 1974b.

Status of Ketamine in Anesthesiology,
edited by E.F. Domino©1990, NPP Books
P.O. Box 1491, Ann Arbor, MI 48106

Ketamine Prolongs the Refractoriness of Neuromuscular Transmission in the Primate

C. Lee, W.-F. Kwan, and S.K. Tsai*

Department of Anesthesiology,
Harbor-UCLA Medical Center
Torrance, CA
and
**Department of Anesthesiology*
National Yang-Ming Medical College
Veterans General Hospital
Taipei, Taiwan

Introduction

Although ketamine may depress neuromuscular transmission both *in vitro* and *in vivo*, little is known about how it depresses neuromuscular transmission *in vivo*. The purpose of this study was to investigate whether ketamine has any effect on the refractoriness of neuromuscular transmission *in vivo*.

Methods

With institutional approval, 7 adult monkeys (Macaca cyclopis, 5-6 kg) were managed as in a clinical pediatric practice. They were studied twice, at least one week apart, once under pentobarbital anesthesia (30 mg/kg i.m. followed by 5 mg/kg/hr by i.v. infusion), and once under halothane anesthesia (0.5-1.0% in 0_2 inhaled). Induction of halothane anesthesia was facilitated by i.m. injection of methohexital (10-15 mg/kg). Following intubation of the trachea without the use of a muscle relaxant, the respiration was controlled with a Harvard Apparatus respiration pump ($PaCO_2$ 30-40 mm Hg). Esophageal temperature was maintained at 35-37°C with a heat lamp and a thermoblanket. An anterior tibial artery was cannulated for blood pressure recording and blood gas determination. Arterial blood pH was maintained at 7.30-7.40. Hydration was maintained with 5% dextrose in water infused at 5 ml/kg/hr.

The ulnar nerve was stimulated at the wrist with a supramaximal rectangular voltage of 0.2 msec duration derived from a Grass S88 stimulator. The evoked compound electromyographic (EMG) response of the first dorsal interosseous muscle was displayed and recorded using the method of Lee *et al.* (1977). The two stimulating electrodes were positioned approximately 2 mm apart. The EMG electrodes were positioned s.c. over the muscle (sensing) and near the tip of the thumb (reference). The grounding electrode was between the stimulating and sensing electrodes. All 5 electrodes were fine platinum needle electrodes made by the Grass Instrument Co., Quincy, MA.

The ulnar nerve was stimulated with twin (paired) pulses, S_1 and S_2, for the two corresponding compound EMG responses of the muscle, R_1 and R_2. Neuromuscular refractoriness was determined by applying twin stimuli of increasingly larger intervals. We used the following interstimulus intervals: 0.5, 0.6, 0.8, 1.0, 1.4, 1.5, 1.6, 1.7, 1.8, 1.9, 2.0, 2.2, 2.4, 2.6, 3.0, 3.4, 3.8, 4.2, 4.6, 5, 6, 7, 8, 9 and 10 msec. After the baseline data were obtained, ketamine was administered at incremental doses of 2, 3, and 5 mg/kg i.v. to make the cumulative total of 2, 5 and 10 mg/kg, and the study was repeated at each dose level. The non-refractory fraction, *i.e.*, the R_2/R_1 value, was plotted as a function of the interstimulus interval. The total refractory period (RI_0), *i.e.*, the largest interstimulus interval when R_2 was still zero, and the half-refractory interval ($RI_{.5}$), *i.e.*, the interstimulus interval when $R_2 = 1/2\ R_1$, were determined (Lee *et al.*, 1977). Results are presented as mean ± SE. The Wilcoxon signed rank and paired t tests were used to evaluate the differences, $P < 0.05$ being regarded as significant.

Results

Halothane anesthesia made the neuromuscular transmission significantly more refractory than observed under pentobarbital anesthesia for all 7 monkeys. Fig. 1 illustrates the increase of the RI_0 and the $RI_{.5}$ in one monkey given ketamine after basal pentobarbital anesthesia. Under both basal anesthetic states, ketamine in a dose dependent manner further increased the refractoriness, causing the refractory curve to shift accordingly. Both the total refractory interval (RI_0) and the half-refractory interval ($RI_{.5}$) were significantly prolonged by ketamine (Table 1). The R_1 was not depressed at any time.

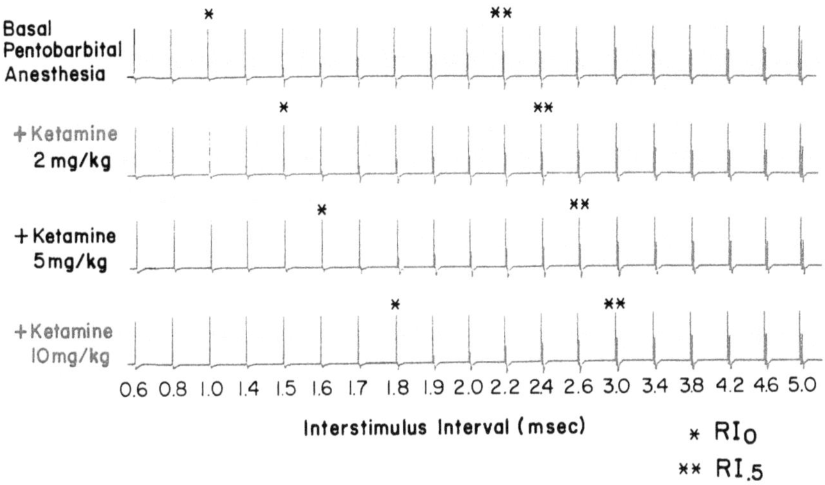

Fig. 1. Ketamine in a dose dependent manner increased the RI_0 and the $RI_{.5}$ in a monkey under basal pentobarbital anesthesia.

TABLE 1. Ketamine increases refractoriness of neuromuscular transmission both under pentobarbital and under halothane anesthesia (N = 7)

	Total Refractory Interval, RI_0 (msec)		*Half Refractory Interval, $RI_{.5}$ (msec)*	
Ketamine Dose (mg/Kg)	*Pentobarbital*	*Halothane*	*Pentobarbital*	*Halothane*
0	1.18±0.14	1.46±0.10†	2.40±0.15	2.80±0.32†
2	1.40±0.18*	1.60±0.13*	2.68±0.18*	3.11±0.31*
5	1.48±0.18**	1.70±0.10**	2.88±0.20**	3.40±0.38**
10	1.66±0.20**	1.82±0.13**	3.00±0.21**	3.90±0.50**

*P<0.05, **P<0.01 comparison with pre-ketamine values
†P<0.05, halothane *vs* pentobarbital

Discussion

Our results indicate that ketamine with or without halothane, increases the refractoriness of neuromuscular transmission without blocking the motor nerve or depressing the neurally evoked muscle twitch. The effect is consistently observable in the therapeutic dose range, in contrast with the other neuromuscular effects of ketamine, which often are controversial under similar experimental or clinical conditions (Johnston *et al.*, 1974; Amaki *et al.*, 1978; Tsai and Lee, 1989). Since transmission between each motor nerve terminal and the muscle cell it innervates is presumed to occur fully or not at all (*all or nothing*), the diminution of the R_2 but not the R_1 indicates that some muscle fibers fail to respond totally to S_2 after responding to S_1 fully. Therefore, RI_0 is the shortest refractory period, and $RI_{.5}$ is the average or median refractory period of all the neuromuscular junctions of the muscle. In other words, our results likely indicate that ketamine blocks the neuromuscular transmission through some endplates shortly after a successful transmission has occurred. This would depress the R_2 beyond the physiological refractoriness and increase the refractoriness as measured over the entire muscle. Epstein and Jackson (1970) studied the neuromuscular refractoriness under diethyl ether, fluroxene, halothane, or methoxyflurane anesthesia in man. Their results with halothane concur with ours, which show that ketamine is similar to halothane. The effect of both of these anesthetics on the neuromuscular refractoriness is dose-dependent, mutually additive, and occurs within the clinical anesthesia dose range.

Neuromuscular blocking relaxants and general anesthetics have different effects on the refractoriness of neuromuscular transmission. Regarding the neuromuscular blocking relaxants, Lee *et al.* (1978a) demonstrated that neuromuscular block by *alpha*-bungarotoxin did not alter the refractoriness of neuromuscular transmission *in vivo* in the cat. This indicates that postjunctional acetylcholine receptor occupation has no effect on the refractoriness itself. By contrast, neuromuscular block by magnesium and neomycin markedly increases the R_2/R_1 ratio and reduces the RI_0 and $RI_{.5}$ (Lee *et al.*, 1979). The seemingly shortened refractoriness is paradoxical and is attributed to the summation of two subthreshold endplate potentials to result in one action potential which is included in the R_2. The second endplate potential is often facilitated in this case. Similarly, the less marked reduction of the RI values by curariform nondepolarizing relaxants (Epstein *et al.*, 1969; Lee *et al.*, 1978b) may be attributed prejunctionally to their negative effect on acetylcholine release. It is not known whether the blockage of the acetylcholine-activated ionic channels by some neuromuscular blocking relaxants has measurable effects on the refractoriness of the neuromuscular transmission. Regarding various general anesthetics, Epstein and Jackson (1970) attributed the increased refractoriness of neuromuscular transmission to depression of the membrane excitability postjunctionally. In support of this theory, Karis *et al.* (1966) demonstrated that the postjunctional membrane was the most sensitive, while the nerve trunk was the least sensitive to general anesthetics. In general, therefore, prejunctional depression of transmitter release (such as by magnesium and neuromuscular blocking agents) paradoxically shortens, while postjunctional depression of membrane excitability (such as by inhalational anesthetics) lengthens the refractory period of neuromuscular transmission *in vivo*.

The mechanism of action by which ketamine prolongs the refractoriness of neuromuscular transmission is not known. Ketamine has prejunctional (Amaki *et al.*, 1978) and postjunctional neuromuscular actions (Maleque *et al.*, 1981; Wachtel, 1988). Since it clearly prolongs the refractoriness of neuromuscular transmission, it probably depresses the postjunctional membrane excitability as a general anesthetic more than it reduces acetylcholine release prejunctionally as a neuromuscular transmission blocker. Maleque *et al.* (1981), using an exact electrophysiological technique to study frog neuromuscular junction *in vitro*, concluded that ketamine blocks neuromuscular transmission by interaction with acetylcholine-activated ionic channels in their open conformation. They also concluded that ketamine had few prejunctional effects. Subsequently, Wachtel (1988) reported that ketamine decreased the open time of single channel currents activated by acetylcholine. Until the ionic channels regain their normal sensitivity to acetylcholine, the endplate will not respond normally to the second motor impulse, and an R_2 evoked shortly after the R_1 will be blocked beyond physiological refractoriness.

In conclusion, ketamine in a systemic i.v. dose of 2-10 mg/kg in a dose-dependent manner prolongs the refractoriness of neuromuscular transmission in the primate. The effect is similar and additive to that of halothane. It may be explained by the postjunctional blocking action of ketamine on the acetylcholine-activated ionic channels. We suggest that the main neuromuscular effect of ketamine *in vivo* is the postjunctional depression of the endplate sensitivity.

Acknowledgements

The authors wish to thank Sandy Adamson for assistance in the preparation of the manuscript and Marlyn Cheng, M.D. for comments on the paper. This work was supported in part by grants from the National Science Council, Academia Sinica, Republic of China (NSC 75-0412-B075-52, NSC 77-0412-B075-60), which enabled S.K. Tsai, M.D. to pursue his Doctor of Philosophy degree from the Institute of Clinical Medicine, National Yang-Ming Medical College, Taipei, Taiwan under the supervision of Chingmuh Lee, M.D. and other guest and in-residence professors. Part of the materials presented herein has been included in a Ph.D. thesis.

References

Amaki, Y., Nagashima, H., Radnay, P.A., and Folder, F.F.: Ketamine interaction with neuromuscular blocking agents in the phrenic nerve-hemidiaphragm preparation of the rat. Anesth. Analg. 57: 238-243, 1978.

Epstein, R.A. and Jackson, S.H.: The effect of depth of anesthesia on the neuromuscular refractory period of anesthetized man. Anesthesiol. 32: 494-499, 1970.

Epstein, R.A., Jackson, S.H., and Wyte, S.R.: The effects of nondepolarizing relaxants and anticholinesterases on the neuromuscular refractory period of anesthetized man. Anesthesiol. 31: 69-76, 1969.

Johnston, R.R., Miller, R.D., and Way., W.L.: The interaction of ketamine with d-tubocurarine, pancuronium and succinylcholine in man. Anesth. Analg. 53: 494-501, 1974.

Karis, J.H., Gissen, A.J., and Nastuk, W.L.: Mode of action of diethyl ether in blocking neuromuscular transmission. Anesthesiol. 27: 42-51, 1966.

Lee, C., de Silva, A.J.C., and Katz, R.L.: Effects of prejunctional and postjunctional neuromuscular block on the refractoriness of neuromuscular transmission. Anesthesiol. 50: S603-S604, 1978a.

Lee, C., de Silva, A.J.C., and Katz, R.L.: Neuromuscular refractoriness during blockage of transmission. Br. J. Anaesth. 50: 1069-1073, 1978b.

Lee, C. Durant, N.N., and Katz, R.L.: Mechanism of neomycin-induced neuromuscular block. Anesthesiol. 51: S285, 1979.

Lee, C., Katz, R.L., Lee, A.S.J., and Glase, B.: A new instrument for continuous recording of the evoked compound electromyogram in the clinical setting. Anesth. Analg. 56: 260-270, 1977.

Maleque, M.A., Warnick, J.E., and Albuquerque, E.X.: The mechanism and site of action of ketamine on skeletal muscle. J. Pharmacol. Exp. Ther. 219: 638-645, 1981.

Tsai, S.K. and Lee, C.: Ketamine potentiates nondepolarizing neuromuscular relaxants in a primate. Anesth. Analg. 68: 5-8, 1989.

Wachtel, R.E.: Ketamine decreases the open time of single-channel currents activated by acetylcholine. Anesthesiol. 68: 563-570, 1988.

Status of Ketamine in Anesthesiology,
edited by E.F. Domino©1990, NPP Books
P.O. Box 1491, Ann Arbor, MI 48106

Effects of Ketamine on Neuronal Activity in the Hippocampal Dentate Area

Y. Kawakami*, E. Maru*, H. Suzuki**, and J. Tatsuno*****

Departments of Physiology and Anesthesiology,***
Tokyo Women's Medical College, Tokyo
*and Department of Physiology****
National Defense Medical College
Saitama, Japan

Introduction

The "dissociative" anesthetics, ketamine (2-o-chlorophenyl-2-methylaminocyclohexanone) and phencyclidine (1-1-phenylcyclohexylpiperidine) have unique actions on the brain. These agents interfere in the proper association of sensory inputs, and cause hallucinations and a dissociation of neocortical and limbic electroencephalograph patterns that are both convulsant and anticonvulsant. These unusual effects have led many investigators to examine their neuronal mechanisms of action.

Ketamine has consistently been shown to depress excitatory transmission at various synapses including monosynaptic and polysynaptic excitation in the spinal cord (Tang and Schroeder, 1973; Chen and Chow, 1975; Lodge and Anis, 1984), acetylcholine mediated transmission in frog sympathetic ganglia (Gallagher *et al.*, 1976) and glutamate-mediated transmission in the hippocampus (Raja and Guyenet, 1982). The depression of cholinergic transmission by ketamine may be due to a decrease in the post-synaptic membrane's sensitivity to acetylcholine (Gallagher *et al.*, 1976). Some findings indicate that ketamine and phencyclidine selectively block neuronal excitation by N-methyl-D-aspartate (NMDA, Anis *et al.*, 1983; Martin and Lodge, 1985; Dunchen *et al.*, 1985; Brady and Swann, 1986; MacDonald *et al.*, 1987). This could account for their depression of polysynaptic excitation in the spinal cord and synaptic excitation in hippocampus, since these synaptic tramsmissions are thought to be mediated by excitatory amino acids.

In contrast to the consistent depression of excitatory synaptic transmission by ketamine, there remains a controversy concerning the effects of ketamine and phencyclidine on brain excitability. Although ketamine and phencyclidine suppress predominantly neuronal discharge in the cerebellum (Marwaha *et al.*, 1980a,b), in the hippocampus (Sinclair and Tien, 1979; Bickford *et al.*, 1981; Raja and Guyenet, 1982), and in the neocortex (Kayama and Iwama, 1972; Duncan *et al.*, 1982), a small number of neurons respond with an increase in firing rate (Mori *et al.*, 1971; Kayama and Iwama, 1972; Bickford *et al.*, 1981). With regard to the bidirectional effects of ketamine or phencycyclidine on neuronal discharge, it is of interest that the (+) isomer of 1-(1-phenylcyclohexyl)-3-methylpiperidine (PCMP) is 4 to 15 fold more potent than the (-) isomer of PCMP in producing depression of hippocampal neuronal discharge, while the (-) isomer of PCMP exerts an excitant effect on neurons that are only inhibited by the (+) isomer (Bickford *et al.*, 1981).

There is also much conflicting evidence concerning the effects of ketamine and phencyclidine on synaptic inhibition. Ketamine was reported to prolong the duration of inhibitory postsynaptic current (or conductance) in hippocampal CA1 pyramidal cells or olfactory cortex neurons (Scholfield, 1980; Gage and Robertson, 1985), and to potentiate the *gamma*-aminobutyric acid (GABA) evoked response in superior cervical ganglion cells (Little and Atkinson, 1984). However, phencyclidine was demonstrated to reduce GABA mediated recurrent inhibition of hippocampal CA1 pyramidal cells in the urethane anesthetized rat or in the rat slice preparation (Stringer and Guyenet, 1982; Bourne *et al.*, 1983).

The present study was initiated in view of these discrepancies in the literature. The effect of ketamine on excitatory synaptic transmission, excitability of granule cells, and recurrent inhibition in the hippocampal dentate area was examined by an analysis of field potentials recorded in freely moving rats.

Methods

Experiment 1

Changes in the efficacy of excitatory transmission in perforant path-dentate granule cell synapses and granule cell excitability were examined in 10 male Wistar rats weighing 350-450 g.

Stimulating and recording electrodes were implanted under pentobarbital anesthesia in the angular bundle through which perforant path fibers traverse and in the dentate hilus, respectively, as illustrated in Fig. 1. The coordinates for the perforant path and dentate hilus electrodes were, relative to bregma, 7.8 mm posterior, 4.0 mm lateral and 3.5 mm

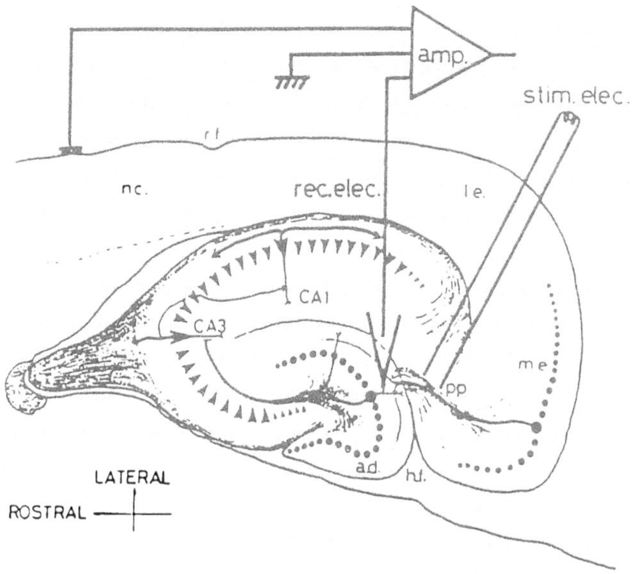

Fig. 1. Schematic drawing of the hippocampal fiber connections and placement of the electrodes. CA: cornu ammonis, a.d.: area dentata, amp.: amplifier, h.f.: hippocampal fissure, l.e.: lateral entorhinal cortex, m.e.: medial entorhinal cortex, n.c.: neocortex, p.p.: perforant path, rec.elec.: recording electrode, r.f.: rhinal fissure, stim.elec.: stimulating electrode.

posterior, 2.0 mm lateral, respectively. The depths of the stimulating and recording electrodes were adjusted to produce a maximum amplitude of the monosynaptic field potential in the dentate hilus. Bipolar polyurethane coated stainless steel wires with a 100 μm diameter, 500 μm distance between their tips were used as stimulating electrodes (MT-Gikenn Co.). Recording electrodes were polyurethane-coated nicrome wires with a 50 μm diameter (MT-Gikenn Co.). Two stainless steel microscrews (1 mm o.d., MT-Gikenn Co.) were implanted in the nasal and frontal bones and served as electrical grounds and indifferent leads. All electrodes were brought together in a 12 pin connector. The electrode assembly was then fixed to the skull with microscrew anchors and acrylic cement.

Pulses of 100 μsec duration were delivered to the perforant path once every 15 sec, while the pulse current was increased stepwise from 80 to 700 μA. The monosynaptic response evoked in the hilus was amplified by a Nihon-Koden VC9 oscilloscope with a frequency range of 0.08 Hz to 10 KHz. The data were stored on an FM magnetic tape (DFR3515, Sony

Corp.) for later analysis. Three field potentials evoked with the same stimulus intensity were averaged by a computer (FM-16β, Fugi-Tsu). Differential values of the averaged response were calculated every 100 μsec. The maximum of the differential values in the first 5 msec from onset of stimulation were designated as the EPSP's maximum rate of rise (or the EPSP slope). The amplitude of the population spikes were determined by measuring the height between onset and peak of the averaged population spike.

Experiments were performed about one week after implantation of the electrodes. During the experimental sessions, the rats moved freely about in a box with an observation window. Ketamine in a dose of 30 (N = 7) or 60 (N = 3) mg/kg was administered i.p. after the 3 successive predrug baseline control recording sessions, The perforant path-dentate field potentials were recorded 5, 15, 30 and 60 min after ketamine injection. The last recording of the field potential was done when motor behavior recovered to the baseline state. However, in experiments with ketamine at a dose of 60 mg/kg, the rats remained in a sedated state for more than 180 min. Therefore, experiments were terminated 180 min after ketamine.

Experiment 2

Alterations in the strength of recurrent inhibition of granule cell discharge following the administration of ketamine were examined in 6 male Wistar rats weighing 370-450 g. The surgical procedure for the electrode implantation was similar to that in Experiment 1.

Paired-pulse depression of the population spikes was measured as an estimate of the strength of recurrent inhibition. A pair of constant-current pulses (300-600 μA) at an interpulse interval of 25-40 msec was delivered to the perforant path at 15 sec intervals, while the stimulus intensity was varied by changing the duration of pulses from 10 to 250 sec by microcomputer control.

After recording the control field potentials, ketamine in a dose of 40 mg/kg was administered i.p. Changes in paired pulse depression were examined 5, 30, 60 and 150 min after ketamine.

Results

1. Effects of ketamine on excitatory synaptic transmission

With increasing stimulus intensity, the EPSP slope became steeper and the superimposed negative population spike appeared. Stimulus-response (S-R) curves were generated by plotting the EPSP slope against

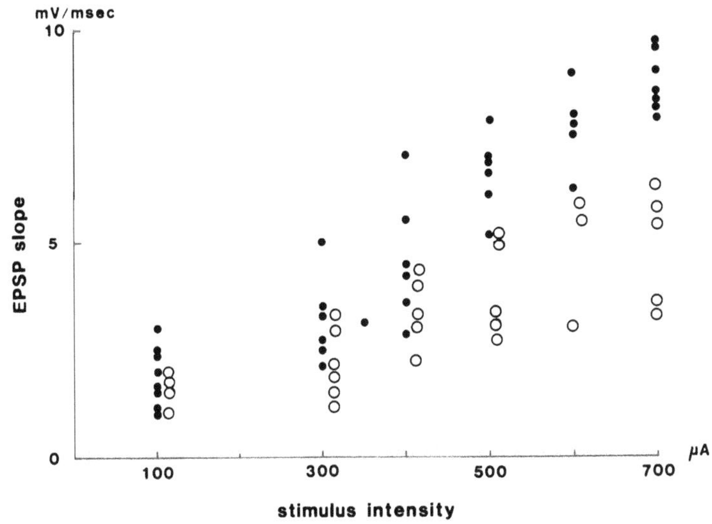

Fig. 2. Effect of ketamine (30 mg/kg, i.p.) on the efficacy of excitatory transmission through perforant path-granule cell synapses. Closed and open circles show the EPSP slopes plotted against the stimulus intensities before and after ketamine injection.

the stimulus intensity. A high correlation coefficient (0.984) was obtained between stimulus intensity and the EPSP slope before ketamine administration.

In all cases, EPSPs were reduced and the slope of the S-R curve declined rapidly after ketamine (30 mg/kg i.p., Figs. 2 and 3). The maximum inhibition of EPSPs was observed between 5 and 30 min after injection. Ketamine, in doses of 30 or 60 mg/kg, depressed the EPSP slope to 70-80% of control value during this period. The depressed EPSPs recovered to the control value between 60 to 90 min after ketamine in a dose of 30 mg/kg (Figs. 4A, 5A), whereas the EPSP depression lasted for at least 180 min after ketamine in a dose of 60 mg/kg.

2. *Effects of ketamine on granule cell excitability*

Associated with the depression of the summated EPSPs, the amplitude of the population spike increased immediately after 30 mg/kg of ketamine in 4 of 7 animals, and after 60 mg/kg of ketamine in all animals tested. The increase in population spike amplitude was maximal between 5-15 min (up to 120-250% of control values). Unlike the EPSPs, the enhanced population spike did not recover to the control values within 60-180 min after ketamine injection (Fig. 4B). In 3 of 7 animals given 30

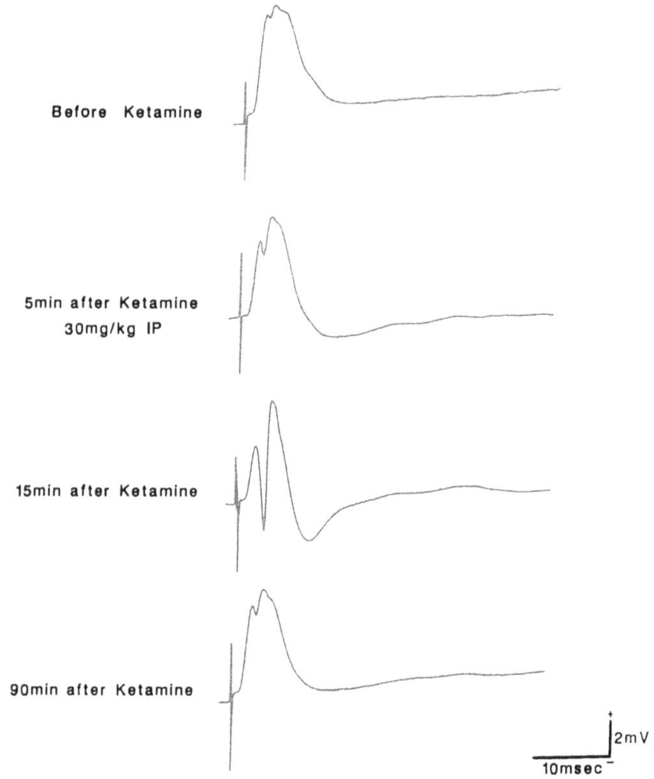

Fig. 3. Example of the changes in the dentate field potential evoked by perforant path stimulation following 30 mg/kg of ketamine i.p. Note that the amplitude of the population spike increased markedly and reversibly after ketamine in spite of a decrease in the EPSP slope.

mg/kg of ketamine, however, a decrease in population spike amplitude was observed (Fig. 5B).

The amplitude of the population spike was plotted against the corresponding EPSP slope in order to estimate the threshold for the generation of the population spike. Regardless of the increase or decrease in population spike amplitude following ketamine, the correlation curve between the population spike and the EPSPs shifted to the left and the slope of the curve increased slightly after ketamine (30 mg/kg, Fig. 4C, 5C). These changes in the correlation curve indicate a decrease in the threshold for generation of the population spike and an increase in granule cell excitability.

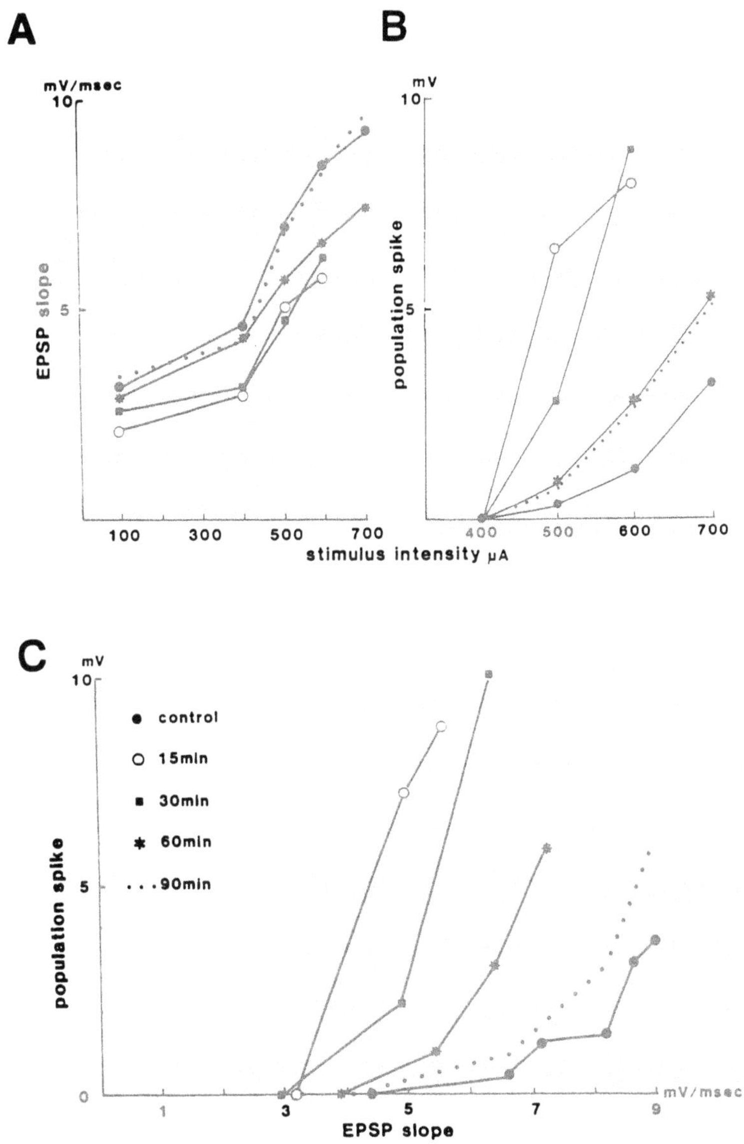

Fig. 4. An example of the changes in the PSPs (A), the population spike (B) and the relationship between them (C) following ketamine (30 mg/kg, i.p.). The population spike amplitude increased reversibly after ketamine injection in spite of a decrease in the EPSP slope. The correlation curve between population spike and EPSP slope shifted to the left and the slope increased slightly after ketamine, indicating a decrease in the threshold for spike generation, *i.e.*, an increase in granule cell excitability.

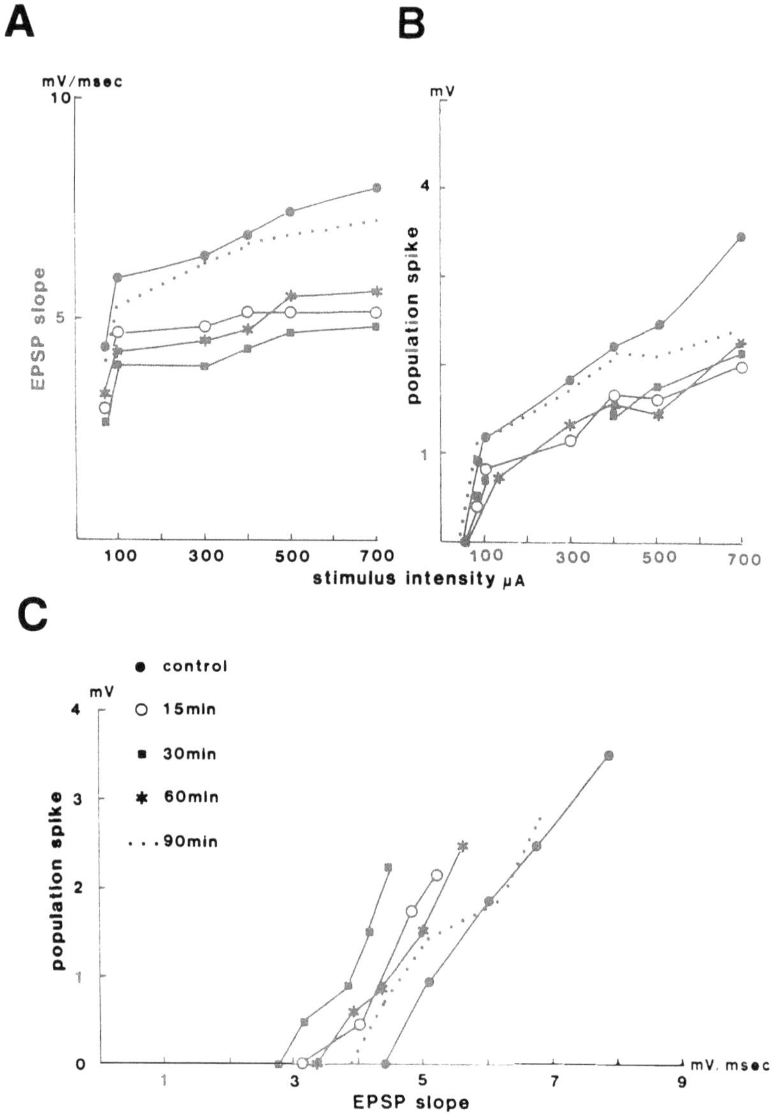

Fig 5. Another example of changes in the EPSPs (A), the population spike (B) and the relationship between them (C) following ketamine (30 mg/kg, i.p.). In contrast to the change in population spike shown in Fig. 4B, the population spike amplitude reversibly decreased after ketamine. This was associated with a decrease in the EPSP slope. The correlation curve between EPSPs and the population spike, however, shifted to the left after ketamine injection in the same manner as in the case shown in Fig. 4C. The change in the correlation curve also indicates a decrease in the threshold for spike generation.

3. Ketamine induced reduction of paired-pulse depression

Paired-pulse stimulation at an interpulse interval of 25-40 msec with low stimulus intensities produced a small potentiation or no inhibition of the population spike amplitude of the second response (PS2) relative to the population spike amplitude of the first response (PS1). As PS1 increased with stronger stimulus intensities, PS2 gradually decreased. In 5 of 6 animals, the strength of the paired pulse depression was reversibly reduced by ketamine (40 mg/kg, i.p., Fig. 6). The reduced paired-pulse

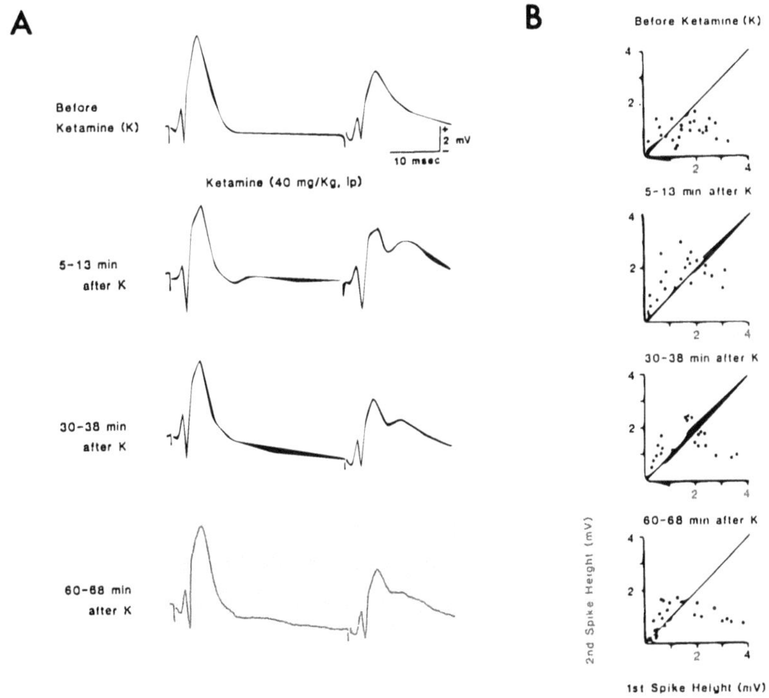

Fig. 6. Examples of changes in the strength of paired-pulse depression as an index of recurrent inhibition following ketamine (40 mg/kg, i.p.). A: Change in the field potential evoked by paired-pulse stimulation at an interpulse interval of 35 msec following ketamine injection. B: Each scatter diagram was generated by plotting the population spike amplitude of the second response against that of the first. As shown in Fig. 6B, the correlation curve moved upward and returned to the predrug control level 60 min after ketamine. These changes following ketamine indicate a reduction of recurrent inhibition.

depression returned to control level within 60-150 min after ketamine injection. The field potentials were selected so that the population spike amplitude of the first responses were almost equal. Note in Fig. 6A that the population spike amplitude of the second response increased reversibly after ketamine.

4. Behavioral changes induced by ketamine

Five min after 30 mg/kg of ketamine i.p., the rats were excited, as demonstrated by their running about the observation box. Ataxia of the extremities appeared progressively, but the animals continued to move in an uncoordinated manner. Finally, complete ataxia of the extremities occurred and the rats became sedated. Motor behavior returned to preinjection levels after 60-180 min. With a dose of 60 mg/kg, complete sedation appeared immediately after injection and lasted for at least 180 min. The criteria for behavioral recovery were the following: (1) disappearance of violent head moving, (2) disappearance of nystagmus, and (3) disappearance of ataxia. The duration of these ketamine induced behavioral changes was almost the same as that of the changes in neuronal activity except for the increase in population spike amplitude observed in some animals.

Discussion

Raja and Guyenet (1982) found that phencyclidine depressed both the EPSPs and population spike of CA1 pyramidal cells evoked by contralateral CA3 stimulation. Ketamine was also shown to decrease the population spike of dentate granule cells induced by perforant path activation. The present study confirms and extends their findings by showing that ketamine depresses excitatory transmission via perforant path-dentate granule cell synapses. Although the effects of ketamine on the sensitivity of perforant path fibers to electrical stimulation and the transmitter release from the fiber endings remain unclear, it is most probable that the decrease in the EPSPs is due, at least in part, to the noncompetitive blockade of NMDA induced postsynaptic activation by ketamine (Anis *et al.*, 1983; Duchen *et al.*, 1985; Martin and Lodge, 1985; Brady and Swann, 1986; MacDonald *et al.*, 1987), since the perforant path-dentate excitatory transmission is thought to be mediated by glutamate (Strom-Mathisen and Iversen, 1979; Cotman and Nadler, 1981).

In the present study, the dentate population spike decreased following ketamine injection in some animals, while an increase in the population spike was observed in others. Raja and Guyenet (1982) demonstrated that phencyclidine consistently reduced the dentate population spike but the relationship between the population spike and EPSPs remained unchanged. In contrast, examination of the correlation curve between the population spike and the EPSPs in the present study showed an increase in granule cell excitability following ketamine, including a decrease in the threshold for the generation of the population spike. The decrease in the dentate population spike after ketamine should, therefore, be attributed to depression of synaptic input represented by the decrease in population EPSPs. There are possible causes for the increase in overall excitability of the granule cells, an increase in intrinsic membrane excitability and/or a reduction of synaptic inhibition. Since ketamine has been shown to have no measurable effect on the resting membrane potential or the input impedance of CA1 pyramidal cells (Duchen *et al.*, 1985; Brady and Swann, 1986), it is more likely that the increase in granule cell excitability is due to a reduction of synaptic inhibition. Previous studies (Stringer and Guyenet, 1982; Bourne *et al.*, 1983) support this hypothesis. Phencyclidine decreased the strength and duration of recurrent inhibition (paired-pulse depression) in the hippocampal CA1 area. Consistent with the findings of the above investigators, the present study showed that ketamine reversibly reduced the strength of the paired-pulse depression of the population spike in the dentate area.

Several previous studies suggested a possible mechanism underlying the reduction of recurrent inhibition after ketamine. It has been shown that ketamine and phencyclidine exert little effect on the inhibition of neuronal discharge produced by GABA in spinal neurons (Anis *et al.*, 1983) and in hippocampal CA1 neurons (Raja and Guyenet, 1982). Moreover, phencyclidine and ketamine prolong the inhibitory postsynaptic current in olfactory cortical neurons and CA1 pyramidal cells (Scholfield, 1980; Gage and Robertson, 1985). Ketamine potentiates the postsynaptic response to GABA in cervical ganglion cells (Little and Atkinson, 1984). These findings suggest an increase in the efficacy of inhibitory synaptic transmission mediated by GABA. Stringer and Guyenet (1982) reported, however, that spontaneous and evoked discharges of interneurons in the CA1 area were depressed by very small doses of phencyclidine, suggesting a decrease in the activity of inhibitory interneurons in the recurrent circuits and, in turn, a decrease in GABA release from interneurons. Thus, ketamine may reduce the discharge of inhibitory interneurons in dentate recurrent circuits. In turn, it produces a decrease in recurrent inhibition of granule cell discharge in spite of an increase in granule cell excitability.

It is unclear whether the decrease in the activity of dentate interneurons is produced by a depressant action of ketamine on excitatory transmission at synapses between interneurons or by its direct depressant action on intrinsic membrane excitability of interneurons. It is evident, however, that ketamine exerts a different depressant action on the dentate recurrent inhibitory circuit from that on the excitatory transmission at the perforant path-granule cell synapses through blockade of NMDA-evoked excitation, since the mossy fibers seem to use neither glutamate nor aspartate as their transmitter (Cotman and Nadler, 1981). Regardless of the mechanism, the reduction of recurrent inhibition and the increase in cellular excitability with ketamine may explain the effects of ketamine in producing electroencephalographic seizure-like activity in the limbic system (Mori *et al.*, 1971).

Summary

The effects of ketamine on excitatory synaptic transmission, cellular excitability, and recurrent inhibition in the hippocampal dentate area were examined by an analysis of field potentials recorded in freely moving rats. The excitatory postsynaptic potentials (EPSPs) of granule cells evoked by perforant path stimulation were clearly reduced in all cases after i.p. administration of ketamine (30 mg/kg). An increase in the amplitude of the population spike of granule cells was observed in 4 of 7 animals. In the other 3 animals, the amplitude of the population spike decreased slightly but did not coincide temporally with the reduction of the EPSPs. The ratio of the population spike amplitude/EPSPs increased after ketamine in all animals, indicating an increase in granule cell excitability. The strength of dentate paired-pulse depression at an interpulse interval of 25-40 msec was reversibly reduced by ketamine (40 mg/kg), indicating a decrease in dentate recurrent inhibition. These results suggest that the enhancement of granule cell excitability produced by ketamine is due to a reduction of recurrent synaptic inhibition.

Acknowledgments

Our grateful thanks are due to Dr. Edward F. Domino (Department of Pharmacology, University of Michigan), Dr. Willie K. Dong (Department of Anesthesiology, University of Washington), and Dr. Hiroshi Ashida (Department of Physiology, National Defense Medical College) for their invaluable suggestions and review of the manuscript.

References

Anis, N.S., Berry, S.C., Burton, N.R. and Lodge, D.: The dissociative anesthetics, ketamine and phencyclidine, selectively reduce excitation of central mammalian neurons by N-methyl-D-aspartate. Br. J. Pharmacol. 79: 565-575, 1983.

Bickford, P.C., Palmer, M.R., Rice, K.C., Hoffer, B.J. and Freedman, R.: Electrophysiological effects of phencyclidine on rat hippocampal pyramidal neurons. Neuropharmacol. 20: 733-742, 1981.

Bourne, G.W., Theoret, Y., Esplin, B. and Capek, R.: Effect of phencyclidine on inhibition in the hippocampal slice. Naunyn Schmiedeberg's Arch. Pharmacol. 323: 168-172, 1983.

Brady, R.J. and Swann, J.W.: Ketamine selectively suppresses synchronized afterdischarges in immature hippocampus. Neurosci. Lett. 69: 143-149, 1986.

Chen, C.F. and Chow, S.Y.: Effects of ketamine on synaptic transmission in cat spinal cord. Neuropharmacol. 14: 147-149, 1975.

Cotman, C.W. and Nadler, J.V.: Glutamate and aspartate as hippocampal transmitters: Biochemical and pharmacological evidence. In Glutamate: Transmitter in the Central Nervous System, ed. by P.J. Roberts, J. Storm-Mathisen and S.R. Johnston, pp. 117-154. John Wiley & Sons Ltd., New York, 1981.

Duchen, M.R., Burton, N.R. and Biscoe, T.J.: An intracellular study of the interactions of N-methyl-D-aspartate with ketamine in the mouse hippocampal slice. Brain Res. 342: 149-153, 1985.

Duncan, G.H., Dreyer, D.A., McKenna, T.M. and Whitsel, B.L.: Dose- and time-dependent effects of ketamine on SI neurons with cutaneous receptor fields. J. Neurophysiol. 47: 677-689, 1982.

Gage, P.W. and Robertson, B.: Prolongation of inhibitory postsynaptic currents by pentobarbitone, halothane and ketamine in CA1 pyramidal cells in rat hippocampus. Br. J. Pharmacol. 85: 675-681, 1985.

Gallagher, J.P., Dun, H., Higashi, H. and Nishi, S.: Actions of ketamine on synaptic transmission in frog sympathetic ganglia. Neuropharmacol. 15: 139-143, 1976.

Kayama, Y. and Iwama, K.: The EEG, evoked potentials, and single-unit activity during ketamine anesthesia in cats. Anesthesiol. 36: 316-328, 1972.

Little, H.J. and Atkinson, H.D.: Ketamine potentiates the responses of the rat superior cervical ganglion to GABA. Eur. J. Pharmacol. 98: 53-59, 1984.

Lodge, D. and Anis, N.A.: Effects of ketamine and three other anesthetics on spinal reflexes and inhibitions in the cat. Br. J. Anesth. 56: 1143-1151, 1984.

MacDonald, J.F., Miljkovic, Z. and Pennefather, P.: Use-dependent block of excitatory amino acid currents in cultured neurons by ketamine. J. Neurophysiol. 58: 251-266, 1987.

Martin, D. and Lodge, D.: Ketamine acts as a non-competitive N-methyl-D-aspartate antagonist on frog spinal cord *in vitro*. Neuropharmacol. 24: 999-1003, 1985.

Marwaha, J., Palmer, M.R., Hoffer, B.J., and Freedman, R.: Phencycldine-induced depressions of cerebellar Purkinje neurons. Life Sci. 26: 1509-1516, 1980a.

Marwaha, J., Palmer, M.R., Woodward, D.J., Hoffer, B.J. and Freedman, R.: Electrophysiological evidence for presynaptic action of phencyclidine on noradrenergic terminals in rat cerebellum. J. Pharmacol. Exp. Ther. 215: 606-613, 1980b.

Mori, K., Kawamata, M., Mitani, H., Yamazaki, Y. and Fujita, M.: A neurophysiologic study of ketamine anesthesia in the cat. Anesthesiol. 35: 373-383, 1971.

Raja, S.N. and Guyenet, P.G.: Action of phencyclidine on synaptic transmission in the hippocampus. Brain Res. 236: 289-304, 1982.

Scholfield, C.N.: Potentiation of inhibition by general anesthetics in neurons of the olfactory cortex *in vitro*. Pflugers Arch. 383: 249-255, 1980.

Sinclair, J.G. and Tein, A.F.: Neuronal responses to ketamine administered microiontophoretically or intraperitoneally in the rat. Gen. Pharmacol. 10: 51-55, 1979.

Stringer, J.L. and Guyenet, P.G.: Effect of phencyclidines on hippocampal pyramidal cells. Brain Res. 252: 343-352, 1982.

Strom-Mathisen, J. and Iversen, L.L.: Uptake of [^{3}H]glutamic acid in excitatory nerve endings: Light and electron microscopic observations in the hippocampal formation of the rat. Neuroscience 4: 1237-1253, 1979.

Tang, A.H. and Schroeder, L.A.: Spinal cord depressant effects of ketamine and etoxadrol in the cat and the rat. Anesthesiol. 39: 37-43, 1973.

Status of Ketamine in Anesthesiology,
edited by E.F. Domino©1990, NPP Books
P.O. Box 1491, Ann Arbor, MI 48106

Ketamine Induced Changes in the Electroencephalogram (EEG) Investigated by Two Dimensional Amplitude Maps

J. Tatsuno, Y. Kawakami*, H. Suzuki and M. Fujita****

Department of Physiology
National Defense Medical College,
Tokorozawa, Saitama
and
Departments of Physiology and Anesthesia***
Tokyo Women's Medical College
Tokyo, Japan

Introduction

The most conspicuous changes in the EEG induced by ketamine were reported as *theta* bursts in adult human subjects (Corssen *et al.*, 1969; Schwartz *et al.*, 1974) and slow wave bursts in children (Rosen and Hagerdal, 1976) and experimental animals (*e.g.*, Massopust *et al.*, 1972). Preceding or concomitant with this slow wave spread, an increase in fast waves was noticed (Schwartz *et al.*, 1974; Mori *et al.*, 1971). The fast wave increase, however, cannot be considered as ketamine specific because many other anesthetics, such as barbiturates, also increase fast waves (Takao, 1988). The differences between ketamine induced fast waves and barbiturate induced fast waves should be researched. However, few reports have addressed this issue (*e.g.*, Tamasy *et al.*, 1975). Although this topic is interesting, it is beyond the scope of this report.

The findings regarding ketamine induced changes in the EEG, herein investigated by two dimensional amplitude maps, are described. This technique has recently been developed to a very sophisticated level due to the progress in computer hardware and software. Two dimensional maps can be generated from multi-channel EEG data with the values of the picture elements in the map calculated by various interpolation methods according to mathematical principles. We used the Unbiased Polynomial Interpolation technique (Ashida *et al.*, 1986) which calculates the value by a polynomial formula. Furthermore, this method gives us polynomial coefficients that are of great importance for an objective evaluation of the pattern differences using Mahalanobis' distance (Tatsuno *et al.*, 1988).

Two dimensional maps of EEG activities of various frequency bands indicate where these activities appear and how they spread over the surface of the brain. The application of this technique to ketamine anesthesia has never been done. By this technique, the amplitude map of the evoked potential data can also be generated, either for amplitude or latency (Tatsuno *et al.*, 1984). The results are not included in this report.

One typical time course of EEG amplitude change during induction of ketamine anesthesia in a male patient is described in detail below through two dimensional maps whose pattern differences were objectively estimated.

METHODS

Subject. A 50 yr old male patient with a body weight of 66 kg was the subject of this report. He lay on an operating table with no premedication and was conscious. Twelve electrodes were placed on his scalp as shown in Fig. 1.

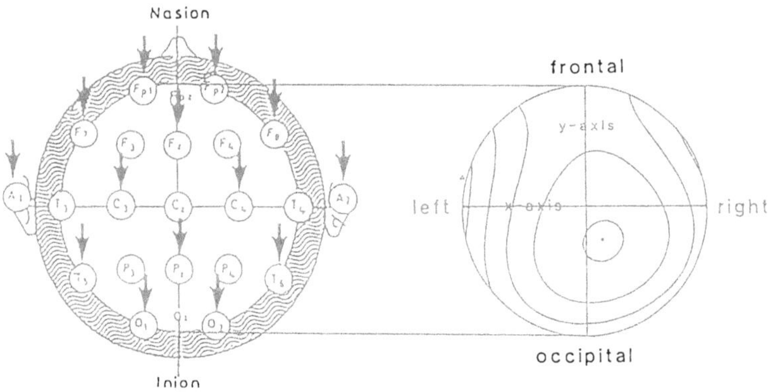

Fig. 1. Electrode position and relation to the generated maps. As noted in this and all subsequent figures, the maps correspond to the inside area within the shaded ring. Up: frontal, down: occipital. Left is the subject's left and right is his right. The Unbiased Polynomial Interpolation method calculates amplitude values F(X,Y). The x and y axises are shown in the map at the right. Numbers on the isopotential lines are mean amplitudes in μV in Figs. 2-8.

The EEG was recorded monopolarly using electrodes connected together on both earlobes as reference (Nihon Koden EEG 7213 TC 0.3, HC off) from twelve locations: Fp_1 Fp_2, F_7, F_8, C_3, C_4, T_5, T_6, O_1, O_2, F_z, P_z according to the International 10-20 method. Control data were recorded for a few min while the patient closed his eyes. A dose of 1 mg/kg of ketamine was administered i.v. in 1 min, and 7 min EEG recordings were made thereafter. All EEG data were stored on an FM magnetic tape (TEAC XR-50, tape speed 2.4 cm/sec). On replaying, the data were A/D converted (Sampling frequency 256 Hz, 12 bits), and the digitalized data were used for further computer processing. Average amplitudes were calculated from 4 sec epochs free from artifact by FFT for 10 frequency bands: *alpha* (8-13 Hz), *beta* (13-25 Hz), *theta* (3-8 Hz), *delta* (1-3 Hz), *alpha* low (8-10 Hz), *alpha* high (10-13 Hz), *beta* low (13-19 Hz), *beta* high (19-25 Hz), *theta* low (3-5 Hz) and *theta* high (5-8 Hz).

Unbiased Polynomial Interpolation calculated values of the picture elements, F(X,Y), in the map from 10 polynomial coefficients of 12 channels of EEG data, such as a_0,a_1,a_2—a_9, appear in the polynomial formula below.

$$F(X,Y) = a_0 + a_1X + a_2Y + a_3X^2 + a_4XY + a_5Y^2 + a_6X^3 + a_7X^2Y + a_8XY^2 + a_9Y^3$$

The X axis denotes the line connecting the ears, and the Y axis denotes the midline of the head. The constant term, a_0, indicates average amplitude of the 4-sec epoch for the frequency band investigated. Four coefficients, a_6, a_7, a_8 and a_9 relate to the global pattern of the map. Mahalanobis'distance of the 4 coefficients (Q4), therefore, indicates the objective pattern differences between the maps of two periods. Statistical significance is shown by the F value which has a linear relationship to Q value (Tatsuno, 1988). Seven periods of 40 sec duration (consisting of 10 epochs of 4 sec each) were chosen during ketamine anesthesia: control period, 1 to 40 sec after the injection (period 1), 41 to 80 sec (period 2), 151 to 190 sec (period 3), 261 to 300 sec (period 4), 341 to 380 sec (period 5), and 401 to 440 sec (period 6).

Typical data generated are given in Table 1 which shows the Q values of the *alpha*, *beta*, and *theta* bands. The larger the Q value, the more remarkable the pattern difference between the two compared periods. The largest value was found in the Q value of the comparison for the *theta* pattern between control and period 4. The difference is statistically significant at the 0.2% level. In the *beta* patterns, the largest difference was between that of periods 2 and 5. Generally Q values of the *beta* bands

TABLE 1. Mahalanobis' distances between two periods in the left and uppermost rows. Q4 values of *alpha*, *beta*, and *theta* bands. The larger the Q value, the more remarkable the pattern difference between the compared periods. Numbers in parentheses are statistically significant, *e.g.*, P = 1.466<2.0000 means the difference is significant at the 2% level.

Alpha 8-13 Hz	***1–40 (per 1)***	***41–80 (per 2)***	***151–190 (per 3)***	***261–300 (per 4)***	***341–380 (per 5)***	***401–440 (per 6)***
Control	1.7243	2.9850	1.8866	4.4234	2.5019	3.0279
	(19.698)	(5.553)	(16.518)	(1.466)	(8.887)	(5.135)
1–40		1.2499	0.6962	1.7813	0.3224	0.2587
		(33.238)	(60.625)	(18.512)	(85.857)	(89.980)
41–80			0.3928	2.4533	1.0182	0.9383
			(81.060)	(9.098)	(42.935)	(46.853)
151–190				1.1811	0.8493	0.4664
				(35.872)	(51.585)	(75.951)
261–300					1.4435	1.2654
					(26.821)	(32.672)
341–380						0.3025
						(87.175)

Beta 13–25 Hz	***1–40 (per 1)***	***41–80 (per 2)***	***151–190 (per 3)***	***261–300 (per 4)***	***341–380 (per 5)***	***401–440 (per 6)***
Control	1.2893	1.5365	0.8834	0.2770	0.9453	0.8297
	(31.818)	(24.204)	(49.726)	(88.826)	(46.497)	(52.680)
1–40		2.3621	1.2227	3.0343	1.9232	3.0959
		(9.993)	(34.256)	(5.104)	(15.879)	(4.810)
41–80			0.5426	1.1184	6.9078	2.4697
			(70.701)	(38.448)	(0.232)	(8.946)
151–190				0.8142	2.6897	1.2796
				(53.558)	(7.161)	(32.162)
261–300					1.4033	0.5898
					(28.041)	(67.516)
341–380						2.8070
						(5.681)

Theta 3–8 Hz	***1–40 (per 1)***	***41–80 (per 2)***	***151–190 (per 3)***	***261–300 (per 4)***	***341–380 (per 5)***	***401–440 (per 6)***
Control	0.2154	0.4983	3.2914	7.4568	2.1411	3.8209
	(92.576)	(73.741)	(3.995)	(0.163)	(12.489)	(2.463)
1–40		0.5316	3.6949	3.7230	1.7123	2.2586
		(71.452)	(2.757)	(2.688)	(19.957)	(11.128)
41–80			4.7619	4.8200	1.7379	5.9887
			(1.111)	(1.060)	(19.408)	(0.437)
151–190				0.8543	2.3902	1.4706
				(51.309)	(9.707)	(26.029)
261–300					1.1108	0.9495
					(38.772)	(46.285)
341–380						1.7441
						(19.277)

were smaller than those of the *theta*, which means that the global pattern changes were more positive in *theta* activity. For the *alpha* band, a significant Q value increase (2.5%) appeared the earliest, and that was between control and period 2, 41 to 80 sec after the injection.

Results

Fig. 2 (control) shows the amplitude maps of the 10 frequency bands mentioned above. The subject was in a relaxed state with his eyes closed. The *alpha* activity was quite dominant on the right occipital area where the maximum amplitude existed. The maximum *beta* activity was also found in the right occipital area. The *theta* activity was on the contrary

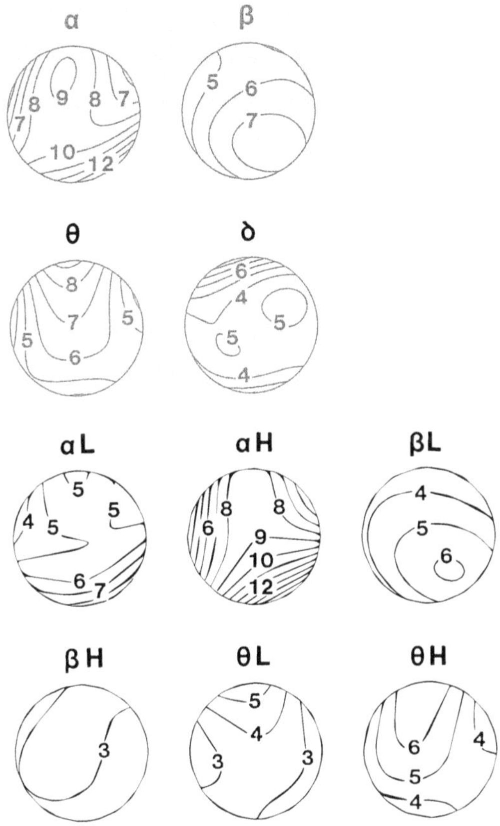

Fig. 2. Control. Amplitude maps of 10 frequency bands in μv. Max *alpha* 14.47; max *beta* 7.63; max *theta* 10.28; max *delta* 9.81.

frontally dominant. The *delta* activity also showed frontal dominance. The pattern of the *alpha* map was mainly determined by *alpha* high activity because the pattern was more similar to the *alpha* map than the *alpha* low map. The pattern of the *beta* low map was more similar to the *beta* map, and the *theta* high was more similar to the *theta* map.

Fig. 3 (period 1) shows the maps just after injection. Although the *alpha* amplitude already decreased, occipital dominance was still observed. The *theta* and *delta* amplitudes increased, but the principal pattern did not change. The *theta* pattern was more similar to the *theta* low pattern.

As seen in Fig. 4 (period 2), in the next 40 sec *alpha* pattern changed markedly. The maximum point moved to the frontal midline area. The

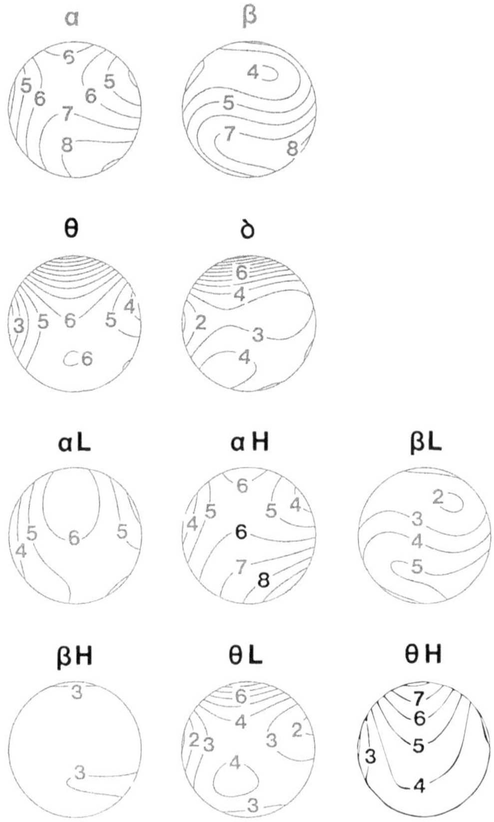

Fig. 3. Period 1, 1-40 sec. Amplitude maps of 10 frequency bands in μv. Max *alpha* 9.19; max *beta* 8.47; max *theta* 14.14; max *delta* 12.33.

maximum point of the *beta* map was also found in the frontal area, but the amplitude increase was small. For *theta* and *delta* maps, the pattern changes were trivial.

Fig. 5 (period 3) shows the maps about 2.5 min after injection. Changes in the *theta* pattern, mainly due to *theta* low activity, were remarkable. The *beta* pattern changed slightly. The maximal zone moved to the frontopolar region, and the amplitude markedly increased.

Fig. 6 (period 4) shows the maps in the period about 4.5-5 min after injection. The global pattern of the *theta* map was still changing, but the amplitude of the activity remained almost the same. The amplitude of the *beta* activity had diminished, and the decrease of *alpha* activity was quite

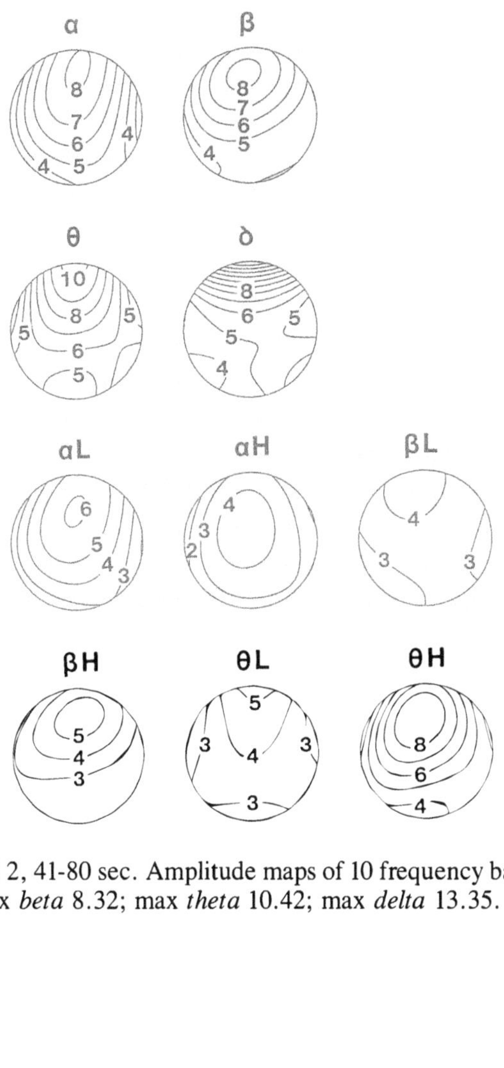

Fig. 4. Period 2, 41-80 sec. Amplitude maps of 10 frequency bands in μv. Max *alpha* 8.20; max *beta* 8.32; max *theta* 10.42; max *delta* 13.35.

clear. These two maps were covered by weak activities (as indicated by numbers on the equipotential lines in the maps).

Fig. 7 (period 5) shows the maps about 6 min after injection. This period revealed an increase in the *theta* frontal and the parietal areas. This secondary increase was characterized by a striking symmetry.

Fig. 8 (period 6) shows the maps about 7 min after injection. The *theta* amplitude again decreased, and the pattern seemed to return to that of the control. The patterns of the *alpha* and *beta* maps, however, were quite different from those in the initial period.

Fig. 9 shows the changes in the constant term of the polynomial coefficients; Fig. 9A for *alpha* band, 9B for *beta* band and 9C for *theta*

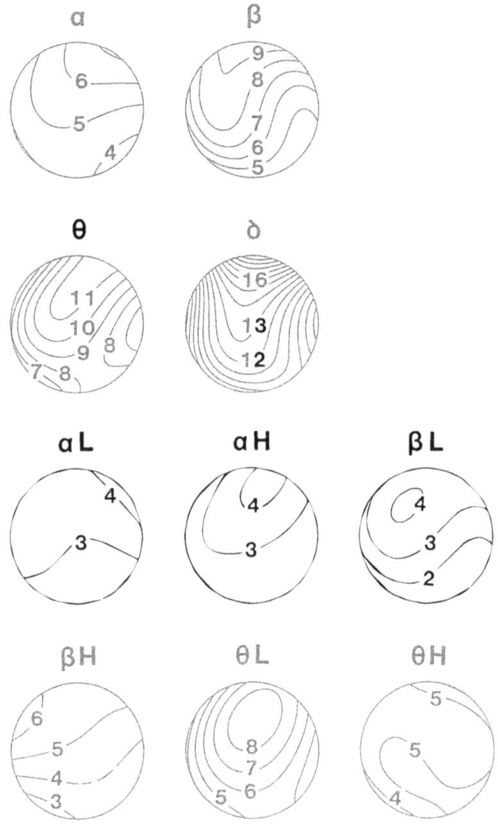

Fig. 5. Period 3, 151-190 sec. Amplitude maps of 10 frequency bands in μv. Max *alpha* 7.18; max *beta* 10.00; max *theta* 11.72; max *delta* 21.98.

band. There seemed to be two phases in the *theta* increase, one appeared soon after injection. The pattern was a little asymmetrical. The other phase appeared a few min later. The pattern was remarkably symmetrical with maximum areas in the frontal and occipital regions. The time course of the *theta* activity was more closely related to the *theta* low rather than the *theta* high.

Discussion

We have previously reported (Tatsuno *et al.*, 1984), that the somatosensory evoked potential by left median nerve stimulation was

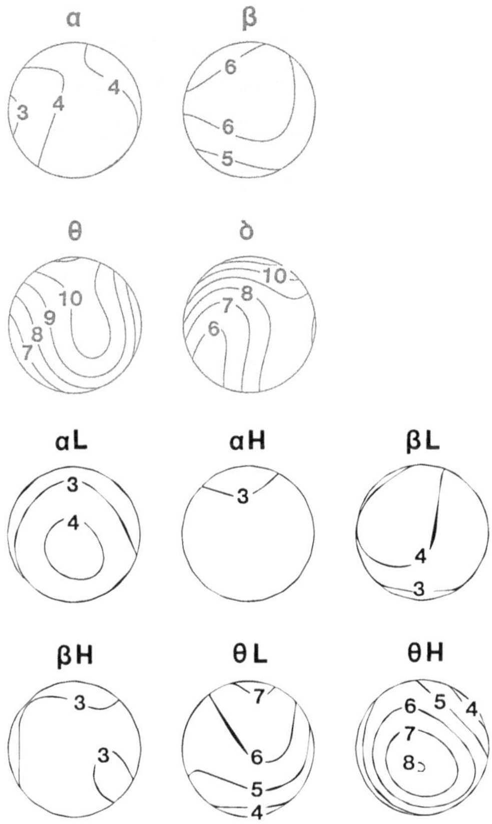

Fig. 6. Period 4, 261-300 sec. Amplitude maps of 10 frequency bands in μv. Max *alpha* 4.85; max *beta* 6.58; max *theta* 11.10; max *delta* 11.80.

topographically distorted during ketamine anesthesia, especially during the *theta* burst period.

Both in the amplitude and the latency maps, the pattern of P40, P60, and N80 became, therefore, obscured in the C6 area. It seemed quite important to investigate the time course of the changes in the background EEG and to investigate the nature of their changes topographically, as is the subject of this report.

It has often been reported that ketamine may precipitate seizure discharges, especially when administered in high doses (Kayama, 1982). In this study, seizure patterns did not appear because low doses of ketamine (*e.g.*, 1 mg/kg) were used.

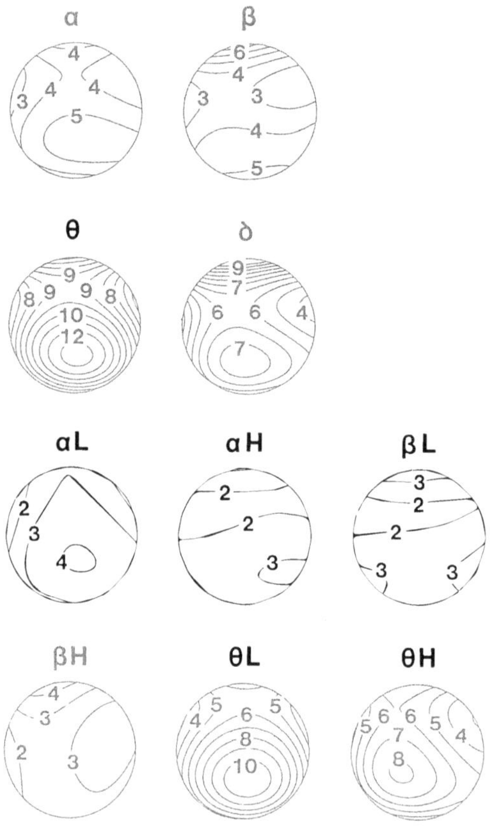

Fig. 7. Period 5, 341-380 sec. Amplitude maps of 10 frequency bands in μv. Max *alpha* 5.56; max *beta* 7.61; max *theta* 13.45; max *delta* 13.90.

It might be argued that the dosage is too small for complete anesthesia. Although the patient was fully unconscious, he sometimes groaned, especially near the end of the induction when the second *theta* increase began to disappear. His state may be concluded as being cataleptic (Winters *et al.*, 1972), and, of course, he never responded to his name being called.

Characteristic topographical changes were observed in many maps. *Alpha* disappearance may be related to the loss of consciousness. The *beta* increase in the initial portion of the induction is not unique to ketamine, but there should be topographical differences between the fast wave patterns. This is a theme for future research. The main findings of

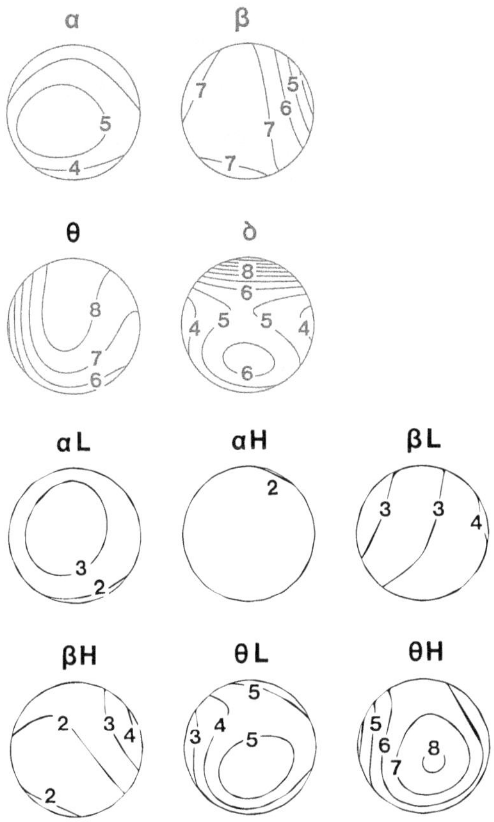

Fig. 8. Period 6, 401-440 sec. Amplitude maps of 10 frequency bands in μv. Max *alpha* 5.94; max *beta* 8.01; max *theta* 8.75; max *delta* 13.05.

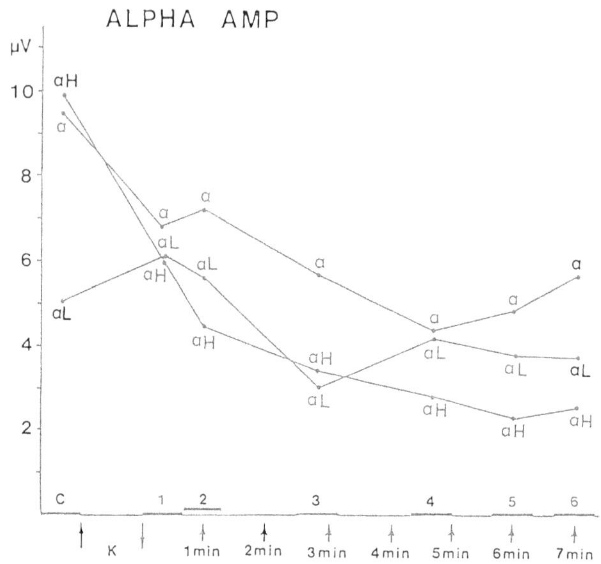

Fig. 9A. Mean amplitude changes in the *alpha* band expressed as the constant term of the polynomial coefficients. Root mean square values are given in 4 sec epochs (in μV). *Alpha* amplitude had already decreased by the end of the injection, and it continued to decrease throughout the period of observation. The time course was more related to *alpha* high rather than to *alpha* low activity. ↑ K ↓ shows the period of injection.

this study were that the *theta* increase appeared twice, and the topographical patterns were different between the two. The pattern of the second increase was completely symmetrical. This pattern difference may be caused by different locations of the generators. For example, the generator of the symmetrical pattern is more likely to exist in the depth of the brain.

These predictions must be confirmed in animal experiments that employ depth electrodes and larger doses of ketamine.

Summary

1. Two dimensional maps of EEG amplitudes were generated for the investigation of EEG changes induced by ketamine. The subject was a 50 yr old male. One mg/kg ketamine was injected i.v. within 1 min.

2. The *theta* activities thus evoked showed increases in amplitude twice, but the patterns of the two were different. The pattern of the secondary increase was remarkably symmetrical.

3. The *beta* activity increased temporarily, preceding a *theta* in-

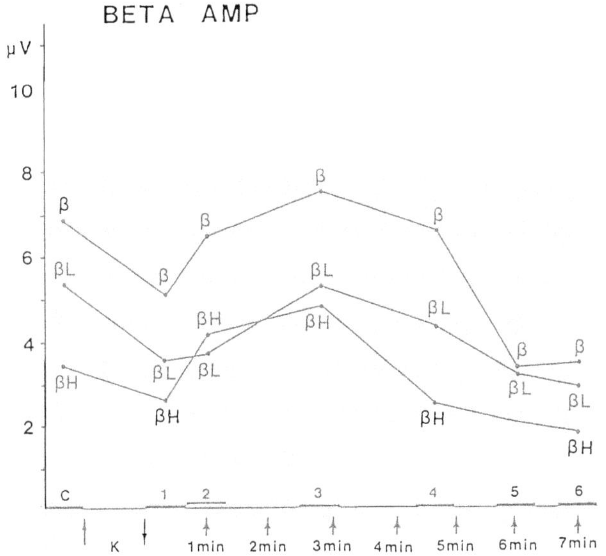

Fig. 9B. Mean amplitude changes in the *beta* band expressed as in the constant term of the polynomial coefficients. Root mean squares are given in 4 sec epochs (in μV). The *beta* increase occurred quickly and then disappeared rapidly before the second increase of *theta*.

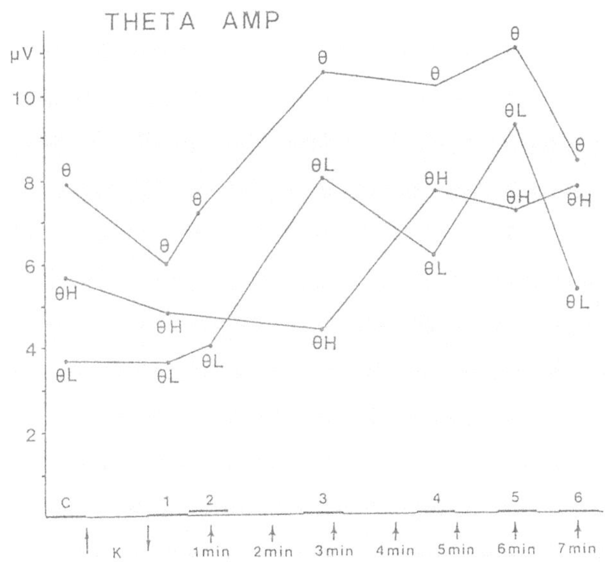

Fig. 9C. Average amplitude changes in the *theta* band expressed as the constant term of the polynomial coefficients. Root mean square values are given in 4 sec epochs (in μV).

crease. The *alpha* decrease occurred earliest and continued throughout the induction for several min.

4. No seizure patterns were observed.

References

Ashida, H., Tatsuno, J., Okamoto, J. and Maru, E.: Field mapping of EEG by unbiased polynomial interpolation. Comput. Biomed. Res. 17: 267-276, 1986.

Corssen, G., Domino, E.F. and Bree, R.L.: Electroencephalographic effects of ketamine anesthesia in children. Anesth. Analg. Curr. Res. 48: 141-147, 1969.

Kayama, Y.: Ketamine and EEG seizure waves: interaction with anti-epileptic drugs. Br. J. Anaesth. 54: 879-883, 1982.

Massopust, L.C., Wolin, L.R. and Albin, M.S.: Electrophysiologic and behavioral responses to ketamine hydrochloride in the rhesus monkey. Anesth. Analg. 51: 329-341, 1972.

Mori, K., Kawamata, M., Mitani, H., Yamazaki, Y. and Fujita, M.: A neurophysiologic study of ketamine anesthesia in the cat. Anesthesiol. 35: 373-383, 1971.

Rosen, I. and Hagerdal, M.: Electroencephalographic study of children during ketamine anesthesia. Acta Anaesth. Scand. 20: 32-39, 1976.

Schwartz, M.S., Virden, S. and Scotte, D.F.: Effects of ketamine on the electroencephalograph. Anaesthesia 29: 135-140, 1974.

Takao, A.: EEG fast waves induced by thiopental, diazepam and successive administration of both drugs studied by means of two dimensional amplitude map. Tokyo Joshi Ikadigaku Zasshi. (J. of Tokyo Women's Medical College) 58: 973-985, 1988.

Tamasy, V., Koranyi, L. and Tekeres, M.: EEG and multiple unit activity during ketamine and barbiturate anaesthesia. Br. J. Anaesth. 47: 1247-1251, 1975.

Tatsuno, J., Ozaki, M., Kawakami, Y., Suzuki, H. and Fujita, M.: Topographic analysis on amplitude changes in somatosensory evoked potential induced by anesthetics (ketamine). Masui (Jap. J. Anesth.) 32: 5108, 1984.

Tatsuno, J., Ashida, H. and Takao, A.: Objective evaluation of differences in patterns of EEG topographical maps by Mahalanobis distance. EEG Clin. Neurophysiol. 69: 287-290, 1988.

Winters, W.D., Ferrar-Allado, T., Guzman-Flores, C. and Alcaraz, M.: The cataleptic state induced by ketamine: A review of the neuropharmacology of anesthesia. Neuropharmacol. 11: 303-313, 1972.

Status of Ketamine in Anesthesiology,
edited by E.F. Domino©1990, NPP Books
P.O. Box 1491, Ann Arbor, MI 48106

Use of Ketamine in Electrophysiological Studies of Midbrain Dopamine Neurons

M.D. Kelland, L.A. Chiodo and A.S. Freeman

Laboratory of Neurophysiology
Center for Cell Biology Sinai Research Institute
and
the Cellular and Clinical Neurobiology Program
Department of Psychiatry
Wayne State University School of Medicine
Detroit, MI

INTRODUCTION

Ketamine and its parent compound phencyclidine (PCP) have been described as producing a "dissociative" state of anesthesia (Corssen and Domino, 1966; Domino *et al.*, 1965). Behavioral and biochemical studies suggest that some of the effects of these compounds may be mediated via dopamine (DA) systems. Thus, PCP induced stereotypy can be blocked by DA antagonists (Marwaha, 1982: Schlemmer *et al.*, 1978). PCP induced increases in locomotor activity are blocked by 6-hydroxydopamine lesion of the ventral tegmental area (A10) DA neurons (French *et al.*, 1985). PCP induced rotational behavior is blocked by DA antagonists (Finnegan *et al.*, 1976). Ketamine induced rotation in rats is similar to that induced by amphetamine (Myslobodsky *et al.*, 1979) and PCP alters DA metabolite levels in mesolimbic, mesocortical and nigro-striatal DA projection areas (Deutch *et al.*, 1987; Nabeshima *et al.*, 1983a). Nabeshima *et al.* (1983b,c) have suggested that the neostriatum serves as a site of DA serotonin integration in the control of PCP induced stereotypy and locomotor activity. In addition, the ability of ketamine and PCP to alter the firing rate of midbrain DA containing neurons themselves has also been examined. Raja and Guyenet (1980) first demonstrated that both ketamine and PCP (administered i.v.) selectively increase the firing rate of slow firing (1-3 spikes/sec) substantia nigra zona compacta (A9) DA neurons as compared to fast firing (4.5-6 spikes/sec) A9 DA neurons. More recent studies have confirmed the ability of PCP to increase the firing rate of both A9 (Freeman and Bunney, 1984) and A10 (Freeman and Bunney, 1984;

French, 1986) DA neurons. However, Freeman and Bunney (1984) also observed inhibition of DA neurons following high doses of PCP. They found no relationship between basal firing rate and DA cell responsiveness. Locally applied PCP typically either inhibits or has no effect on the firing rate of midbrain DA neurons (Freeman and Bunney, 1984; French, 1986: Marwaha, 1982).

It is noteworthy that the aforementioned electrophysiological studies were conducted in chloral hydrate (CH) anesthetized rats except for Marwaha (1982) who used urethane. Several studies have demonstrated that the anesthetic condition of rats alters the responsiveness of midbrain DA neurons to both DA agonists (Kelland *et al.*, 1989) and antagonists (Bunney *et al.*, 1973; Mereu *et al.*, 1983, 1984). In locally anesthetized, paralyzed rats, DA neurons exhibit a greater degree of burst, firing activity, and they require higher doses of the direct acting D2 DA agonist quinpirole to effect inhibition of cell firing (Kelland *et al.*,1989). Given that ketamine and PCP are themselves anesthetics, we felt it was necessary to address two issues. First, what effect, if any, does ketamine induced anesthesia have on the basal activity and/or pharmacological responsiveness of nigrostriatal DA neurons? The present study will also show that ketamine induced anesthesia alters the ability of electrical stimulation of the pedunculopontine tegmental nucleus (PPN) to excite nigrostriatal DA cell firing. Second, what are the effects of ketamine and PCP on these cells in locally anesthetized, paralyzed rats (*i.e.* in the absence of general anesthesia)?

Methods

Surgical and Recording Procedures

Standard extracellular single unit recording techniques were used to sample the activity of nigrostriatal DA neurons in rats, as previously described (Bunney *et al.*, 1973). Briefly, male Sprague-Dawley rats were anesthetized with either ketamine (100 mg/kg) or CH (400 mg/kg) and placed in a stereotaxic instrument (Activational Systems, Inc., SAS 1450). The skull overlying the substantia nigra was removed (from bregma: posterior 4.3 to 6.3 mm, lateral 0.0 to 3.0 mm; Paxinos and Watson, 1986). A lateral tail vein was cannulated for i.v. administration of drugs. In some experiments, the animals were paralyzed with gallamine triethiodide (25 mg/kg, i.v.). All experiments carried out in paralyzed animals were in strict accordance with the "Guiding Principles in the Care and Use of Animals" approved by the Council of the American Physiologic Society. The rats were first anesthetized with a mixture of halothane and room air. The anesthesia was maintained by dropping halothane onto a cone placed over the animal's snout, and all surgery was performed under temporary halothane anesthesia. All incision sites and blunt pressure points were infiltrated with 2% mepivacaine HCl. A tracheotomy was performed, the trachea intubated with a 13 gauge cannula and the cannula connected to an Edco rodent respirator (Model 804). At the end of the surgical procedure, gallamine triethiodide was administered via the tail vein, resulting in complete paralysis of all skeletal muscle and the cessation of spontaneous respiration. All animals were respired with room air at a rate which maintained the expired CO_2 concentration at 3.5-4.0% as continuously monitored by a Biochem International $ETCO_2$ Monitor (Lifespan 100).

Neuronal signals were sampled through a single barrel glass micropipette filled with 2 M NaCl containing 2% pontamine sky blue dye (*in vitro* impedances at 135 Hz, 3-6 megohms). DA containing neurons located within the substantia nigra zona compacta were identified on the basis of previously described extracellular electrophysiological criteria (Bunney *et al.*, 1973). All DA neurons included for analysis were shown to be nigrostriatal DA neurons by means of antidromic activation (Guyenet and Aghajanian, 1978).

Electrical stimulation of the PPN was performed by inserting a concentric electrode (SNE-100, Rhodes Medical Instruments) into the PPN (from bregma: posterior 7.8 mm, lateral 1.9 mm, ventral 7.3 mm: Paxinos and Watson, 1986) and delivering constant-current square wave pulses (0.3 mA, 300 sec duration) by a digital pulse generator and coupled stimulus-isolation unit (World Precision Instruments, Anapulse Stimulator 301-T).

Drug Administration

Injectable ketamine HCl (QUAD Pharmaceuticals) was diluted in 0.9% NaCl. Phencyclidine HCl (Sigma) and quinpirole HCl (Lilly) were freshly dissolved in 0.9% NaCl. Chloral hydrate (Sigma) was dissolved in distilled H_2O. Drug doses refer to the weight of the respective salt. Ketamine (0.25-16.0 mg/kg), PCP (0.25-8.0 mg/kg) and quinpirole (1-512 g/kg) were administered in cumulative, exponentially increasing doses every 90 sec via a lateral tail vein.

Results

Ketamine vs Chloral Hydrate Anesthesia

Nigrostriatal DA neurons sampled in ketamine anesthetized rats exhibited a greater degree of burst firing activity as compared to CH anesthetized animals (Table 1). The degree of burst firing in ketamine anesthetized rats was comparable to that seen previously in locally anesthetized, paralyzed rats (Kelland *et al.*, 1989).

Significantly higher doses of quinpirole were required to inhibit nigrostriatal DA cell firing in ketamine anesthetized rats ($ED_{50} = 20.9 \pm 0.2$ μg/kg: N = 8) as compared to CH anesthetized rats ($ED_{50} = 5.6 \pm 0.4$ μg/kg; N = 8; Fig. 1A). As seen previously (Kelland *et al.*, 1988, 1989), there was a significant positive correlation between the basal firing rate of the DA neurons and the ability of quinpirole to effect inhibition of cell firing in CH anesthetized rats (Fig. 1B). Likewise, there was a positive correlation between basal firing rate and ED_{50} in ketamine anesthetized animals (Fig. 1B). There was no statistical difference between the slopes of the regression lines shown in Fig. 1B.

Electrical stimulation of the PPN in CH anesthetized rats failed to alter nigrostriatal DA cell firing rate (43 cells sampled in 12 rats). In locally anesthetized, paralyzed rats, however, PPN stimulation elicited both short latency and longer latency excitations of these cells (Fig. 2; Table 2). The short latency, possibly monosynaptic excitations occurred in 26% of the cells. There also appeared to be two distinct groups of longer latency responses: a medium latency group exhibited by 43% of the cells,

TABLE 1. Influence of ketamine or CH anesthesia on nigrostriatal DA cell basal activity[1]

	CH Anesthesia	*Ketamine Anesthesia*
All Cells	N = 19	N = 21
Firing rate (per sec)	3.7 ± 0.4	4.7 ± 0.4
Conduction velocity (m/sec)	0.48 ± 0.01	0.47 ± 0.03
% Spikes in bursts	15.0 ± 5.0	28.0 ± 5.0*
Bursting Cells[2]	47%	81%**
Number of bursts	60.6 ± 8.0	50.1 ± 6.7
% Spikes in bursts	31.0 ± 6.0	34.0 ± 6.0
Spikes per burst	2.5 ± 0.2	3.5 ± 0.5
Interspike interval (msec)	66.9 ± 4.0	69.8 ± 3.5
Interburst interval (sec)	3.2 ± 1.0	3.2 ± 1.0
Postburst inhibition (msec)	456.7 ± 51.2	338.0 ± 24.1***

Data presented as mean ± S.E.
[1]500 action potentials were recorded as the baseline for each cell.
[2]Burst firing analysis was performed as previously described (Chiodo *et al.*, 1984; Grace and Bunney, 1984; Kelland *et al.*, 1989).
*$t(38) = 1.81$; approached significance at $P<0.1$
**Chi square = 4.95; $P<0.05$
***$t(24) = 2.39$; $P<0.05$

and a diffuse group of long latency excitations exhibited by 31% of the cells. Some cells exhibited more than one type of response. We have also examined the ability of PPN stimulation to excite nigrostriatal DA cell firing rate in a few ketamine anesthetized animals. A total of 10 cells were

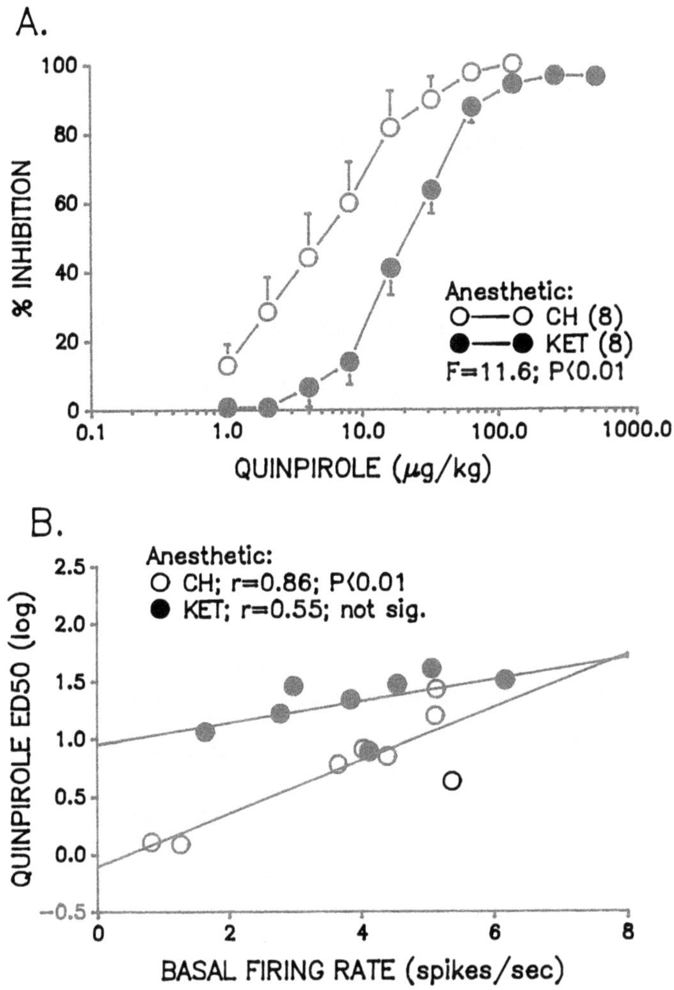

Fig. 1. Effects of CH anesthesia as compared to KET anesthesia on the responsiveness of nigrostriatal DA neurons to quinpirole administration. A. Dose response curves illustrating that signifciantly higher doses of quinpirole were required to effect either 50% or total inhibition of cell firing (ANCOVA). B. Scatter plots demonstrating the positive correlation between basal firing rate and ED_{50}. The slopes of the regression lines are not significantly different.

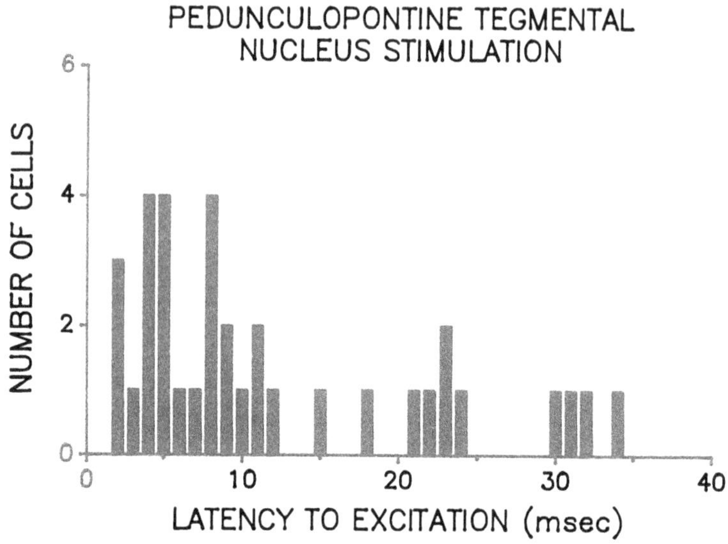

Fig. 2. Bar graph demonstrating three apparent types of excitatory responses seen in nigrostriatal DA neurons following PPN stimulation. The first two major peaks represent possible mono- and disynaptic excitations (see Table 2 for mean values), whereas the much longer latencies to excitation involve an unknown number of synaptic junctions.

sampled, with 3 cells exhibiting short latency excitations, 3 cells exhibiting medium latency excitations, and 4 cells were unaffected (Table 2).

Ketamine and PCP effects in CH Anesthetized vs Paralyzed Rats

In CH anesthetized rats, PCP increased the firing rate of nigrostriatal DA neurons at lower doses (maximal excitation: 27 ± 11 % at 1.0 mg/kg) and decreased their firing rate at higher doses (maximal inhibition: 36 ± 8 % at 8 mg/kg, Fig. 3). In contrast, ketamine failed to alter the firing rate of nigrostriatal DA neurons (Fig. 3).

In locally anesthetized, paralyzed rats, PCP elicited only the high dose inhibition (maximal effect: 30 ± 11 % at 8 mg/kg) of cell firing rate (Fig. 4). As was the case in CH anesthetized animals, ketamine was without effect in paralyzed rats (Fig. 4).

Discussion

The basal activity of nigrostriatal DA neurons in ketamine anesthetized rats resembles the high degree of burst firing seen in locally anesthe-

TABLE 2. PPN stimulation induced excitation of DA neurons in different anesthetic conditions

	CH Anesthesia	*Ketamine Anesthesia*	*Paralyzed*
Short latency	0/43	3/10	9/35
Latency (msec)	—	3.0 ± 0.6	3.8 ± 0.6
Duration (msec)	—	2.3 ± 0.3	5.3 ± 0.8
Medium latency	0/43	3/10	15/35
Latency (msec)	—	14.0 ± 1.5	8.1 ± 0.8
Duration (msec)	—	5.3 ± 2.4	12.1 ± 1.6
Long latency	0/43	0/10	11/35
Latency (msec)	—	—	24.5 ± 2.1
Duration (msec)	—	—	19.3 ± 2.4
No Effect	43/43	4/10	11/35

Latency and duration data are presented as means ± S.E. The observation of multiple latency responses and the proportion of cells exhibiting these responses is in general agreement with Scarnati *et al.* (1984, 1986).

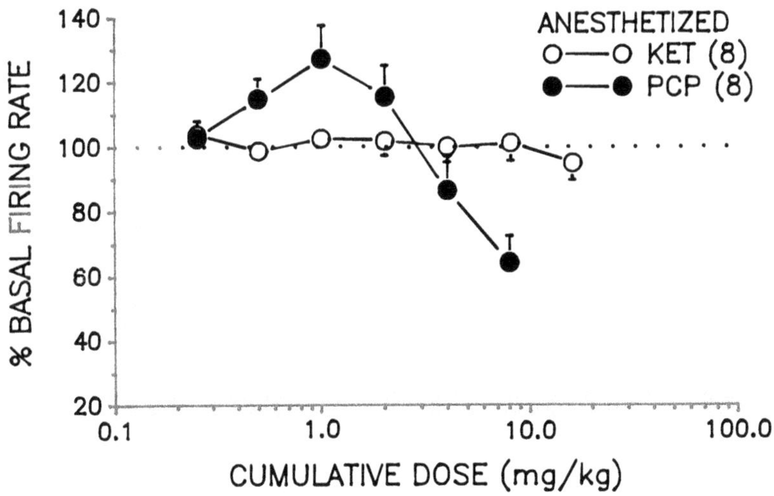

Fig. 3. Dose response curves illustrating the effects of ketamine and PCP on nigrostrial DA cell firing rate in CH anesthetized rats.

tized, paralyzed (Kelland *et al.*, 1989) and awake, freely moving rats (Freeman and Bunney, 1987) but not in CH anesthetized rats (present study and Kelland *et al.*, 1989). The responsiveness of these neurons to quinpirole in ketamine anesthetized rats is also more similar to the re-

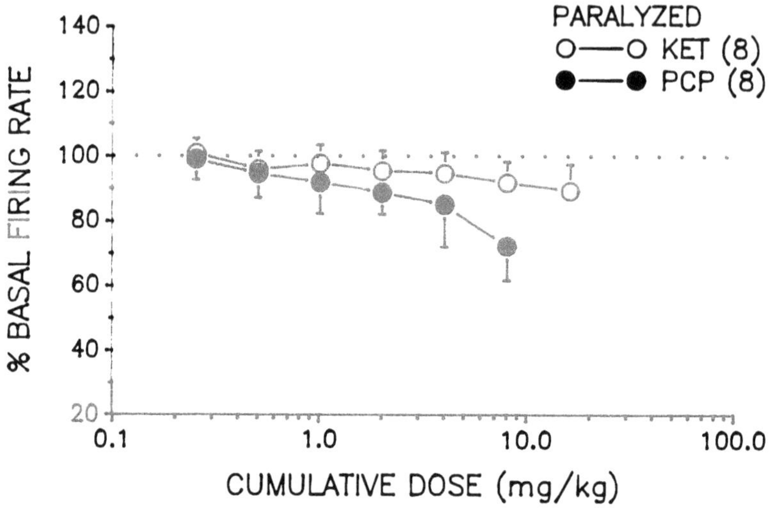

Fig. 4. Dose response curves illustrating the effects of ketamine and PCP on nigrostriatal DA cell firing rate in locally anesthetized, paralyzed rats.

sponsiveness of DA neurons in paralyzed as compared to CH anesthetized animals (Kelland *et al.*, 1989). Furthermore, CH appears to block the responsiveness of nigrostriatal DA neurons to the excitatory effects of PPN stimulation. These data would appear to support studies which have demonstrated that ketamine exerts its anesthetic actions primarily on diffuse thalamoneocortical systems (Miyasaka and Domino, 1968: Virtue *et al.*, 1967). Therefore, since ketamine exerts limited influences on brainstem neuronal systems, this anesthetic may provide a more appropriate preparation than CH anesthesia in which to study certain electrophysiological properties of midbrain DA neuronal systems.

Ketamine failed to alter the firing rate of nigrostriatal neurons in either CH anesthetized or paralyzed rats. Based on Raja and Guyenet's observations that ketamine and PCP preferentially excite slowly firing DA neurons (1980), we examined the effects of ketamine on DA cells which fired slowly (<4 spikes/sec) or rapidly (>4 spikes/sec) (see Kelland *et al.*, 1988). Although there was a tendency towards weak excitation of more slowly firing neurons, there was no significant difference between the effects of ketamine on slow as compared to fast DA neurons. Preliminary data from our laboratory also suggest that ketamine has no effect on DA neurons *in vitro* in the midbrain superfused slice preparation (Freeman, unpublished observations). Further investigation will be necessary in order to address these apparent discrepancies.

PCP caused a biphasic excitation/inhibition of nigrostriatal DA neurons, and again there was a nonsignificant trend toward greater excitation of the slowly firing subgroup of DA cells. In paralyzed animals however, PCP failed to excite nigrostriatal DA cell firing rate, though PCP retained its ability to inhibit these neurons. Thus, it is suggested that the ability of PCP to excite DA neurons involves some mechanism which is expressed only in anesthetized preparations.

This study has demonstrated that ketamine anesthesia does not appear to alter the basal activity or the responsiveness of nigrostriatal DA neurons, whereas general anesthetics such as CH do (Kelland *et al.*, 1989). In addition, ketamine and PCP cause little or no effects on the firing rate of these cells in paralyzed rats. Therefore, dissociative anesthesia may provide a useful preparation for the study of midbrain DA electrophysiology when conditions of anesthesia are a matter of concern and the use of the locally anesthetized, paralyzed preparation is not possible.

Acknowledgements

The authors thank Drs. D.K. Pitts and C. Rouillard for their comments regarding this work and Ms. J. Rubin for technical assistance. This research was supported, in part, by grants MH42136 (ASF), MH41557 (LAC), and by the Sinai Research Institute. M.D. Kelland is a Tourette Syndrome Association Postdoctoral Research Fellow.

References

Bunney, B.S., Walters, J.R., Roth, R.H., and Aghajanian, G.K.: Dopaminergic neurons: Effect of antipsychotic drugs and amphetamine on single cell activity. J. Pharmacol. Exp. Ther. 185: 560-571, 1973.

Chiodo, L.A., Bannon, M.J., Grace, A.A., Roth, R.H., and Bunney, B.S.: Evidence for the absence of impulse-regulating somatodendritic and synthesis-modulating nerve terminal autoreceptors on subpopulations of midbrain dopamine neurons. Neurosci. 12: 1-16, 1984.

Corssen, G. and Domino, E.F.: Dissociative anesthesia: Further pharmacologic studies and first clinical experience with the phencyclidine derivative CI-581. Anesth. Analg. 45: 29-40, 1966.

Deutch, A.Y., Tam, S.-Y., Freeman, A.S., Bowers, Jr., M.B., and Roth, R.H.: Mesolimbic and mesocortical dopamine activation induced by phencyclidine: Contrasting pattern to striatal response. Eur. J. Pharmacol. 134: 257-264, 1987.

Domino, E.F., Chodoff, P. and Corssen, G.: Pharmacologic effects of CI-581, a new dissociative anesthetic in man. Clin. Pharmacol. Ther. 6: 279-291, 1965.

Finnegan, K.T., Kanner, M.I., and Meltzer, H.Y.: Phencyclidine-induced rotational behavior in rats with nigrostriatal lesions and its modulation by dopaminergic and cholinergic agents. Pharmacol. Biochem. Behav. 5: 651-656, 1976.

Freeman, A.S. and Bunney, B.S.: The effects of phencyclidine and N-allylnormetazocine on midbrain dopamine neuronal activity. Eur. J. Pharmacol. 104: 287-293, 1984.

Freeman, A.S. and Bunney, B.S.: Activity of A9 and A10 dopaminergic neurons in unrestrained rats: Further characterization and effects of apomorphine and cholecystokinin. Brain Res. 405: 46-55, 1987.

French, E.D.: Effects of phencyclidine on ventral tegmental A10 dopamine neurons in the rat. Neuropharmacol. 25: 241-248, 1986.

French, E.D., Pilapil, C. and Quirion, R: Phencyclidine binding sites in the nucleus accumbens and phencyclidine induced hyperactivity are decreased following lesions of the mesolimbic dopamine system. Eur. J. Pharmacol. 116: 1-9, 1985.

Grace, A.A. and Bunney, B.S.: The control of firing pattern in nigral dopamine neurons: Burst-firing. J. Neurosci. 4: 2877-2890, 1984.

Guyenet, P.G. and Aghajanian, G.K.: Antidromic identification of dopaminergic and other output neurons of the substantia nigra. Brain Res. 150: 69-84, 1978.

Kelland, M.D., Freeman, A.S., and Chiodo, L.A.: SKF 38393 alters the rate-dependent D2-mediated inhibition of nigrostriatal but not mesoaccumbens dopamine neurons. Synapse 2: 416-423, 1988.

Kelland, M.D., Freeman, A.S., and Chiodo, L.A.: Chloral hydrate anesthesia alters the responsiveness of identified midbrain dopamine neurons to dopamine agonist administration. Synapse 3: 30-37, 1989.

Marwaha, J.: Candidate mechanisms underlying phencyclidine-induced psychosis: An electrophysiological, behavioral, and biochemical study. Biol. Psychiat. 17: 155-198, 1982.

Mereu, G., Casu, M., and Gessa, G.L.: (-)- Sulpiride activates the firing rate and tyrosine hydroxylase activity of dopaminergic neurons in unanesthetized rats. Brain Res. 264: 105-110, 1983.

Mereu, G., Fanni, G., and Gessa, G.L.: General anesthetics prevent dopaminergic neuron stimulation by neuroleptics. In Catecholamines, Part B: Neuropharmacology and Central Nervous System-Theoretical aspects, ed. by E. Usdin, A. Carlsson, A. Dahlström, and J. Engel, pp. 353-358, Alan R. Liss, Inc., New York, 1984.

Miyasaka, M. and Domino. E.F.: Neuronal mechanisms of ketamine-induced anesthesia. Int. J. Neuropharmacol. 7: 557-573, 1968.

Myslobodsky, M., Ackermann, R.F., Mansour, R. and Golovchinsky, V: Ketamine-induced rotation and its interaction with naloxone in rats. Brain Res. 172: 191-195, 1979.

Nabeshima, T., Hiramatsu, M., Amano, M., Furukawa, H., and Kameyama, T.. Effects of acute and chronic administration of phencyclidine on the levels of dopamine and metabolites in discrete brain areas of mouse. Res. Comm. Sub. Abuse 4: 273-286, 1983a.

Nabeshima, T., Yamada, K., Yamaguchi, K., Hiramatsu, M., Furukawa, H., and Kameyama, T.: Effect of lesions in the striatum, nucleus accumbens and medial raphe on phencyclidine induced stereotyped behaviors and hyperactivity in rats. Eur. J. Pharmacol. 91: 455-462, 1983b.

Nabeshima, T., Yamaguchi, K., Yamada, K., Hiramatsu, M., Furukawa, H., and Kameyama, T.: Phencyclidine-induced stereotyped behaviors in rats following specific neurotoxin lesions of the striatum. Eur. J. Pharmacol. 93: 229-234, 1983c.

Paxinos, G. and Watson, C.: The Rat Brain in Stereotaxic Coordinates, 2nd Ed., Academic Press, New York, 1986.

Raja, S.N. and Guyenet, P.G.: Effects of phencyclidine on the spontaneous activity of monoaminergic neurons. Eur. J. Pharmacol. 63: 229-233, 1980.

Scarnati, E., Campana, E., and Pacitti, C.: Pedunculopontine evoked excitation of substantia nigra neurons in the rat. Brain Res. 304: 351-361, 1984.

Scarnati, E., Proia, A., Campana, E., and Pacitti, C.: A microiontophoretic study on the nature of the putative synaptic neurotransmitter involved in the pedunculopontine-substantia nigra pars compacta excitatory pathway of the rat. Exp. Brain Res. 62: 470-478, 1986.

Schlemmer, Jr., R.F., Jackson, J.A., Preston, K.L., Bederka, Jr., J.P., Garver, D.L., and Davis, J.M.: Phencyclidine induced stereotyped behavior in monkeys: Antagonism by pimozide. Eur. J. Pharmacol. 52: 379-384, 1978.

Virtue, R.W., Alanis, J.M., Mori. M., Lafargue, R.T., Vogel, J.H.K.,and Metcalf, D.R.: An anesthetic agent: 2-orthochloro-phenyl, 2-methylamino cyclohexanone HCl (CI-581). Anesthesiol. 28: 823-833, 1967.

Status of Ketamine in Anesthesiology,
edited by E.F. Domino©1990, NPP Books
P.O. Box 1491, Ann Arbor, MI 48106

Effects of Ketamine on Electromyographic Responses Following Transcranial Magnetic Stimulation in Primates

R.F. Ghaly, J.L. Stone and J. A. Aldrete

Department of Anesthesiology and Critical Care, Division of Neurosurgery/ Department of Surgery, Cook Country Hospital and Hektoen Institute for Medical Research, Chicago, IL

Introduction

Electromyographic (EMG) response recording after transcranial magnetic stimulation (TMS) is a new clinical tool for testing the descending motor pathways of the nervous system (Barker *et al.*, 1985; Levy, 1987). Extracranial stimulation to produce motor evoked potentials (MEPs) can be accomplished using either a pulsed electric current or a pulsed magnetic field (Barker *et al.*, 1985; Levy, 1987). Magnetic stimulation is preferred over electrical stimulation because the former is electrodeless, painless, and appears noninjurious (Barker *et al.*, 1985). Anesthetic agents are known to variably suppress sensory evoked potentials (Grundy, 1985). In order to study the utility of MEPs following TMS under anesthesia, we decided to investigate the effects of incremental doses of ketamine on magnetic induced MEPs in primates. We wanted to examine if ketamine, which is known to produce motor system activation, will potentiate and hence maintain measurable MEP responses during deep anesthesia. The present study investigated the cumulative dose effect of ketamine on MEPs after TMS in primates.

Materials and Methods

Ten normal cynomolgus monkeys (Macaca fuscata) weighing 5 to 6 kg were used in this experiment. After premedication with atropine (0.04 mg/kg), all animals were intubated following ketamine HCl 10 mg/kg i.m. and ventilated with room air. Electrocardiogram, arterial blood pressure, rectal temperature and endtidal CO_2 were continuously monitored. A peripheral i.v. catheter was inserted. The core temperature was maintained at 36.5-37°C and endtidal CO_2 was at 34-45 mm Hg. EMG responses were recorded from the distal forelimb and hindlimb flexor muscles using Grass needle EEG electrodes and a Nicolet Pathfinder II unit. The active electrode was placed s.c. at the muscle site and the reference electrode 7 cm distally. The filter settings were 150 Hz-8 KHz. Novametrix Mag-Stim 200 was used for TMS, producing a maximum magnetic power of 1.5 Tesla via a flat coil. The stimulating coil was positioned over the animal's head (as described previously by Ghaly *et al.*, 1988) such that a potential of maximal amplitude could be recorded. When the animal was lightly anesthetized, baseline EMG responses were recorded following 1.5 Tesla TMS. The threshold for forelimb and hindlimb muscle excitation was also identified. Eight incremental ketamine doses (50 mg/kg total dose) were administered with 15 to 20 min between each dose. After 5 to 8 min of each ketamine dose injection, the EMG responses were recorded and magnetic intensity threshold was determined. The EMG tracings were stored on floppy disks and printed on paper. The peak latency and peak-to-peak amplitude of EMG waveforms were studied using one way analysis of variance (ANOVA) with repeated measures and Dunnett's posthoc test. The dose response relationship was examined utilizing linear regression analysis. Statistical significance was defined for P values <0.05. All animals were observed for gross neurological, behavioral, or seizure disorders over a one year period.

Results

EMG responses from the upper and lower limb following TMS were consistently recorded in all animals under various ketamine doses (Fig. 1). The baseline threshold intensity was 0.76 Tesla (± 0.08) for forelimb and 0.88 Tesla (± 0.014) for hindlimb muscles. There were no significant changes noted following ketamine injections. The optimal scalp stimulation site was unchanged during ketamine anesthesia. Significant latency prolongation was observed after administration of >20 mg/kg total ketamine dose, and was dose dependent (Fig. 2). Amplitude depression was noted after a ketamine dose of ≥ 15 mg/kg, but was not statistically significant (Fig. 2). The technique was well tolerated by all animals with no gross complications noted.

Discussion

The present study demonstrated that EMG responses following TMS were well preserved during deep ketamine anesthesia (50 mg/kg total

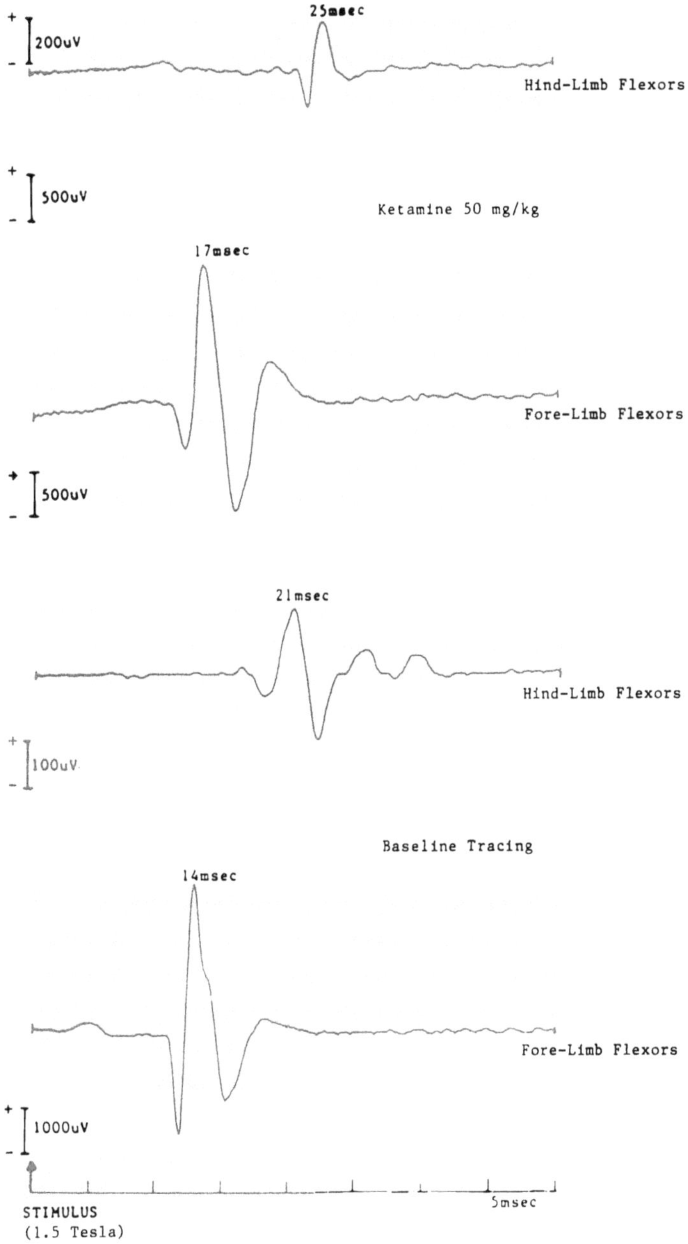

Fig. 1. Contralateral EMG waveforms recorded from the forelimb and hindlimb flexor muscles in response to transcranial magnetic stimulation in a monkey before (bottom) and after receiving ketamine 50 mg/kg i. v. total cumulative dose (top).

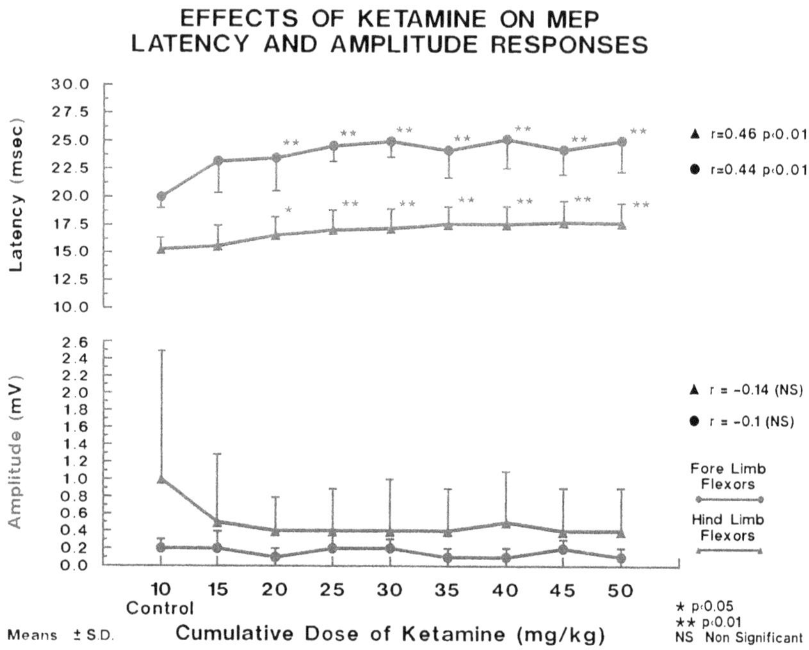

Fig. 2. Cumulative dose effects of ketamine on extracranial magnetic induced motor evoked potentials (MEPs) in primates using 1.5 Tesla.

dose). This effect may indeed reflect the state of motor neuronal excitability induced by ketamine (Kayama and Iwama, 1972; Massopust *et al.*, 1972; Winters *et al.*, 1972). Massopust *et al.* (1972) reported that ketamine induced excitatory effects on the extrapyramidal and limbic systems in monkeys with some enhancement of spontaneous electrical activity. Kayama and Iwama (1972) found that ketamine potentiated the electric shock induced evoked potential of the sensorimotor cortex in cats. Ketamine can produce spontaneous head, ocular, and extremity movements. Zsigmond and Domino (1980) observed an increase in muscle tone and catecholamine release following ketamine, in contrast to marked depression by thiamylal sodium injection.

We demonstrated in a previous study that thiamylal, which is a central depressant agent, caused a detrimental effect on MEP in contrast to ketamine (Ghaly *et al.*, 1988). Therefore, we postulate that ketamine maintains the excitability of motor neuronal pathways to electrical and magnetic stimulation, possibly through its stimulant effect on the motor system. It seems from this study that ketamine is an excellent anesthetic supplement to be used when intraoperative MEP recording is desired. Ketamine doses ≤20 mg/kg produced minimal alteration of the MEP responses. The technique appears to be safe and simple in the subhuman primate model. Although we feel this is a step towards noninvasive intraoperative MEP utilization, further observations are needed before it is applicable to humans.

ACKNOWLEDGEMENTS

The authors wish to extend their very appreciative and sincere thanks to Lisa for preparation of this manuscript.

REFERENCES

Barker, A.T. and Jalinous, R.: Non-invasive magnetic stimulation of human motor cortex. Lancet 1: 1106-1107, 1985.

Ghaly, R.F., Stone, J.L. and Adrete, J.A.: Motor evoked potentials (MEP) following transcranial magnetic stimulation in monkeys anesthetized with nitrous oxide, ketamine, and thiamylal sodium. Anesthesiol. 69: A606, 1988.

Grundy, B.L.: Evoked potential monitoring. In Monitoring in Anesthesia and Critical Care Medicine, ed. by C.D. Blitt, pp 345-411, Churchill Livingstone, New York, 1985.

Kayama, Y. and Iwama, K.: The EEG, evoked potentials, and single-unit activity during ketamine anesthesia in cats. Anesthesiol. 36: 316-328, 1972.

Levy, W.J.: Clinical experience with motor and cerebellar evoked potential monitoring. Neurosurg. 20: 169-182, 1987.

Massopust, L.C., Wolin, L.R., and Albin, M.S.: Electrophysiologic and behavioral responses to ketamine hydrochloride in the rhesus monkey. Anesth. Analg. 51: 329-341, 1972.

Winters, W.D., Ferrar-Allado, T., Flores, C.G. and Alcaraz, M.: The cataleptic state induced by ketamine: A review of the neuropharmacology of anesthesia. Neuropharmacol. 11: 304-315, 1972.

Zsigmond, E.K. and Domino, E.F.: Clinical pharmacology and current uses of ketamine. In: Trends in Intravenous Anesthesia, ed. by J.A. Aldrete and T.H. Stanley, pp 283-328, Year Book Medical Publisher, Chicago London, 1980.

Status of Ketamine in Anesthesiology,
edited by E.F. Domino©1990, NPP Books
P.O. Box 1491, Ann Arbor, MI 48106

Ketamine Analgesia in Rats May Be Mediated by an Interaction with Opiate Receptors

D.J. Smith, G.M. Pekoe, P.J. Monroe, L.L. Martin, M.E.Y. Cabral and T. Crisp

Departments of Anesthesiology and Pharmacology
West Virginia University Health Sciences Center
Morgantown, WV

Ketamine produces an analgesic response in rodents that is detectable using a variety of nociceptive tests. These include the writhing test (Ryder *et al.*, 1978; Wiley and Downs, 1982), tail flick test initiated either by hot water (Lakin and Winters, 1978; Lawrence and Livingston, 1980) or by radiant heat (Fratta *et al.*, 1980; Pekoe and Smith, 1982; Smith *et al.*, 1980; Wiley and Downs, 1982), and the hot plate test (Vargiu *et al.*, 1978). It appears that the analgesia is mediated, in part, by neuronal opioid systems. Not only has ketamine analgesia been found to be sensitive to the narcotic antagonist, naloxone (Fig. 1A and B), but it has also been demonstrated that in mice the development of tolerance to the opioid receptor mediated analgesic effect of morphine results in cross tolerance to ketamine (Finck *et al.*, 1988). On the other hand, opioid mechanisms may not be the only CNS processes involved in ketamine's antinociceptive action. Some investigators (Fratta *et al.*, 1980; Wiley and Downs, 1982) found it difficult to antagonize ketamine analgesia with narcotic antagonists, while others have shown that, in addition to opioid antagonists, antagonists of other neurotransmitter systems attenuate analgesia (Pekoe and Smith, 1982). Given the wide variety of neurotransmitter systems affected by this complex drug (White *et al.*, 1982; this volume), it is not surprising that ketamine may involve several neuronal systems in its actions, and that perhaps some differences may be observed as a consequence of the balance between such systems in various experimental models. However, in this report, only the evidence for an opioid link in ketamine's analgesic action is reviewed.

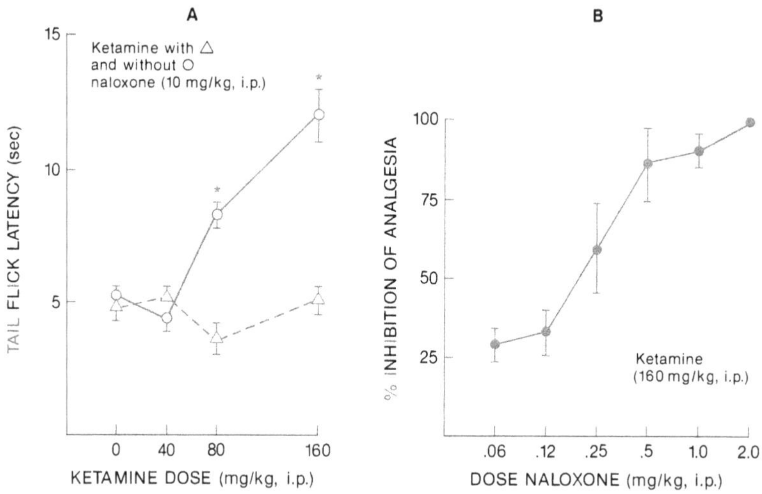

Fig. 1. Ketamine's analgesic action is inhibited by narcotic antagonists. Analgesia is defined as an increase in the latency of the tail flick reflex initiated by exposure of the tail to heat from a light source. In most studies in this report, a Model 33 Analgesia Meter (IITC, Inc., Landing, NJ) was used; the rat's tail was blackened with India ink, and a 10 sec cut off time was used. In panel A, 15 sec was used as the cut off time. Naloxone was administered 10 min prior to ketamine, and the tail flick latency was determined 5-10 min post ketamine when the response is maximal.

Unlike its antinociceptive action, the anesthetic action of ketamine does not appear to involve opioid mechanisms and is not altered by narcotic antagonists. Smith *et al.* (1985) have found that while the influence of ketamine on the latency of tail flick reflex (TFL) is reversed by the administration of naloxone, this narcotic antagonist does not affect the duration of the loss of the righting reflex (Table 1), nor is the qualitative appearance of anesthetic depth changed. Others have found, however, that ketamine anesthesia may be attenuated by a variety of non-opioid neurochemicals including, 1) adrenergic drugs (Hatch and Ruch, 1974), 2) thyrotropin releasing hormone (Bhargava, 1981), and 3) cholinergic agonists (cholinesterase inhibitors, Lawrence and Livingston, 1979; Leeuwin *et al.*, 1984). Thus, it seems that the neurochemical basis for the anesthetic effect of ketamine is clearly dissociable from its opioid mediated analgesic action.

Several studies, using radioligand binding assays and rat brain membranes, have provided evidence to suggest that ketamine's opioid actions may be associated with a direct interaction of the drug with opioid recep-

TABLE 1. Influence of naloxone on ketamine analgesia[a] and anesthesia[b]

	Ketamine (160 mg/kg, i.p.)	*Ketamine and Naloxone (3 mg/kg, i.p.)*
Predrug (TFL in sec)	2.69 ± 0.14	2.60 ± 0.09
Postdrug (TFL at 14 min)	6.14 ± 1.2*	3.72 ± 0.66**
Righting reflex (duration in min)	61.80 ± 9.0	75.00 ± 3.90

[a]Ketamine and naloxone were administered simultaneously, and the tail flick test was conducted 15 min later. N = 9 animals in each group.
[b]Anesthesia was defined as a loss of righting reflex.
*Significantly elevated over predrug (baseline) TFL ($P < 0.05$).
**Significantly less than postdrug latency in animals receiving ketamine alone ($P < 0.05$).

tors. Finck and Ngai (1982) and Smith *et al.* (1980, 1987) have shown that ketamine effectively competes with binding sites labeled by a variety of ^{3}H opioid ligands including ^{3}H-naloxone, dihydromorphine, ethylketocyclazocine, [D-Ala^2,D-Leu^5]enkephalin, and racemic N-allylnormetazocine (Fig. 2 and Table 2). Compared to classical narcotics like morphine that have binding affinities in the nM range, ketamine exhibits a weak affinity with K_i's in the mid μM range.

The interaction of ketamine with opioid binding sites labeled by ^{3}H-naloxone was stereospecific with the levorotatory free base from an enriched mixture of the isomers (*i.e.*, contained ≥80% levorotatory ketamine and the remainder as the dextrorotatory isomer) exhibiting an IC_{50}

TABLE 2. Inhibitory binding affinity constants (K_i) for ketamine and morphine at sites for various opioid radioligands

	Ki values[a]	
	Ketamine	*Morphine*
[^{3}H]dihydromorphine	26.8 ± 2.7 μM	2.7 ± 0.3 nM
[^{3}H]DADLE	101.0 ± 9.0 μM**	10.0 ± 0.6 nM**
[^{3}H]ethylketocyclazocine	85.2 ± 26.0 μM	—
[^{3}H]N-allylnormetazocine	66.0 ± 10.0 μM	5.6 ± 1.9 nM[b] 106.0 ± 75.0 μM

[a]K_i, inhibitory binding affinity constants obtained from competitive binding curves analyzed by LIGAND (Munson and Rodbard, 1980). Values were derived from at least 5 experiments run in triplicate and are presented with ± S.E.
[b]Biphasic displacement curve was observed with a B_{max} for the high affinity site of 14.7 ± 2.4 fmol/mg tissue and the low affinity site of 6.3 ± 0.86 fmol/mg tissue.
**Value is significantly different ($P < 0.05$) from the value obtained for the inhibition of [^{3}H]dihydromorphine.

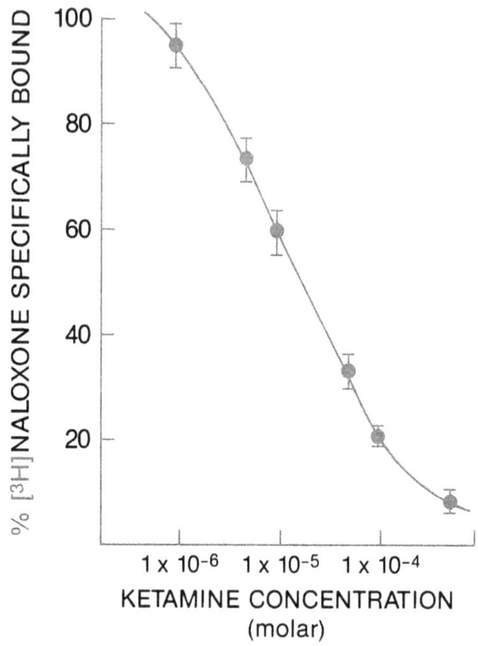

Fig. 2. Ketamine competes for opioid binding sites. Assay was conducted by adding 1.8 ml of a brain [brain-cerebellum] membrane fraction in 0.05 M Tris-HCl buffer (pH 7.7) to tubes containing 0.05 ml of [^{3}H]naloxone (1.4 nM final concentration), 0.05 ml of the appropriate drug dilution and additional buffer to bring the final volume to 2 ml. Levallorphan (1 μM) was used to determine the degree of nonspecific [^{3}H]naloxone binding. All tubes were incubated at 25°C for 20 min.

of 7.0 ± 0.98 μM, while the dextrorotatory enriched mixture had an IC_{50} of 23.8 ± 1.7 μM (Smith *et al.*, 1980). Furthermore, ketamine's interaction with these sites was found to be sensitive to the sodium ion, with the drug's potency being reduced 6 fold by the inclusion of 100 mM Na^+ in the incubation medium. This "sodium shift" was intermediate between that reported for opioid agonists (> 16) and antagonists (0). It is indicative of the interaction of partial opioid agonists or compounds that have prominent *kappa* or *sigma* opioid receptor activity with opioid receptors (Chang *et al.*, 1980).

Regardless of its weak affinity at opioid receptors, ketamine has been found to effectively compete in rats for opioid binding sites labeled *in vivo* by ^{3}H-naloxone (Smith *et al.*, 1987). Analgesic doses (80-120 mg/kg) of the drug administered i.p. produced a dose dependent inhibition of

TABLE 3. Ketamine competes for [^{3}H]naloxone binding *in vivo*[c]

Dose (mg/kg,i.p.)	*Specific binding[b] of [^{3}H]naloxone (1μg/kg)* Brain (-cerebellum)	*Spinal Cord*	*Cerebellum (nonspecific)[a]*
Saline	673 ± 96	308 ± 70	628 ± 52
40	703 ± 81	294 ± 44	635 ± 30
80	530 ± 74	244 ± 48	556 ± 40
120	459 ± 71**	172 ± 38**	562 ± 39
160	528 ± 104	180 ± 39**	613 ± 74

[a]The accumulation of [^{3}H]naloxone was not reduced by excess (1 mg) cold naloxone, and cerebellum was used as non-specific binding.
[b]Specific binding (fmol radioligand/g tissue).
[c][^{3}H]naloxone, 1μg/kg (30 mCi/kg) was administered via the tail vein. Tissue was homogenized 15 min later in 1.0 N HCl. Supernatants were assayed for tritium. Ketamine was simultaneously administered (i.p.) with the radioligand (i.v.).

^{3}H-naloxone binding in both brain and spinal cord tissue (Table 3). In the brain, the reduction was most marked in the hippocampus, thalamus, striatum and cortex. It was also shown that these doses of ketamine yielded concentrations in brain and spinal cord that were in the range required to compete for opioid binding *in vitro* (Smith *et al.*, 1987). For example, a 120 mg/kg dose i.p. resulted in a peak accumulation that occurred at 15 min postinjection. The value was about 50 μg/g in both brain and spinal cord and was calculated to be about 200 μM, assuming equal distribution, and 1 gm of tissue being equivalent to 1 ml volume. Thus, even with its weak potency, ketamine reaches concentrations *in vivo* that should be sufficient to cause analgesia via opioid receptor interactions.

In order to verify that the interaction of ketamine at opioid receptors would result in the initiation of an opioid receptor mediated response, the drug was studied in the longitudinal smooth muscle-myenteric plexus preparation of the guinea pig ileum, a bioassay system for opiates. Smith *et al.* (1982) determined that similar to morphine, ketamine produced a concentration dependent inhibition of the electrically induced twitch response of the ileum (Fig. 3). The inhibition was attenuated by naloxone, but the antagonist appeared to be about 3 times less effective against ketamine than it was against morphine. For example, the concentration of ketamine required for 50% inhibition of the response in the absence of naloxone was 68.9 ± 5.9 μM. In the presence of a fixed concentration of naloxone (10 nM), the IC_{50} for ketamine was about 3 times greater, while morphine was required in concentrations that were 8 times higher.

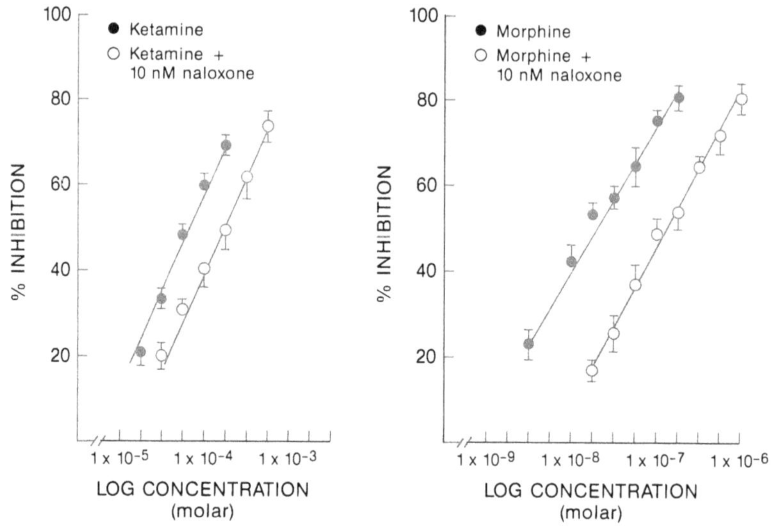

Fig. 3. Inhibitory action of ketamine and morphine in the ileum: Reversibility by naloxone. Inhibition of the electrically induced contraction of the longitudinal muscle-myenteric plexus preparation of the guinea pig ileum. The tissue was bathed in Kreb's solution, and a concentration inhibition curve to drug was obtained. The tissue was then bathed in Kreb's solution containing 10 nM naloxone, and the exposure to drug was repeated 1 hr later. After rinsing the tissue in Kreb's solution without naloxone (30 min - 1 hr), a single concentration of drug was tested to verify tissue responsiveness. The data are expressed as mean ± S.E. of 8 experiments.

Finck and Ngai (1982) extended these observations by determining that the action of ketamine in the ileum was stereospecific, with the levorotatary free base being most effective. They also demonstrated that only the levorotatory isomer was reversible by naloxone. Moreover, the nonopioid action of the dextrorotatory isomer of ketamine on the contractile response may have been associated with a mild nonspecific depressant action of the drug on the ileum. In support of this suggestion, Smith's group observed an inhibition of contractile responses to ACh and histamine when 1 mM racemic ketamine was used.

Several attempts have been made to distinguish sites in the rat central nervous system that may be associated with the opioid mediated analgesic action of ketamine (Pekoe and Smith, 1982; Smith *et al.*, 1985; Tung and Yaksh, 1981). Intrathecal (i.t.) administration of the drug in doses ranging from 0.3-3.0 μmols has been shown to induce a naloxone reversible analgesic effect that was clearly detected using the rat tail flick test (Figs.

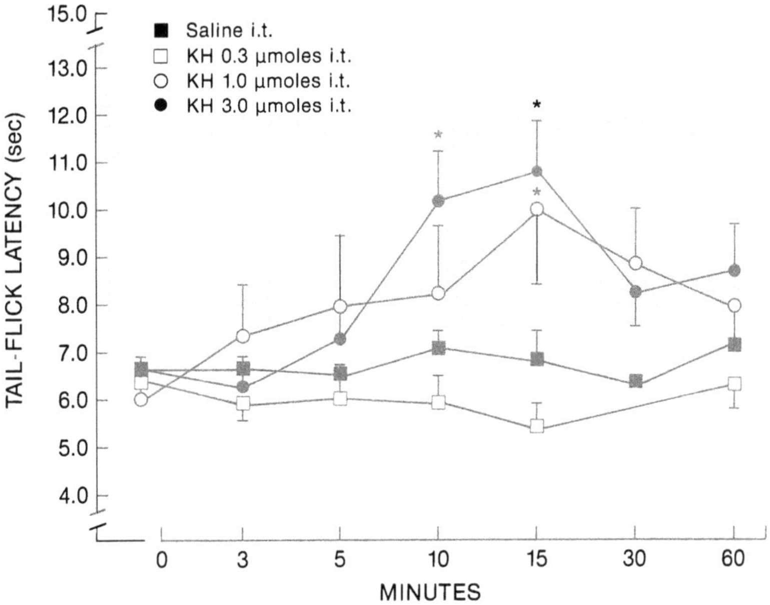

Fig. 4. Ketamine produces an analgesic reaction when administered intrathecally. Ketamine was administered in 10 μl of saline followed by a 5 μl saline flush using an infusion pump. A predrug baseline and postdrug cut off of 6-7 and 15 sec was used, respectively.

4 and 5). Doses of naloxone required to inhibit the effect of ketamine were greater [IC_{50} (C.I.); 1.48 (0.16-8.80) mg/kg, s.c.] than those needed to antagonize 10 nmols of i.t. morphine [0.025 (0.0037-0.106)mg/kg, s.c.], perhaps suggesting that ketamine produces its effect through interaction with an opioid receptor other than the one preferred by morphine. This observation is consistent with results obtained in the ileum, where naloxone was also less effective against ketamine than it was against morphine (Fig. 4). Moreover, unlike morphine, ketamine has been found to be ineffective as an agonist when administered supraspinally by either i.c.v. administration (10 μmols) or by microinjection (0.3 μmols) into the opioid-sensitive periaqueductal gray (PAG) region of the rat brain. On the other hand, it was found to act antagonistically to morphine in the PAG where it appears that *mu* opioid receptors (Smith *et al.*, 1988; Jensen and Yaksh, 1986) may be responsible for the analgesic actions of narcotics.

The naloxone reversibility of ketamine's actions in the intact rat and in the guinea pig ileum, as well as in the rat spinal cord, is compelling evidence that opioid receptor interactions are involved in the analgesic response to the anesthetic. On the other hand, several lines of evidence

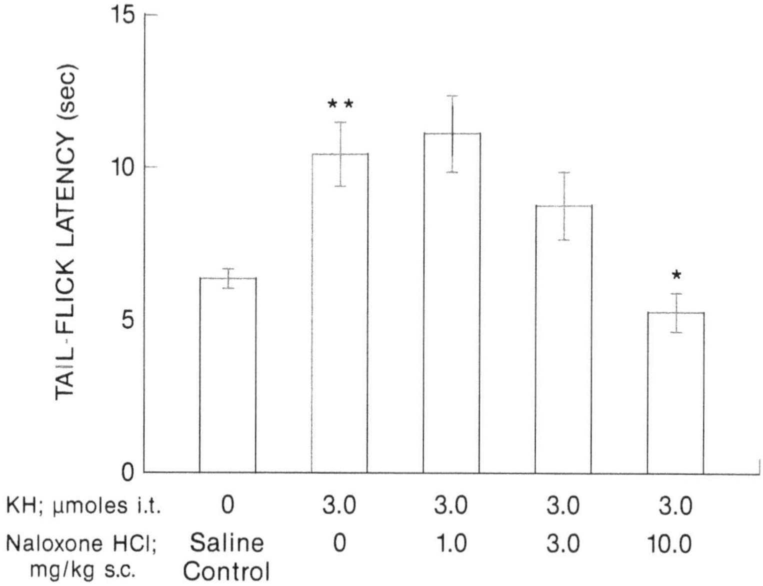

Fig. 5. Ketamine's spinal cord action is reversible by naloxone. Naloxone (s.c.) and ketamine (i.t.) were administered simultaneously, and the tail flick test was conducted 15 min later.

lead to the conclusion that the opioid receptor involved is not the same type as that activated by narcotics like morphine. Firstly, the apparent difference in the potency of naloxone as an antagonist of ketamine compared to morphine strongly suggests that the receptors involved differ in their affinity for the antagonist. Thus, at least two separate receptor populations would seem to be mediating the individual responses to these two types of opioid agonists. Secondly, the inability of ketamine to induce analgesia by an action in the PAG may indicate that it has limited agonistic actions at the *mu* receptor subtype through which morphine like narcotics act and which appears to be the only subtype involved in the activation of descending pain inhibitory pathways from this brain site (Smith *et al.*, 1988). In fact, the antagonistic action of ketamine against morphine may indicate that it acts primarily as an antagonist at *mu* sites. This inhibitory effect may be similar to that observed with several other opioid analgesics that seem to have agonist actions through other opioid receptor subtypes (*i.e.*, benzomorphans at *kappa* and *sigma* opioid receptors) yet act as antagonists or, at best, partial agonists at *mu* sites.

The type of opioid receptor associated with ketamine's actions is yet to be determined. However, some evidence is accumulating to suggest that a *kappa* site could be involved. This includes the prominent spinal component in the action of the drug and a "Na shift" in radioligand binding assays that is in the range observed for *kappa* drugs like ethylketocyclazocine. In addition, the inability of ketamine to antagonize the action of morphine in the ileum is also a characteristic shared by *kappa* drugs (Hutchinson *et al.*, 1975). Antagonism of morphine by ketamine in the PAG but not in the ileum is not as inconsistent as it may appear, since the *mu* subtype involved in the response to morphine in the ileum may be a mu_2 (Gintzler and Pasternak, 1983) and unaffected by ketamine whereas the type in the PAG appears to be a mu_1 subtype (Bodnar *et al.*, 1987).

In conclusion, although opioid receptors appear linked to ketamine analgesia in the rodent, additional studies will be necessary to define the subtype involved and its locations within the central nervous system.

Acknowledgements

The authors would like to thank Jeanette Perrotti, Jay Amedro, Jim Adams, Joannie Scalzitti, Rena Bouchal, and Amy Mansell for their excellent technical assistance in various phases of this research. Appreciation is also extended to Richette Sigley for preparation of the manuscript. This work was supported in part by NIH grant GM 30002, NIH 5 T 32 GM 07039 and the Department of Anesthesiology.

References

Bhargava, H.N.: Antagonism of ketamine-induced anesthesia and hypothermia by thyrotropin releasing hormone and cyclo (hispro). Neuropharmacol. 20: 699-702, 1981.

Bodnar, R.J., Williams, C.L., Less, S.J. and Pasternak, G.W.: Role for the high affinity μ_1 opioid binding site in central opiate and opioid analgesia. Abstr. Soc. Neurosci. 13: 1016, 1987.

Chang, K.-J., Hazum, E. and Cuatrecasas, P.: Possible role of distinct morphine and enkephalin receptors in mediating actions of benzomorphan drugs (putative *kappa* and *sigma* agonists). Proc. Natl. Acad. Sci. USA 77: 4469-4473, 1980.

Finck, A.D. and Ngai, S.H.: Opiate receptor mediation of ketamine analgesia. Anesthesiol. 56: 291-297, 1982.

Finck, A.D., Samaniego, E. and Ngai, S.H.: Morphine tolerance decreases the analgesic effects of ketamine in mice. Anesthesiol. 68: 397-400, 1988.

Fratta, W., Casu, M., Balestrieri, A., Loviselli, A., Biggio, G. and Gessa, G.L.: Failure of ketamine to interact with opiate receptors. Eur. J. Pharmacol. 61: 389-391, 1980.

Gintzler, A.R. and Pasternak, G.W.: Multiple *mu* receptors: Evidence for mu_2 sites in the guinea pig ileum. Neurosci. Lett. 39: 51-56, 1983.

Hatch, R.C. and Ruch, T.: Experiments on antagonism of ketamine anesthesia in cats given adrenergic, serotonergic and cholinergic stimulants alone and in combination. Am. J. Vet. Res. 35: 35-39, 1974.

Hutchinson, R.C., Kosterlitz, H.W., Leslie, F.M., Waterfield, A.A., and Terenius, L.: Assessment in the guinea-pig ileum and mouse vas deferens of benzomorphans which have strong antinociceptive activity but do not substitute for morphine in the dependent monkey. Br. J. Pharmacol. 55: 541-546, 1975.

Jensen, T.S. and Yaksh, T.L.: Comparison of the antinociceptive action of the *mu* and *delta* opioid receptor ligands in the periaqueductal gray matter, medial and paramedial ventral medulla in the rat as studied by the microinjection technique. Brain Res. 372: 301-312, 1986.

Lakin, M.L. and Winters, W.D.: Behavioral correlates of naloxone inhibition of analgesia induced by various CNS excitatory drugs in rats. Proc. W. Pharmacol. Soc. 21: 27-30, 1978.

Lawrence, D. and Livingston, A.: The effect of physostigmine and neostigmine on ketamine anesthesia and analgesia. Br. J. Pharmacol. 67: 426P, 1979.

Lawrence, D. and Livingston, A.: A comparison of the analgesic activity of ketamine using two different methods of assessment. Br. J. Pharmacol. 70: 189P, 1980.

Leeuwin R.S., van der Wal, J.K. and Spanger, W.: Interactions of cholinesterase inhibitors and glucocorticoids with ketamine and pentobarbitone-induced general anesthesia in the rat: Possible effects on central cholinergic activity. Br. J. Pharmacol. 82: 339-347, 1984.

Munson, P.J. and Rodbard, D.: LIGAND: A versatile computerized approach for characterization of ligand binding systems. Analyt. Biochem. 107: 220-239, 1980.

Pekoe, G.M. and Smith, D.J.: The involvement of opiate and monoaminergic neuronal systems in the analgesic effects of ketamine. Pain 12: 57-73, 1982.

Ryder, S., Way, W.L. and Trevor, A.J.: Comparative pharmacology of the optical isomers of ketamine in mice. Eur. J. Pharmacol. 49: 15-23, 1978.

Smith, D.J., Bouchal, R.L., de Sanctis, C.A., Monroe, P.J., Amedro, J.B., Perrotti, J.M., and Crisp, T.: Properties of the interaction between ketamine and opiate binding sites *in vivo* and *in vitro*. Neuropharmacol. 26: 1253-1260, 1987.

Smith, D.J., Pekoe, G.M., Martin, L.L., and Coalgate, B.: The interaction of ketamine with the opiate receptor. Life Sci. 26: 789-795, 1980.

Smith, D.J., Perrotti, J.M., Crisp, T., Cabral, M.E.Y., Long, J.T., and Scalzitti, J.M.: The opiate receptor is responsible for descending pain inhibition originating in the periaqueductal gray region of the rat brain. Eur. J. Pharmacol. 156: 47-54, 1988.

Smith, D.J., Perrotti, J.M., Mansell, A.L., and Monroe, P.J.: Ketamine analgesia is not related to an opiate action in the periaqueductal gray region of the rat brain. Pain 21: 253-265, 1985.

Smith, D.J., Westfall, D.P., and Adams, J.D.: Assessment of the potential agonistic and antagonistic properties of ketamine at opiate receptors in the guinea-pig ileum. Neuropharmacol. 21: 605-611, 1982.

Tung, A.S. and Yaksh, T.L.: Analgesic effect of intrathecal ketamine in the rat. Reg. Anesth. 6: 91-94, 1981.

Vargiu, L., Stefanni, E., Musinu, C., and Saba, G.: Possible role of brain serotonin in the central effects of ketamine. Neuropharmacol. 17: 405-408, 1978.

White, P.F., Way, W.L., and Trevor, A.J.: Ketamine — its pharmacology and therapeutic use. Anesthesiol. 56: 119-136, 1982.

Wiley, J.N. and Downs, D.A.: Lack of antagonism by naloxone of the analgesic and locomotor stimulant actions of ketamine. Life Sci. 31: 1071-1075, 1982.

Status of Ketamine in Anesthesiology,
edited by E.F. Domino©1990, NPP Books
P.O. Box 1491, Ann Arbor, MI 48106

A Pharmacological Analysis of the Interaction of Ketamine with *Kappa* Opiates

K. Ramabadran*, M. Bansinath, H. Turndorf, and M.M. Puig

Department of Anesthesiology
New York University Medical Center
School of Medicine
New York, NY

Introduction

The anesthetic properties of ketamine, a phencyclidine derivative, differ from other general anesthetics and, hence, ketamine has been classified as a "dissociative anesthetic" (Corssen and Domino, 1966). Several *in vivo* studies have implicated opiate mechanisms in the mode of action of ketamine (Fidecka, 1987; Finck *et al.*, 1988; Smith *et al.*, 1980; Winters *et al.*, 1988). Most of these studies have used naloxone antagonism as the principal evidence to implicate opiate receptors. Both biochemical and behavioral evidence for the existence of multiple opiate receptors is now well established. Naloxone is more a *mu* rather than a *delta* or *kappa* receptor antagonist and has no effect on *sigma* receptors. The role of opiate receptor subtypes other than *mu* in the pharmacodynamics of ketamine has not been extensively investigated.

The results of *in vitro* radioligand binding study indicates that the order of affinity of ketamine for opiate binding sites is *mu* > *sigma* > *kappa* > *delta* (Smith *et al.*, 1987). Biochemical evidence also exists for a common *sigma* opiate and phencyclidine binding site (Zukin and Zukin, 1983). Furthermore, a moderate binding to *sigma* opiate sites for the putative *kappa* agonist, U-50488H has been shown (Tam, 1983). Taken together, these *in vitro* experiments suggest a possible *in vivo* interaction of ketamine and *kappa* opiates.

---

*Present address: Dept. 426, AP-9A, Abbott Laboratories, Abbott Park, IL 60064

The perioperative period, during which ketamine is clinically used, is often associated with altered glucose homeostasis. We have recently investigated the implications of hyperglycemia on the pharmacodynamics of opiates (Bansinath *et al.*, 1988, 1989a, b; Ramabadran *et al.*, 1989a,b). These results suggest that hyperglycemia significantly modifies the pharmacodynamics of opiates. Since opiate mechanisms are implicated in the mode of action of ketamine, an assessment of the role of hyperglycemia as a factor affecting the pharmacodynamics of ketamine is of specific interest.

This paper presents our preliminary results aimed at: 1) an analysis of the *in vivo* interactions of *kappa* opiates with ketamine, and 2) the evaluation of the thermonociceptive reactions as affected by ketamine in normoglycemic, acute and chronic hyperglycemic conditions.

Materials and Methods

Animals

Male Swiss Webster mice weighing 25-30 g (Taconic Farms, PA) were housed 5 per cage in a room with controlled temperature (22 ± 2°C), humidity, and artificial light (06:30-1900 hr). A minimum of 10 animals was used per group. The animals had free access to food and water, and were used after a minimum of 4 days acclimation to the housing conditions. To avoid the diurnal and seasonal variations, all experiments were conducted between 09:00 and 17:00 hr, March through May.

Hyperglycemic mice. Acute and chronic hyperglycemia were induced according to previously reported methods (Bansinath *et al.*, 1989a). Briefly, acute hyperglycemia was induced by i.p. dextrose (5 g/kg) injection along with s.c. ketamine injections. Chronic hyperglycemia (diabetes) was induced by an i.p. injection of 200 mg/kg streptozocin (Sigma Chemical Co., St. Louis, MO) dissolved in 0.01 M citrate buffer at a pH of 4.0-4.5 and administered 7-8 days before the experimental day. Control animals received vehicle alone. Blood samples were collected from the retro-orbital sinus to measure blood glucose levels. The induction of diabetes was confirmed by measurement of blood glucose levels with Ames Dextrostix and a reflectance colorimeter (Accu-chek II, Boehringer Mannheim Diagnostics, Indianapolis, IN). On the day of the experiment, streptozocin treated animals had blood sugar levels of 480 ± 20 mg/dl, while citrate buffer treated mice had sugar levels of 178 ± 15 mg/dl. At 10 min following dextrose injection, the time point at which post drug nociceptive reactions were assessed, the blood sugar levels were 320 ± 20 mg/dl.

Drugs

Ketamine hydrochloride, naloxone hydrochloride (Sigma Chemical Co., St. Louis, MO), *trans*-(+)-3,4-dichloro-N-methyl-[2-(1-pyrrolidinyl)cyclohexyl]-benzeneacetamide methane sulfonate hydrate (U-50488H; Upjohn Co., Kalamazoo, MI), (±)-*trans*-N-methyl-N-[2-(1-pyrrolidinyl)cyclohexyl[benzo[b]-thio-phene-4-acetamide (PD 117,302; Warner Lambert/Parke Davis, Ann Arbor, MI) were dissolved in sterile water just before use and were injected s.c. in a volume of 10 ml/kg. (-)-(1R,5R,9R)-5,9-Diethyl-2-(3-furylmethyl)-2'-hydroxy-6,7-benzomorphan (MR 2266; Boehringer Ingelheim, Ingelheim-am-Rhein, FRG) was dissolved in acidified pyrogen free water. Animals in the control group received the respective vehicle injections.

Hot plate test

A hot plate analgesia meter (model 35D, IITC, Landing, NJ) was used with its surface temperature maintained at 60 ± 0.5° C. Accuracy of the temperature setting was monitored and verified using a surface thermometer. After placing the mouse on the hot plate, the reaction times for paw licking and the escape attempt (jumping) were recorded in sec (Ramabadran *et al.*, 1989a). A cut off time of 120 sec was used.

Tail immersion test

The details of the tail immersion test procedure used were essentially similar to those published earlier (Ramabadran *et al.*, 1989c). Briefly, using a circulating immersion water heater (catalog #13-874-170, Fisher Scientific, Pittsburgh, PA), a constant temperature of 50 ± 0.2°C was maintained in the water bath in which the terminal 3 cm of the animal's tail was immersed. The nociceptive end point was characterized by a violent jerk of the tail (tail flick/withdrawal). During nociceptive reaction measurements, the animals were briefly immobilized (25-30 sec) by gentle wrapping in chux. Baseline latencies were determined twice, 5 min apart, and averaged to give a single predrug latency. Postdrug latencies were measured 10 min after ketamine injection. In order to minimize tissue injury due to repeated exposure of the heat stimulus, a cut off time of 15 sec was imposed. The postdrug latencies were calculated as a percentage of the respective animal's control latency.

Measurement of colonic temperature

The temperature measurements were done at an ambient temperature of 22 ± 0.2°C. Colonic temperatures of mice were measured using a telethermometer (Yellow Spring Instrument Inc. Model 43 TD, Yellow Springs, OH) and thermistor probe (Model #402). The probe was inserted 3.5 cm deep into the rectum and temperature was recorded when a constant reading was obtained (Bansinath *et al.*, 1986, 1989a). While the temperature measurements were made, the animals were gently restrained (45-60 sec) in chux. The predrug temperature for each mouse was measured twice, 15 min apart and the readings were averaged to obtain the basal temperature of the respective animal. The net change in temperature 30 min after drug administration was obtained by subtracting postdrug measurement for each mouse from its initial preinjection temperature.

Measurement of the duration of loss of righting reflex (LRR)

The method used to assess the duration of loss of righting reflex was essentially similar to that published earlier (Bansinath *et al.*, 1982a). In all three successive trials, the inability or ability of the animal to right itself within 5 sec when placed on its back was taken as the criterion for the loss and return of the righting reflex, respectively.

Measurement of gastrointestinal transit

Gastrointestinal transit was measured by the charcoal meal test as described previously (Bansinath *et al.*, 1988; Ramabadran *et al.*, 1988). Prior to testing, the animals were fasted for 20-24 hr with free access to water. They were given, soon after the s.c. drug administration, 0.25 ml of a suspension of charcoal meal (10% charcoal in 5% gum acacia). The animals were sacrificed 40 min later by cervical dislocation. The abdomen was opened and the intestine from the pyloric junction to the caecal end removed. The distance travelled by the charcoal meal as well as the total length of the intestine was measured. Gastrointestinal transit was expressed as the percentage of the distance travelled by the charcoal relative to the total length of the small intestine.

Maximal electroshock seizure (MES) test

The test procedure adopted was based on our earlier reports (Bansinath *et al.*, 1982b; Ramabadran *et al.*, 1980). Drug and test naive mice were used. Thirty min after ketamine administration and 15 min after naloxone or MR 2266 administration, the animals were subjected to trans-auricular MES (shock parameters: 150 V, 50 pulses per sec, 2 sec). The convulsive stimulus was delivered using a Grass stimulator (Model S48) coupled with a stimulus isolation unit (Model SIU 5A). A minimum of 30 mice were used for each treatment group. Absence of the tonic hindlimb extension was considered as the criterion of protection against MES. The percentage of animals protected after each treatment group was calculated.

Data analysis

The data are presented as group means (± S.E.). The statistical significance of the data was expressed by ANOVA followed by the Newman-Keuls test, where appropriate, using a computer program (CSS 1987). The ED_{50} and 95% confidence limits were calculated according to the method of Litchfield and Wilcoxon using a computer program (Tallarida and Murray, 1987).

RESULTS

Hot plate test

Dose effects of ketamine on jump latency are illustrated in Fig. 1. Ketamine injection resulted in significant changes in licking ($F_{5,107}$ = 10; P <0.0001) and jumping ($F_{5,107}$ = 40.1; P <0.0001) latencies when tested 10 min after the drug administration. Post hoc comparison indicated that 20 and 40 mg/kg doses of ketamine increased the jumping latency significantly (P <0.05), while only the highest dose of ketamine increased the

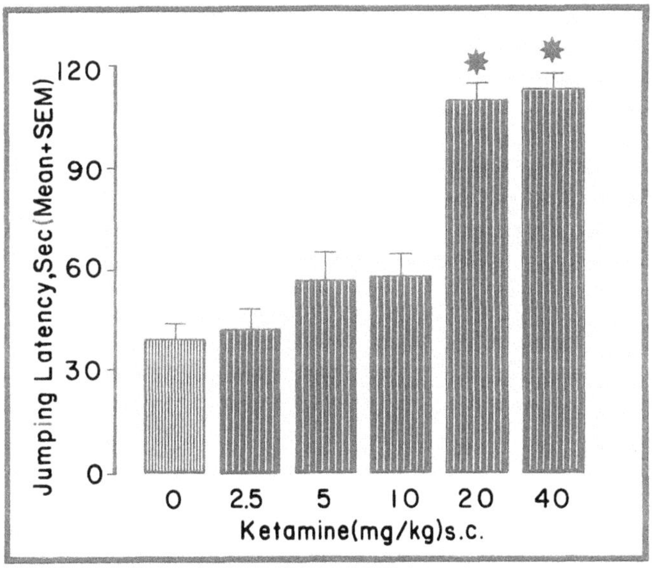

Fig. 1. Dose response relationship of ketamine on jumping latency in the hot plate test (60°C). *P <0.05 when compared with vehicle treated group (0). Each bar represents mean ± S.E. (N ≥ 10).

licking latency when compared to the vehicle treated group. When placed on the hot plate, the animals injected with ketamine in doses of 10 mg/kg and above elicited signs of exaggerated agitation, as manifested by aimless running along the wall of the restraining cylinder.

The effect of the combination of ketamine (10 and 20 mg/kg) and the *kappa* antagonist, MR 2266 (3 and 10 mg/kg), on jumping latency is shown in Fig. 2. ANOVA indicated a significant effect for the dose of ketamine ($F_{2,82}$ = 95.2; P <0.0001) but not for ketamine x MR 2266 interaction ($F_{4,82}$ = 0.55; P = 0.7).

The results of the effects of the combination of the *kappa* agonist, PD 117,302, with a subthreshold dose of ketamine (2.5 mg/kg) are presented in Table 1. The dose of PD 117,302 ($F_{3,72}$ = 7.2; P <0.0001) had a significant effect on the jumping latency. However, ketamine treatment did not influence the results ($F_{3,72}$ = 1.03; P = 0.4).

The effects of ketamine on the reaction latencies in normoglycemic, acute, and chronic hyperglycemic groups are presented in Table 2. ANOVA of the jumping latencies indicated significant effects for the dose of ketamine ($F_{5,231}$ = 52.6;P <0.0001) and the glycemic conditions ($F_{2,231}$

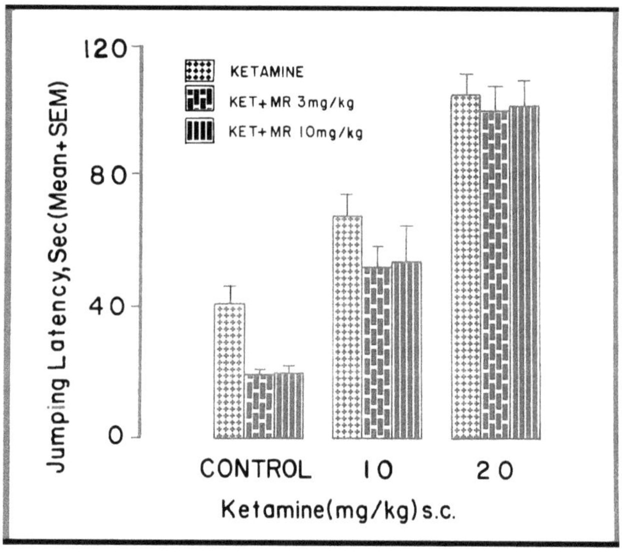

Fig. 2. Effects of MR 2266 (MR) and ketamine (KET) combination on jumping latency in the hot plate test. The increase in jumping latency in ketamine (10 and 20 mg/kg) treated groups are significantly (P <0.05) higher when compared with their respective controls.

TABLE 1. Comparison of the effects of PD 117,302 alone and its combination with ketamine in the hot plate test

Group	Dose mg/kg	N	Reaction Latency (sec) Licking	Jumping
PD 117,302				
	0	10	5.2±0.6	63.0±7.1
	1	10	5.7±0.7	58.9±6.8
	3	10	6.3±0.5	80.3±8.2
	10	10	12.6±1.5*	93.5±9.6*
PD 117,302 + Ketamine (2.5 mg/kg)				
	0	10	6.0±1.1	53.8±8.7
	1	10	5.4±0.7	68.7±8.8
	3	10	8.7±0.7	67.1±8.6
	10	10	22.2±2.6*	97.0±12*

*P <0.05 when compared with the respective control(0) group

TABLE 2. Comparison of the effects of ketamine in normoglycemic, acute and chronic hyperglycemic mice in the hot plate test

Group	Dose mg/kg	N	Reaction Latency (sec) Licking	Jumping
Normoglycemic				
	0	36	4.92 ± 0.22	39.57 ± 3.48
	2.5	15	4.56 ± 0.36	42.85 ± 5.29
	5	16	3.72 ± 0.24	57.20 ± 8.29
	10	15	4.16 ± 0.41	58.11 ± 6.18
	20	16	3.76 ± 0.21	110.83 ± 4.54*
	40	15	7.77 ± 1.04*	113.82 ± 4.23*
Acute Hyperglycemic				
	0	25	5.82 ± 0.39	57.20 ± 4.64
	2.5	10	4.21 ± 0.38	59.78 ± 9.71
	5	9	4.50 ± 0.34	75.58 ± 10.2
	10	10	3.60 ± 0.21	76.45 ± 10.3
	20	10	3.84 ± 0.40	111.50 ± 3.98*
	40	10	5.50 ± 0.40	119.50 ± 0.51*
Chronic Hyperglycemic				
	0	10	4.67 ± 0.37	55.70 ± 11.5
	2.5	10	4.63 ± 0.46	50.60 ± 9.33
	5	10	4.89 ± 0.32	58.30 ± 8.28
	10	11	4.57 ± 0.49	65.30 ± 9.95
	20	11	7.23 ± 1.57*	103.30 ± 5.55*
	40	10	11.54 ± 1.49*	115.40 ± 3.95*

*P<0.05 when compared with the respective control (0) group

= 5.7; $P < 0.005$). However, the ketamine dose x hyperglycemic condition interaction was not significant ($F_{10,231} = 0.6$; $P = 0.82$). In ketamine (20 and 40 mg/kg) treated mice, both licking and jumping reaction latencies were significantly ($P < 0.05$) increased when compared with respective controls.

Tail immersion test

Tail withdrawal latencies 10 min after injecting increasing doses of ketamine are depicted in Fig. 3. Ketamine significantly ($F_{5,87} = 7.8$; $P < 0.0001$) decreased the response latencies, and doses of 5 mg/kg and above produced tail rigidity.

The mean basal tail flick latencies in normoglycemic, acute, and chronic hyperglycemia mice are presented in Fig. 4. ANOVA indicated significant variation ($F_{2,210} = 14.2$; $P < 0.0001$) in the reaction latencies. The tail flick latencies were significantly lower ($P < 0.05$) in chronic hyperglycemic mice when compared with their normoglycemic counterparts.

The effects of ketamine on the reaction latencies in the normoglycemic, acute, and chronic hyperglycemic groups are presented in Table 3. ANOVA indicated a significant effect for the dose of ketamine ($F_{5,195} = 6.96$; $P < 0.0001$) and for the glycemic state ($F_{2,195} = 9.5$, $P < 0.0001$). However, the interaction of ketamine dose x glycemic state was

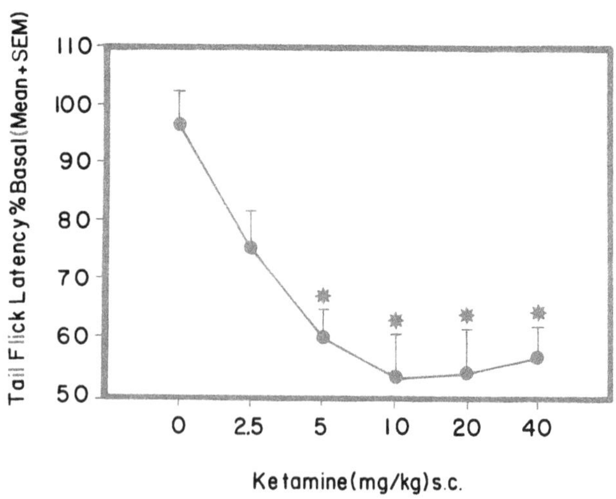

Fig. 3. Dose response relationship of ketamine on tail flick latency in the tail immersion test (50°C). *$P < 0.05$ when compared with vehicle treated group (0). Each bar represents mean ± S.E. (N≥10).

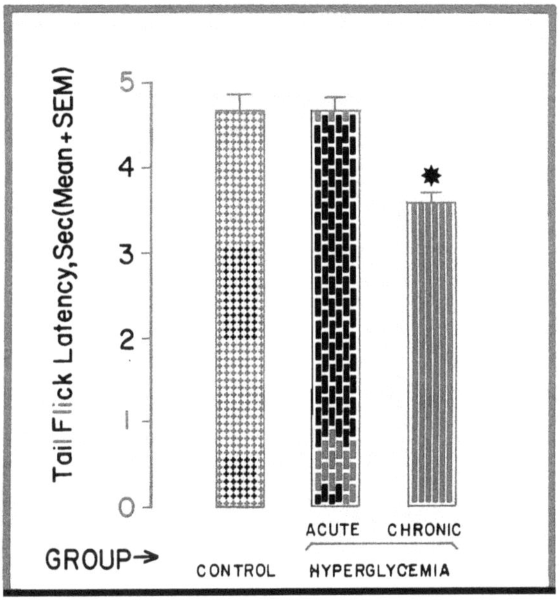

Fig. 4. Basal tail flick latency in normoglycemic controls, acute and chronic hyperglycemic groups. *P <0.05 when compared with normoglycemic controls. Each bar represents ± S.E. (N≥20).

not significant ($F_{10,195}$ = 0.82; P = 0.6). Post hoc comparison indicated that ketamine effects on tail flick reactions were attenuated in chronic hyperglycemic mice.

Effect on colonic temperature

The *kappa* agonist, PD 117,302 induced a dose related hypothermic response (Fig. 5). ANOVA indicated a significant effect for the dose of PD 117,302 ($F_{3,80}$ = 81.2; P <0.001), combination of ketamine (20 mg/kg; $F_{1,80}$ = 20.4; P <0.001) and for the interaction of dose of PD 117,302 x ketamine treatment ($F_{3,80}$ = 2.65; P < 0.05). The hypothermic response of the *kappa* agonist was augmented by ketamine.

The hypothermic response of U-50488H and the effect of the ketamine (20 mg/kg) combination on this response are shown in Table 4. ANOVA indicated a significant effect for the dose of U-50488H ($F_{3,72}$ = 10.4; P <0.0001) and for the interaction of ketamine x dose of the *kappa* agonist ($F_{3,72}$ = 8.5; P <0.0005). As with the results from PD 117,302 treated groups, ketamine treated mice showed an augmented hypothermic response to U-50488H.

TABLE 3. Comparison of the effects of ketamine in normoglycemic, acute, and chronic hyperglycemic mice in the tail immersion test

Group	*Dose mg/kg*	*N*	*Tail Flick Latency % of basal*
Normoglycemic	0	19	96.2 ± 6.1
	2.5	15	75.4 ± 6.2*
	5	15	60.0 ± 4.6*
	10	15	53.5 ± 7.2*
	20	15	53.9 ± 7.3*
	40	24	56.8 ± 5.0*
Acute Hyperglycemic	0	10	94.9 ± 12.6
	2.5	10	90.0 ± 10.9
	5	10	65.1 ± 13.6*
	10	10	46.3 ± 6.8*
	20	10	50.9 ± 7.1*
	40	10	53.6 ± 8.3*
Chronic Hyperglycemic	0	10	108.1 ± 14.9
	2.5	10	80.2 ± 12.0
	5	10	99.1 ± 15.4
	10	10	79.7 ± 15.1
	20	10	80.8 ± 12.2
	40	10	84.2 ± 10.0

*P <0.05 when compared with the respective control (0) group

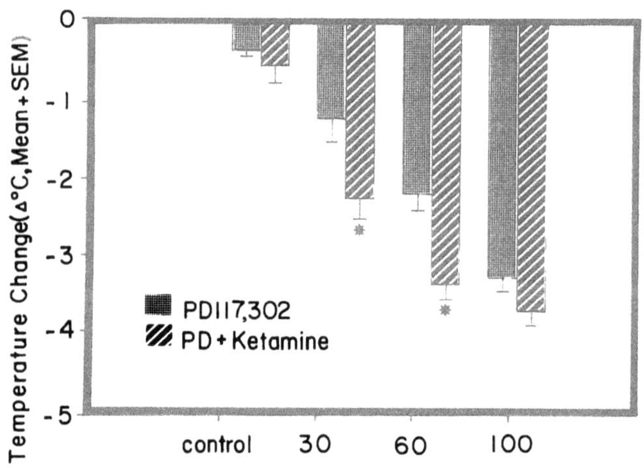

Fig. 5. Effects of PD 117,302 (PD 30, 60, 100 mg/kg) and ketamine (20 mg/kg) combination on colonic temperature in mice. *P <0.05 when compared with the respective dose of *kappa* agonist treated group (N ≥ 10).

TABLE 4. Comparison of the effects of U-50488H alone and its combination with ketamine on colonic temperature

Group	*Dose mg/kg*	*N*	*Basal*	*Postdrug*	*Delta*
U-50488H					
	0	10	37.9±0.14	37.5±0.10	-0.43±0.07
	30	10	37.7±0.11	36.7±0.23	-0.97±0.21
	60	10	37.5±0.09	36.7±0.25	-0.76±0.27
	100	10	37.7±0.01	36.6±0.21	-1.16±0.20
U-50488H + Ketamine (20 mg/kg)					
	0	10	37.9±0.09	37.3±0.27	-0.59±0.31
	30	10	37.4±0.11	37.8±0.17	0.37±0.17*
	60	10	37.5±0.13	36.1±0.20	-1.45±0.24*
	100	10	37.8±0.14	36.2±0.15	-1.61±0.23

*P<0.05 when compared with that of the corresponding dose of *kappa* agonist alone

Effect on righting reflex

The *kappa* agonist, U-50488H, in doses of 30, 60, and 100 mg/kg induced behavioral depression as manifested by a decrease in locomotor activity. However, none of the animals injected with any of the above doses of U-50488H lost their righting reflex. Furthermore, up to 40 mg/kg of ketamine also failed to induce loss of righting reflex.

The effect of the combination of a fixed dose of ketamine (20 mg/kg) with increasing doses of U-50488H on the duration of loss of the righting reflex is presented in Fig. 6. ANOVA indicated a significant effect for the dose of *kappa* agonist ($F_{2,27}$ = 5.27; P <0.02).

Effect on gastrointestinal transit

The percent of the gut traversed by the test meal in vehicle and increasing doses of ketamine treated mice (2.5, 5, 10, 20, and 40 mg/ kg), were 89±2.74, 87±2.7, 81±3.2, 85±2.6; 83± 3.0, and 86±3.8 respectively. ANOVA indicated that there were no significant differences between the groups ($F_{5,56}$ = 1.04; P = 0.39).

The antitransit effect of different doses of U-50488H *per se* and in combination with ketamine (40 mg/kg) are shown in Fig. 7. ANOVA indicated a significant effect for the dose of the *kappa* agonist ($F_{3,70}$ = 46.12; P <0.0001) but not for the *kappa* agonist x ketamine interaction ($F_{3,70}$ = 0.69; P = 0.56).

The antitransit effects of different doses of PD 117,302 *per se* and in combination with ketamine (40 mg/kg) are shown in Fig. 8. As in the

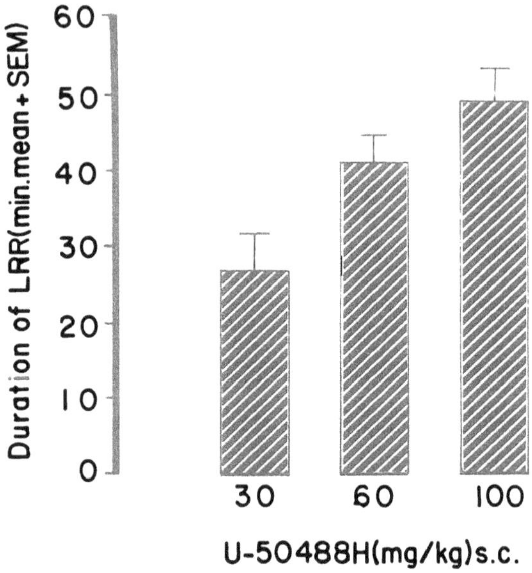

Fig. 6 Dose related effect of U-50488H on the duration of loss of the righting reflex (LRR) with a fixed dose of ketamine (20 mg/kg). Ketamine was administered s.c. with U-50488H (N = 10).

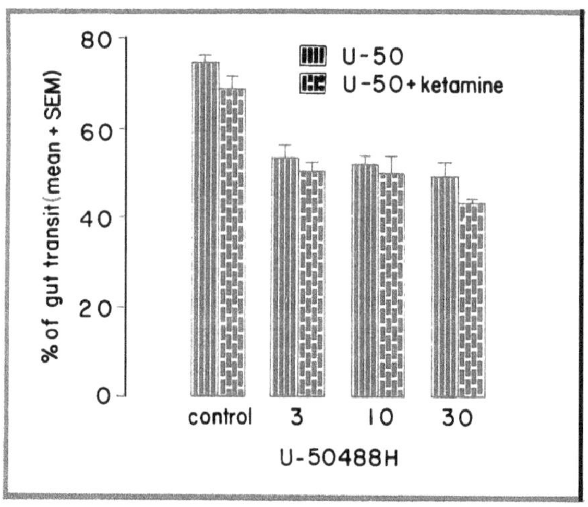

Fig. 7. Inhibition of charcoal meal transit induced by U-50488H (U-50) alone and in combination with ketamine (40 mg/kg). Control groups received vehicle alone. The numbers (3, 10, and 30) in the abscissae represent dose of *kappa* agonist in mg/kg (N ≥ 10).

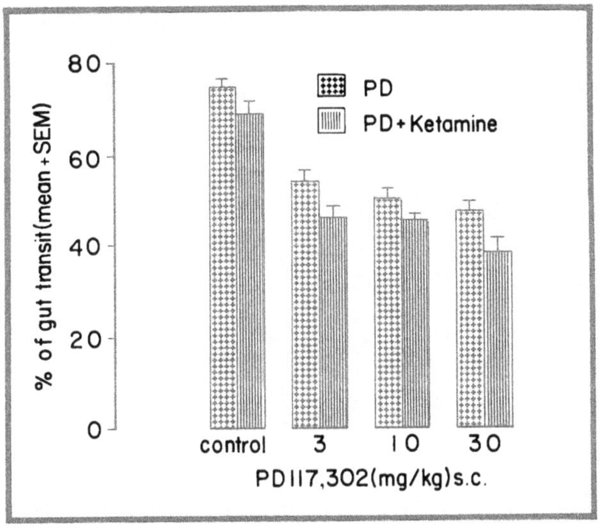

Fig. 8. Inhibition of charcoal meal transit induced by PD 117,302 (PD) alone and in combination with ketamine (40 mg/kg). Control groups received vehicle only. The numbers (3, 10, and 30) in the abscissae represent dose of *kappa* agonist in mg/kg (N ≥ 10).

case of U-50488H, ANOVA indicated a significant effect for the dose of the *kappa* agonist ($F_{3,63}$ = 69.87; P <0.0001) but not for the *kappa* agonist x ketamine interaction ($F_{3,63}$ = 0.36; P = 0.79).

Maximal electroshock seizure (MES) test

Ketamine produced a dose related anticonvulsant effect (Fig. 9; Chi-square for 4 degrees of freedom = 9.48; calculated = 3.22). The ED_{50} (95% confidence limits) was 2.06 (1.29-3.3). The percentage of animals showing abolition of tonic extensor phase in groups of mice injected with ketamine (10 mg/kg) alone or in combination with either naloxone (10 mg/kg) or MR 2266 (1 mg/kg), respectively, were 77, 83, and 93. Neither of the opiate antagonists blocked the anticonvulsant effect of ketamine.

Discussion

The present investigation indicates that when subthreshold doses of ketamine and *kappa* agonists are combined, the animals lose their righting reflex, suggesting a synergism between *kappa* opiate agonists and ketamine. Similar conclusions are possible when the results on colonic temperature are considered. Being a chemical analog, ketamine has an

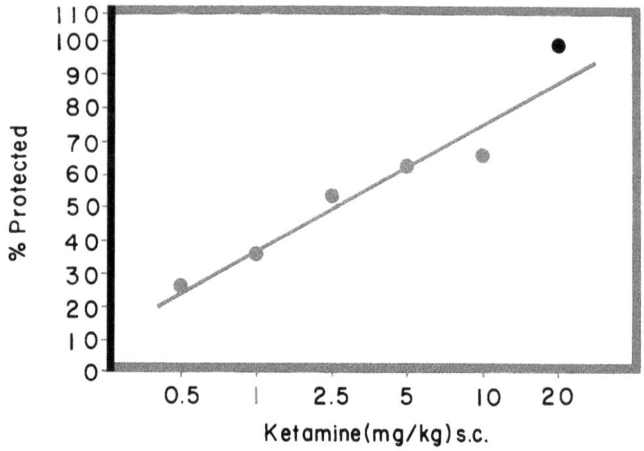

Fig. 9. Anticonvulsant effects of different doses of ketamine in the maximal electroshock seizure test. Each point represents the % of animals showing abolition of the tonic extensor phase (% protected; N $\geq$ 30 per dose).

affinity for phencyclidine binding sites. Hence, these *in vivo* data support the earlier *in vitro* evidence of a common opiate and phencyclidine receptor (Zukin and Zukin, 1983). However, the findings from the hot plate test, maximal electroshock seizure, and gastrointestinal transit studies do not support the above conclusions. Considering the *in vitro* binding characteristics of phencyclidine and *sigma* opiate agonists, it was proposed that the *sigma* and phencyclidine receptors may be distinct, although they have some similar properties (Tam, 1983). Therefore, when the entire pharmacological profile of the interaction between ketamine and *kappa* opiates is considered, present results are in favor of the *in vitro* evidence regarding the existence of distinct *sigma* opiate and phencyclidine binding sites sharing some common properties. Similar conclusions had been drawn earlier when the amino acid antagonism characteristics of *kappa* opiate agonists and ketamine were compared (Parsons *et al.*, 1986).

Ketamine has been shown to inhibit polysynaptic reflexes to a greater extent than monosynaptic reflexes (Anis *et al.*, 1983). Some studies propose that ketamine may activate both analgesic and antanalgesic systems (Pekoe and Smith, 1982). Furthermore, ketamine was reported to act as an antagonist in small doses, when catalepsy induced by morphine was used as a test parameter (Hance *et al.*, 1989). The tail flick is predominantly a monosynaptic spinal reflex under a tonic inhibitory influence of the endogenous opioid systems (Ramabadran *et al.*, 1989c). Therefore, the enhanced nociceptive reflex following ketamine administration in the tail immersion test may be explained on the basis of one or more of the following mechanisms: 1) a lack of an inhibitory effect on the monosynaptic reflex, 2) activation of an endogenous hyperalgesic system, and 3) opiate antagonistic effect at spinal levels.

The observed decrease in basal tail withdrawal latencies in streptozocin treated mice confirms our earlier findings (Ramabadran *et al.*, 1989a). Chronic hyperglycemia was shown to attenuate the hyperalgesic response of naloxone (Ramabadran *et al.*, 1989a) but not that of yohimbine (Bansinath *et al.*, 1989c). Present data on ketamine in the tail immersion test extend these observations on the differential effects of hyperglycemia on the descending tonic inhibitory spinal thermonociceptive mechanisms.

Inhibition of gastrointestinal transit is one of the well known classical effects of opiates. Both *mu* and *kappa* opiate receptors have been implicated in antitransit effects. An earlier report indicated that ketamine enhanced gastrointestinal transit (Takahashi *et al.*, 1987). However, with the protocol used in the present study, no effect of ketamine on gut motility could be observed over a wide range of doses. Furthermore, ketamine did not modify the antitransit effect of the *kappa* opiate agonist U-50488H and PD 117,302. These results indicate that *in vivo* gut inhibitory mechanism(s) are among those where *kappa* receptors cannot be implicated in the mode of action of ketamine. Similarly, the anticonvulsant activity of ketamine against maximal electroshock seizures also appears to be independent of opiate receptor mediated mechanisms, since naloxone and MR 2266 did not modify the action of ketamine.

In conclusion, the present results suggest that ketamine does not appear to mediate its effects through *kappa* opiate receptors. However, it augments some but not all of the pharmacological effects of *kappa* opiate agonists. *Kappa* opiate agonists are considered to be effective supplements to anesthesia without the liability of the side effects of other available opiate analgesics. Therefore, further studies are warranted to characterize the *in vivo* interactions of ketamine with *kappa* opiate agonists and to elucidate the mechanism(s) of such interactions.

ACKNOWLEDGEMENTS

The authors would like to thank Drs. P.F. Von Voigtlander, J. Hughes and H. Merz for their generous gifts of U-50488H, PD 117,302, and MR 2266, respectively. The assistance of Dr. C.K. Tang and Mr. Mark Lovitz in the preparation of the manuscript is gratefully acknowledged.

References

Anis, N.A., Berry, S.C., Burton, N.R., and Lodge, D.: The dissociative anaesthetic, ketamine and phencyclidine, selectively reduce excitation of central mammalian neurones by N-methyl-D-aspartate. Brit. J. Pharmacol. 79: 565-575, 1983.

Bansinath, M., Bose, A.C., Hema, S., and Guruswami, M.N.: Interaction of metamizol with some hypnotics in rats. Arch. Int. Pharmacodyn. 260: 14-27, 1982a.

Bansinath, M., Hema, S., Bose, A.C., and Guruswami, M.N.: Assessment of anticonvulsant and central depressant activity of *Cerbera odollam* in mice. Fitoterapia 53: 53-56, 1982b.

Bansinath, M., Matwyshyn, G.A., and Bhargava, H.N.: The binding of ^{3}H(3-MeHis^2) thyrotropin releasing hormone to brain membranes and temperature response to thyrotropin releasing hormone in different strains of mice. Neuropharmacol. 25: 923-926, 1986.

Bansinath, M., Ramabadran, K., Turndorf, H., and Puig, M.M.: Effects of acute and chronic hyperglycemia on morphine-induced inhibition of gastrointestinal transit in mice. Pharmacol. 37: 281-285, 1988.

Bansinath, M., Ramabadran, K., Ramanathan, S., Turndorf, H., and Puig, M.M.: Effects of acute and chronic hyperglycemia on morphine-induced hypothermia in mice. In Thermoregulation: Research and Clinical Applications, P. Lomax and E. Schonbaum, ed., pp. 139-144, Karger, Basel, 1989a.

Bansinath, M., Ramabadran, K., Turndorf, H., and Puig, M.M.: Hyperglycemia does not modify the pupillary effects of μ and κ agonists in mice. J. Ocular Pharmacol. 5: 33-43, 1989b.

Bansinath, M., Ramabadran, K., Turndorf, H., and Puig, M.M.: Effect of yohimbine on nociceptive threshold in normoglycemic and streptozotocin-treated hyperglycemic mice. Pharmacol. Biochem. Behav. 33: 459-463, 1989c.

Corssen, G. and Domino, E.F.: Dissociative anesthesia: Further pharmacologic studies and first clinical experience with the phencyclidine derivative CI-581. Anesth. Analg. 45: 29-40, 1966.

CSS: Complete statistical system with graphics and data management. Release 1A, Version B384, Statsoft Inc., Tulsa, OK, 1987.

Fidecka, S.: Opioid mechanisms of some behavioral effects of ketamine. Pol. J. Pharmacol. Pharm. 39: 353-360, 1987.

Finck, A.D., Samaniego, E., and Ngai, S.H.: Morphine tolerance decreases the analgesic effects of ketamine in mice. Anesthesiol. 68: 397-400, 1988.

Hance, A.J., Winters, W.D., Quam, D.D., Benthuysen, J.L., and Cadd, G.G.: Catalepsy induced by combination of ketamine and morphine: Potentiation, antagonism, tolerance and cross-tolerance in the rat. Neuropharmacol. 28: 109-116, 1989.

Parsons, C.G., Martin, D., Franklin, R.J.M., Wood, J.L., and Headley, P.M.: Do *kappa* opioids mimic *sigma* agonists as amino acid antagonists? Neuropharmacol. 25: 217-220, 1986.

Pekoe, G.M. and Smith,D.J.: The involvement of opiate and monoaminergic neuronal systems in the analgesic effects of ketamine. Pain 12: 57-73, 1982.

Ramabadran, K., Bansinath, M., Hema, S., Karanth, S., and Guruswami, M.N.: Assessment of taurine for anticonvulsant activity. Ind. J. Exp. Biol. 18: 1035-1037, 1980.

Ramabadran, K., Bansinath, M., Turndorf, H., and Puig, M.M.: Stereospecific inhibition of gastrointestinal transit by k opioid agonists in mice. Eur. J. Pharmacol. 155: 329-331, 1988.

Ramabadran, K., Bansinath, M., Turndorf, H., and Puig, M.M.: The hyperalgesic effect of naloxone in streptozotocin-diabetic mice. Psychopharmacol. 97: 169-174, 1989a.

Ramabadran, K., Bansinath, M., Turndorf, H., and Puig, M.M.: Hyperglycemia as a factor affecting k opiate agonist-induced inhibition of the gastrointestinal transit in mice. J. Pharm. Pharmacol. 41: 496-498, 1989b.

Ramabadran, K., Bansinath, M., Turndorf, H., and Puig, M.M.: Tail immersion test for evaluation of nociceptive reaction in mice: Methodological considerations. J. Pharmacol. Methods 21: 21-31, 1989c.

Smith, D.J., Bouchal, R.L., DeSanctis, C.A., Monroe, P.J., Amedro, J.B., Perrotti, J.M., and Crisp, T.: Properties of the interaction between ketamine and opiate binding sites *in vivo* and *in vitro*. Neuropharmacol. 26: 1253-1260, 1987.

Smith, D.J., Pekoe, G.M., Martin, L.L., and Colgate, B.: The interaction of ketamine with opiate receptors. Life Sci. 26: 789-795, 1980.

Takahashi, R.N., Morato, G.S., and Rae, G.A.: Effects of ketamine on nociception and gastrointestinal motility in mice are unaffected by naloxone. Gen. Pharmacol. 18: 201-203, 1987.

Tallarida, R.J. and Murray, R.B.: Manual of pharmacological calculations with computer programs, 2nd Ed., Springer-Verlag, New York, 1987.

Tam, S.W.: Naloxone-inaccessible *sigma* receptor in rat central nervous system. Proc. Natl. Acad. Sci. (USA) 80: 6703-6707, 1983.

Winters, W.D., Hance, A.J., Cadd, G.G., Quam, D.D., and Benthuysen, J.L.: Ketamine- and morphine-induced analgesia and catalepsy. I. Tolerance, cross-tolerance, potentiation, residual morphine levels and naloxone in the rat. J. Pharmacol. Exp. Ther. 244: 51-57, 1988.

Zukin, R.S. and Zukin, S.R.: A common receptor for phencyclidine and the *sigma* opiates. In Phencyclidine and Related Arylcyclohexylamines: Present and Future Applications, J.-M. Kamenka, E.F. Domino and P. Geneste, eds., pp. 107-124, NPP Books, Ann Arbor, 1983.

Status of Ketamine in Anesthesiology,
edited by E.F. Domino©1990, NPP Books
P.O. Box 1491, Ann Arbor, MI 48106

Spinal Analgesic Mechanisms of Ketamine: Antagonism by Naloxone

K. Hanaoka, M. Tagami, M. Nagase, Y. Ide, and H. Yamamura

Department of Anesthesiology
University of Tokyo
Tokyo, Japan

Introduction

In the last decade, specific opiate receptors have been found in the central nervous system. Recent work has shown that the analgesic actions of certain general anesthetic agents are antagonized by naloxone, suggesting that those agents release opiate like substances at opiate receptor sites in the pain pathways.

The purpose of this study was to investigate the effects of ketamine on single unit activity of cells in Rexed lamina V (Rexed, 1952) of the feline lumbar spinal cord and to determine if naloxone would antagonize these effects.

Methods

Details of the experimental methods have been reported elsewhere (Kitahata *et al.*, 1971). Procedures specific to the present investigation are as follows: A total of 31 cats of either sex, weighing 2.5 to 4.0 kg, were divided into groups given ketamine hydrochloride alone (12), ketamine-naloxone (9), and naloxone alone (10). Ethrane, nitrous oxide and oxygen anesthesia were used for tracheostomy, cannulation of the femoral artery and vein, and lumbar laminectomy. Each animal was rendered decerebrate by bilateral electrolytic lesions placed in the midbrain reticular formation, and the spinal cord was transected at the T12-L1 level. Anesthesia was then discontinued and the animal was given pancuronium bromide and ventilated with 100% oxygen using a volume cycled ventilator connected to a non-rebreathing system. Femoral artery pressure, endotracheal pCO_2, EKG, pulse rate, and rectal and spinal cord temperatures were recorded continuously on a polygraph. These parameters were kept within the normal physiological range. Arterial blood gas analyses were performed from time to time and kept in the range of pO_2-300 to 600 torr, pCO_2-35 to 45 torr, and pH-7.30 to 7.45.

A glass rod platinum sheathed microelectrode with a 1 to 2 μm exposed tip was then inserted into the lumbar spinal cord near the L7 root entry zone using a hydraulic microdrive. Neurons were characterized by their evoked responses to cutaneous pinching stimuli and by their spontaneous firing patterns. As a microelecrode was passed ventrally through the dorsal column at a depth of about 2000 μm from the cord dorsum, cells in lamina V displayed a spontaneous activity of bursts followed by steady firing, responding primarily to high threshold stimuli with graded responses. The Rexed laminae are illustrated below in Fig. 1.

In this study, all lesions made were found and all physiological characteristics were anatomically correlated. Signals were recorded through a WP Instruments Inc. preamplifier on magnetic tape and displayed simultaneously on a cathode-ray oscilloscope.

1) Ketamine hydrochloride alone (12 cats). Single units were observed for about 30 min after isolation to obtain a stable firing pattern and to control the effect of transient tissue distortion produced by insertion of

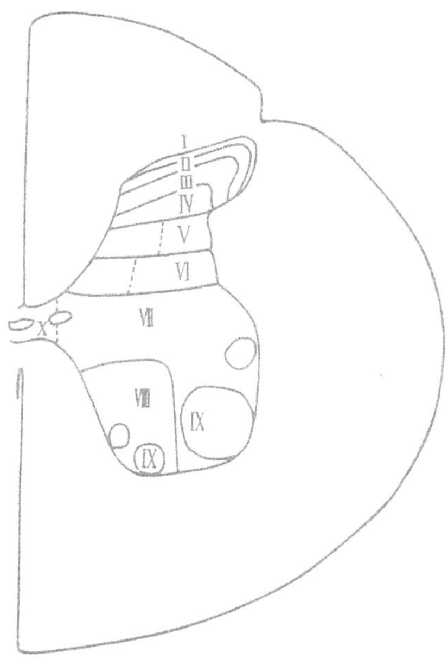

Fig. 1. Rexed laminae of feline lumbar spinal cord.

the microelectrode. The spontaneous and evoked activities of each single unit were counted electronically and instantaneous frequencies displayed on the polygraph.

A pinching method, using the Nihon Kohden quantitative pain stimulating system, was used for the investigation of evoked activity. A 10 min control period was then recorded, after which the effect of 5 mg/kg of ketamine i.v. was studied upon spontaneous and evoked activities. The changes in spontaneous and evoked activities caused by pinching the center of the receptive field were investigated every 5 min until recovery of single unit activity.

The receptive field characteristics of lamina V cells were studied before, during, and at the time of recovery from the effects of ketamine. At the conclusion of each experiment, electrolytic lesions were placed through the recording microelectrode by passing a d.c. current of 20 to 50 μa for 60 sec. After fixation with 10% formalin, the spinal cord was sectioned in 30 μm slices and stained with cresyl violet to study the cytoarchitecture of the spinal cord. Data were analyzed using a NEC PC-9801 VM computer. The significance of the mean values obtained during the control period, during the administration of ketamine, and during the recovery period was assessed by the Student's paired t-test.

2) Ketamine-naloxone (9 cats). Details of experimental methods have been described above. Procedures specific to the investigation of this group were as follows: After a 10 min control period, 5 mg/kg i.v. of ketamine was administered. Five min after ketamine, 0.1 mg/kg i.v. of naloxone was administered.

The significance of the mean values obtained during the control period, during the administration of ketamine and naloxone, and during the recovery period was assessed by the Student's paired t-test. The data obtained in the ketamine-naloxone animals were compared to those from animals given ketamine alone.

3) Naloxone alone (10 cats). Details of experimental methods were similar to those described above. Procedures specific to the investigation of this group were as follows: A 10 min control period was recorded, after which the effect of 0.1 mg/kg of naloxone i.v. upon spontaneous and evoked activity was studied for 60 min.

RESULTS

The salient features of the physiological characterization of the lamina of the dorsal horn utilized in this study were reported previously

(Kitahata *et al.*, 1971). In the present study, the cells in Rexed lamina V responded primarily to high threshold peripheral cutaneous stimuli, deep squeezing, pinching, and the application of high intensity heat or ethyl chloride. Their spontaneous single unit activity was characterized by bursts followed by steady firing. Their average frequencies were 19.7 ± 3.6 (mean ± 1 S.E.)/sec in the ketamine alone group, 20.7 ± 4.6 (mean ± 1 S.E.)/sec in the ketamine-naloxone group, and 19.7 ± 4.1 (mean ± 1 S.E.)/sec in the naloxone alone group.

1) Ketamine alone. The effect of ketamine on spontaneously and evokedly firing lamina V cellular activity, expressed as percent decrease from the control values, and the time course are shown in Figs. 2 and 3 and Table 1.

Significant suppression of the spontaneous and evoked activities of neurons in Rexed lamina V was demonstrated 5 min after 5 mg/kg of ketamine i.v. ($P<0.05$).

2) Ketamine-naloxone. Five min after the administration of 5 mg/kg of ketamine i.v., significant suppression of the spontaneous and evoked activities of neurons in Rexed lamina V was observed ($P<0.05$). Three min after 0.1 mg/kg of naloxone i.v., a significant antagonistic effect was seen ($P<0.05$), as shown in Figs. 4 and 5 and Table 1.

3) Naloxone alone. Naloxone in a dose of 0.1 mg/kg i.v. had no

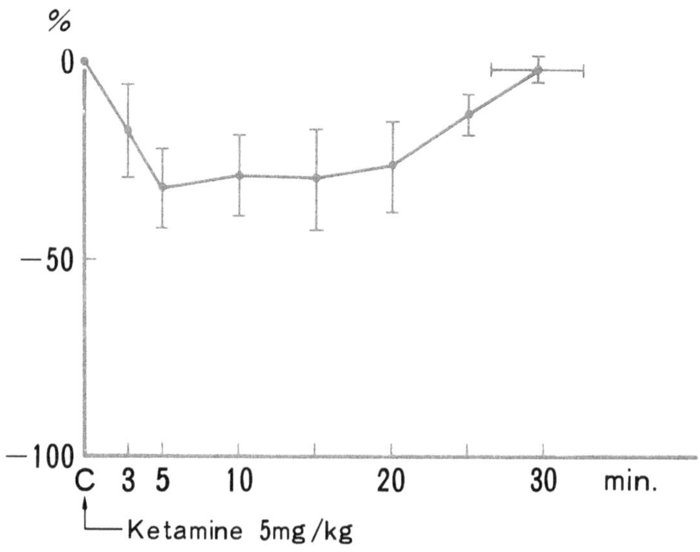

Fig. 2. Effect of ketamine on spontaneously firing lamina V cellular activity expressed as percent decrease from control.

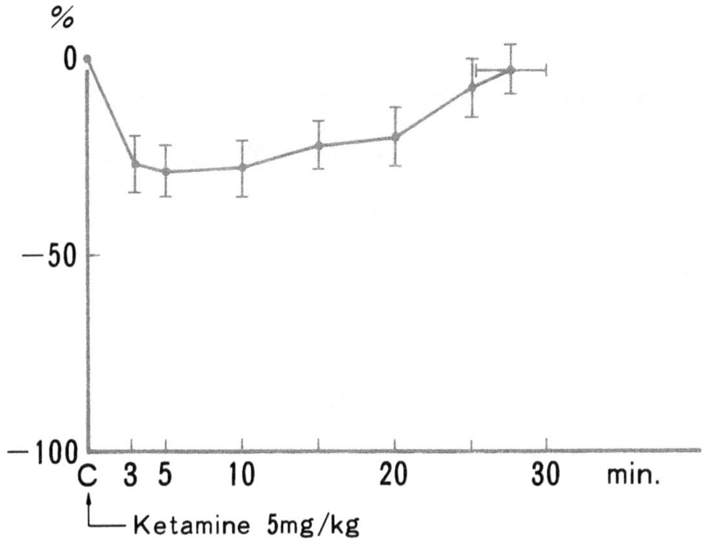

Fig. 3. Effect of ketamine on evoked firing lamina V cellular activity expressed as percent decrease from control.

TABLE 1. Percentage decreases from control of single unit activity produced by ketamine alone and ketamine-naloxone

	Control (%)	*5 min (%)*	*10 min (%)*
Ketamine			
Spontaneous	0	-32.2*	-28.7*
Evoked	0	-28.9*	-27.8*

	Control (%)	*5 min (%)*	*3 min after naloxone*	*5 min after naloxone*
Ketamine-Naloxone				
Spontaneous	0	-28.6*	- 6.6+	-11.6+
Evoked	0	-30.2*	-10.0+	- 6.0+

* (P<0.05) vs. control
+ (P<0.05) vs. 5 min in ketamine-naloxone

effect on the spontaneous and evoked activities of cells in Rexed lamina V, as shown in Figs. 6 and 7. These results indicate that naloxone reversed the depressant effect of ketamine on lamina V cellular activity in cats.

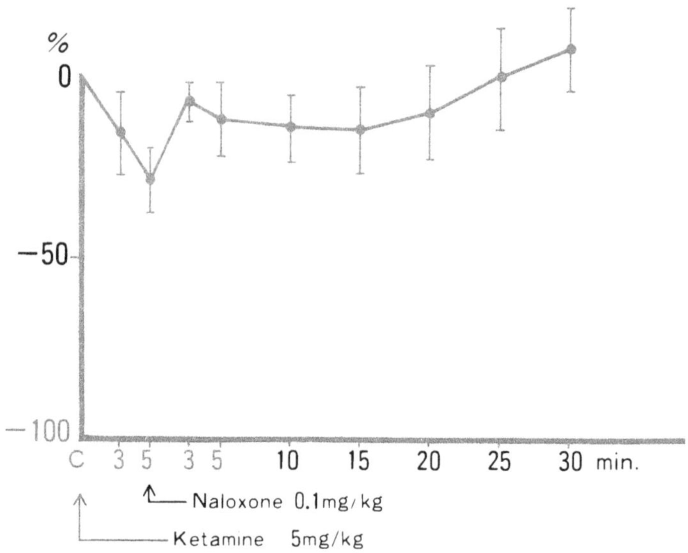

Fig. 4. Effect of ketamine-naloxone on spontaneously firing lamina V cellular activity expressed as the percent decrease from control. Note that a significant antagonistic effect was observed after naloxone.

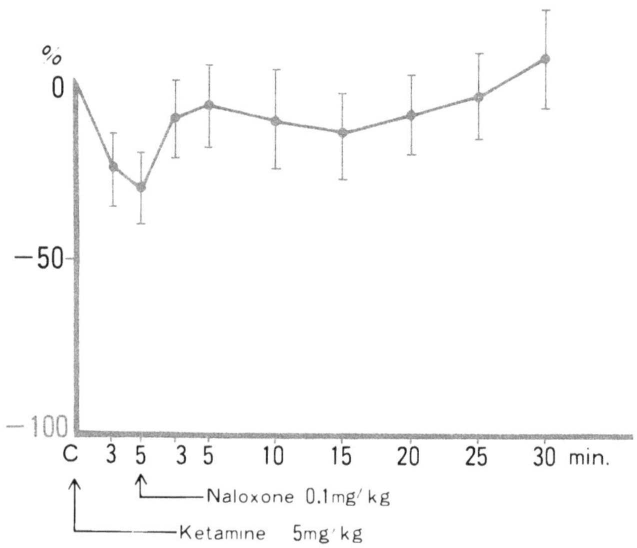

Fig. 5. Effect of ketamine-naloxone on evoked firing lamina V cellular activity expressed as the percent decrease from control. Note that a significant antagonistic effect was seen after naloxone.

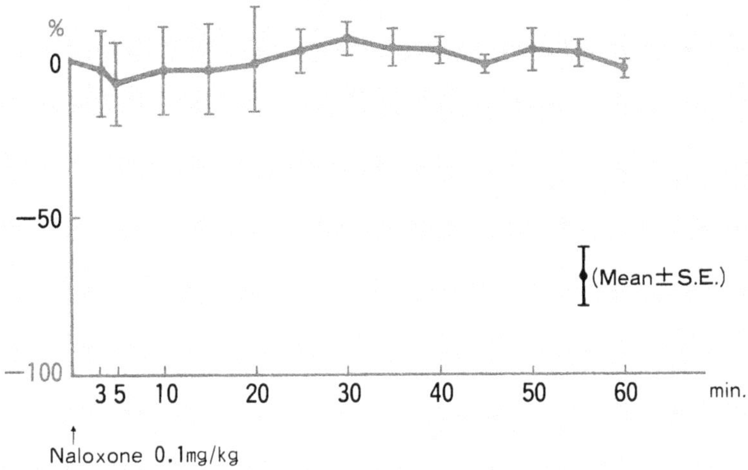

Fig. 6. Effect of naloxone alone on spontaneously firing lamina V cellular activity expressed as the percent decrease from control.

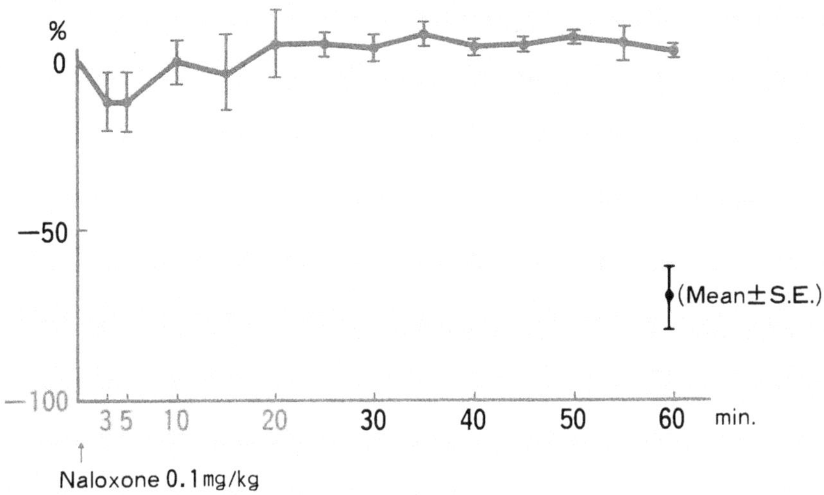

Fig. 7. Effect of naloxone alone on evoked firing lamina V cellular activity expressed as the percent decrease from control.

Discussion

The neurophysiological basis of the analgesic action of ketamine has been controversial with regard to an opiate action. At the spinal level, there are reports that systemically administered ketamine has a significant suppressive effect in spinal animals (Conseiller *et al.*, 1972; Tang and

Schroeder, 1973; Kitahata *et al.*, 1973) as well as when it is given intrathecally (Ahuja, 1983). The present study also showed that ketamine suppressed single units in Rexed lamina V which respond to noxious stimuli.

Recent work using binding assays (Smith *et al.*, 1980; Finck and Ngai, 1982) has shown that ketamine may interact directly with opiate receptors to produce its opiate like actions. Some studies have shown that naloxone, a specific opiate antagonist, reversed the depressant effect of ketamine (Smith *et al.*, 1982; Little *et al.*, 1983; Okuda, 1986). In contrast, other reports indicate that ketamine has no affinity for specific opiate receptors and that its depressant effect is not antagonized by naloxone (Fratta *et al.*, 1980; Wiley and Downs, 1982; Smith *et al.*, 1985).

We have shown that ketamine in a dose of 5 mg/kg i.v. significantly suppressed the spontaneous and evoked activities of cells in Rexed lamina V and that such depressed activity recovered after 0.1 mg/kg i.v. of naloxone. Naloxone in a dose of 0.1 mg/kg i.v. alone did not show any effect on lamina V cellular activity. Therefore, it is clear that the depressant effect of ketamine on cells in lamina V is antagonized by naloxone.

It should be noted that the antagonistic effect of naloxone was incomplete. This is partially explained by nonspecific opiate mechanisms such as monoaminergic neuronal processes (Ylitalo *et al.*, 1976; Azzaro and Smith, 1977; Vargiu *et al.*, 1978; Martin *et al.*, 1982). We have shown previously the effect of morphine on spontaneous and evoked firing single unit activity of cells in Rexed lamina V (Hanaoka *et al.*, 1978). According to that study, the suppressive effects of morphine (0.5 mg/kg) on spontaneous and evoked activity were somewhat greater than those of 5 mg/kg of ketamine. Naloxone in a dose of 0.02 mg/kg was enough to reverse the suppressive effect of 2.0 mg/kg of morphine on activity in lamina V. However, in the present study, 0.1 mg/kg of naloxone did not completely reverse the suppressive effect of ketamine. These results suggest that the suppressive effect of ketamine is not completely due to an opiate mechanism.

In conclusion, the present study indicates that ketamine acts, in part, through an opiate like mechanism. Whether it does so by releasing a humoral substance or by a direct effect on opiate receptors is not known.

Acknowledgements

The authors would like to thank Mrs. Shigemi Kobayashi for preparing this manuscript. This work was supported by a grant in aid for scientific research (B) NO 59480321.

References

Ahuja, B.R.: Analgesic effect of intrathecal ketamine in rats. Br. J. Anaesth. 55: 991-995, 1983.

Azzaro, A.J. and Smith, D.J.: The inhibitory action of ketamine HCl on [^{3}H] 5-hydroxytryptamine accumulation by rat brain synaptosomal rich fractions: Comparison with [^{3}H] catecholamine and [^{3}H] aminobutyric acid uptake. Neuropharmacol. 16: 349-356, 1977.

Conseiller, C., Bonoist, J.M., Hamann, K.F., Millard, M.C., and Besson, J.M.: Effects of ketamine (CI-581) on cell responses to cutaneous stimulations in lamina IV and V in the cat's dorsal horn. Eur. J. Pharmacol. 18: 346-352, 1972.

Finck, A.D. and Ngai, S.H.: Opiate receptor mediation of ketamine analgesia. Anesthesiol. 56: 291-297, 1982.

Fratta, W., Casu, M., Balesteieri, A., Loviselli, A., Biggio, G., and Gessa, G.L.: Failure of ketamine to interact with opiate receptors. Eur. J. Pharmacol. 61: 389-391, 1980.

Hanaoka, K., Ohtani, M., Toyooka, H., Dohi, S., Ghazi-Saidi, K., Taub, A., and Kitahata, L.M.: The relative contribution of direct and supraspinal descending effects upon spinal mechanisms of morphine analgesia. J. Pharmacol. Exp. Ther. 207: 476-484, 1978.

Kitahata, L.M., Taub, A., and Satoh, I.: Lamina-specific suppression of dorsal horn unit activity by nitrous oxide and by hyperventilation. J. Pharmacol. Exp. Ther. 176: 101-108, 1971.

Kitahata, L.M., Taub, A., and Kosaka, Y.: Lamina-specific suppression of dorsal horn activity by ketamine hydrochloride. Anesthesiol. 38: 4-11, 1973.

Little, H., Alexander, K.L., Gargan, M.F., and Widdison, A.L.: Ketamine and the guinea-pig ileum: Possible opiate agonist and antagonist action and effects of peptidase inhibition. J. Pharmacol. Exp. Ther. 225: 206-212, 1983.

Martin, L.L., Bouchal, R.L., and Smith, D.J.: Ketamine inhibits serotonin uptake *in vivo*. Neuropharmacol. 21: 113-118, 1982.

Okuda, T.: Comparison of direct and indirect depressant actions of ketamine on dorsal horn cells in rabbits. Neuropharmacol. 25: 433-440, 1986.

Rexed, B.: The cytoarchitectonic organization of the spinal cord in the cat. J. Comp. Neurol. 96: 415-495, 1952.

Smith, D.J., Pekoe, G.M., Martin, L.L., and Coalgate, B.: The interaction of ketamine with the opiate receptor. Life Sci. 26: 789-795, 1980.

Smith, D.J., Perrotti, J.M., Mansell, A.L., and Monroe, P.J.: Ketamine analgesia is not related to an opiate action in the periaqueductal gray region of the rat brain. Pain 21: 253-265, 1985.

Smith, D.J., Westfall, D.P., and Adams, J.D.: Assessment of the potential agonistic and antagonistic properties of ketamine at opiate receptors in the guinea pig ileum. Neuropharmacol. 21: 605-611, 1982.

Tang, A.H. and Schroeder, L.A.: Spinal cord depressant effects of ketamine and etoxadrol in the cat and the rat. Anesthesiol. 39: 37-43, 1973.

Vargiu, L., Stefanini, E., Musinu, C., and Saba, G.: Possible role of brain serotonin in the central effects of ketamine. Neuropharmacol. 17: 405-408, 1978.

Wiley, J.N. and Downs, D.A.: Lack of antagonism by naloxone of the analgesic and locomotor stimulant actions of ketamine. Life Sci. 31: 1071-1075, 1982.

Ylitalo, P., Saarnivaara, L., and Ahtee, L.: Effect of ketamine anaesthesia on the content of monoamines and their metabolites in the rat brain. Acta Anaesth. Scand. 20: 216-220, 1976.

Status of Ketamine in Anesthesiology,
edited by E.F. Domino©1990, NPP Books
P.O. Box 1491, Ann Arbor, MI 48106

The Analgesic Effect of Ketamine: Evidence for a Non-opioid, PCP Receptor Mediated Mechanism

A. Maurset*, E. Ratti Moberg, and I. Øye

Department of Pharmacology
Oslo University School of Medicine
Oslo, Norway

Introduction

The analgesic action of ketamine in subanesthetic doses was observed in early studies in human volunteers (Domino *et al.*, 1965). Most subsequent investigations on the action of ketamine in humans focus on its anesthetic properties, whereas relatively few studies deal with its action as an analgesic in sub-anesthetic doses. Based on studies in animals, both opioid (Smith *et al.*, 1980; Finck and Ngai, 1982) and non-opioid (Fratta *et al.*, 1980; Takahashi *et al.*, 1987) mechanisms for ketamine analgesia have been suggested. The present investigation was initiated in order to examine the pharmacological mechanisms involved in low dose ketamine analgesia.

Methods and Results

Evidence for a Non-Opioid Analgesic Mechanism

In order to assess the possible role of opioid mechanisms in ketamine analgesia, we compared the analgesic effect of ketamine with that of the opioid meperidine (pethidine) in experimental and postoperative pain in human volunteers and in the presence and absence of the narcotic antagonist naloxone (Maurset *et al.*, 1989). The pain was recorded on a visual analogue scale (VAS) running from 0 (no pain) to 100 mm (unbearable pain). Drugs were given i.v. through an indwelling cannula according to a double blind, crossover protocol.

Experimental ischemic pain was induced by the post-exercise tourni-

*During the time of this work, A.M. was attached to the Joint Norwegian Medical Service, HQ Defense Command, Norway.

quet method. Briefly, the subjects exercised their forearm muscles for 2 min by compressing a hand grip strengthener. Maximum effort was encouraged, resulting in a slowing of compressions and exhaustion. After the exercise, a sphygmomanometer cuff was rapidly inflated to shut off the blood supply to the arm. Naloxone in a dose of 1.6 mg or placebo was given in the contralateral arm 5 min prior to induction of ischemia. Ketamine (0.3 mg/kg) or meperidine (pethidine, 0.7 mg/kg) was infused during the first 2 min of ischemia. The results are shown in Fig. 1. Naloxone reversed the analgesic effect of meperidine, but did not alter ketamine analgesia.

Postoperative pain was studied in patients who had their impacted 3rd molar teeth surgically removed on prophylactic indication, under local anesthesia without premedication. When postoperative pain had reached at least 50 on the VAS scale, naloxone (1.6 mg) or placebo followed by either ketamine (0.3 mg/kg) or meperidine (pethidine 0.7

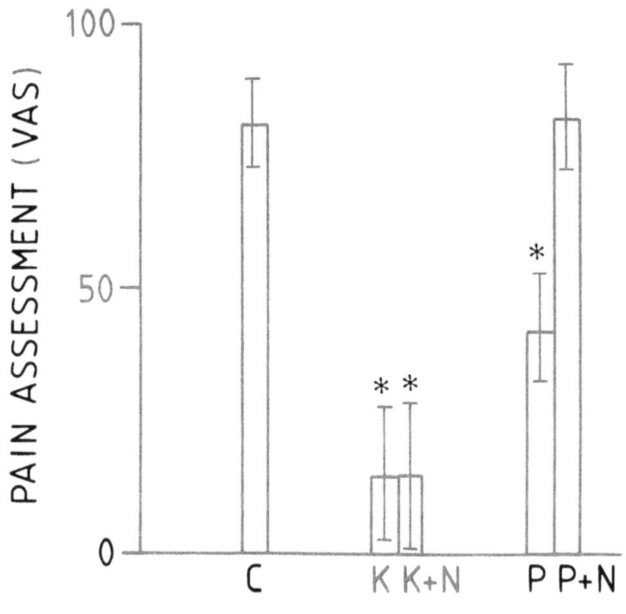

Fig. 1. Pain assessment on a 100 mm visual analogue scale (VAS) after 5 min of ischemia in the left arm. The bars represent mean values ± S.E. of pain assessment by 6 subjects. Control values (C), ketamine 0.3 mg/kg (K), ketamine 0.3 mg/kg preceded by 1.6 mg naloxone (K+N), pethidine 0.7 mg/kg (P), and pethidine 0.7 mg/kg preceded by 1.6 mg naloxone (P+N). Asterisks denote values significantly different from C ($P<0.05$). (Reproduced from Maurset *et al.*, 1989 with permission from the publisher.).

mg/kg) was given as described above for experimental ischemic pain. Fig. 2 shows the reduction in pain score after ketamine with and without naloxone. Naloxone failed to inhibit ketamine analgesia in this pain model. In contrast, the effect or meperidine was inhibited (but not completely blocked) by naloxone (Fig. 3). The results of these studies indicate that the analgesic effect of ketamine in subanesthetic doses in man is mediated by a non-opioid mechanism.

Evidence for a PCP receptor mediated mechanism

Receptor binding studies have shown that ketamine and related drugs bind to PCP as well as *sigma* binding sites, both of which must be considered as putative pharmacological receptors mediating at least some of the characteristic effects of ketamine (Weissmann *et al.*, 1988). In order to test the role of these two receptors for the analgesic effect of ketamine, we took advantage of the fact that ketamine has an asymmetric carbon atom. We separated the two ketamine enantiomers by crystallization with tartaric acid and tested their relative order of analgesic potency

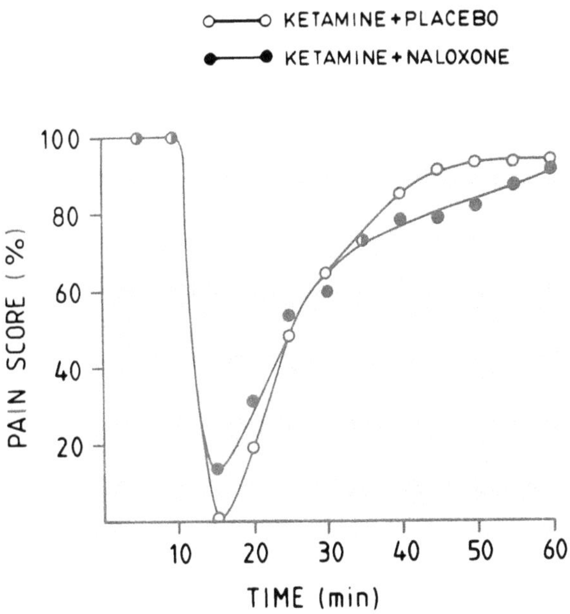

Fig. 2. Effect of ketamine 0.3 mg/kg preceded by 1.6 mg/kg naloxone or placebo on postoperative pain. The figure shows pain score in percent, 100 percent being the pain assessed by each individual patient on the VAS scale before drugs were given. Naloxone (1.6 mg/kg) or placebo were given at 5 min, ketamine at 10 min. Each point represents mean values for 6 subjects:

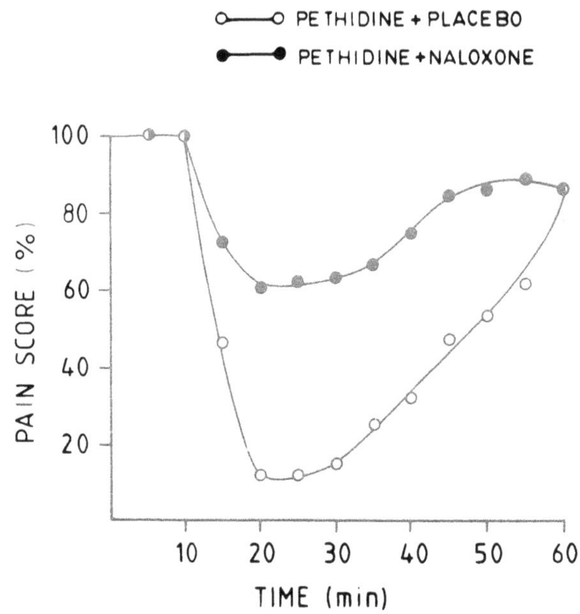

Fig. 3. Effect of pethidine 0.7 mg/kg preceded by 1.6 mg naloxone or placebo on postoperative pain. The figure shows pain score in percent, 100 percent being the actual pain assessed by each individual patient on the VAS scale before drugs were given. Naloxone (1.6 mg/kg) or placebo was given at 5 min and pethidine at 10 min. Each point is the mean value from 6 patients. (Reproduced from Maurset *et al.*, 1989 with permission from the publisher.)

in human volunteers as well as their relative affinities for PCP and *sigma* receptors.

The analgesic potency of (S)-ketamine and (R)-ketamine was examined using the post-exercise ischemic pain test described above. Six healthy male volunteers participated in the study, which was carried out in a double blind cross-over fashion. The results are shown in Fig. 4. As seen from the figure, both ketamine enantiomers had a dose dependent analgesic effect in this pain model. The ED_{50} for the analgesic action of (R)-ketamine is approximately 0.5 mg/kg, whereas the ED_{50} for (S)-ketamine is between 0.1 mg/kg and 0.15 mg/kg. (S)-ketamine thus appears to be about 4 times more potent than (R)-ketamine as an analgesic agent.

The affinities of (S)-ketamine and (R)-ketamine for PCP and sigma receptors were examined in guinea pig brain homogenates. *Sigma* sites were labeled with + (^{3}H)SKF-10,047 in the presence of MK-801 (in order

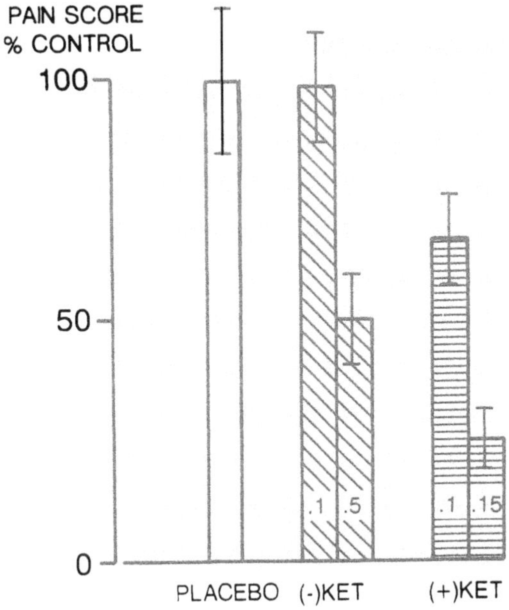

Fig. 4. Pain assessment on a 100 mm visual analogue scale (VAS) after 5 min post-exercise ischemia in the left arm. The bars represent mean values ± S.E. of pain reduction as percent of control experiments for each subject (placebo). Hatched bars: (R)-ketamine (-ket) 0.1 and 0.5 mg/kg i.v. Slashed bars: (S)-ketamine (+ket) 0.1 and 0.15 mg/kg i.v. The difference between the two doses of each drug is significant ($P < 0.01$).

to mask PCP receptor binding), and the PCP sites were labeled with (^{3}H)TCP in the presence of haloperidol (in order to mask *sigma* receptor binding). The K_i values obtained are listed in Table 1. As seen from the table, (S)-ketamine has about 4 times higher affinity for the PCP receptor than (R)-ketamine. The relative order of PCP receptor affinity thus correlates positively to the relative order of analgesic potency when the two

TABLE 1. The relative affinities of (S)-ketamine and (R)-ketamine for PCP and *sigma* receptors. The figures are mean values of 3 triplicate experiments ± S.E.

	Inhibition Constant (μmol/1)	
	PCP Receptor	Sigma *Receptor*
(S)-Ketamine	0.6 (±0.5)	145 (±7.3)
(R)-Ketamine	2.0 (±0.17)	35 (±7.4)
MK-801	0.007 (±0.002)	—
Haloperidol	—	0.24 (±0.15)

ketamine enantiomers are compared. On the other hand, a negative correlation between *sigma* site affinity and analgesic potency was found. The correlation studies thus support the view that PCP binding sites, but not *sigma* binding sites, are pharmacological receptors mediating the analgesic action of low dose ketamine in humans.

Discussion

In the central nervous system, PCP receptors are localized together with the NMDA type of receptors for the excitatory amino acid transmitter glutamate (Maragos *et al.*, 1986). Ketamine inhibits synaptic transmission at this receptor (Anis *et al.*, 1983) and (S)-ketamine was a more potent inhibitor when the two enantiomers were compared (Lodge *et al.*, 1983). The molecular requirements for inhibition by PCP receptor ligands of synaptic transmission at the NMDA receptor correlates with *in vivo* behavioral actions of PCP-like drugs (see Quirion *et al.*, 1988). These findings indicate that at least some of the effects of ketamine are due to PCP receptor mediated inhibition of the NMDA subtype of glutamate receptors.

Our present study shows a positive correlation between PCP receptor binding and analgesic potency when the two chiral forms of ketamine are compared. Enantiomers are, by definition, non-superimposable mirror images with identical physical chemical properties. They may differ in affinity to receptors and enzymes, but it is unlikely that enzyme dependent pharmacokinetic differences are responsible for the order of analgesic potency described above. Our findings, therefore, strongly indicate that the analgesic effect of low dose ketamine is due to PCP receptor mediated blockade of transmission at the NMDA type of glutamate receptors.

The hypothesis that ketamine analgesia is due to PCP receptor mediated blockade of transmission at the NMDA type of excitatory amino acid synapses does not preclude that other pharmacological mechanisms are involved in the action of ketamine, particularly at higher doses. Previous studies of the anesthetic properties of ketamine enantiomers in humans indicate that the excitatory phenomena on emergence from anesthesia are more pronounced for (R)-ketamine (White *et al.*, 1980). In view of the receptor affinities reported above (Table 1), this indicates that a non-PCP, possibly *sigma* receptor mediated pharmacological mechanism is responsible for the excitatory phenomena observed at higher doses.

Species differences are important for the pharmacology of ketamine

(McCarthy *et al.*, 1965). Whereas analgesia in humans was found after doses as low as 0.1 mg/kg i.v., and 2 mg/kg i.v. is a common dose for surgical anesthesia in humans, doses of approximately 50 mg/kg and 150 mg/kg, respectively, are necessary in rats. At these high doses, the general membrane stabilizing action of ketamine, involving several different ion channels, are likely to be involved. Thus, several pharmacological mechanisms may contribute to the effects of ketamine. The experimental data presented in this report are in accordance with the hypothesis that low dose ketamine analgesia is due to PCP receptor mediated inhibition of excitatory amino acid transmission at NMDA synapses.

Acknowledgements

The authors would like to thank Ms. Aase Holmen and Ms. Mette Enger for expert assistance in the binding studies. This work was supported by Hydro Pharma Norway A/S.

References

Anis, N.A., Berry, S.C., Burton, N.R., and Lodge, D.: The dissociative anesthetics, ketamine and phencyclidine, selectively reduce excitation of central mammalian neurones by N-methylaspartate. Br. J. Pharmacol. 79: 565-575, 1983.

Domino, E.F., Chodoff, P., and Corssen, G.: Pharmacologic effects of CI-581, a new dissociative anesthetic in man. Clin. Pharmacol. Ther. 6: 279-291, 1965.

Finck, A.D. and Ngai, S.H.: Opiate receptor mediation of ketamine analgesia. Anesthesiology 56: 291-297, 1982.

Fratta, W., Casu, M., Balestrieri, A., Loviselli, A., Biggio, G., and Gessa, G.L.: Failure of ketamine to interact with opiate receptors. Eur. J. Pharmacol. 61: 389-391, 1980.

Lodge, D., Anis, N.A., and Burton, N.R.: Effects of optical isomers of ketamine on excitation of cat and rat spinal neurones by amino acids and acetylcholine. Neurosci. Lett. 29: 282-286, 1982.

Maragos, W.F., Chu, D.C.M., Greenamyre, T., Penney, J.B., and Young, A.B.: High correlation between the localization of (^{3}H) TCP binding and NMDA receptors. Eur. J. Pharmacol. 123: 173-174, 1986.

Maurset, A., Skoglung, L.A., Hustveit, O., and Oye, I.: Comparison of ketamine and pethidine in experimental and postoperative pain. Pain 36: 37-41, 1989.

McCarthy, D.A., Chen, G., Kaump, D.J., and Ensor, C.: General anesthetic and other pharmacological properties of 2-(o-chlorophenyl)-2-(methylamino)cyclohexanone HCl (CI-581). J. New Drugs 5: 21-33, 1965.

Quirion, R., Chicheportiche, R., Contreras, P.C., Johnson, K.M., Lodge, D., Tam, S.W., Woods, J.H., and Zukin, S.R.: A comment on the classification and nomenclature of phencyclidine and *sigma* receptor sites. Reply from Quirion *et al.*, TINS 11: 388-389, 1988.

Smith, D.J., Pekoe, G.M., Martin, L.L., and Coalgate, B.: The interaction of ketamine with the opiate receptor. Life Sci. 26: 789-795, 1980.

Takahashi, R.N., Morato, G.S., and Rae, G.A.: Effects of ketamine on nociception and gastrointestinal motility in mice are unaffected by naloxone. Gen. Pharmac. 18: 201-203, 1987.

Weissman, A.D., Su, T.-P., Hedreen, J.C., and London, E.D.: *Sigma* receptors in post-mortem human brains. J. Pharmacol. Exp. Ther. 247: 29-33, 1988.

White, P.F., Ham, J., Way, W.L., and Trevor, A.J.: Pharmacology of ketamine isomers in surgical patients. Anesthesiology 52: 231-239, 1980.

Status of Ketamine in Anesthesiology,
edited by E.F. Domino©1990, NPP Books
P.O. Box 1491, Ann Arbor, MI 48106

Effects of Ketamine and Combination with Acetylpromazine, Diazepam, or Butorphanol on Visceral Nociception in the Cat

D.C. Sawyer†*, R.H. Rech*, and R.A. Durham†

Departments of Small Animal Clinical Sciences† and
*Pharmacology and Toxicology**
College of Veterinary Medicine
Michigan State University
East Lansing, MI

INTRODUCTION

Pain is a complex physiological phenomenon usually difficult to recognize and interpret in animals. Pain may be inferred from clear clinical signs such as lameness, dysphagia, dysuria, and behavioral responses such as vocalization, frequent changes in positions, or thrashing about in a cage. In situations when a noxious stimulus does not cause functional impairment to normal activities, pain may be much less apparent and demonstrated only by subtle behavioral changes such as a pained facial expression, mild restlessness, or an unnatural resting position. Differences in the effects of analgesics between animal species further complicate the problem. Opiate agonists such as fentanyl, meperidine, morphine, and oxymorphone exert their effects by stimulating all central and peripheral opiate receptors. In the dog, analgesia is usually accompanied by mild to profound sedation. In early studies, low dose morphine was shown to produce similar analgesic effects in the cat to those seen in the dog (Davis and Donelly, 1968; Watts *et al.*, 1973; Heavner, 1970). However, larger doses of opiates may cause stimulatory effects in the cat, demonstrated by mydriasis, apprehension, hypersalivation, foaming at the mouth, or excitement, thereby virtually precluding the use of these drugs for analgesia in this species. Further, when tranquilizers are used alone or in combination with opiates in the cat, analgesia will not be provided or augmented (Sawyer *et al.*, to be published).

Ketamine has been a very useful drug for chemical restraint, anesthesia induction, or surgical anesthesia, administered either alone or in combination with other drugs in a large number of animal species, including the cat, in doses ranging from 10 to 45 mg/kg of body weight (Short, 1987; Azar and Ozomek, 1973; White *et al.*, 1982). To avoid marked cardiovascular responses and unpleasant emergence reactions associated with ketamine, tranquilizers such as acetylpromazine or diazepam are often combined with this agent (Green *et al.*, 1981; Manziano and Manziano, 1978; Tobin, 1982). Because of the adverse effects of opioid agonists in the cat, ketamine has been suggested for use for post surgical analgesia at doses lower than those recommended for other purposes. However, some authors question the ability of ketamine to provide adequate visceral analgesia in these animals (Short, 1987; Sawyer, 1982; Wright, 1982).

Compounds such as butorphanol, levallorphan, nalbuphine, nalorphine, and pentazocine produce both agonist and antagonist activity and thus are classified as agonist-antagonist analgesics (Jaffe and Martin, 1985). They produce their responses by binding to the opiate receptors but they either exert no action, indicative of competitive antagonists, or they produce variable agonistic effects as would be expected from other opiate agonists such as morphine. Of this group, butorphanol appears to have the strongest opiate agonist receptor activity and provides long term analgesia in the cat compared to the effects of nalbuphine and pentazocine (Jaffe and Martin, 1985; Sawyer and Rech, 1987).

Recently, we have developed a method to measure threshold responses to visceral stimulation in the unrestrained cat (Sawyer and Rech, 1987). Since the distension of the colon is considered to produce pain as the only sensory consequence (Sawyer *et al.*, 1984; Guyton, 1986), the subject's reaction was taken to be a nociceptive response. In order to avoid emotional irritability and conditioning of avoidance, the stimulus to the colon was maintained at threshold levels and presented infrequently interspersed with many subthreshold challenges. This method for evaluating visceral pain responses was adapted from a method developed for the horse (Muir, 1982; Pippi and Lumb, 1979). We have included scoring techniques of behavioral variables to allow for an estimation of sedative effects as well. With the use of this method, we assessed the effectiveness of ketamine alone and in combination with diazepam, acetylpromazine, or butorphanol to promote visceral analgesia in the cat.

Methods

Healthy, neutered female domestic cats were approved for use in these studies by the Michigan State University All University Committee on Animal Facilities and Care. Cats were kept in individual cages in a room without other animals.

For stimulation of visceral receptors, a 12F Foley catheter with a 42 ml balloon incorporated was inserted approximately 7 cm into the colon. The free end of the catheter was then secured to the tail with self-adherent wrap. Each cat was then placed in a 71 x 71 x 117 cm plexiglas enclosure and allowed to move about freely. Ambient air was then injected rapidly into the balloon with a large syringe. Response to colonic balloon inflation was recorded by a blinded observer and levels of visceral stimulation to elicit a minimum response were determined during training sessions for each cat. A positive response to balloon inflation was achieved if the cat elicited a strain, as if preparing to defecate, which was usually accompanied by panting or heavy breathing. If a higher than minimum threshold stimulus was given, the cat defecated the balloon. It was then replaced and the volume of air to be injected into the balloon was decreased at 3 ml increments in order to determine the level at which the strain responses would be observed. During 50% of the training sessions, less than 0.5 ml of sterile water (SW) was also given i.v. Prior to each drug study, control values were obtained subsequent to the injection of SW in a femoral vein and the drug to be studied was given. Ketamine (Ketaset, Fort Dodge Laboratories Inc., Fort Dodge, IA 50501) alone was tested at 2.0, 4.0 and 8.0 mg/kg. In addition, we injected butorphanol (Torbugesic Injection, Bristol Laboratories, Evansville, IN 47721) at 0.025, 0.05, 0.1, 0.2, 0.4, and 0.8 mg/kg; acetylpromazine (PromAce, Fort Dodge Laboratories Inc., Fort Dodge, IA 50501) at 0.025, 0.05, and 0.1 mg/kg; and diazepam (Valium, Hoffmann-LaRoche Inc., Nutley, NJ 07110) at 0.1, 0.2, and 0.4 mg/kg. For all combinations, drugs were drawn up into two separate syringes and mixed in one syringe prior to injection: ketamine/diazepam at 2.0/0.2, 4.0/0.2, and 8.0/0.2 mg/kg; ketamine/acetylpromazine at 2.0/0.1, 4.0/0.1, and 8.0/0.1 mg/kg; and ketamine/butorphanol at 2.0/0.1, 4.0/0.1, and 8.0/0.1 mg/kg. All doses were given i.v.

Ten min following injection, minimum threshold response was determined. When there was a positive response, the balloon was deflated and testing was terminated for that interval. If there was no response, the balloon was deflated and reinflated with an additional 3 ml of air. This procedure was repeated until a positive response was observed or until a maximum of 42 ml of air was injected into the balloon.

To avoid conditioned responses, 1 to 5 repetitive predictable negative stimuli were carried out prior to and following the threshold response. An increase in balloon volume above control level was considered indicative of analgesia. Duration of analgesia was determined as the interval between onset of the increase from control threshold response and return to control values. In addition, studies were terminated when values did not return to control within 360 min. Respiratory and pulse rates (beats/min) were recorded along with any behavioral changes or sedative effects induced by the drugs. These were graded as follows: 0 = no perceptible change; 1 = very slight sedation; 2 = mild sedation; 3 = moderate sedation; and 4 = marked sedation (Sawyer *et al.*, 1984).

Ten cats were used as test subjects in these studies. However, each cat did not receive the same drug treatment. The butorphanol group (N = 8) and the ketamine/butorphanol group (N = 7) were dissimilar, therefore, the ANOVA was done for independent groups. The 6 animals in the ketamine, ketamine/acetylpromazine, and ketamine/diazepam groups were all the same cats and were similar. Thus, the ANOVA for repeated measures was used. Balloon volume, pulse rate, and respiratory rate were analyzed using Tukey's test to determine the significant differences ($P<0.05$) between the treatment group means.

Results

The magnitude of analgesia provided by ketamine is expressed as a percent change from control in balloon volume (Fig. 1). Balloon volume increased following ketamine injection, indicating that there was a mild

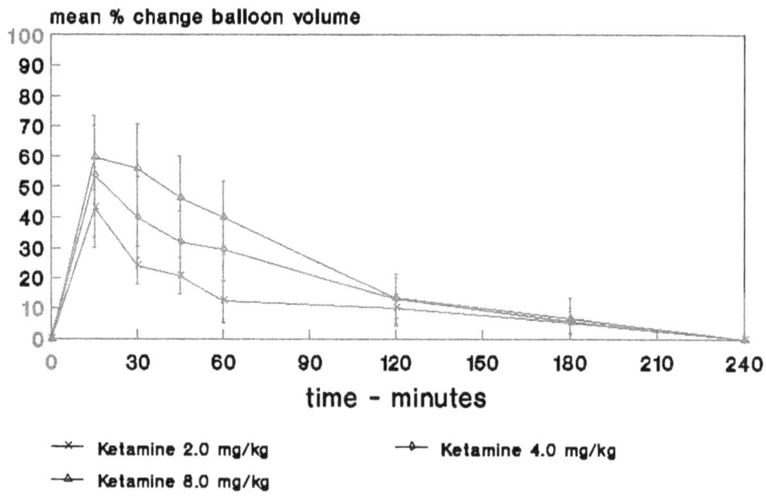

Fig. 1. Magnitude of analgesia following injection of ketamine in 6 cats at 2.0, 4.0, and 8.0 mg/kg expressed as percent change from control in balloon volume. M ± S.E.

degree of visceral analgesia provided by ketamine at all 3 doses (Fig. 1). However, there were no significant differences between doses, so that definitive evidence of a dose response pattern was not available.

Acetylpromazine alone did not increase balloon volume and, when it was combined with ketamine, the response to visceral nociceptor stimulation was not different from ketamine alone (Fig. 2). The same was true with the combination of ketamine and diazepam (Fig. 3), although we did not evaluate the effects of diazepam alone.

Butorphanol increased balloon volume at all 6 doses, with the greatest degree of analgesia provided by 0.1 mg/kg i.v. (Sawyer and Rech, 1987). We selected this dose to combine with the 3 doses of ketamine and found that there were no significant differences between ketamine alone, butorphanol alone, or the 3 doses of ketamine/butorphanol (Fig. 4).

Ketamine alone and ketamine/acetylpromazine provided essentially the same duration of effect with no significant difference between the 3 doses (Fig. 5). Comparisons between the 3 levels of ketamine/acetylpromazine showed that mean values at the 8.0/0.1 mg/kg dose represented the longest duration of effect, lasting 125 ± 22 min. Ketamine/diazepam responses did not differ significantly from those of ketamine/acetylpromazine, although there was a trend toward a shorter duration of effect when diazepam was added to ketamine (Fig. 6). However, these

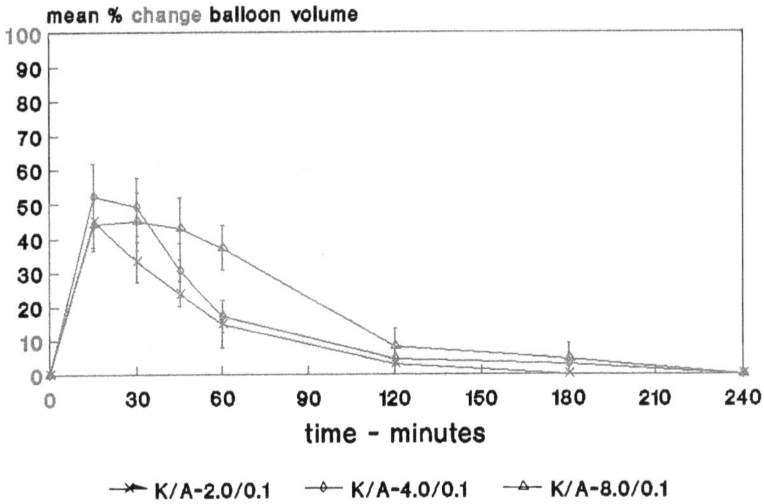

Fig. 2. Magnitude of analgesia following injection of ketamine/ acetylpromazine in 6 cats at 2.0/0.1, 4.0/0.1, and 8.0/0.1 mg/kg expressed as percent change from control in balloon volume. M ± S.E.

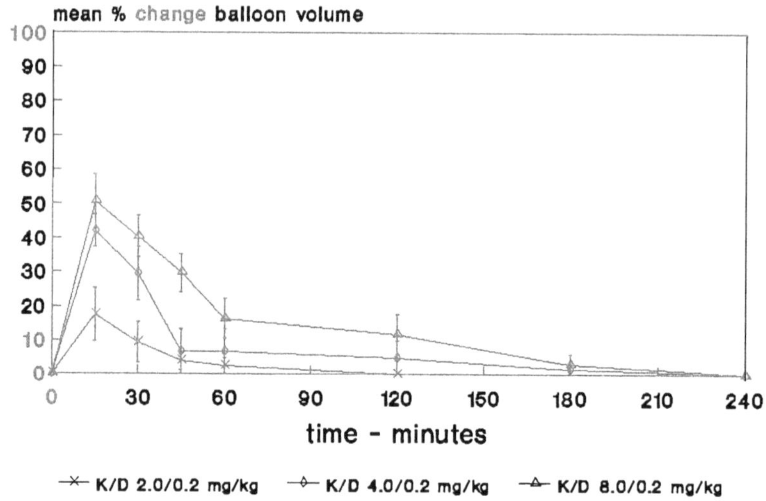

Fig. 3. Magnitude of analgesia following injection of ketamine/ diazepam in 6 cats at 2.0/0.2, 4.0/0.2, and 8.0/0.2 mg/kg expressed as percent change from control in balloon volume. M ± S.E.

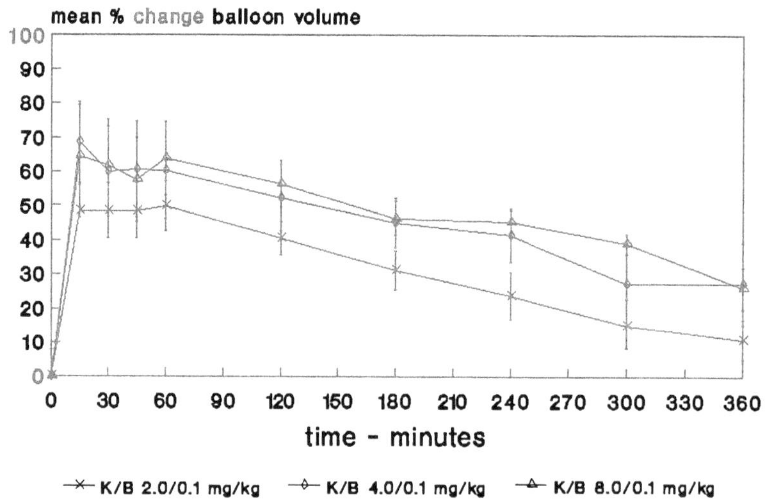

Fig. 4. Magnitude of analgesia following injection of ketamine/ butorphanol in 7 cats at 2.0/0.1, 4.0/0.1, and 8.0/0.1 mg/kg expressed as percent change from control in balloon volume. M ± S.E.

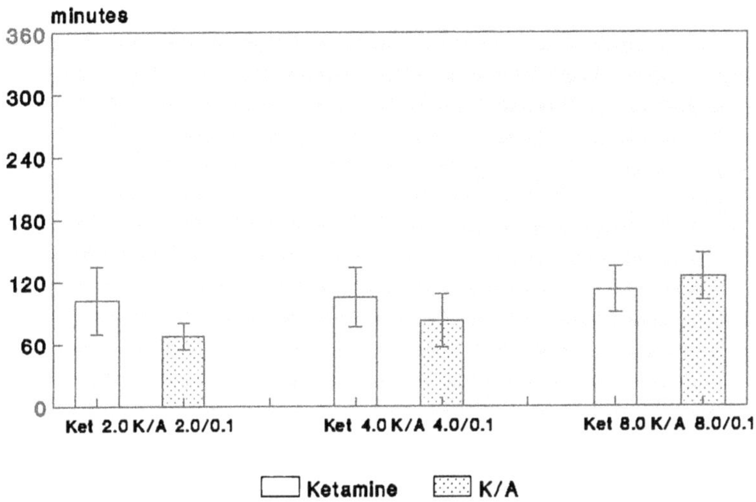

Fig. 5. Duration of visceral analgesia following injection of ketamine in 6 cats at 2.0, 4.0, and 8.0 mg/kg compared to the duration of visceral analgesia following injection of ketamine/ acetylpromazine in 6 cats at 2.0/0.1, 4.0/0.1, and 8.0/0.1 mg/kg i.v. M ± S.E.

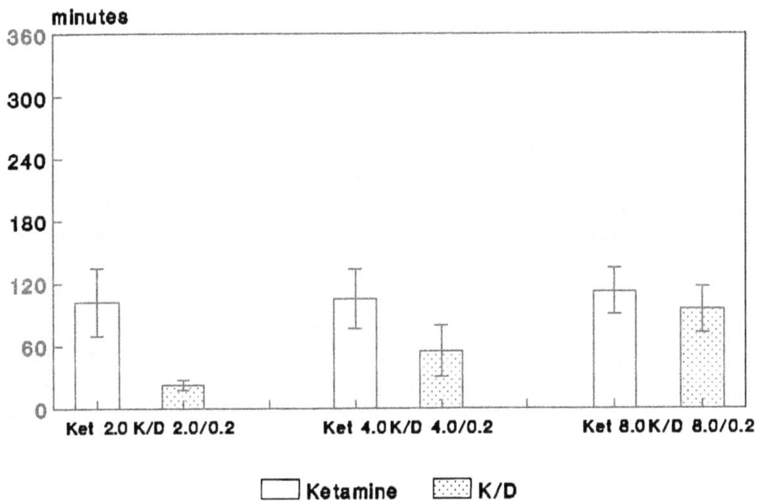

Fig. 6. Duration of visceral analgesia following injection of ketamine in 6 cats at 2.0, 4.0, and 8.0 mg/kg compared to the duration of visceral analgesia following injection of ketamine/ diazepam in 6 cats at 2.0/0.2, 4.0/0.2, and 8.0/0.2 mg/kg i.v. M ± S.E.

differences between ketamine alone and the combinations were not significant. In contrast to the other treatments, butorphanol alone (0.1 mg/kg) provided a long lasting effect, with a mean duration of analgesia of 348 ± 11 min (Fig. 7). The combination of butorphanol with ketamine did not significantly increase duration of analgesia, suggesting that the predominant influence was that of butorphanol.

Marked sedation at all dosage levels of ketamine was observed, with the most prominent effect provided by ketamine/acetylpromazine (Table 1).

There were no significant differences with duration, thus we selected variables recorded at 60 min for comparison. There were no significant differences in the degree of sedation provided by ketamine alone, ketamine/acetylpromazine, or ketamine/ butorphanol. Diazepam decreased the sedative effects of ketamine about 50%. Cats were not sedated by butorphanol.

There was a trend for pulse rate to increase following ketamine alone and with all 3 drug combinations, but these changes were not significant (Table 2). Pulse rate was not significantly changed by butorphanol alone and the values taken at 60 min at 0.1 mg/kg are also included in Table 2.

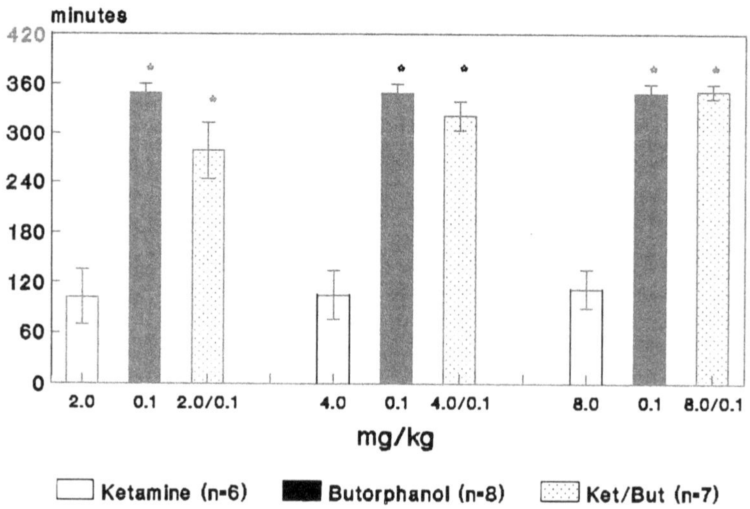

Fig. 7. Duration of visceral analgesia following injection of ketamine in 6 cats at 2.0, 4.0, and 8.0 mg/kg compared to the duration of visceral analgesia following injection of butorphanol in 8 cats at 0.1 mg/kg and with the duration of visceral analgesia following injection of ketamine/butorphanol in 7 cats at 2.0// 0.1, 4.0/0.1, and 8.0/0.1 mg/kg i.v. M ± S.E. *Significant difference ($P < 0.05$) from ketamine alone.

TABLE 1. Sedation level at 60 min postdrug injection compared to predrug control time period

Drug	*Control*	*60 min*
Ket-8.0 m/kg	0	3.2 ± 0.2
K/A-8.0/0.1 mg/kg	0	3.5 ± 0.2
K/B-8.0/0.1 mg/kg	0	2.4 ± 0.5
K/D-8.0/0.2 mg/kg	0	1.5 ± 0.5
But-0.1 mg/kg	0	0

Sedation level was defined on a 0-4 scale: 0 = no perceptible change; 1 = very slight sedation; 2 = mild sedation; 3 = moderate sedation; and 4 = marked sedation

TABLE 2. Pulse rates (beats/min) at 60 min compared to the predrug control time period

Drug	*Control*	*60 min*
Ket-8.0 mg/kg	165.3 ± 3.8	200.7 ± 8.3
K/A-8.0/0.1 mg/kg	162.7 ± 5.1	186.7 ± 14.4
K/B-8.0/0.1 mg/kg	149.7 ± 3.1	172.0 ± 5.3
K/D-8.0/0.2 mg/kg	168.7 ± 5.6	182.7 ± 10.1
But-0.1 mg/kg	165.5 ± 3.8	170.5 ± 3.0

Data are M ± S.E. in beats/min

TABLE 3. Respiratory rates (breaths/min) by 60 min compared to the predrug control time period

Drug	*Control*	*60 min*
Ket-8.0 mg/kg	48.0 ± 5.3	50.7 ± 2.7
K/A-8.0/0.1 mg/kg	42.7 ± 6.2	50.7 ± 6.7
K/B-8.0/0.1 mg/kg	40.0 ± 4.1	36.0 ± 2.6
K/D-8.0/0.2 mg/kg	47.3 ± 5.3	44.5 ± 4.6
But-0.1 mg/kg	63.0 ± 4.4	50.5 ± 3.7

Data are M ± S.E. in breaths/min

Respiratory rate did not change with ketamine and additional changes were not induced by acetylpromazine, diazepam, or butorphanol (Table 3).

Two cats reacted adversely in response to ketamine. One appeared to hallucinate at all 3 doses while the other reacted adversely only to the high dose. All cats hypersalivated subsequent to ketamine (slight to moderate) during these studies. Two of the 8 cats showed discomfort upon injection of the 8.0 mg/kg dose.

No discomfort was observed following injections of butorphanol, but mydriasis was produced at all doses. Five of the 8 cats appeared minimally apprehensive for 52 ± 26 min following i.v. injection at 0.4 and 0.8 mg/kg of butorphanol. At all other doses, they became very affectionate, rubbing and purring throughout each study. The cats did not purr following the injection of ketamine but did purr with the ketamine/butorphanol at intervals beyond 120 min.

Discussion

Ketamine is a safe, rapidly acting parenteral anesthetic and analgesic agent which has been in clinical use for more than 20 years in animal and human patients (Sadove *et al.*, 1971). Although there have been many neurophysiologic investigations relating to the effects of ketamine on central nervous system activity, its exact mechanism and site of analgesic action in brain remain unclear. Ohtani and colleagues (1979) demonstrated that ketamine suppresses activity in single neurons in the nucleus reticularis gigantocellularis following high intensity electrical stimulation of peripheral neurons. The extent of suppression of the nucleus reticularis gigantocellularis neurons by ketamine was greater than that induced by comparable doses of neurons in the dorsal horn of the lumbar spinal cord. Thus, they concluded that ketamine's effect on activity in the nucleus reticularis gigantocellularis was more likely related to the analgesic action of the drug than actions at the spinal level. In addition, ketamine has been shown to displace narcotics from opioid receptors in rats (Finck and Ngai, 1979) and a portion, though not all, of the analgesic effects of ketamine may be reversed with naloxone. These and many other studies support the hypothesis that ketamine may exert activity on both *mu* and *kappa* opioid mechanisms, though an action at *sigma* receptors is usually emphasized (Maurset *et al.*, 1988; Smith *et al.*, 1980; Vincent *et al.*, 1979; Zukin and Zukin, 1988; Johnson, 1987).

It is also interesting to speculate that this study supports the concept that ketamine acts, in part, at *kappa* opioid receptors. In previous studies from this laboratory, the increase in balloon volume provided by butorphanol was reversed by naloxone. However, we did not antagonize the effect of ketamine alone or ketamine/butorphanol with naloxone in the cat. Balloon volume did not increase when butorphanol was added to ketamine and one might reason that ketamine somehow occludes the analgesic response to butorphanol.

The results of our study demonstrate that ketamine increased the threshold response to nociceptor stimulation, thus providing visceral analgesia in the cat without adverse side effects. The degree of analgesia was similar to that provided by butorphanol but there was no increase in the analgesic response with increasing doses of ketamine. Even at the highest dose of ketamine (8 mg/kg i.v.), animals appeared to be anesthetized but still responded to colonic distention. Certainly the analgesia provided by ketamine was not profound, which would suggest that this drug would be more effective for surgery and postoperative analgesia for procedures involving the skeleton and extremities than for abdominal procedures in the cat (Sawyer, 1982; Haskins *et al.*, 1975; Short, 1987).

It was not surprising to find that acetylpromazine did not provide analgesia when tested alone, nor did it augment the analgesic effects of ketamine. We found the same to be true for diazepam, although we did not investigate its possible analgesic effects alone. Haskins *et al.* (1986) found that diazepam did not tranquilize dogs when given alone and was frequently associated with exuberant behavior. We have seen this effect clinically in cats as well and did not want to replicate this response in these animals. The few episodes of adverse responses with ketamine were found to be minor and the hypersalivation usually produced by ketamine can be offset with an anticholinergic such as atropine.

Acknowledgements

Technical assistance was provided by Susan Eberhardt, Jennifer Feddeler, Cindy Franklin, Carol Lawton, Steve Stelma, Marlee Langham, and Elaine Striler. The help provided by Dr. Greg Fink for data processing and statistical analysis is greatly appreciated.

This study was funded by grants from Bristol Laboratories, the M.S.U. College of Veterinary Medicine, and Michigan State University.

References

Azar, I. and Ozomek, E.: The use of ketamine for abdominal tubal ligation. Anesth. Analg. Curr. Res. 52: 39-42, 1973.

Davis, L.E. and Donelly, E.J.: Analgesia drugs in the cat. J. Am. Vet. Med. Assoc. 153: 1161-1167, 1968.

Finck, D.A. and Ngai, S.H.: A possible mechanism of ketamine induced analgesia. Anesthesiol. 51: S34, 1979.

Green, C.J., Knight, J, Precious, S., and Simpkin, S.: Ketamine alone and combined with diazepam and xylazine in laboratory animals: A 10 year experience. Lab. Animals 15: 163-170, 1981.

Guyton, A.C.: Textbook of Medical Physiology, pp. 598, W.B. Saunders, Philadelphia, 1986.

Haskins, S.C., Peiffer, R.L., and Stowe, C.M.: A clinical comparison of CT 1341, ketamine, and xylazine in cats. Am. J. Vet. Res. 36: 1537-1543, 1975.

Haskins, S.C., Farver, T.B., and Patz, J.D.: Cardiovascular changes in dogs given diazepam and diazepam-ketamine. Am. J. Vet. Res. 47: 795-798, 1986.

Heavner, J.E.: Morphine for postsurgical use in cats. J. Am. Vet. Med. Assoc. 156: 1018-1019, 1970.

Jaffe, J.H. and Martin, W.R.: Opioid analgesics and antagonists. In The Pharmacological Basis of Therapeutics, A.G. Goodman, L.S. Goodman, T.W. Rall, and F. Murad, ed., pp. 520-524, MacMillan Publishing, New York, 1985.

Johnson, K.M., Jr.: Neurochemistry and neurophysiology of phencyclidine. In Psychopharmacology: The Third Generation of Progress, H.Y. Meltzer, ed., pp. 1581-1588, Raven Press, New York, 1987.

Manziano, C.F. and Manziano, J.R.: The combination of ketamine HCl and acetylpromazine maleate as a general anesthetic in dogs. Vet. Med./Sm. Anim. Clin. pp. 727-730, June, 1978.

Maurset, A., Skoglund, L.A., and Øye, I.L.S.: The analgetic action of ketamine in humans is non-opioid and mediated by PCP receptors. In *Sigma* and Phencyclidine-Like Compounds as Molecular Probes in Biology, E. Domino and J.-M. Kamenka, eds., pp. 541-544, NPP Books, Ann Arbor, 1988.

Muir, W.W.: Evaluation of butorphanol as an analgesic in balloon induced equine colic model. Equine Colic Symposium, University of Georgia, Athens, GA, September, 1982.

Ohtani, M., Hirosato, K., Kitahata, L., Taub, A., Hidenori, T., Hanaoka, K., and Dohi, S.: Effects of ketamine on nociceptive cells in the medial medullary reticular formation of the cat. Anesthesiol. 51: 414-417, 1979.

Pippi, N.L. and Lumb, W.F.: Objective tests of analgesic drugs in ponies. Am. J. Vet. Res. 40: 1082-1086, 1979.

Sadove, M.S., Shulman, M., Hatano, S., and Fevold, N.: Analgesic effects of ketamine administered in subdissociative doses. Anesth. Analg. Curr Res. 50: 452-457, 1971.

Sawyer, D.C.: The Practice of Small Animal Anesthesia, pp 103, W.B. Saunders Co., 1982.

Sawyer, D.C. and Rech, R.H.: Analgesia and behavioral effects of butorphanol, nalbuphine, and pentazocine in the cat. J. Am. Anim. Hosp. Assoc. 23: 438-446, 1987.

Sawyer, D.C., Rech, R.H., Hartman, D., and Gilmour, M.: A model to evaluate analgesic drugs in the cat. Proceedings, Scientific Meetings, Am. Col. Vet. Anes., New Orleans, October 12, 1984.

Short, C.E.: Dissociative Anesthesia. In Principles and Practices of Veterinary Anesthesia, C.E. Short, ed., pp 163, Williams and Wilkins, Baltimore, 1987.

Smith, D.J., Westfall, D.P., and Adams, J.D.: Ketamine interacts with opiate receptors as an agonist. Anesthesiol. 53: S5, 1980.

Tobin, H.A.: Low dose ketamine and diazepam. Arch. Otolaryngol. 108: 439-444, 1982.

Vincent, J.P., Kartalowski, B., Geneste, P., Kamenka, J.-M., and Lazdunski, M.: Interaction of phencyclidine ("angel dust") with a specific receptor in rat brain membranes. Proc. Natl. Acad. Sci. USA 76: 4678-4682, 1979.

Watts, S.J., Slocombe, F.R., Harbison, W.D., and Stewart, G.A.: Assessment of analgesia and other effects of morphine and thiambutene in the mouse and cat. Aust. Vet. 49: 525-529, 1973.

White, P.F., Way, W.L., and Trevor, A.: Ketamine—Its pharmacology and therapeutic uses. Anesthesiol. 56: 119-139, 1982.

Wright, M.: Pharmacologic effects of ketamine and its use in veterinary medicine. J. Am. Vet. Med. Assoc. 180: 1462-1471, 1982.

Zukin, R.S. and Zukin, S.R.: Phencyclidine, *sigma* and NMDA receptors: Emerging concepts. In *Sigms* and Phencyclidine-Like Compounds as Molecular Probes in Biology, E.F. Domino and J.-M. Kamenka, eds., pp 407-424, NPP Books, Ann Arbor, MI, 1988.

Status of Ketamine in Anesthesiology,
edited by E.F. Domino©1990, NPP Books
P.O. Box 1491, Ann Arbor, MI 48106

Neuropharmacological Effects of Ketamine: Gross Behavior, EEG, Unit Activity, Wake-Sleep, Kindling, and Interactions with Diazepam and Propranolol

W.D. Winters

Department of Pharmacology, School of Medicine
University of California Davis, California

Introduction

Phencyclidine (Sernyl), the parent compound of ketamine, was introduced as an anesthetic agent in 1957 (Greifenstein *et al.*, 1958). The drug induced an initial amnesia, then analgesia, catalepsy, anesthesia, and convulsions (Luby *et al.*, 1959). During emergence, phencylidine induced a high incidence of acute psychotic reactions and, thus, was never approved for clinical use. The behavior described, as well as the EEG progression, was similar to those of agents which induced a progression of CNS excitation up to generalized seizures (Winters *et al.*, 1969).

The search for analogs which had less propensity for inducing seizures and severe emergence phenomena resulted in the development of ketamine (Ketalar, Ketaject). Along with lesser potency, this agent was reported to induce seizures less frequently, to have a shorter duration of action, and to cause fewer severe emergence phenomena (Domino *et al.*, 1965). The principal disadvantage of ketamine was reported to be adverse psychic effects during emergence, such as changes in mood, body image, affect, and hallucinations. Some of the hallucinations were sufficiently frightening to the subjects that they preferred not to repeat the drug. Domino *et al.* (1965) noted that, in some subjects, ketamine induced an alarming rise in systolic and diastolic blood pressure and heart rate, along with sweating, lacrimation, hyperactive tendon reflexes, and a rise in blood glucose levels. In addition, many of the protective reflexes were maintained during catalepsy. EEG studies demonstrated a hypersynchronous slow wave pattern during catalepsy similar to that seen with phencyclidine and other agents which induce a continuum of CNS excitation (Winters *et al.*, 1969).

Assessment of the activated CNS in an immobile subject can be confusing and may lead one to assume that the subject is depressed rather than hyperexcited. Therefore, to examine the ketamine induced level of CNS excitability, we utilized neuropharmacological techniques involving the placement of electrodes in various parts of the brain, and examination of the brain wave activity during control and ketamine induced states. Correlation of EEG patterns, reticular formation multiple-unit activity, response to sensory stimuli, and gross behavior formed the basis for examination of the ketamine induced states. Studies were undertaken in the unrestrained cat using these parameters with chronically implanted cortical and subcortical electrodes. These studies included examination of: ketamine induced neuropharmacological actions, the influence of ketamine on wake-sleep cycles, the attenuating influence of diazepam and propranolol on ketamine induced catalepsy, the epileptoid EEG waveform during and after consecutive daily low (ataxic) and high (cataleptic) doses of ketamine, and the dose-response relationship of ketamine in amygdaloid kindled seizures.

Methods

Adult Female Cats

Chronic cortical and subcortical electrodes were implanted in each animal during pentobarbital anesthesia using sterile surgical techniques. The animals were fully recovered in 1 to 2 weeks, and baseline wake-sleep cycles were established for each cat. The behavioral criteria for each level of drug induced excitability were based on the assessment of the general activity, posture, and responsiveness to auditory and tactile stimulation. EEG recording techniques have been described in detail previously by Winters *et al.* (1967, 1969). Ketamine was administered i.p. at a dose of 15 to 40 mg/kg and post-drug observations were obtained. Twenty-four hr wake-sleep cycles were determined by evaluation of the EEG, multiple unit activity, and EMG, as described previously by Winters (1964).

Studies involving attenuation of ketamine induced catalepsy were performed about 1 week after a test dose of ketamine (25 mg/kg) was administered. The cats were pretreated with saline, 0.25 or 3 mg/kg of diazepam, or 1-2 mg/kg propranolol, followed 10 to 60 min later by the challenge dose of 25 mg/kg of ketamine.

Adult Male Rats—Sprague-Dawley

Chronic daily ketamine. Stainless steel electrodes were placed chronically into the amygdala, hippocampus, and cerebral cortices. The rats were allowed to recover for 7-10 days before EEG recordings were begun. One group received daily injections of 80 mg/kg i.p. ketamine (a sub-cataleptic dose). A second group received a daily injection of 30 mg/kg i.p. ketamine (ataxia for 40-500 min), and a control group received 0.9% NaCl i.p. All of the injections were given between 11 a.m. and 1 p.m. daily. Behavioral manifestations, the latencies to the development of ataxia or catalepsy, and the duration of such effects were noted. In each animal, EEG recordings were made once every 3-5 days, prior to and after the drug or saline administration. Animals received a daily dose of drug for 1, 2 or 3 months.

Kindled seizures. Twisted stainless steel wires were implanted in the amygdala for electrical stimulation, and monopolar screw electrodes were placed over the motor cortex and frontal sinus for recording the EEG. The induction and maintenance of kindled seizures were assessed utilizing standard techniques reported in detail previously by Bowyer *et al.* (1981, 1983). Dose-response relationships of ketamine were recorded for kindling, utilizing the gross behavioral response and spike frequency of the afterdischarge as criteria.

Results

Female Cats—Behavior

Following a 15 to 40 mg/kg dose of ketamine, there was a rapid appearance of motor excitability and ataxia within 2 to 4 min. With the lowest dose (15-20 mg/kg), the cats then lay in bizarre positions but were responsive to noxious stimuli (catatonia), and within 30-70 min were again ataxic for the next 10 hr. A moderate dose (25 mg/kg) induced a 45 min period of catalepsy (loss of the righting reflex and immobility with no response to noxious stimuli), followed by ataxia and a return to relative control states in 50 hr. The highest dose (40 mg/kg) induced 80 min of catalepsy followed by ataxia and a return to control after 50 hr. Thus, the 15 and 20 mg/kg doses did not induce a state of catalepsy, whereas the 25 and 40 mg/kg doses did.

EEG

The EEG patterns were related to the above-noted behavioral changes (Fig. 1). During motor excitation, the pattern was characteristic of an alert EEG with low voltage, fast waves—desynchronized. During

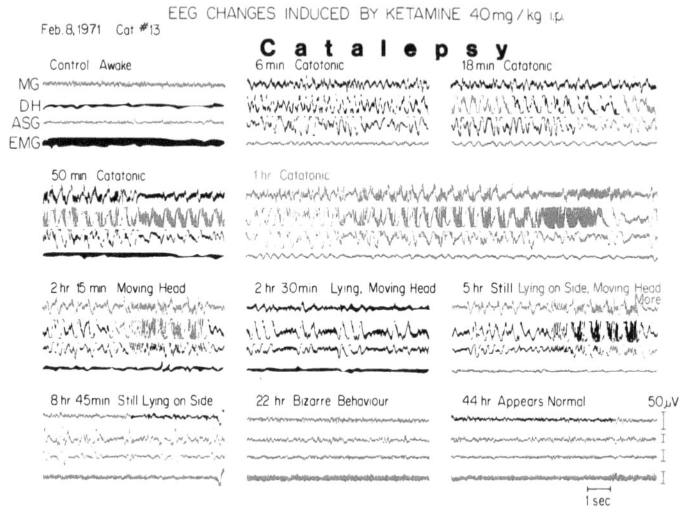

Fig. 1. EEG progression following ketamine 40 mg/kg i.p. MG, medial geniculate; DH, dorsal hippocampus; ASG, cortex; and EMG, neck muscle, in the female cat.

ataxia with bizarre postures, there was intermittent and then continuous hypersynchrony (2.5 cycles per sec). During catalepsy, the pattern was a continuous 2.5 cycles per sec hypersynchrony with spikes. Of note was the appearance of a seizure discharge in the dorsal hippocampus during catalepsy following the cataleptic-inducing doses of ketamine. The discharges did not spread to adjoining areas of cortex, and no gross behavioral manifestations of epilepsy were noted. A similar discharge was noted by Ferrar-Allado *et al.*, (1973) in a human temporal lobe epileptic with electrodes in the hippocampus for diagnostic procedures. This subject, likewise, had no observable gross manifestations of seizure activity.

Reticular Multiple Unit Activity

Ketamine induced an elevated basal amplitude and fluctuation of the reticular formation unit activity (Fig. 2), as previously noted with other cataleptoid agents.

Wake-Sleep Cycles

Observations of the daily wake-sleep cycles of these cats were examined prior to and following ketamine. There was almost no REM sleep during the first day following ketamine in a dose of 40 mg/kg. Instead there was 1 hr of catalepsy followed by 18 hr of hallucinoid activity during emergence and no REM sleep until 23 hr post-drug (Table 1).

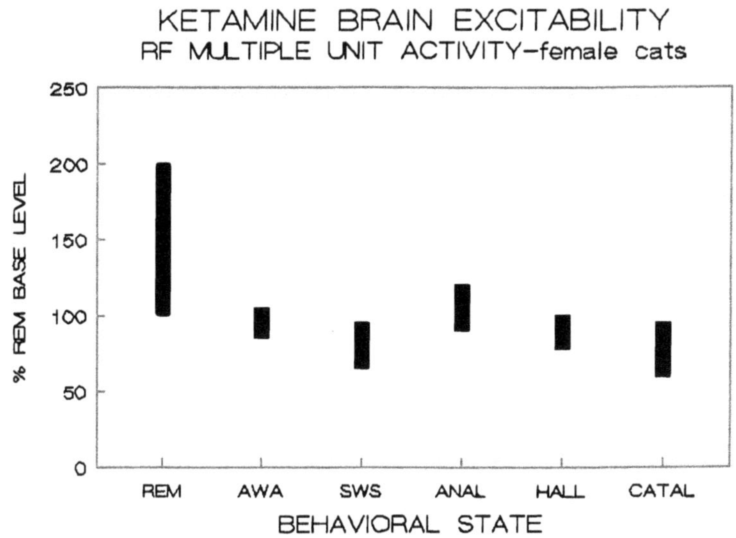

Fig. 2. Reticular neuronal activity during REM,dream sleep; AWA, awake; SWS, slow wave sleep; and following ketamine 25-40 mg/kg, ANAL, analgesia; HALL, hallucinatory; and CATAL, catalepsy in the female cat.

TABLE 1. Duration of ketamine induced behavior in female cats

State	*15 mg/kg*	*20 mg/kg*	*25 mg/kg*	*40 mg/kg*
Induction				
Ataxia	7 min	5 min	4 min	4 min
Catatonia	30 min	70 min	3 min	1 min
Catalepsy	0	0	45 min	80 min
Emergence				
Ataxia	9.5 hr	—	30 hr	31 hr
Normal	10 hr	—	50 hr	50 hr
1st REM	16 hr	—	20 hr	23 hr

Ketamine Interaction With Propranolol or Diazepam

The effects of diazepam or propranolol on ketamine induced catatonia and hypersynchrony can be seen in Table 2. There is no significant difference in the duration of catalepsy or the number of hypersynchronous waves at the high dose of diazepam, whereas propranolol (1-2 mg/kg) was partially effective in blocking ketamine induced hypersynchrony. Propranolol and 0.25 mg/kg of diazepam partially reduced the duration of

TABLE 2. Propranolol or diazepam: interaction with 25 mg/kg of ketamine in the cat

Drug	*mg/kg*	*% Duration Ketamine Effect* *Hypersynchrony*	*Catalepsy*
Propranolol	1-2	30	45
Diazepam	0.25	60	64
Diazepam	3	110	470

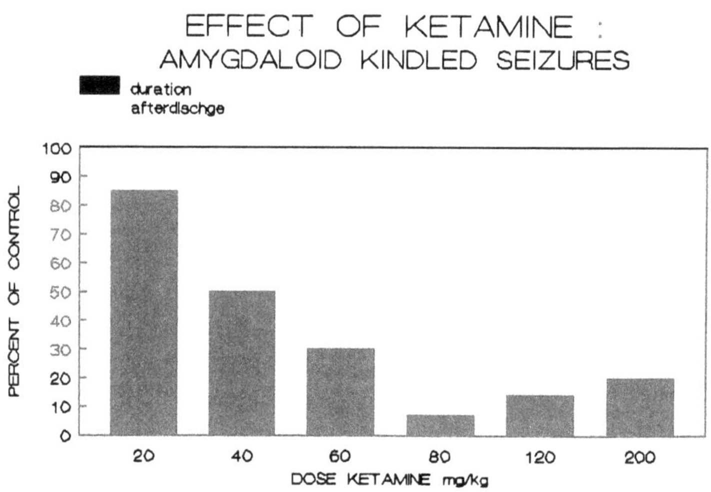

Fig. 3. Effect of ketamine on kindled amygdaloid seizure afterdischarges in the male rat.

catalepsy, whereas diazepam (3 mg/kg) markedly prolonged the duration (Table 2).

Rat Kindled Seizures

As can be noted in Fig. 3, there was a U-shaped dose-response effect. A dose of 20 to 80 mg/kg of ketamine induced a progressive dose related reduction in amygdaloid afterdischarge. A cataleptic dose of 200 mg/kg showed an increase in afterdischarges and the EEG changed from hypersynchronous activity to high frequency bursts with periods of electrical silence. Two of 7 rats died at this dose and 1 died shortly after a brief spontaneous seizure (Bowyer and Winters, 1981).

Discussion

The term dissociative anesthesia was proposed by Miyasaka and Domino (1968), based on the finding that the thalamoneocortex had slow waves but the hippocampus was normal during ketamine anesthesia induced by a dose of 16 mg/kg i.p. in the cat. This is not in agreement with our data, which showed that during the cataleptic state induced by ketamine, EEG seizure wave activity was noted in the hippocampus. Since ketamine induces surgical anesthesia during the cataleptic state, this state does not fit their premise since these authors made their observations at a dose which does not induce cataleptic anesthesia in the cat. This is probably the explanation for our differences in evaluating the hippocampal activity. Perhaps a more appropriate term to describe the ketamine induced anesthetic state would be the "cataleptic-anesthetic state."

The behavioral, EEG, and reticular unit data clearly indicate that ketamine induces actions similar to those of other CNS excitatory agents such as phencyclidine, LSD, and mescaline, rather than inducing CNS depression. From our wake-sleep data, we conclude that the so-called emergence dreaming is actually emergence hallucinations since REM sleep is, in fact, depressed or absent during the first 12 to 23 hr of emergence.

Our studies showed a progression of ketamine induced behavior, EEG, and changes in wake-sleep cycles which are based on dose, time, and frequency of administration. Clearly, this emphasizes the need for paying attention to these issues when attempting to elucidate the mechanisms of action and clinical usefulness of ketamine. Other factors influencing ketamine actions are discussed in greater depth in another chapter (Winters and Hance, this volume). Our data also show a clear dose related U-shaped response to ketamine in terms of protection from amygdaloid kindled seizure activity. Sub-cataleptic doses of ketamine are clearly anticonvulsant, whereas cataleptic doses are pro-convulsant.

The appearance of a ketamine induced progression of EEG patterns characteristic of epileptiform waveforms is of significance. The seizure pattern noted in the limbic structures has also been reported in humans (Ferrar-Allado *et al.*, 1973). These phenomena suggest that ketamine is not the agent of choice for assisting in diagnostic neurological procedures. The misdiagnosis of iatrogenic epilepsy in a patient would be tragic, but would also put the subject with temporal lobe pathology at risk since ketamine may trigger further, more profound seizures. Furthermore, use of this agent as an emergency anti-convulsant treatment must be done cautiously and should be employed only by persons who understand these relationships and exercise extreme care.

Ketamine induced EEG hypersynchrony during behavioral catalepsy was partially blocked by propranolol, whereas neither dose of diazepam was effective; in fact, diazepam prolonged the duration of catalepsy. Propranolol is of questionable value and diazepam is of little value in reversing ketamine action. On the other hand, in terms of "taming ketamine", *i.e.*, reducing stimulation of cardiovascular functions, emergence delirium, and induced seizure activity, the combination of compounds such as diazepam, phenobarbital, or midazolam seems logical and worthy of further evaluation. An alternate approach to attenuating ketamine actions was reported by Winters *et al.* (1986; see also other chapter in this volume), who showed that the specific opioid antagonist, naloxone, reversed the ketamine induced analgesia or catalepsy. Blocking emergence delirium with naloxone probably is not practical since this would also attenuate the analgesic action of both ketamine and opioid analgesic supplements.

References

Bowyer, J.F. and Winters, W.D.: The effects of various anesthetics on amygdaloid kindled seizures. Neuropharmacol. 20: 199-209, 1981.

Bowyer, J.F., Albertson, T.E., Winters, W.D., and Baselt, R.C.: Ketamine-induced changes in kindled amygdaloid seizures. Neuropharmacol. 22: 887-894, 1983.

Domino, E.F., Chodoff, P., and Corssen, G.: Pharmacologic effects of CI-581, a new dissociative anesthetic, in man. Clin. Pharmacol. Ther. 6: 279-291, 1965.

Ferrar-Allado, T., Brechner V.L., Dymond, A., Cozen, H., and Crandall, P.: Ketamine-induced electroconvulsive phenomena in the human limbic and thalamic regions. Anesthesiol. 38: 333-344, 1973.

Greifenstein, F.E., DeVault, M., Yoshitake, J., and Gajewski, J.E.: A study of a 1-aryl cyclohexylamine for anesthesia. Anesth. Analg. 37: 283, 1958.

Luby, E., Cohen, B.D., Rosebaum, G., Gottlieb, J.S., and Kelly, R.: Study of new schizophrenomimetic drug. Sernyl. Arch. Neurol. Psychiat. 81: 363, 1959.

Miyasaka, M. and Domino, E.F.: Neuronal mechanisms of ketamine induced anesthesia. Int. J. Neuropharmacol. 7: 557-573, 1968.

Winters, W.D. Comparison of the average cortical and subcortical evoked response to clicks during various stages of wakefulness, slow wave sleep, and rhombencephalic sleep. EEG Clin. Neurophysiol. 17: 234-245, 1964.

Winters, W.D. and Hance, A.J.: Factors influencing ketamine induced analgesia and catalepsy. This volume, 1989.

Winters, W.D., Hance, A.J., Cadd, G.G., and Lakin, M.L.: Seasonal and sex influences on ketamine-induced analgesia and catalepsy in the rat: A possible role for melatonin. Neuropharmacol. 25: 1099-1101, 1986.

Winters, W.D., Mori, K., Spooner, C.E., and Kado, R.T.: Correlation of reticular and cochlear multiple unit activity with evoked responses during wakefulness and sleep. I. EEG Clin. Neurophysiol. 23: 539-545, 1967.

Winters, W.D., Mori, K., Wallach, M.B., Marcus, R.J., and Spooner, C.E.: Reticular multiple unit activity during a progression of states induced by CNS excitants. III. EEG Clin. Neurophysiol. 27: 514-522, 1969.

Status of Ketamine in Anesthesiology,
edited by E.F. Domino©1990, NPP Books
P.O. Box 1491, Ann Arbor, MI 48106

Factors Influencing Ketamine Induced Analgesia and Catalepsy

W.D. Winters and A.J. Hance

Department of Pharmacology
University of California School of Medicine
Davis, CA

Introduction

Winters (1976) has previously described three diverse progressions of drug-induced anesthetic states; one characterized by profound CNS depression of neuronal activity induced by barbiturates and halothane (stages I, III, IV), a second characterized by progressive CNS activation induced by phencyclidine, ketamine, enflurane, trichlorethylene, *alpha*-chloralose and *gamma*-hydroxybutyrate (stages I, II, catalepsy, convulsions), and a third characterized by changes from an excitatory to a depressant progression as with diethyl ether (stages I, II, III, IV). Studies on ketamine were instituted when the drug was in clinical trial. Initially, we showed (Winters *et al.*, 1972) that the gross behavior and neurophysiology of ketamine were similar to the parent compound phencyclidine (PCP), except that PCP was more potent and had a greater predisposition to induce grand mal seizures. Subsequently (Winters, 1976, Winters *et al.*, 1986, 1988), the dose and time related continuum of the effects of ketamine, *i.e.*, analgesia, hallucinations, catatonia, catalepsy and seizures, were studied. These studies revealed various factors which influence the action of ketamine. The present review will collate these findings in an attempt to enhance our overall understanding of the character and mechanisms of action, focusing primarily on the observed responses to ketamine. The neurophysiological studies were previously described in depth (see Spooner and Winters, 1966; Winters, 1976; Winters *et al.*, 1967, 1969, 1972; Geidt *et al.*, 1978), and are reviewed elsewhere in this volume. Thus, the present report will deal primarily with the more recent ketamine studies in which analgesia and catalepsy were examined in the chick, rat and cat.

Methods

Male DeKalb Warren chicks obtained 4 hr posthatched, male and female Sprague-Dawley rats, and female mongrel cats were utilized in these studies. Chicks were either intact, pinealectomized, or hypophysectomized. Rats were either intact, pinealectomized, or hypophysectomized. The cats were intact or pinealectomized. The animals were housed in a low noise, lighting, and temperature regulated room with food and water supplied *ad libitum*. Most of the studies utilized a 12 hr on-off light cycle. Unless specifically stated, all studies were performed 4 hr after lights were on during the winter months.

Analgesia was assessed in rats by measuring the tail flick latency differences (TFLD) between pre- and post-drug states, when the tail was placed in a beaker of water warmed to 55°C (Winters *et al.*, 1986, 1988).

Catalepsy was quantified by measuring the latency to, and the duration of, the loss of the righting reflex (DLRR) in an immobile (catatonic) rat. The character of the rigidity and the presence of diuresis and/or ataxia on recovery were likewise noted (Winters *et al.*, 1972, 1986, and 1988).

Tolerance was examined by administering the same dose of ketamine on consecutive days and measuring the % difference compared with the Day 1 value (TFLD or DLRR) (Winters *et al.*, 1988; Hance *et al.*, 1989; Benthuysen *et al.*, 1989a, b).

Opioid interactions. Various doses of morphine, fentanyl, sufentanil, alfentanil, butorphanol, nalbuphine and naloxone, were studied alone or in combination with various doses of ketamine (Winters *et al.*, 1988; Hance *et al.*, 1989; Benthuysen *et al.*, 1989b).

Ketamine enantiomers were compared with the racemic mixture (Benthuysen *et al.*, 1989a). Except for these studies, all others were done utilizing the racemic mixture (50/50, Ketalar, Bristol Labs.).

Results

Dose-response relationships

Analgesia was noted in a dose range of 30 to 50 mg/kg in female rats, but was not attainable at any dose prior to catatonia in the male rat (Fig. 1). Catatonia was noted between 50 to 55 mg/kg and catalepsy was apparent at 60 mg/kg and above in the female rat and at slightly higher doses in the male (Fig. 2; Winters *et al.*, 1972, 1988).

Ketamine enantiomers

The S(+) isomer of ketamine was approximately twice as potent as the R(-) isomer in both the rat and cat, although the racemic mixture was similar in potency to the S(+) isomer (Fig. 3; Benthuysen *et al.*, 1989a).

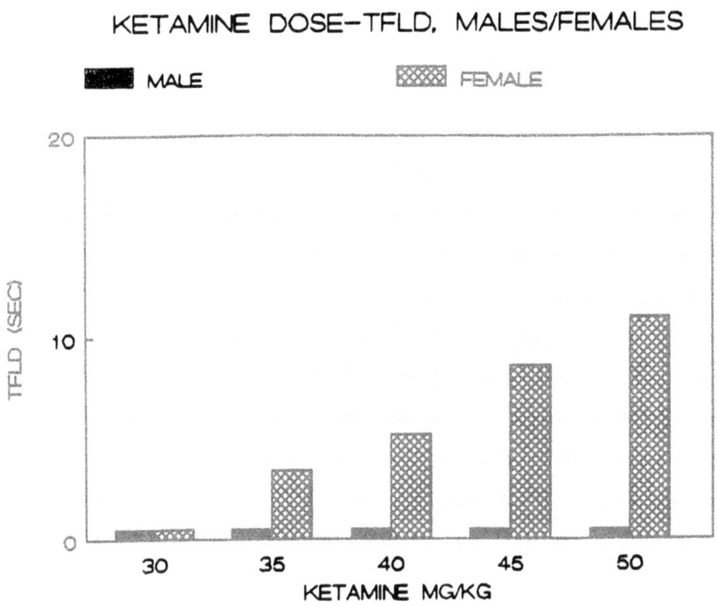

Fig. 1. Mean tail flick latency difference with increasing doses of ketamine.

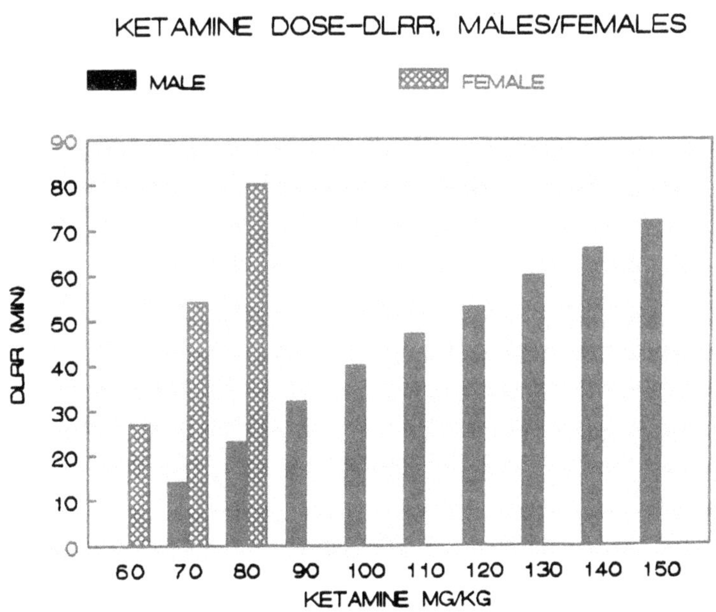

Fig. 2. Mean duration loss of righting reflex with increasing doses of ketamine.

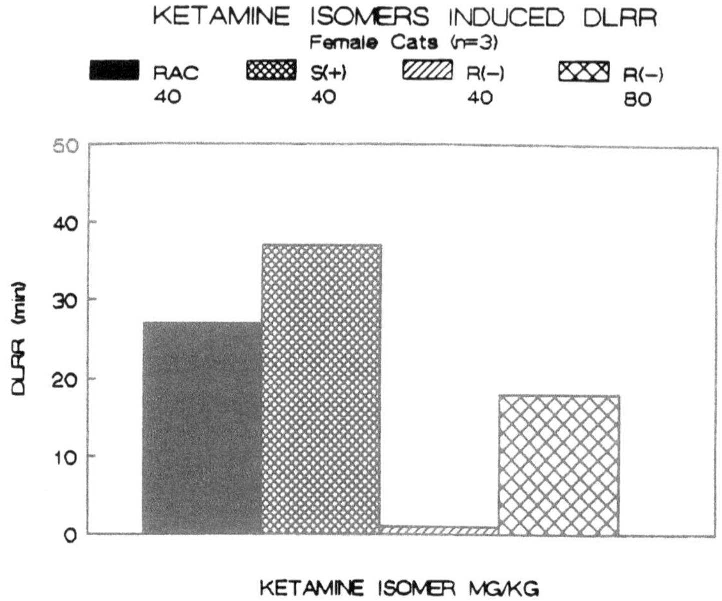

Fig. 3. Effect of isomers of ketamine on the righting reflex.

Pineal relationships

Placing opaque lenses over the eyes of female cats during the light hours increased the cataleptic potency of ketamine (Winters *et al.*, 1973). Pinealectomy blocked this augmentation as well as the augmented cataleptic response noted in the chick and rat when ketamine was given during the dark hours (Figs. 4 and 5; Winters *et al.*, 1973, 1986; Geidt *et al.*, 1978).

Pretreatment of rats with β-adrenergic agonists, or the melatonin precursors serotonin or N-acetyl serotonin, induced an augmented ketamine catalepsy in the intact rat, but not in the absence of the pineal. Melatonin and dopamine were both effective in augmenting the effects of ketamine in the presence or absence of the pineal gland, whereas in the hypophysectomized rat, melatonin no longer augmented the ketamine response, while dopamine still induced an augmentation (Fig. 5).

Seasonal variation

There were differences in the ketamine actions noted in studies performed during different months of the year. The data were re-evaluated on the basis of the time of day and the month in which the study was performed. A strong relationship between the ketamine effect and the

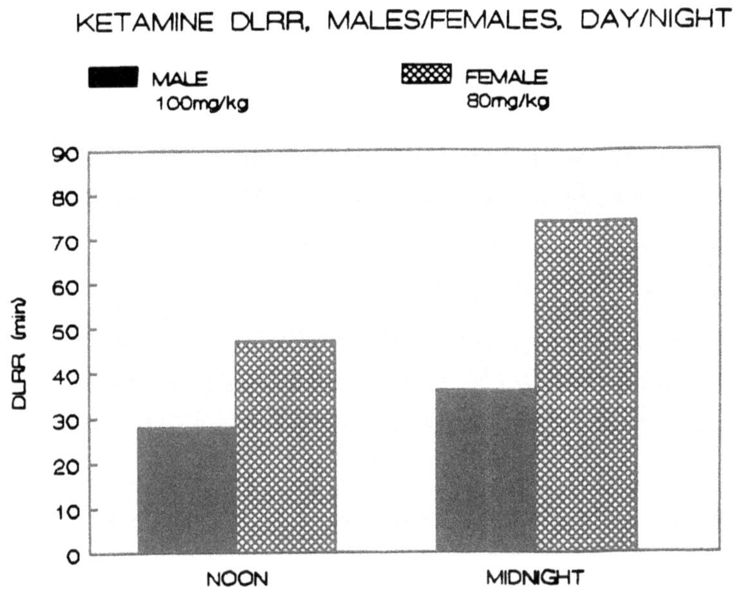

Fig. 4. Effect of the circadian cycle of rats on the duration of loss of the righting reflex.

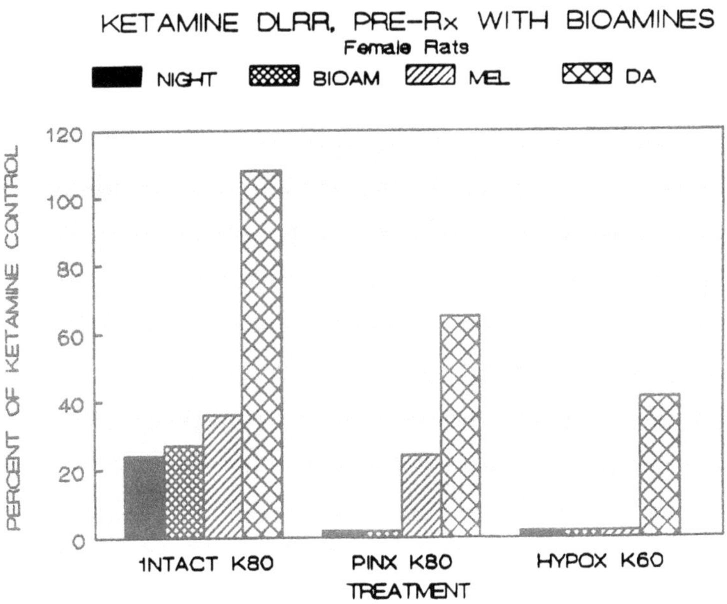

Fig. 5. Effects of various treatments on ketamine induced loss of the righting reflex.

time of day or the month of the year was observed, which confirmed a significant circadian and seasonal cycle for both the analgesic and cataleptic responses to ketamine (Winters *et al.*, 1986). Peak responses were noted during the dark rather than daylight hours (Figs. 4 and 5) and during the winter rather than the summer months (Table 1). These findings correlated with the observed peak analgesic action of melatonin noted during the winter rather than the summer months.

Opioid interactions

Ketamine induced analgesia was blocked by the specific opioid antagonist, naloxone (Winters *et al.*, 1988). The approximate ED_{50} for inducing analgesia and catalepsy induced by morphine and ketamine and the relationship of these agents to naloxone antagonism are shown in Table 2 (Winters *et al.*, 1988). Combinations of various doses of ketamine and morphine (Hance *et al.*, 1989), or fentanyl, sufentanil, alfentanil, butorphanol, nalbuphine (Benthuysen *et al.*, 1989a,b) were examined. Small doses of a combination of ketamine with these opioids resulted in an augmented ketamine response, whereas, a low dose of ketamine and a high dose of morphine resulted in a diminished cataleptic response (Table 3).

Tolerance was noted with daily administration of ketamine or the opioid agonists (Fig. 6; Winters *et al.*, 1986; Hance *et al.*, 1989; Benthuysen *et al.*, 1989b). Cross tolerance was noted for morphine in ketamine tolerant rats. However, ketamine induced catalepsy was aug-

TABLE 1. Seasonal variation-ketamine in female rats

Season	*Analgesia 45 mg/kg*	*Catalepsy 80 mg/kg*
	TFLD sec	*DLRR min*
Winter (D.J.F.)	6.2	68
Summer (J.J.A.)	2.1	36

TABLE 2. Effects of ketamine and morphine on analgesia, catalepsy and naloxone inhibition in the rat

		Control ED_{50} mg/kg		*Naloxone ID_{50} mg/kg*	
Drug	*Sex*	*Analgesia*	*Catalepsy*	*Analgesia*	*Catalepsy*
Morphine	F	5	40	0.007	0.67
Ketamine	F	40	70	6.8	25.0
Ketamine	M	na	130	—	—

TABLE 3. Ketamine-morphine combinations

Ketamine mg/kg	*Morphine mg/kg*	*Latency min*	*DLRR min*	*Rigidity*	*Ataxia and Diuresis*
0	50	7.0	183	LP	—
15	40	4.4	69	LP	—
20	20	8.2	82	LP	—
25	18	4.4	163	LP	—
45	10	3.9	159	SM	+ +
80	0	2.4	89	SM	+ +

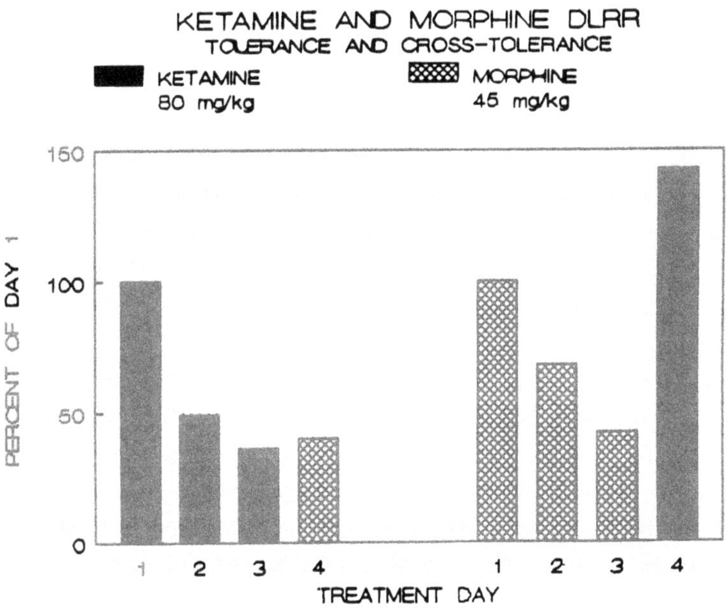

Fig. 6. Effect of daily dosing of ketamine and morphine in female rats.

mented in morphine tolerant rats, probably due to the large residual morphine level in the brain 24 hr after the last morphine cataleptic dose (Table 4).

Discussion

In our laboratory, animal studies showed that ketamine induced analgesia (TFLD) and catalepsy (DLRR) were augmented by the following: S(+) or racemic mixtures of ketamine, female rats, opaque lenses over the eyes, darkness (night-time), winter months (Dec./Jan./Feb.), β-adre-

TABLE 4. Levels of free morphine in plasma and brain after i.p. administration

		Morphine Levels	
		Plasma *ng/ml*	*Brain* *ng/g*
24 hr after 3 daily doses	45 mg/kg	26	16
24 hr after 1 dose	45 mg/kg	52	16
1 hr after 1 dose	2 mg/kg	59	18

nergic agonists (isoproterenol, norepinephrine, dopamine), melatonin precursors (serotonin and N-acetyl serotonin), melatonin, opioid agonists (morphine, fentanyl, alfentanyl, sufentanil) or agonist/antagonists (butorphanol and nalbuphine), hypophysectomy, and diazepam. Conversely, ketamine induced analgesia and catalepsy were decreased by the following: daylight hours (light), summer months (June, July, Aug.), pinealectomy, β-adrenergic blockers (propranolol), physostigmine, and opioid antagonists (naloxone). One to 4 days of repeated daily doses induced tolerance; longer daily doses (9 days or more) kindled epileptic hippocampal and amygdaloid foci (Manohar *et al.*, 1967).

The factors influencing the induced ketamine actions involve multiple levels of interaction of CNS systems. We hypothesize that during dark hours or stress, β-adrenergic agonists are released which stimulate the pineal to synthesize and release melatonin. This melatonin activates an opioid system controlling analgesia, and probably a second opioid-dopamine system which is involved in catalepsy. To date, we know of no studies which correlate pineal or melatonin activity to the NMDA receptor. These melatonin induced actions augment the ketamine induced effects. While there are hints that ketamine has weak direct binding affinities for the *mu* opioid receptor, and is likewise involved at the NMDA, *kappa* and *sigma* receptors, the body of knowledge at the present time does not lend itself to a simple, single model which explains the multiple actions of ketamine in the intact CNS. We anticipate that the continued studies will further elucidate the mechanisms underlying the factors which significantly influence ketamine actions on the CNS.

Our studies suggest several interesting points which should be explored in greater depth in patients, *e.g.*, the significant differences in potency and efficacy of ketamine with respect to females *vs* males, night *vs* day, winter *vs* summer months and the data indicating that small doses of opioid in combination with low doses of ketamine induce a profound augmentation of catalepsy. In addition, the development of tolerance to daily doses of ketamine in contrast to an augmentation when ketamine was administered to morphine tolerant rats is of concern. Understanding these relationships could reduce potential confusion in clinical circumstances where these combinations may occur. In addition, the data showing that multiple doses of ketamine were capable of inducing hippocampal epileptic foci are of concern. These foci can induce future flashbacks and/or seizure disorders. We are especially concerned with multiple dosing of pediatric patients where the CNS is in the early stages of development and most vulnerable to insult. Further, the EEG patterns induced by ketamine are similar to the EEG patterns noted in patients suffering from clinical epilepsy. Ketamine should not be used when patients are being evaluated for CNS pathology by the use of EEG recordings.

The risk-benefits for the clinical use of ketamine must be considered on the basis of the patient population under consideration, the skill and prior knowledge of the clinician, an understanding of the factors modifying ketamine action and the conditions in which ketamine is to be utilized. We have no concerns when ketamine is used by clinicians who are fully knowledgeable of the scope of pharmacological effects induced by this substance. *"There are no harmless substances, there are only harmless ways of using substances"* (Dr. Emil Mrak, former Chancellor at the University of California, Davis).

Acknowledgements

The authors wish to thank the following collaborators for their contributions to various portions of the above mentioned studies: Drs. Benthuysen, Spooner, Mori, Wallach, Guzman-Flores, Alcaraz, Cervantes, Lakin, Manohar, Cadd, and Quam.

References

Benthuysen, J.L., Hance, A.J., Quam, D.D., and Winters, W.D.: Comparison of ketamine isomers on catalepsy in the rat and brain electrical activity and behavior in the cat. Neuropharmacol. In press, 1989a.

Benthuysen, J.L., Hance, A.J., Quam, D.D., and Winters, W.D.: Synthetic opioids with morphine and ketamine: Catalepsy, cross-tolerance and the interactions in the rat. Neuropharmacol. In press, 1989b.

Giedt, W.R., Lakin, M.L., and Winters, W.D.: Diurnal response to ketamine and-hydroxybutyrate and its possible relationship to pineal indoleamines. Neuropharmacol. 17: 221-228, 1978.

Hance, A.J., Winters, W.D., Quam, D.D., Benthuysen, J.L., and Cadd, G.G.: Catalepsy induced by combinations of ketamine and morphine: Potentiation, antagonism, tolerance and cross tolerance in the rat. Neuropharmacol. 28: 109-116, 1989.

Manohar, S., Maxwell, D., and Winters, W.D.: Development of EEG seizure activity during and after chronic ketamine administration in the rat. Neuropharmacol. 6: 65-80, 1967.

Spooner, C.E., and Winters, W.D.: Neuropharmacological profile of the young chick. Int. J. Neuropharmacol. 5: 217-236, 1966.

Winters, W.D.: Effects of drugs on the electrical activity of the brain: Anesthetics, pp. 413-426, In Annual Review of Pharmacology and Toxicology, ed. by H.W. Elliott. Ann. Rev. Inc., Palo Alto, CA, 1976.

Winters, W.D., Alcaraz, M., Cervantes, M.-Y., and Guzman Flores, C.: The synergistic effect of reduced visual input on ketamine action: The possible role of the pineal gland. Neuropharmacol. 12: 407-416, 1973.

Winters, W.D., Ferrar-Allado, T., Guzman-Flores, C., and Alcaraz, M.: The cataleptic state induced by ketamine: A review of the neuropharmacology of anesthesia. Neuropharmacol. 11: 303-315, 1972.

Winters, W.D., Hance, A.J., Cadd, G.G., and Lakin, M.L.: Seasonal and sex influences on ketamine induced analgesia and catalepsy in the rat: A possible role for melatonin. Neuropharmacol. 25: 1095-1101, 1986.

Winters, W.D., Hance, A.J., Cadd G.G., Quam, D.D., and Benthuysen, J.L.: Ketamine- and morphine-induced analgesia and catalepsy. I. Tolerance, cross-tolerance, potentiation, residual morphine levels and naloxone action in the rat. J. Pharmacol. Exp. Ther. 244: 51-57, 1988.

Winters, W.D., Mori, K., Wallach, M.B., Marcus, R.J., and Spooner, C.E.: Reticular multiple unit activity during a progression of states induced by CNS excitants. III. EEG Clin. Neurophysiol. 27: 514-522, 1969.

Winters, W.D., Mori, K., Spooner, C.E., and Bauer, R.O.: The neurophysiology of anesthesia. Anesthesiol. 28: 65-80, 1967.

Status of Ketamine in Anesthesiology,
edited by E.F. Domino©1990, NPP Books
P.O. Box 1491, Ann Arbor, MI 48106

Pharmacokinetics and Pharmacodynamics of Ketamine Following Intravenous, Intramuscular and Rectal Administration to Conditioned Foxhounds

J.-P. Jantzen, D. Hilley, and A.H. Giesecke

Department of Anesthesiology
University of Texas Southwestern Medical School
at Dallas, Dallas, TX

Introduction

The phencyclidine derivative ketamine is a potent analgesic introduced into clinical practice in 1964. However, certain hemodynamic and central nervous side effects limited its applicability and made it one of the more controversial drugs in anesthesia (White *et al.*, 1982). This controversy is reflected by fluctuations in the interest paid to the drug in medical literature. The time course of ketamine related publications listed in Medline is shown in Fig. 1. Medline entries peaked in the mid-seventies, coinciding with the drug's approval in the United States as well as with an increase in the number of reported complications. The latter may have contributed to the subsequent decrease of annual related publications. The development of ketamine-benzodiazepine combinations ("ataranalgesia", "tranquanalgesia") was associated with a second peak in entries, again followed by a gradual decline.

The incidence of undesirable side effects was reported to be lower with enteral routes of administration (St. Maurice *et al.*, 1979; Cetina, 1982; Idvall *et al.*, 1983). This, and the increasing popularity of ketamine in experimental animal research (Wright, 1982), encouraged us to investigate the pharmacology of ketamine in dogs following three different routes of administration.

Methods

Five "conditioned foxhounds" with a mean weight of 27 kg (24.5-29.1) were randomly assigned to receive ketamine (25 mg kg^{-1}) by

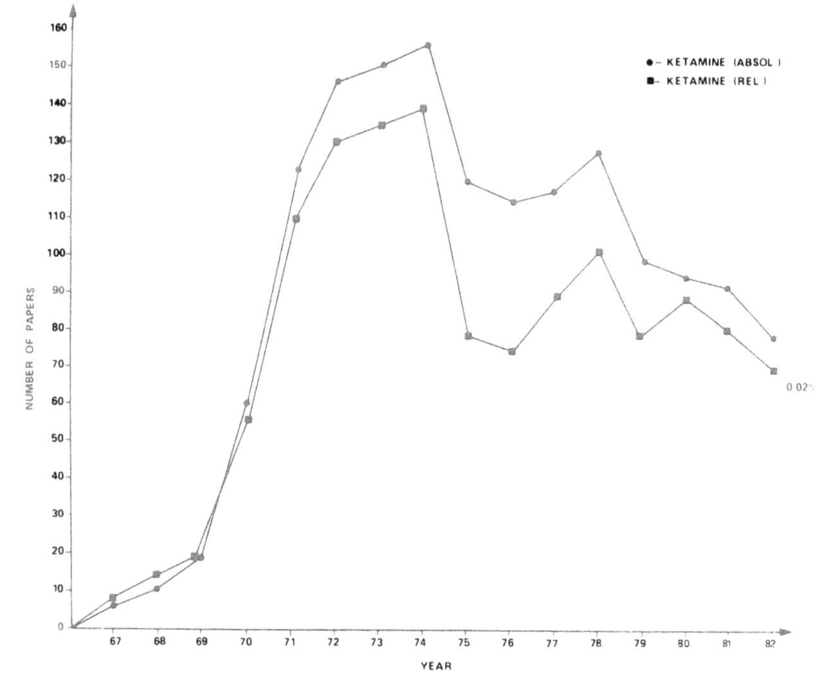

Fig. 1. Medline entries of ketamine related publications, 1963-1983. Absolute numbers and percentage of total entries are given.

either the i.v., i.m., or rectal route. All routes were used in every dog on different days. Thus, every subject acted as its own control. A minimum of three weeks was allowed between injections. The i.v. injection was over 60 sec in order to avoid major circulatory irritation. The i.m. injection was into the right gluteal muscle. Rectal administration was through a 20G Teflon cannula with the drug deposited directly proximal to the anal sphincter. All experiments were carried out under spontaneous breathing of room air. Monitoring was by Doppler measurement of arterial blood pressure (Arteriosonde Roche™). An i.v. line was started in the forelimb and locked with heparinized 0.9% NaCl. Blood samples were taken from this line for analysis, which was performed by gas chromatography (Foerster *et al.*, 1978), at the following time intervals: 0 (control), 1, 3, 5, 10, 15, 20, 30, 40, 60, 90 and 120 min after drug administration and after 24 hr.

The distribution half life ($t_{1/2}\,\alpha$) calculation following the i.v. route was based on plasma levels at the 1, 3, 5 min intervals. Bioavailability of i.m. and rectally administered ketamine was derived from the integral of an area-under-curve (AUC) as percentage of $AUC_{i.v.}$. Correlation between plasma levels and analgesia was evaluated with the minimal square method, intergroup differences were assessed by the Chi square test.

Analgesia was tested at each time interval with two methods, a pin prick to the gingiva, representing superficial pain, and a paw pinch, representing deep pain. Tolerance to a painful stimulus was rated as analgesia.

The protocol was approved by the Ethics Committee of the University of Texas Animal Resources Center (UTHSCD).

RESULTS

Plasma samples at control (C) and at 24 hr did not contain ketamine. Plasma concentrations and analgesia for all routes of administration are shown in Figs. 2 and 3. Pharmacokinetic data are presented in Table 1. Intravenous administration gave reliable analgesia and reproducible plasma levels in all subjects. Following i.m. administration, analgesia proved satisfactory in 4 subjects and lasted longer than after i.v. injection. Rectal administration was followed by scattered peak plasma levels, on the average at 40 min. Analgesia was poor in 4 subjects. The correlation coefficients for plasma concentration *vs* analgesia were 0.69, 0.52 and 0.30 for i.v., i.m., and rectal administration, respectively. With respect to analgesia, differences between routes of application were statistically significant ($P \leq 0.01$).

DISCUSSION

The pharmacokinetic data for the parenteral routes of administration obtained in this study are in agreement with those reported in the literature (Kaka and Hayton, 1980). Analgesia following i.v. and i.m. administration was satisfactory, but its correlation with plasma concentration was poor. When administered rectally, bioavailability depends upon the site of absorption and on the pH of the local milieu (Jantzen *et al.*, 1986). Consequently, uncertainties associated with local pH climate and type of venous drainage render bioavailability unpredictable. The low plasma levels following rectal administration thus reflect poor bioavailability associated with this route. This appears to be the reason for the unsatisfactory analgesia. The analgesic threshold concentration for ketamine in dogs (3.0 mg kg^{-1}) was never reached after rectal administration. That some degree of analgesia was achieved could be ascribed to the analgesic

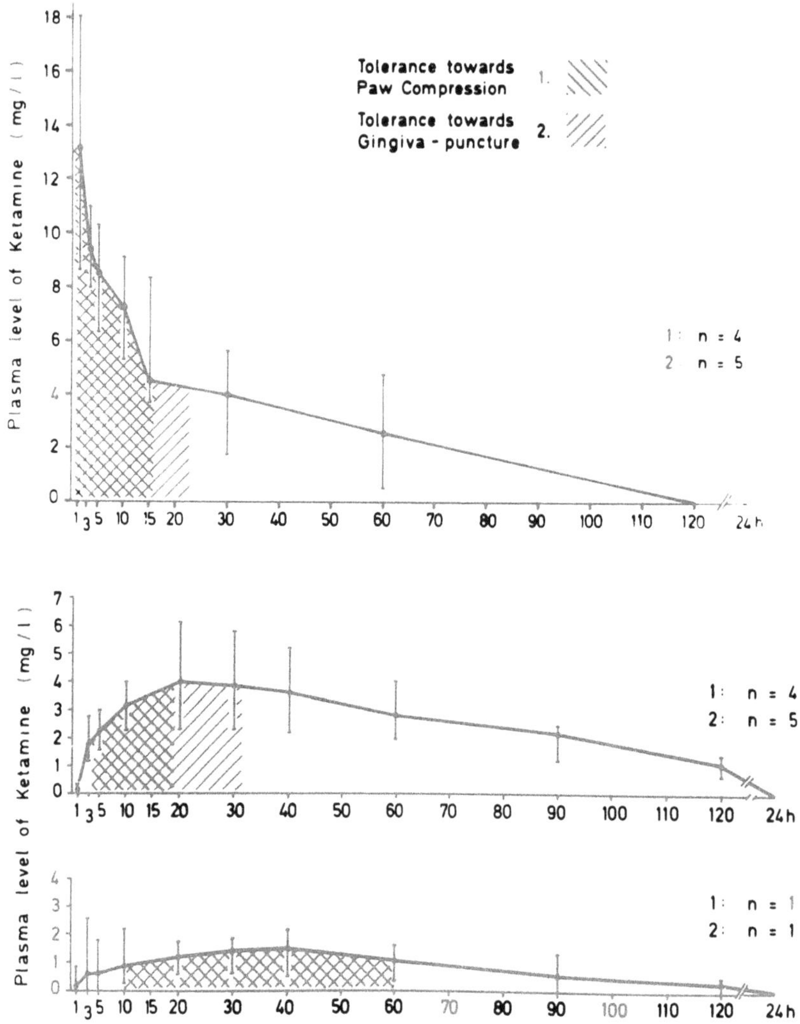

Fig. 2. Ketamine plasma concentrations and analgesic effect following i.v. (top), i.m. (middle) and rectal (bottom) administration. Crosshatched areas represent the mean analgesic time range of those dogs showing tolerance to either pain test.

properties of the metabolites, resulting from first-pass-metabolism (Grant *et al.*, 1981).

Conclusions

Ketamine may be administered to dogs by the i.v., i.m., and rectal routes without causing major hemodynamic or respiratory side effects.

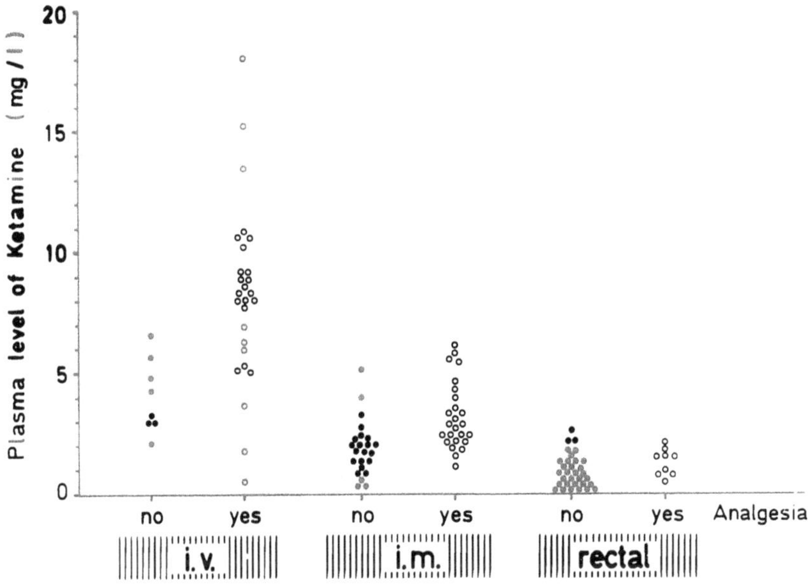

Fig. 3. Individual sample concentrations of ketamine according to the route of administration and analgesic effect (gingiva puncture).

TABLE 1. Pharmacokinetic Data

	i.v.	*i.m.*	*rectal*
Cmax (min)	1	20	40
$t_{1/2}\alpha$ (min)	6	—	—
$t_{1/2}\beta$ (min)	55	52	43
Bioavailability	100%	90%	30%

When administered i.v. or i.m., ketamine (25 mg kg^{-1}) provides surgical anesthesia for approximately 15 min. This dosage, however, does not produce satisfactory analgesia when given rectally. Whether this problem of poor bioavailability can be overcome by an increase in dosage, or by other means of enhancing bioavailability, requires further investigation.

References

Cetina, J.: Schonende Narkoseeinleitung bei Kindern durch orale oder rektale Ketamin-Dehydrobenzperidol-Applikation. Anaesthesist 31: 277, 1982.

Foerster, E., Hatchett, D. and Garriott, J.C.: A rapid, comprehensive screening procedure for basic drug in blood or tissue by gas-chromatography. J. Anal. Toxicol. 2: 50, 1978.

Grant, I.S., Nimmo, W.S., Clements, J.A.: Pharmacokinetics and analgesic effects of i.m. and oral ketamine. Br. J. Anaesth. 53: 805, 1981.

Idvall, J., Holasek, J. and Stenberg, P.: Rectal ketamine for induction of anesthesia in children. Anaesthesia 38: 60, 1983.

Jantzen, J.P., Erdmann, K., Witton, P.K. and Klein, A.M.: Der Einfluss des rektalen pH-Wertes auf die Resorption von Methohexital. Anaesthesist 35: 496, 1986.

Kaka, J. and Hayton, W.L.: Pharmacokinetics of ketamine and two metabolites in the dog. J. Pharmacokinet. Biopharm. 82: 193, 1980.

St. Maurice, C., Laguenie, G., Couturier, C. and Goutail-Flaud, F.: Rectal ketamine in paediatric anaesthesia. Br. J. Anaesth. 51: 573, 1979.

White, P., Way, W.L. and Trevor, A.J.: Ketamine–its pharmacology and therapeutic use. Anesthesiol. 56: 119, 1982.

Wright, J.: Pharmacologic effects of ketamine and its use in veterinary medicine. J. Am. Vet. Med. Assn. 180: 1462, 1982.

Status of Ketamine in Anesthesiology,
edited by E.F. Domino©1990, NPP Books
P.O. Box 1491, Ann Arbor, MI 48106

Interspecies Pharmacokinetics of Ketamine

J.L. Pedraz, J.M. Lanao, and A. Dominguez-Gil

Department of Practical Pharmacy, Faculty of Pharmacy
University of Salamanca
Salamanca, Spain

INTRODUCTION

One of the great challenges in pharmacology today is the development of methods that will allow one to predict from results obtained in experimental animals the pharmacodynamic and pharmacokinetic behavior in humans of new molecules endowed with pharmacological activity.

Comparison of the pharmacokinetic behavior of a drug in different animal species can be tackled from two different points of view (Mordenti, 1986); first, from an allometric, and second, from a physiological viewpoint. In the allometric approach, the plasma levels of a given drug in different animal species are adjusted to a pharmacokinetic model (compartmental or non-compartmental). The parameters obtained are fitted to an exponential equation of the type $Y = aB^x$, where B is body weight and Y is the pharmacokinetic parameter considered. Later, calculation of the value of this in man is done by substituting the weight by a mean value of approximately 70 kg in the previous equation.

In the physiological approach, a physiological model is designed in which the pharmacokinetic parameters are substituted with physiological variables. Having defined the model, the corresponding mass balance is calculated and the resulting differential equations are solved simultaneously. Extrapolation to man is then carried out by substitution of each of the values of the physiological, biochemical, or anatomical parameters of the species assayed by the values corresponding to these parameters in human beings.

The development of such methods has allowed investigators to obtain more information from fewer experiments and has proved to be of great use in drug design and the screening of new molecules. It has also increased safety in design, carrying out Phase I assays, and reduced the cost of research on new molecules with pharmacological potential.

Material and Methods

The present study was begun with pharmacokinetic data obtained from experiments carried out at our laboratory and a review of the literature in such a way that would fulfill the following conditions:

1. Ketamine had to be administered i.v., since its absorption through other routes is erratic and incomplete (Grant *et al.*, 1981).

2. The doses administered did not exceed 15 mg/kg in order to avoid the phenomenon of nonlinearity.

3. The plasma levels had to be fitted to a two compartment kinetic model in order to carry out the allometric analysis of different parameters.

After reviewing the literature, and in agreement with these criteria, only satisfactory data for the rat (Adams *et al.*, 1980), rabbit (Pedraz *et al.*, 1985), dog (Kaka *et al.*, 1980), and man (Pedraz *et al.*, 1987) were found.

The method used in the analysis of ketamine, together with calculation of its pharmacokinetic parameters corresponding to the kinetic model employed, are described in the literature just quoted. Data relating to rabbit and man were obtained from studies carried out in our laboratory.

Ketamine concentrations were related to the weight of each of the species and the doses administered. This permitted introduction of a new series of coordinates and the possibility of superimposing the plasma ketamine levels in the different species analyzed. To do so, the corresponding allometric relationships between clearance and the distribution volume were established to obtain the following equations:

$$Vd = aB^{\alpha_1} \qquad Cl = bB^{\alpha_2}$$

If the correlation obtained in both expressions is good, it is possible to normalize the plasma levels, dividing each concentration by the relationship between the dose and the weight raised to the exponent of the allometric equation of the distribution volume (α_1). In addition, chronological time should be converted to a new scale of pharmacokinetic time; chronological time divided by weight raised to the difference between the allometric exponents of the distribution volume and the plasma clearance (α_1-α_2).

Using these transforms, one can obtain a new plot known as the Dedrick complex plot (Boxembaum and Ronfeld, 1983) in which the new time unit is the Apolysychron, *i.e.*, the time over which each of the species considered has eliminated the same fraction of drug and has cleared the same plasma volume per kg of body weight.

Ketamine is a drug that is principally eliminated by biotransformation (Chang and Glazko, 1974). Only about 5% of the dose administered is collected in the urine in an unaltered state. Accordingly, ketamine plasma clearance can be thought of as being the same as metabolic clearance with no important errors being involved. Furthermore, if one accepts that the extrahepatic metabolism of ketamine is zero, or at least is negligible, the metabolic clearance would be the same as the hepatic clearance. In view of the great liposolubility of this compound, the well-stirred model (Pang and Rowland, 1977) can be accepted as a physiological model of hepatic disposition that is valid for ketamine. Hence, it is possible to calculate the intrinsic metabolic parameters of ketamine with the following expression:

$$\text{Cluint} = (\text{Cl-Qh})/[(\text{fu}(\text{Qh-Cl})]$$

where Qh is hepatic blood flow, which in turn can be calculated from the expression:

$$\text{Qh} = 0.0554 \text{ B}^{0.894}$$

The term fu is the fraction unbound to plasma proteins. It is assumed that this is linear throughout the working concentration range and similar in all species, with a value of 0.5 (Dayton *et al.*, 1983). Cl is the plasma clearance.

The Maximum Potential Lifespan (MPL) for each of the species was calculated according to the following expression:

$$\text{MPL} = 10.839 \text{ Brain Weight}^{0.636} \text{ B}^{-0.225}$$

Results and Discussion

Fig. 1 shows the time course of the plasma levels of ketamine in the different species chosen. The physiological parameters and the main pharmacokinetic parameters of ketamine in these species are given in Tables 1 and 2.

The elimination half-life of ketamine ranges between 17.3 min for the rat and 176.4 min for man. Alterations in half-life were proportional to the weight of the species. It was possible to obtain a linear relationship between both parameters for comparative purposes, as shown in Fig. 2.

Something similar occurred with the distribution volumes. The dis-

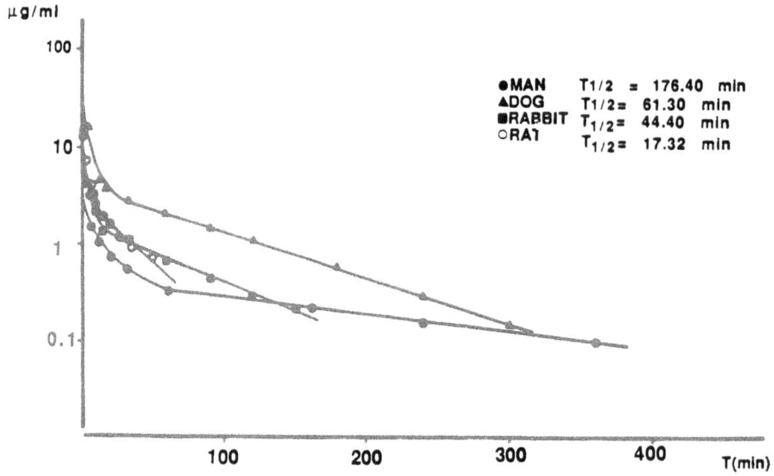

Fig. 1. Time course of plasma ketamine concentrations in 4 different species of animals.

TABLE 1.

Species	*Weight (Kg)*	*Brain (Kg)*	*Qh (l/min)*	*MPL (years)*	*Dose (mg/Kg)*
Man	62.5	1.500	2.23	95.80	2.0
Dog	19.1	0.070	0.77	18.44	15.0
Rabbit	2.6	0.010	0.13	7.93	10.0
Rat	0.4	0.002	0.02	4.20	7.5

TABLE 2.

Species	$T_{1/2}$ *(min)*	Vβ *(l)*	*Clp (l/min)*	*Cluint (l/min)*	*Cluint (l/MPL)* 10^8
Man	176.4	276.7	1.20	5.19	2.613
Dog	61.3	66.1	0.61	5.87	0.568
Rabbit	44.4	10.5	0.11	1.43	0.059
Rat	17.3	0.8	0.02	0.18	0.004

tribution volume corresponding to the slow disposition phase has values ranging between 272.7 l in man and 0.80 l in the rat. However, when this parameter is expressed as a function of body weight, the values obtained are much more homogeneous among the different species, proving to be around 4 l/kg. These findings point to the existence of a relationship

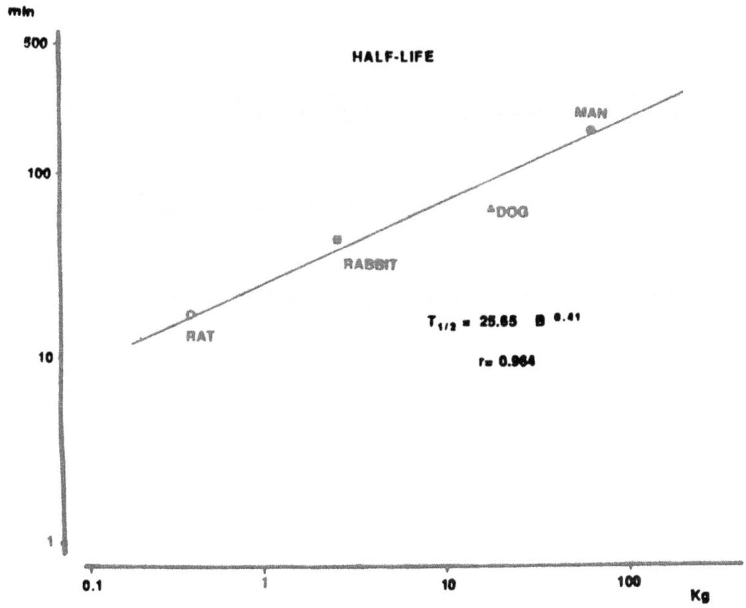

Fig. 2. Linear relationship between mean body weight of 4 different species and the elimination half-life of ketamine.

between the distribution volume and the weight of each of the species considered, as may be seen in Fig. 3. On a double logarithmic plot, this shows the distribution volume against the weight of each species. A straight line was obtained with a correlation coefficient of 0.996.

The existence of this kind of relationship for the parameters defining the elimination and distribution characteristics of the drug analyzed here suggests that the concentrations of drug in the different species chosen could also be correlated as a function of weight and dose administered.

Fig. 1 shows that there is a considerable difference between the time course of the plasma levels of ketamine obtained after ketamine administration to different species. However, if the above considerations are true, all species should obey the same kind of dynamics in the distribution and elimination of the drug. Accordingly, although the processes appear to occur at different rates when measured on the chronological scale, when this time is transformed into an intrinsic or biological scale, one obtains superimposition in the time course of the plasma levels of the drug in the different species studied. This can be seen in Fig. 4. In this plot, the scales of the axes have been transformed as a function of the weight of each species, the dose administered, and the exponentials of the al-

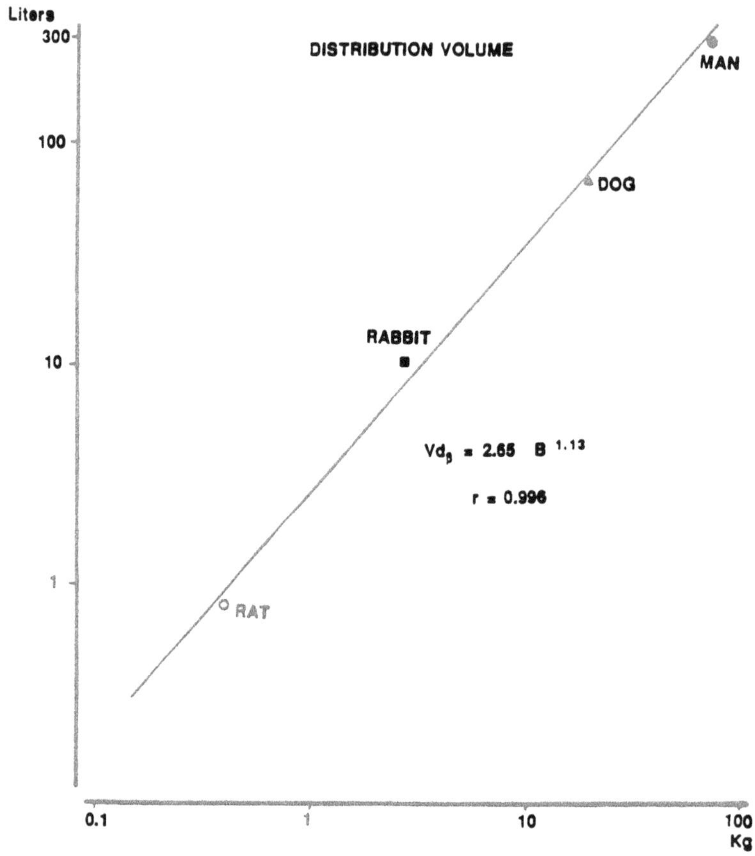

Fig. 3. Linear relationship between mean body weight of 4 different species and the volume of distribution of ketamine.

lometric equations of clearance and distribution volumes. In this way, a new biological time unit, known as the apolysychron, is obtained. According to this new scale, the elimination half-life of ketamine would be equivalent 30.66 apolysychrons. Thus, it may be concluded that all of the animal species tend to clear ketamine over the same period of biological time.

In agreement with these findings, some authors have developed the theory of absolute metabolic quantity (Boxenbaum, 1984) in which all animals would have the same amount of vital energy. Therefore, according to this theory, the maximum period of chronological lifespan would be defined by the rate of utilization of this energy. Thus, those animals with a shorter lifespan, generally those smaller in size, would use this

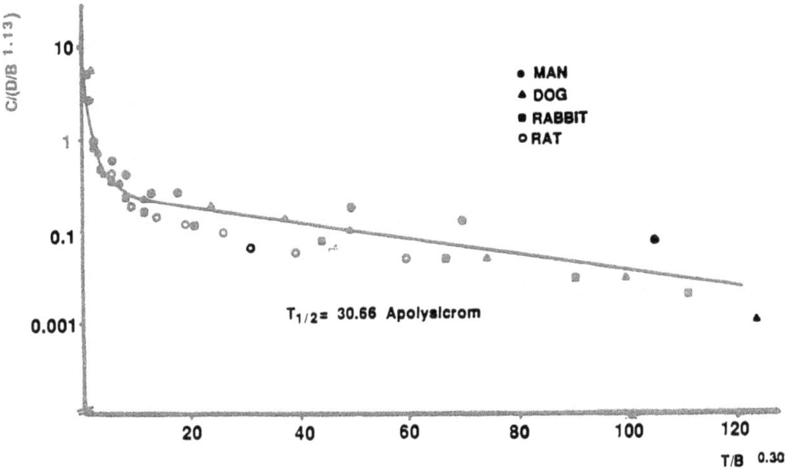

Fig. 4. Superimposition of plasma ketamine time course for 4 different species when transformed into a biological scale.

energy faster than those that live longer. This would explain why the former tend to clear drugs faster than the latter when this parameter is measured in terms of chronological time.

Fig. 5 shows the relationship between ketamine plasma clearance and the mean body weights of different species. It may be seen that there is a good correlation between the clearances found for the rat, rabbit and dog, whereas the corresponding value for man is less than predicted. This again supports the demonstrated fact that man biotransforms drugs and xenobiotics more slowly than other species (Brodie, 1964). Since metabolic processes are subject to numerous variables, it is preferable to work with, and make comparisons with, intrinsic parameters in which the variability due to factors such as hepatic blood flow and plasma protein binding have been eliminated.

Fig. 6 shows the relationship between the intrinsic clearances of ketamine calculated by the above described method and the mean weight of the species studied. Again a good correlation can be seen between the values of this parameter and the weight of the rat, rabbit, and dog, while the value obtained for man is approximately 7-fold smaller than what would theoretically be attributed to this species. Similar results have been reported by Boxenbaum (1980) for antipyrine, some benzodiazepines and phenytoin. This has been attributed to a loss in the biotransformation capacity of man for drugs and xenobiotics.

This theory has not been accepted by all scientists since when the

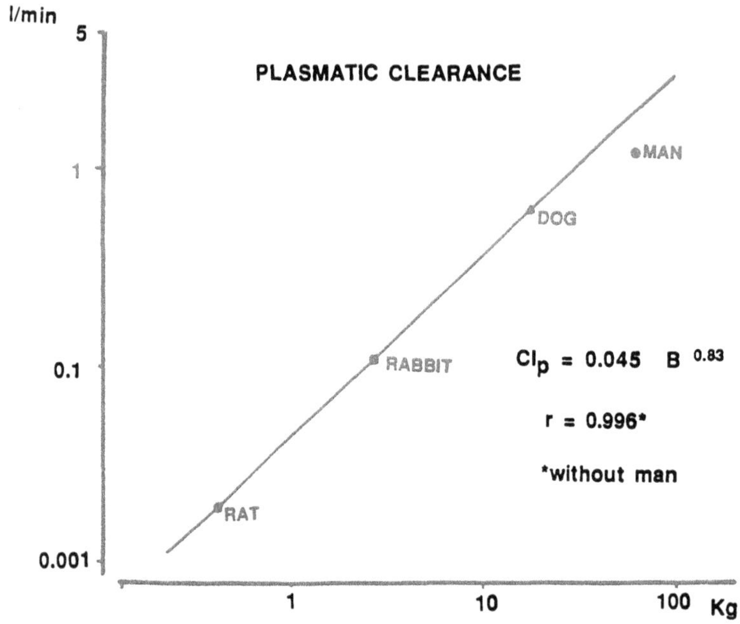

Fig. 5. Plasma clearance of ketamine in 4 different species as a function of mean body weight.

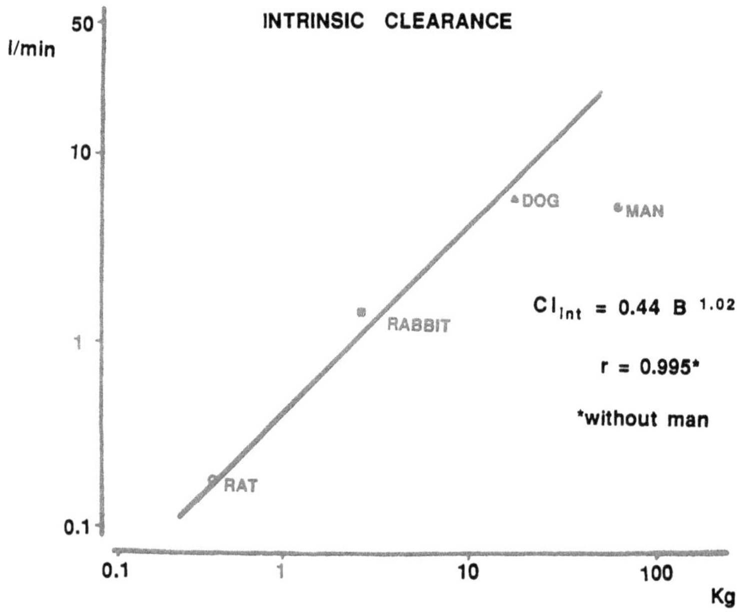

Fig. 6. Intrinsic clearance of ketamine in 4 different species plotted as a function of mean body weight.

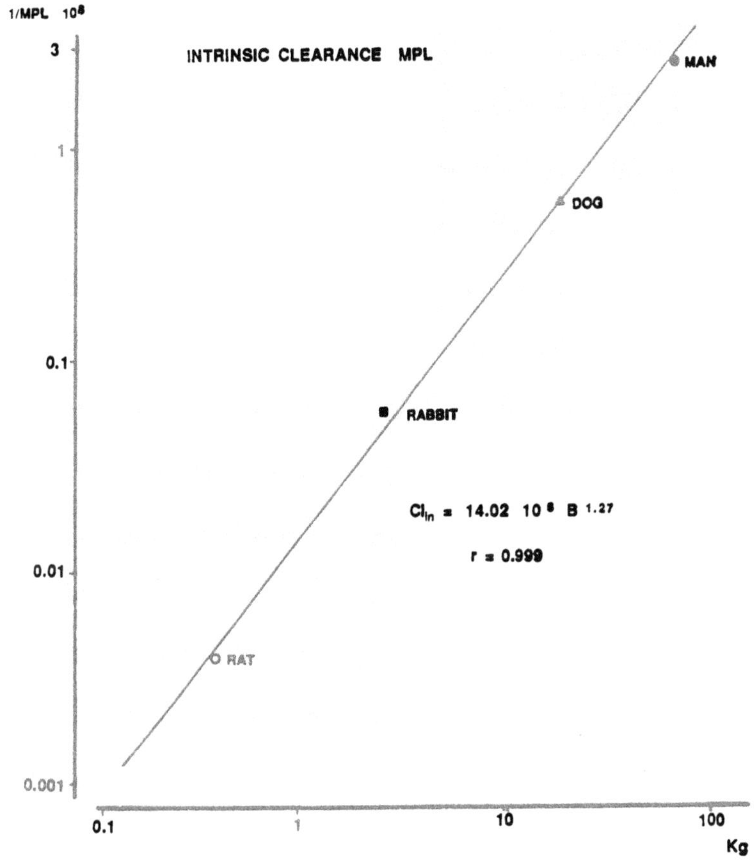

Fig. 7. Intrinsic clearance of ketamine plotted on a double blind logarithmic scale as a function of mean body weight of 4 different species.

intrinsic clearance is represented by the MPL on a double logarithmic scale, as can be seen in Fig. 7, excellent linearity is observed between the data of all species, with a correlation coefficient of 0.999.

These results led Yates and Kugler (1986) to offer an alternative explanation for the lack of linearity in the parameters in man. This is known as the phenomenon of neoteny. According to this theory, man shows a delay in his development compared to the rest of mammals, which accounts for such types of anomalous behavior.

Summary

The pharmacokinetic behavior of ketamine in rat, rabbit, dog and man were analyzed using allometric equations. The data employed were results obtained in our laboratory and from a review of the literature. In all the species studied, the time course of plasma ketamine can be fitted to an open two-compartment kinetic model. The elimination half-life had values ranging between 17.3 and 176.4 min for man. These modifications in the half-life were proportional to the mean weight (B) of the species. The following relationship was obtained between both parameters: $T_{1/2} = 25.65B^{0.41}$ (r = 0.964).

The distribution volume of the slow disposition phase (Vd_β) ranged between 275.7 l in man to 0.811 l in the rat. When this parameter was expressed as a function of weight, the values obtained for the different species were much more homogeneous, ranging around 4 l/kg. These results reflect the existence of a relationship between the volume of distribution and the mean weight of each species analyzed: $Vd_\beta = 2.65B^{1.33}$ (r = 0.996). Thus, the concentrations of ketamine are a function of weight and the dose administered. It is possible to superimpose the time course of the ketamine levels in the different species using a Dedrick plot in which all the species have a single half-life value corresponding to 30.66 Apolysychrons.

When the relationship between clearance (Cl) and weight was analyzed, it was observed that human subjects deviate by approximately 20% compared to the other species. Similar results were found when the values of intrinsic clearance (Cl_{int}) were used. However, when the intrinsic clearance was corrected as a function of the maximum potential lifespan (MPL), an excellent correlation between both parameters was obtained: $Cl_{int} \times MPL = 14.01 \times 10^8 B^{1.27}$ (r = 0.999).

These results confirm the validity of allometric studies in the prediction of pharmacokinetic parameters and their possible application in the phase I clinical trials.

REFERENCES

Adams, H.D., Glen, J.B. and Hayte, P.A.: Pharmacokinetics in laboratory animals of ICl 35 868, a new anaesthetic agent. Br. J. Anaesth. 52: 743-746, 1980.

Boxenbaum, H.: Interspecies variation in liver weight, hepatic blood flow and antipyrine intrinsic clearance. J. Pharmacokin. Biopharm. 8: 165-176, 1980.

Boxenbaum, H. and Rodfeld, R.: Interspecies pharmacokinetics scaling and the Dedrick plots. Am. J. Physiol. 245: R768-R775, 1983.

Boxenbaum, H.: Interspecies pharmacokinetics scaling and the evolutionary-comparative paradigm. Drug Metab. Rev. 15: 1071-1121, 1984.

Brodie, B.: Of mice, microsomes and man. Pharmacologist, 6: 12-26, 1964.

Chang, T. and Glazko, A.J.: Biotransformation and disposition of ketamine. Int. Anesthesiol. Clinics 12: 157-177, 1974.

Dayton, P.G., Stiller, R.L., Cook, D.R. and Perel, J.M.: The binding of ketamine to plasma proteins: Emphasis on human plasma. Eur. J. Clin. Pharmacol. 24: 825-831, 1983.

Grant, I.S., Nimmo, W.S. and Clements, J.A.: Pharmacokinetics and analgesic effects of IM and oral ketamine. Br. J. Anaesth. 53: 805-810, 1981.

Kaka, J.S. and Hayton, W.S.: Pharmacokinetics of ketamine and two metabolites in the dog. J. Pharmacokin. Biopharm. 8: 193-202, 1980.

Mordenti, J.: Man versus beast: pharmacokinetic scaling in mammals. J. Pharm. Sci. 75: 1028-1040, 1986.

Pang, K.S. and Rowland, M.: Hepatic clearance of drugs 1. Theoretical considerations of a "Well Stirred" model and a "Parallel Tube" model. Influence of hepatic blood flow, plasma and blood cell binding and the hepatocellular enzymatic activity on hepatic drug clearance. J. Pharmacokin. Biopharm. 5: 625-653, 1977.

Pedraz, J.L., Lanao, J.M. and Dominguez-Gil, A.: Kinetics of ketamine and its metabolites in rabbits with normal and impaired renal function. Eur. J. Drug Metab. Pharmacokin. 10: 33-39, 1985.

Pedraz, J.L., Lanao, J.M., Calvo, M.B., Muriel, C., Hernandez-Arbeiza, J. and Dominguez-Gil, A.: Pharmacokinetics and clinical evaluation of ketamine administered by i.v. and epidural routes. Int. J. Clin. Pharmacol. 25: 77-80, 1987.

Yates, F.E. and Kugler, P.N.: Similarity principles and intrinsic geometries: contrasting approaches to interspecies scaling. J. Pharm. Sci. 75: 1019-27 1986.

Status of Ketamine in Anesthesiology,
edited by E.F. Domino©1990, NPP Books
P.O. Box 1491, Ann Arbor, MI 48106

Plasma Ketamine: Relation to Brain Concentrations and the Hippocampal Electroencephalogram

D.J. Gole*, J. French, J. Houser*** and E.F. Domino**

Department of Pharmacology
University of Michigan
Ann Arbor, MI

Introduction

The electroencephalogram (EEG) has been widely used to study various general anesthetic agents. However, its use in relationship to plasma pharmacokinetics has been limited in both man and various animals. In view of the fact that our laboratory was able to chemically assay ketamine, as well as to study its EEG effects, we decided to test the hypothesis that the plasma pharmacokinetics of ketamine would be closely related to its EEG changes. Therefore, a study was initiated using adult male rats. Electrodes were placed in the hippocampus, an area in the brain with a high concentration of N-methyl-D-aspartate (NMDA) and phencyclidine receptors.

Methods

EEG studies

All electrodes were chronically implanted in 6 adult male Sprague-Dawley rats under pentobarbital anesthesia about 2 weeks prior to the onset of drug testing. Staggered bipolar recording configurations were used at each site such that one tip of the hippocampal electrode was 0.8 mm above the other tip to obtain maximal differential amplification of the

Present Address:
*Mediventure, 655 Phoenix, Ann Arbor, MI 48104
**USAFSAM/VNB, Brooks AFB, TX 78235-5301
***Central Research, Pfizer Inc., Eastern Point Rd., Groton, CT 06340

EEG signal. Stereotaxic zero was used as the reference (Pellegrino *et al.*, 1979) with the incisor bar set at 5 mm above the interaural line.

The hippocampal electrodes were directed at 3.2 mm anterior, 3.0 mm lateral, and the deepest tip at 2.2 mm above the zero line. The dorsal CA_1 site in the hippocampus reacts with a large amplitude field potential when it is perforated with an electrode, and this pattern was generally observed during electrode implantation. This activity and the predominance of rhythmic 6-8 Hz activity in the hippocampal EEG from all the rats were considered evidence that the hippocampal electrodes were located in the correct sites prior to histology.

All electrodes and pedestals were purchased from the Plastic Products Co. (Roanoke, VA) and consisted of 0.125 mm stainless steel wires (Model #E363/3), insulated with Formvar varnish except for 0.5 mm at the recording tip, and twisted together such that the electrode sockets could be fed into the pedestal (Model #MS363). A self-curing acrylic mixture (Plastic Products Co.) was used to hold the pedestal and electrode array to 3, 0-80 self-tapping anchor screws embedded in the calvarium. During a recording session, each rat was placed in a Nalgene chamber 29 cm deep by 30 cm in diameter and was tethered to the recording cable (Plastic Products Co., Model #363) attached to a miniature electrical swivel commutator (Harvard Apparatus, Model #56-8188) which allowed the animal unobtrusive movements. A videocassette recorder over the chamber was used to record the ongoing behavior and the associated brain electrical activity (A.R. Vetter Co., Model #420-C). Data also were simultaneously collected on polygraph paper (Grass Instruments, Model #7C) and FM magnetic tape (Honeywell Co., Model #5600C).

Plasma brain levels

Rats were injected with ketamine (30 mg/kg) through catheters previously inserted into the tail or jugular vein. The rats were then killed by decapitation at 1, 2, 6, 10, 20, 30 min, 1, 2, 4, 6, 8, 10, 12, and 24 hr. The body blood was collected, centrifuged at 3500 rpm and the plasma layer removed and frozen until the day of the assay. After the blood collection, the brains were dissected and homogenized (10% w/v). These samples were also frozen until the day of the assay. For the EEG studies, implanted rats were also injected with ketamine (30 mg/kg) through cannulated tail veins. Recordings were taken at the same time points listed above.

Chemical analysis

The flow diagram of the extraction and analysis procedure of ketamine from the rat, plasma and brain samples is shown in Table 1. The *o*-

TABLE 1. Flow diagram for the extraction and analysis of ketamine in plasma and brain

Extraction

For the standard curve ketamine HC1 0-1 μg
in water was added to plasma or brain

To 0.4-3 ml of plasma or 10% brain homogenate was added
0.625 μg of CL-394 in 1 ml of 0.1N HC1 in 0.9% HC1;
0.6 ml of 15% NaOH,
mix 4 ml of methylene chloride

Shake for 20 min at 89-100 oscillations min^{-1}

Centrifuge, 3500 rev min^{-1} (20 min)

Aspirate top aqueous layer, add 300 mg of anhydrous Na_2SO_4

Centrifuge, 3500 rev min^{-1} (20 min)

Decant methylene chloride layer into another test tube,
add 1 drop of 0.1% methanolic HCl solution,
evaporate contents of the test tube to dryness under N_2

Dissolve residue in 100 μl of toluene containing
0.1% N,N-dimethylenethanolamine, volume for analysis (3 μl)

GC conditions

Injection port temp.: 250° C
Splitless mode
Columns: Fused-silica capillary column with cross-linked
methyl silicone bonded phase
Oven temp.: Initial: 100° C, 3 min
Linear increase @ 240° C/min
Final: 250° C, 3 min
Carrier gas: Helium, rate 2 ml/min

MS conditions

Mass selective detector: 195° C
Direct interface
Selected ion mode

Sample: Volume 3 μl, concentration, 0-25 ng/μl
IS: *o*-Br-ketamine (CL-394)
RT: Ketamine 7.54 min; IS 7.98 min
Detection Limit: 15 pg/μl of injected sample

Br analog (CL-394) of ketamine was used as an internal standard (IS). The ketamine and the IS were obtained as a gift from the Warner Lambert Company. All other chemicals used were of analytical reagent grade.

Analytical instrumentation

An HP 5890 gas chromatograph equipped with a mass selective detector with a direct interface was used for sample analysis. A high performance fused silica capillary column with crossed linked methyl silicone bonded phase (12 mm length x 0.2 mm i.d. x 0.33 m thickness) was found suitable for separation of these compounds. Each sample was injected into the GC using a splitless mode with an HP 7363A autosampler. The column head pressure of the carrier gas was 5 psi. Data acquisition was done on an HP 9000 series computer. All of the quantitative analyses were performed in a selected ion mode. The fragment m/e180 was the base peak for ketamine, and the ions which were monitored selectively were as follows: 180.0, 181.0, 181.1, 182.0, 182.1, 183.0, and 183.1. The base peak for an internal standard was m/e 224 and the ions which were monitored selectively were as follows: 223.95, 224.05, 224.95, 225.05, 225.95, 226.05, 226.95, and 227.05. The detection limit of the present assay procedure was 50 pg and was found to be linear up to 75 ng.

Computer analysis

The recorded analog EEG data was first passed through a tuneable high pass filter (Frequency Devices). Analog to digital conversion was accomplished by a 12 bit (2.4 mV/bit) Dash-8 input board (Metrobyte, Taunton, MA) installed in an IBM-AT work station equipped with an Intel 80287 math coprocessor microchip. Software was custom designed around a high speed Fourier transformation routine (Cooper, 1981) based on the Cooley-Tukey bit inversion algorithm and programmed in Turbo-87 Pascal.

EEG power spectral density analysis was conducted on the activity in 5 frequency bands: 1-4 Hz, 4-8 Hz, 8-12 Hz, 12-20 Hz and 20-40 Hz. These parameters were obtained from each band: 1) the dominant frequency, defined as the frequency associated with the largest power value, 2) cumulative power, defined as the sum of all the power values in a band, and 3) percent power, defined as a ratio of all the power values in a band relative to power values in the entire 40 Hz spectrum. Six samples, each consisting of 1024 digitalized points and representing 10 sec of analog data, were obtained for each time point post ketamine for each rat. The samples were individually Fourier transformed and averaged to obtain a single spectrum for each time point after dosing. Spectral density parameters were extracted from each average power spectrum and archived in data files for subsequent statistical evaluation.

Results

Hippocampal EEG power following ketamine

As illustrated in Figs. 1 and 2, there was a marked increase in hippocampal *beta* and *delta* power after the administration of 30 mg/kg i.v. ketamine which rapidly diminished within 1 hr and was almost normal in 2 hr.

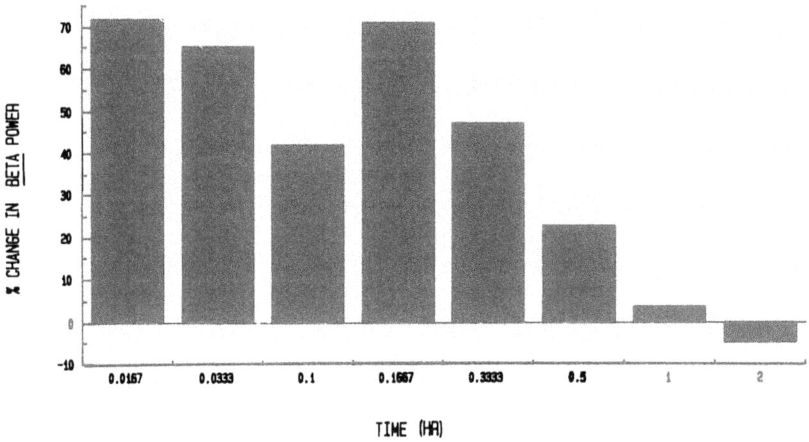

Fig. 1. Percent change in hippocampal *beta* power over time.

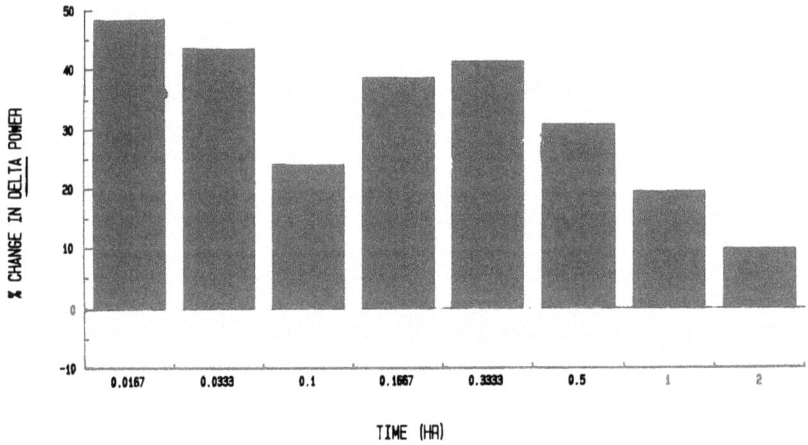

Fig. 2. Percent change in hippocampal *delta* power over time.

Relation of percent change in hippocampal EEG power and plasma and brain ketamine concentration

In general, the greatest increases in hippocampal EEG power occurred when ketamine plasma and brain concentrations were high. This is due to a very marked increase in *beta* and *delta* power. This is illustrated in Figs. 3 and 4.

It should be noted that brain ketamine concentrations are greater than plasma concentrations for most concentrations (>5×10^3 and <10^5 ng/gm or ml) of relevance to anesthesia. Especially impressive is the very close

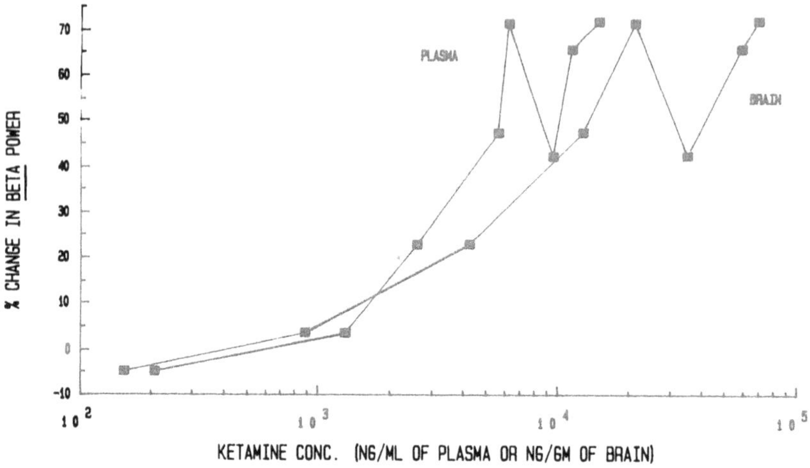

Fig. 3. Relation of percent change in hippocampal *beta* power to plasma and brain ketamine concentrations.

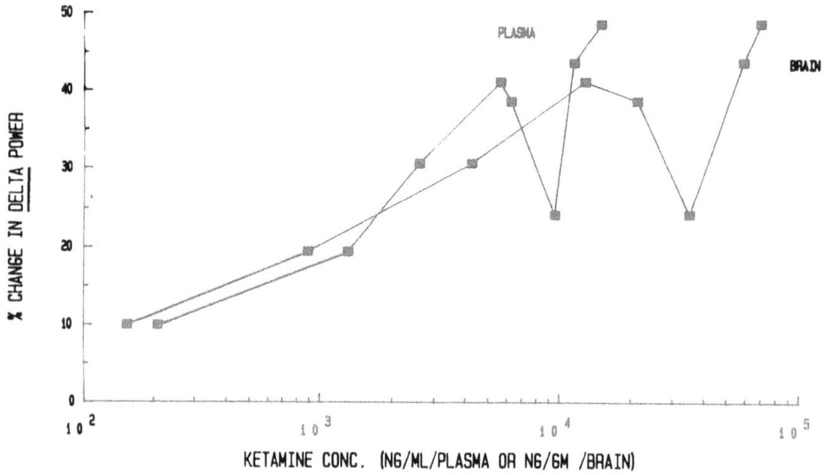

Fig. 4. Relation of percent change in hippocampal *delta* power to plasma and brain ketamine concentrations.

correlation (r = 0.99) between plasma and brain ketamine levels over the 2 hr period of study. This is illustrated in Fig. 5.

Discussion

Just as in humans, ketamine is a relatively short acting anesthetic in rats. Marietta *et al.* (1976) reported that 30 mg/kg i.v. ketamine in rats

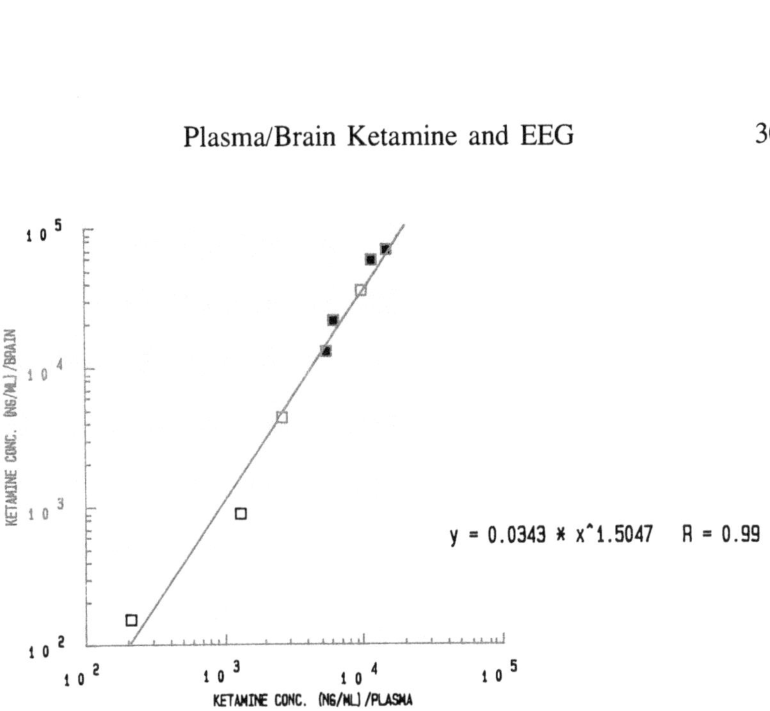

Fig. 5. Correlation of plasma and brain ketamine concentrations.

produced a mean ± S.E. loss of the right reflex of 8.0 ± 1.7, ataxia for 27.2 ± 5.0, and analgesia for 29.1 ± 3.4 min. Leung and Baille (1986) reported that 40 mg/kg i.v. ketamine caused a mean ± S.E. loss of the righting reflex of 7.11 ± 0.96 and an increase in spontaneous locomotor activity of 24.6 ± 4.5 min. Hence, the dose of ketamine used in the present study (30 mg/kg i.v.) was effective but short acting. Both groups of investigators mentioned showed that brain ketamine concentrations were greater than plasma concentrations 10 to 60 min after injection. The present study confirms this fact. Furthermore, rat brain and plasma levels are highly correlated (r = 0.99), indicating that the concentration of ketamine in plasma can be used as an index of brain ketamine concentration.

Considerable evidence suggests that phencyclidine (PCP) agonists, including ketamine, share unique behavioral and EEG properties. For example, in subanesthetic doses in rodents these agents produce hyperactive circling, head swaying, and other stereotypic behaviors, and an increase in neocortical slow wave activity in the EEG (Domino *et al.*, 1983; Mattia and Moreton, 1986; Young *et al.*, 1988). Although PCP is known to produce a persistent increase in the incidence of the atropine sensitive, low frequency (4-8 Hz) activity in the hippocampal EEG (Leung, 1985; Vanderwolf and Leung, 1981), it is not known if ketamine or other PCP agonists share this effect.

Young *et al.* (1988) have shown a very close regional distribution of

N-methyl-D-aspartate (NMDA) and PCP receptor binding sites in rat brain using [^{3}H] glutamate and [^{3}H] TCP. The greatest density of binding sites was in the hippocampus, especially the CA1 area. Therefore, in the present study we placed bipolar EEG electrodes in this area with one tip directed toward the CA1 stratum radiatum and the other at the upper portion of the dentate gyrus. It is quite noteworthy that, as expected, hippocampal EEG power (*beta* and *delta*) reflected brain and plasma ketamine concentrations.

References

Cooper, J.W. In: Pascal For Scientists, pp. 200-217, John Wiley and Sons, Inc., New York, 1981.

Domino, E.F., Fukuda, N., and Simonić, A.: Comparative electroencephalographic and gross behavioral effects of phencyclidine, related substances and various centrally acting drugs in Macaca mulatta. In J.-M. Kamenka, E.F. Domino, and P. Geneste, eds., Phencyclidine and Related Arylcyclohexylamines: Present and Future Applications, pp. 369-395, NPP Books, Ann Arbor, 1983.

Leung, L.W.: Spectral analysis of hippocampal EEG in the freely moving rat: Effects of centrally active drugs and relations to evoked potentials. EEG Clin. Neurophysiol. 60: 1, 65-77, 1985.

Leung, L.Y. and Baillie, T.A.: Comparative pharmacology in the rat of ketamine and its two principal metabolites, norketamine and (Z)-6-hydroxynorketamine. J. Med. Chem. 29: 2396-2399, 1986.

Maragos, W.F. and Penney, J.B.: Regional localization of NMDA and TCP binding in mammalian brain. In Domino, E.F. and Kamenka, J.-M., eds., *Sigma* and Phencyclidine-Like Compounds as Molecular Probes in Biology, pp. 269-276, NPP Books, Ann Arbor, 1988.

Marietta, M.P., White, P.F., Pudwill, C.R., Way, W.L., and Trevor, A.J.: Biodisposition of ketamine in the rat: Self-induction of metabolism. J. Pharmacol. Exp. Therap. 196: 536-544, 1976.

Mattia, A. and Moreton, J.E.: Electroencephalographic (EEG) power spectra and behavioral correlates in rats given phencyclidine. Neuropharmacol. 25: 763-769, 1986.

Pellegrino, L.J., Pellegrino, A.S., and Cushman, A.J.: A stereotaxic atlas of the rat brain. Plenum Press, New York, 1979.

Vanderwolf, C.H. and Leung, L.W.: Hippocampal rhythmical slow activity: A brief history and the effects of entorhinal lesions and phencyclidine. In W. Seifert, ed., Neurobiology of the Hippocampus, pp. 275-301, Academic Press, London, 1981.

Status of Ketamine in Anesthesiology,
edited by E.F. Domino©1990, NPP Books
P.O. Box 1491, Ann Arbor, MI 48106

Computer Supported Infusion Profiles for Long Lasting Anesthesia with Ketamine-Midazolan (Computer Tranquanalgesia-CTA)

H.P. Kreuscher, J.P. Braune, and M.D. Lechner*

Department of Anesthesiology
Städt Kliniken Osnabrück
and
**Department of Physical Chemistry*
Osnabrück University
Osnabrück, F.R. Germany

INTRODUCTION

Tranquanalgesia (TA) is the term for a technique we created in 1976 (Kreuscher *et al.*, 1977). Our aim was to compare this method with other combinations of ketamine and several other drugs, avoiding side effects like cardiovascular stimulation and psychotomimetic disorders. A special term was needed for this technique to indicate that, in contrast to other drug combinations with ketamine, TA is a standardized method with defined components as a mixture of ketamine with diazepam (TA I) or with midazolam (TA II), respectively. TA is induced with a solution of both ketamine and diazepam or midazolam in 0.9% NaCl, 5% dextrose, or another crystalline water infusion (Lechner and Kreuscher, 1989). TA involves a continuous i.v. drip technique which is used to obtain effective demand controlled blood and tissue levels of the two drugs. TA has the property of reproducibility and the feature of easy and safe administration. The rationale of the method, developed in the late 1960s, was to make ketamine acceptable and useful for particular anesthetic and operative purposes. Meanwhile, both TA techniques are standard in many anesthesiology departments in Europe, especially in the eastern countries, as well as overseas. TA is well accepted for short therapeutic or diagnostic interventions like reposition of bone fractures, incisions, wound surgery, dressing in burns, uterine curettage, endoscopy including cystoscopy, bronchoscopy, laparoscopy, etc., anesthesia in medical disasters, and as a supplement in unsatisfactory regional techniques. The method is simple and flexible enough to change, if necessary, to any other anesthetic technique. The following was used:

Prescription for TA I-ketamine 250 mg, diazepam 50 mg 0.9% NaCl 500 ml.

Prescription for TA II-ketamine 250 mg, midazolam 30 mg, 0.9% NaCl 500 ml.

Dosage

Induction. TA I and TA II are started with a maximal drop rate (20 drops/ml) until 2 ml/kg of body weight are given.

Maintenance. A total of 60-80 drops/min (3-4 ml/min) are given, up to a maximum of 500 ml. In average cases about 150 to 180 ml of the solution are needed for short interventions like uterine curettage.

The i.v. TA drip can be given alone or, as we recommend, with additional inhalation of N_2O/O_2. The induction period of approximately 5 min can be shortened by the administration of 0.2 mg/kg of etomidate. Muscle relaxants can be given, if needed. The patient should be intubated if this is necessary due to ventilatory demand. Vital parameters measured under both TA I and TA II remain in normal range. The recovery period during the patient's stay in the recovery unit is comparable to that after common general anesthetics but shorter in the follow up period after TA II (Kreuscher, 1977, 1982). The introduction of midazolam, which is water soluble and has a half life comparable to that of ketamine allowed further development in TA techniques for long lasting operational procedures as well as for analgosedation in intensive care situations. The experiences with TA for thoracotomy by Dr. Peter Harris of Derby, England (personal communication) stimulated us to proceed with our investigation in order to obtain data concerning the cardiovascular, respiratory, and adrenergic endocrine systems, and central nervous activity during major surgeries under TA II. These parameters must be observed if one wants to judge the properties and ability of an anesthetic for a particular patient and the indicated surgery (Bormann *et al.*, 1985). Long term TA II for surgeries of more than one hour required alteration of the dosage, observing the pharmacodynamic and pharmacokinetic properties of the administered drugs with regard to initial loading, distribution, and inactivation or excretion.

Methods

Twenty randomized patients (9 male, 11 female, mean age 56 yr, mean weight 68.9 kg) were anesthetized for one of the following major operations: vagotomy, osteosynthesis, Wertheim's, mastectomy, Whipple's choledocho-duodenostomy, hemicolectomy, femoropopliteal bypass, partial liver resection, laparotomy, gastrectomy, sigmoidectomy, or bowel amputation.

Anesthetic procedure

Premedication. A dose of 0.5 mg atropine i.v. was given before induction of anesthesia.

Induction. A dose of 0.2 mg/kg etomidate and 1 mg/kg succinylcholine was given followed by endotracheal intubation for ventilation with N_2O/O_2 1:3 l/min maintaining normal CO_2.

Maintenance of anesthesia was carried out by means of computer controlled TA II N_2O/O_2 2:1 l/min and skeletal muscle relaxation with pancuronium chloride.

Control parameters included arterial blood pressure, heart rate, blood gas analysis, EEG, EKG, blood glucose, plasma cortisol, epinephrine, and norepinephrine.

The time schedule for obtaining control measures or blood samples is shown in Fig. 1.

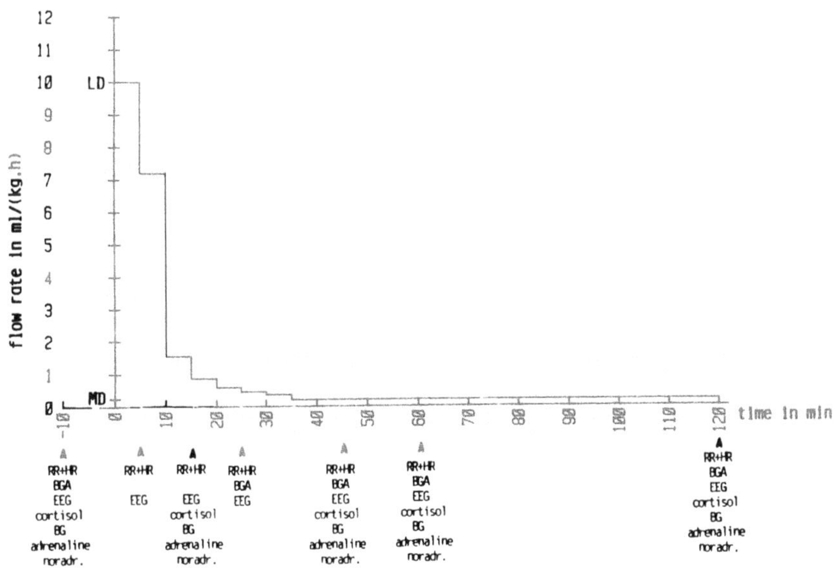

Fig. 1. Computer controlled infusion profile for 250 mg ketamine and 30 mg midazolam in a 500 ml solution. LD = loading dose (10 ml/kg/hr); MD = maintenance dose (0.2 ml/kg/hr).

The plasma concentrations (Cp) for anesthesia used were: ketamine (Wieber *et al.*, 1975, Fig. 2); midazolam (Crevoisier *et al.*, 1981, Fig. 3).

Our aim was to obtain effective plasma concentrations of both ketamine and midazolam in a clinically acceptable time schedule. Thus we designed the infusion profile with three steps: 1) loading dose-5 min 10 ml/kg/hr, 2) approximate exponential decrease over 30 min (see Fig. 1), down to 3) maintenance dose-0.2 ml/kg/hr. Using this schedule, we calculated the behavior of plasma concentration curves for both ketamine and midazolam, as shown in Fig. 4.

Technical setup

The infusion pump (IMED 929) was controlled by a CODIC computer, whose hardware and software were designed by Stoffregen (1985). The computer was programmed with individual data of a particular patient including body weight, height, sex, age, and dosage parameters as mentioned above. Blood pressure was measured indirectly by means of a CRITICON-DINAMAP. EEG monitoring was done by computer frequency analysis with LIFESCAN.

Laboratory techniques

Ketamine and midazolam levels were measured by HPLC on stored, deep frozen plasma after thawing. A volume of 0.5 ml of plasma was

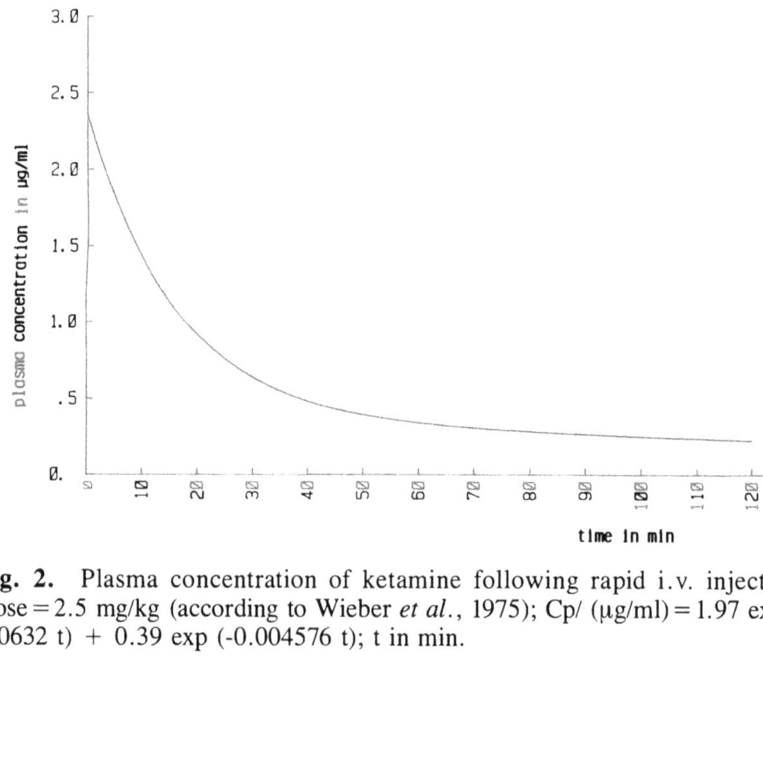

Fig. 2. Plasma concentration of ketamine following rapid i.v. injection. Dose = 2.5 mg/kg (according to Wieber *et al.*, 1975); Cp/ (µg/ml) = 1.97 exp (-0.0632 t) + 0.39 exp (-0.004576 t); t in min.

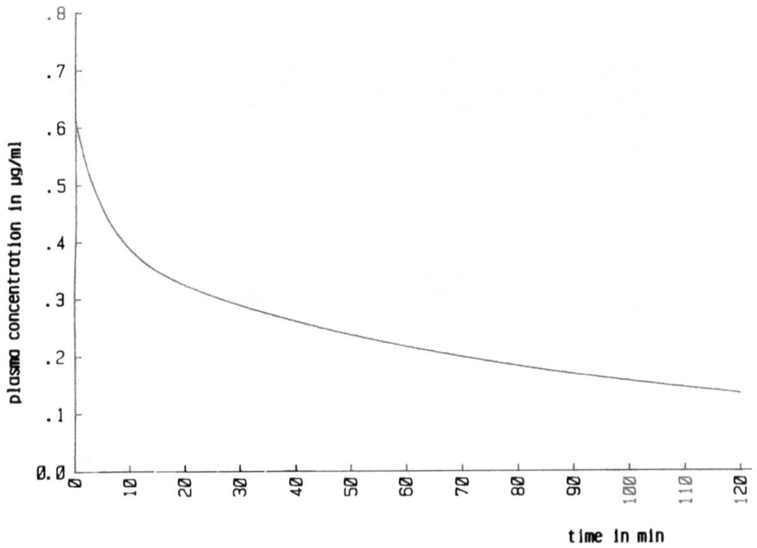

Fig. 3. Plasma concentration of midazolam following rapid i.v. injection; Dose = 0.18 mg/kg (according to Crevoisier *et al.*, 1981); Cp/(µg/ml) = 0.215 exp (-0.191 t) + 0.222 exp (-0.0168 t) + 0.174 exp (-0.00418 t); t in min.

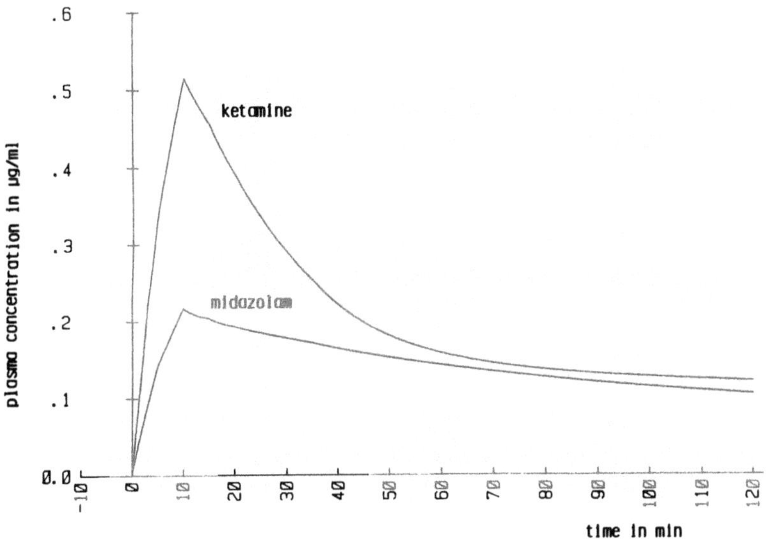

Fig. 4. Plasma concentration of ketamine and midazolam according to a computer controlled infusion profile. Calculated from the pharmacokinetic parameters of Figs. 2 and 3.

mixed with 50 μl NaOH (concentration-1 mol/l) and 4 ml diethyl ether. The solution was centrifuged for 5 min at 800 g. The ether layer was transferred and evaporated to dryness at 34°C. Then 0.5 ml of the eluent was added and 0.1 ml was injected onto the column. The HPLC measurements were done with an HPLC 414 pump, an injection system Rheodyne 7125, and a UV detector UVIKON 714 from Kontron Analytical, Munich, F.R. Germany. Peak integration was done with a computer. The HPLC conditions were: column μ-Bondapak, C18, 10 μm, 250 x 5 mm; injection volume 20 μl; flow rate 0.5 ml/min; wavelength of detector 215 nm; solvent (mobile phase) Na acetate (0.01 mol/l)/acetic acid/water (pH 4.0), and methanol (25:75 V/V).

Calibration was performed with pure midazolam obtained from Hoffmann-La Roche AG, Grenzach-Wyhlen (FRG) and ketamine obtained from Parke Davis and Co., Munich, F.R. Germany. These were prepared in different concentrations in the infusion solution as described above. The calibration curves were linear in the concentration range of interest (Lechner and Kreuscher, 1989). Cortisol was determined by a radioimmunoassay method (RIA) with iodine as the marker (coated tube method). Catecholamines were determined by HPLC, according to the method of Boos *et al.* (1987). The other substances were determined by the usual clinical laboratory methods.

Results

Plasma concentrations of ketamine. The values obtained were close to the calculated concentration curve (Fig. 5).

Plasma concentrations of midazolam. The values obtained were close to the calculated concentration curve (Fig. 6).

Arterial pH. There were no significant changes (Fig. 7).

Mean arterial blood pressure. There were no significant changes (Fig. 8).

Heart rate. There were no significant changes (Fig. 9).

$PaCO_2$. There were no significant changes (Fig. 10).

$PaCO_2$. There was a significant increase caused by inhalation of a mixture with oxygen concentrations over atmospheric values (Fig. 11).

Blood glucose. There was significant increase after 60 and 120 min (Fig. 12).

Cortisol in plasma. The values remained in the normal range (Fig. 13).

Plasma epinephrine. There were no significant changes (Fig. 14).

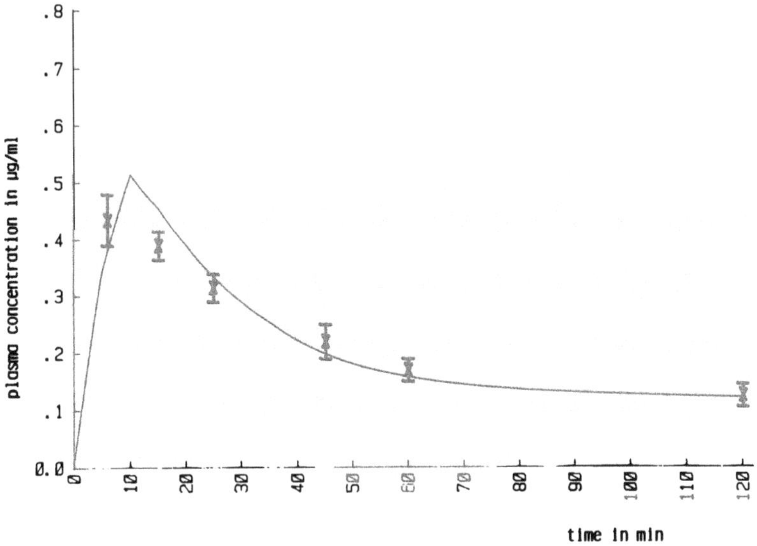

Fig. 5. Plasma concentration of ketamine according to a computer controlled infusion profile. —— = calculated from the pharmacokinetic parameters. I = median $\tilde{x}$ and interquartil distance I_{50} (N = 18).

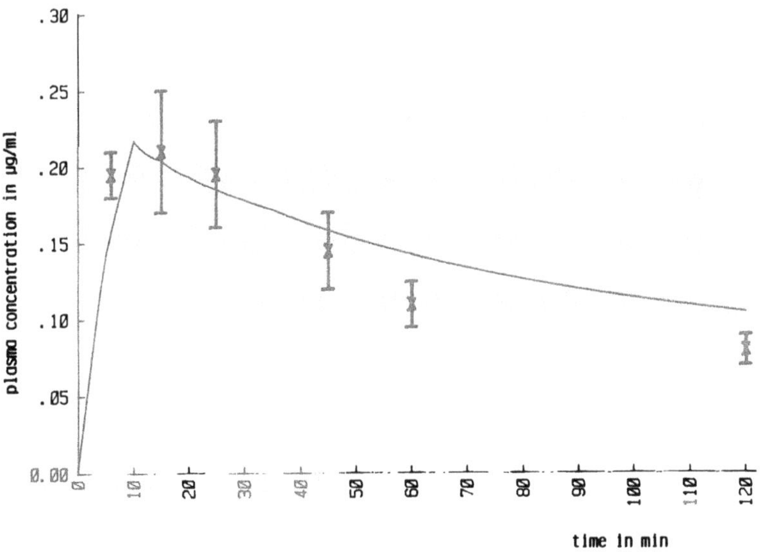

Fig. 6. Plasma concentration of midazolam according to a computer controlled infusion profile. —— = calculated from the pharmacokinetic parameters. I = median $\tilde{x}$ and interquartil distance I_{50} (N = 18).

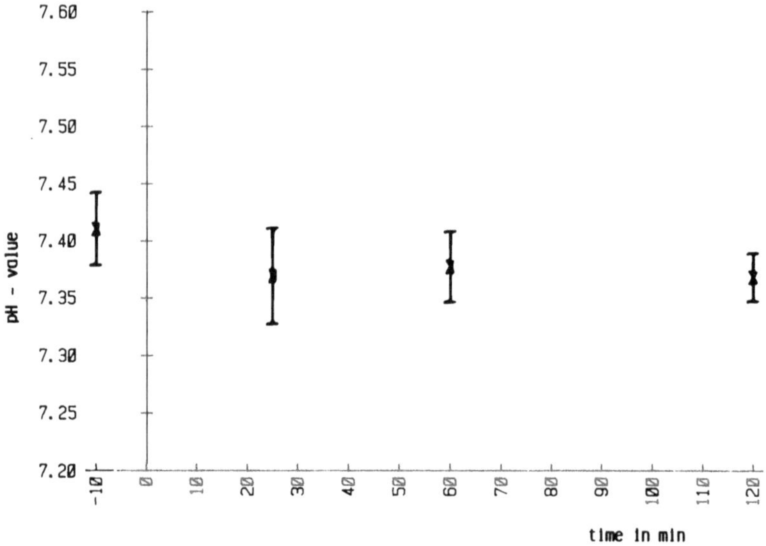

Fig. 7. pH of arterial blood (N = 20).

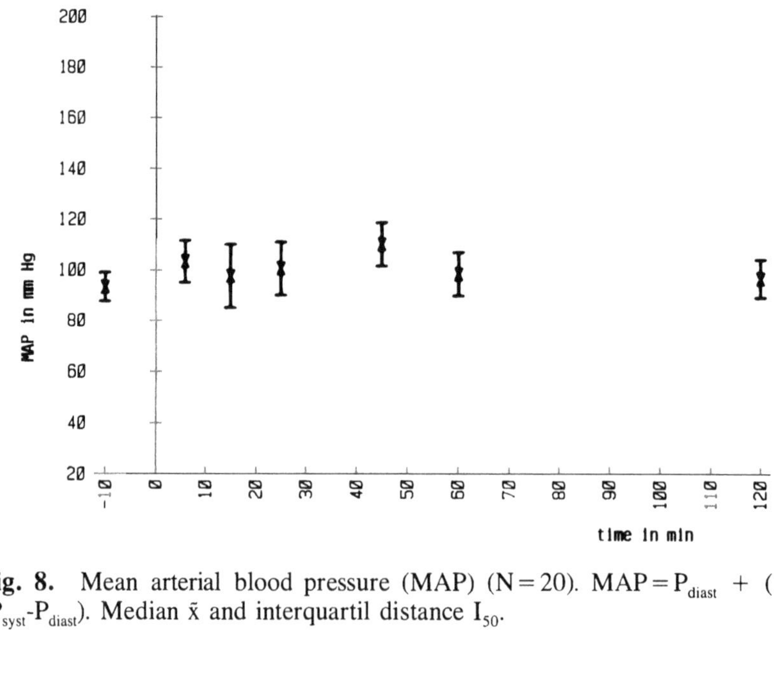

Fig. 8. Mean arterial blood pressure (MAP) (N = 20). MAP = P_{diast} + (1/3) (P_{syst}-P_{diast}). Median $\tilde{x}$ and interquartil distance I_{50}.

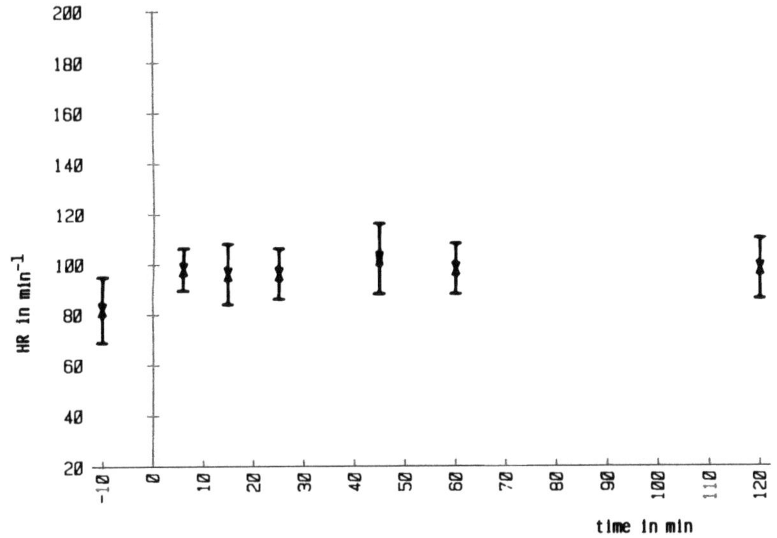

Fig. 9. Heart rate/min (N = 20). Median $\tilde{x}$ and interquartil distance I_{50}.

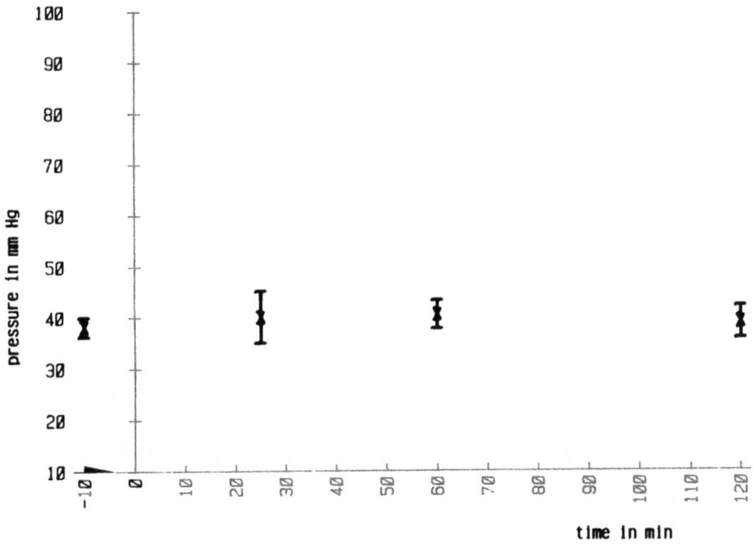

Fig. 10. $PaCO_2$ in arterial blood (N = 20). Median $\tilde{x}$ and interquartil distance I_{50}.

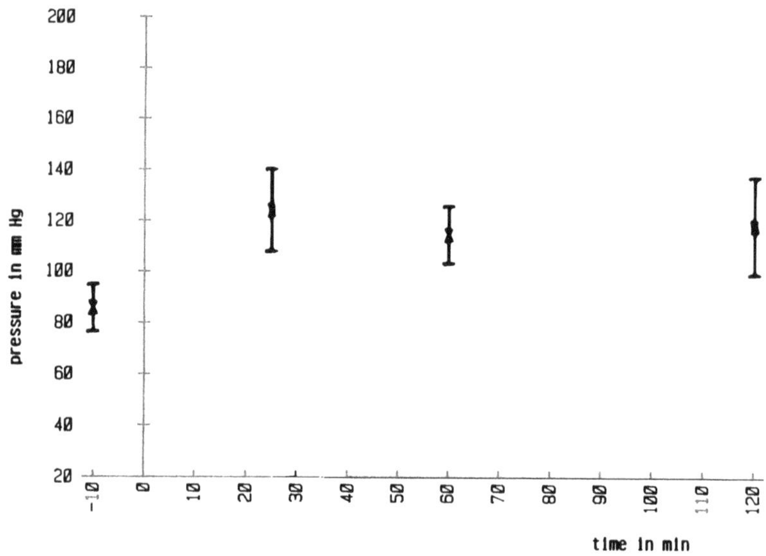

Fig. 11. $PaCO_2$ in arterial blood (N = 20). Median $\tilde{x}$ and interquartil distance I_{50}.

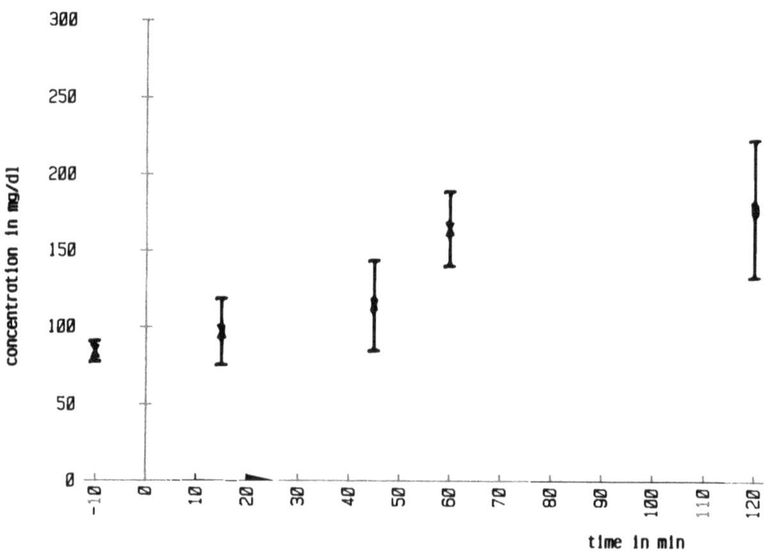

Fig. 12. Blood glucose (N = 20). Median $\tilde{x}$ and interquartil distance I_{50}.

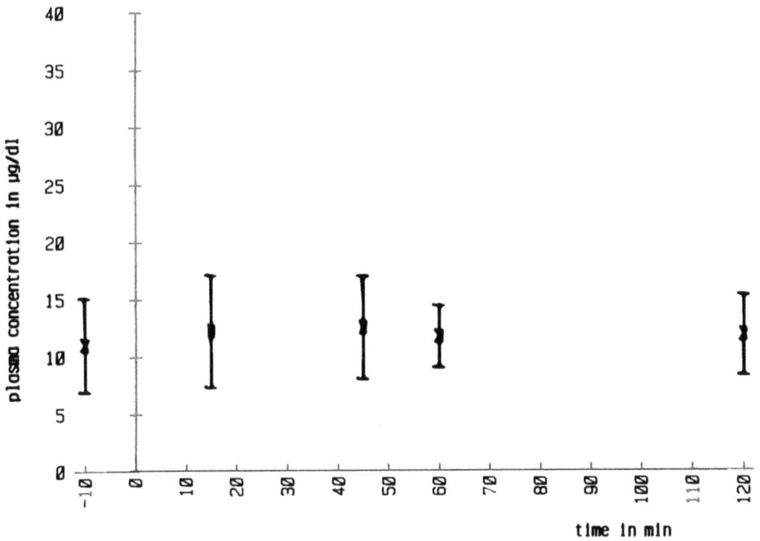

Fig. 13. Plasma concentration of cortisol (N = 19). Median x̃ and interquartil distance I_{50}. Normal: 5-25 µg/dl.

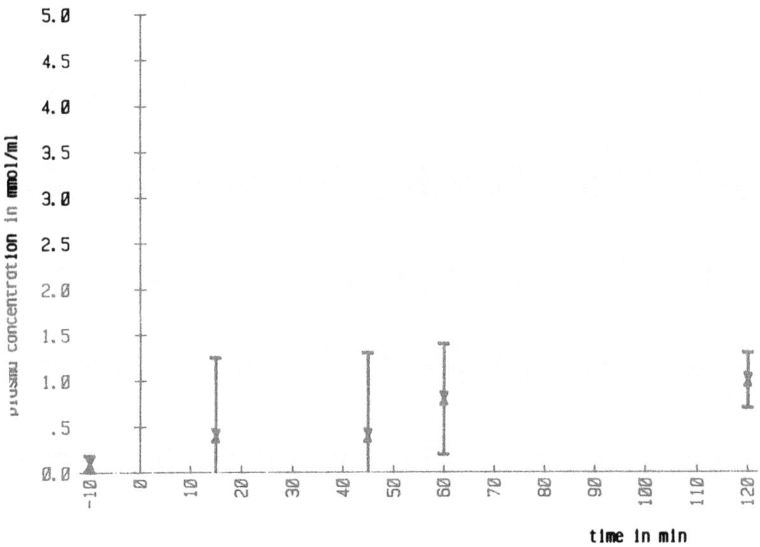

Fig. 14. Plasma concentration of epinephrine (N = 9). Median x̃ and interquartil distance I_{50}. Normal: below 0.27 mmol/ml.

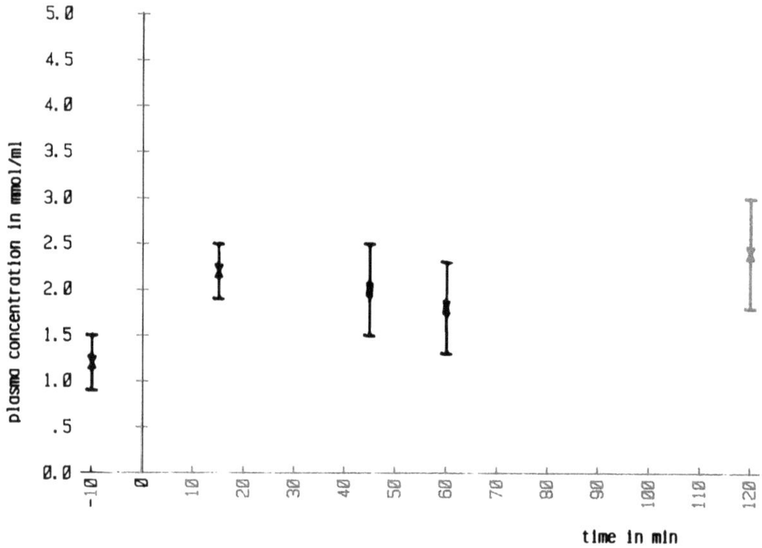

Fig. 15. Plasma concentration of norepinephrine (N = 9). Median x̃ and interquartil distance I_{50}. Normal: below 1.5 mmol/ml.

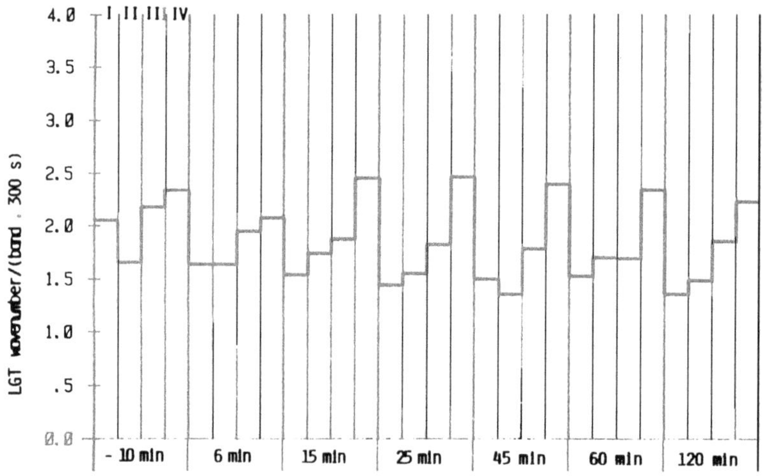

Fig. 16. EEG frequency analysis by LIFESCAN® during computerized tranquanalgesia (CTA, N = 19). Medians of the averages of the registered wave numbers per frequency band and analysis period (300 sec) are shown. I = 0.5-3 Hz (δ); II = 3-8 Hz (θ); III = 8-12 Hz (α); IV = 12-30 Hz (β).

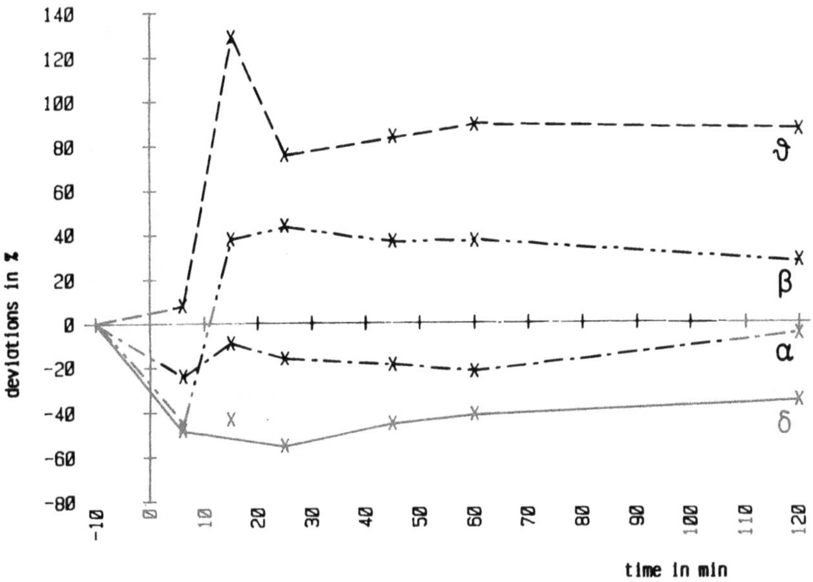

Fig. 17. EEG frequency analysis by LIFESCAN® during CTA (N = 19). Average of the deviation in percent of the registered wave number per frequency band and analysis period (300 sec) are shown.

Plasma norepinephrine. There was an initial small increase which remained constant throughout the measuring period (Fig. 15).

EEG frequency analysis. There was an increase in EEG *theta* and *beta* activity, and a decrease in *alpha* and *delta* activity occurred after reaching steady state. It remained unchanged throughout the measuring period (Figs. 16 and 17).

Discussion and Conclusions

One goal for the use of i.v. drip techniques for long lasting anesthesia or analgosedation in intensive care situations is to reach stabile concentrations of the active drug in plasma as well as in tissues. Intermittent (bolus) applications will not produce these conditions and can trigger undesirable reactions in the autonomic nervous system. The aim of modern anesthesia is a stabile state of the central and autonomic nervous systems, as well as protection against nociceptive stimulation due to surgery. This state should be reached with a minimum of drugs without marked depression of the central nervous system. Most general anesthetics have strong hypnotic and poor analgesic properties. The simultaneous use of relatively high doses of hypnotic, analgesic, and skeletal muscle relaxant drugs in general anesthesia avoids hyperactivity of the adrenergic system as measured by catecholamine release (stress).

The results of the data obtained in our study with computerized TA (CTA) show stabile behavior of the parameters representative of desirable as well as for undesirable reactions on trauma. The necessary amount of ketamine and midazolam to produce a satisfactory anesthetic state during the operative procedures was extremely small (ketamine 0.4 mg/kg/hr, midazolam 0.05 mg/kg/hr). The recovery time of the patients in this study was short and they showed no psychotomimetic or physical emergence reactions.

References

Boos, K.S., Wilmers, B., Sauerbrey, R., and Schlimme, E.: Development and performance of an automated HPLC analyzer for catecholamines. Chromatographic 24: 363-370, 1987.

Bormann v., B., Sturm, G., Kling, D., Scheld, H.H., Boldt, J., and Hempelmann, G.: Wertigkeit endokriner Stressparameter. Anaesthesist 34: 280-286, 1985.

Crevoisier, C., Eckert, M., Heizmann, P., Thurneysen, D.J., and Ziegler, W.H.: Relation entre l'effect clinique et la pharmacocinetique du midazolam après administration i.v. et i.m. Arzneimittelforschung 31(II): 2211-2115, 1981.

Kreuscher, H.: Erfahrungen mit der Tranquanalgesie. In Erlanger Anästhesieseminar, Rügheimer, E., ed., Verlag Medizin Media, Bubenreuth, 1977.

Kreuscher, H.: Fortschritte der Tranquanalgesie. In Ketanest und Benzodiazepin-Kombination in der Anästhesie, Langrehr, D., ed., Perimed-Verlag (Erlangen), 1982.

Kreuscher, H. and Huebner: Tranquanalgesia: Intravenous anesthesia procedure with diazepam and ketamine. In Clinical Use of Ketamine in Intravenous Drip Infusion, Selected Proceedings of the Sixth World Congress of Anaesthesiology, Mexico City, Mexico, April 24-30, 1976, Excerpta Medica, 1977.

Lechner, M.D. and Kreuscher, H.: Physikalische Kompatibilität von Ketamin mit Diazepam und Midazolam in Infusionslösungen. Anäesthesist 38: 418-420, 1989.

Stoffregen, J.: Das therapeutische System CODIC. Anästh. Intensivth. Notfallmed. 4: 210-212, 1985.

Wieber, J., Gugler, R., Hengstmann, J.H., and Dengler, H.J.: Pharmacokinetics of ketamine in man. Anaesthesist 24: 260-263, 1975.

Status of Ketamine in Anesthesiology,
edited by E.F. Domino©1990, NPP Books
P.O. Box 1491, Ann Arbor, MI 48106

Ketamine for Intravenous Regional Anesthesia

Z. Durrani, A.P. Winnie, and E.K. Zsigmond

Department of Anesthesiology
University of Illinois
Chicago, IL

INTRODUCTION

Cardiac arrest has occurred after unintentional or intentional deflation of the tourniquet following the use of i.v. regional anesthesia with all of the currently used amide type local anesthetic agents (Kennedy *et al.*, 1965; Cox, 1964; Heath, 1984). Unfortunately, the ester type local anesthetic agents, which have a several fold greater safety margin than amide type local anesthetics, have a too short duration of action to be clinically useful for i.v. regional anesthesia. These agents are hydrolyzed by plasma cholinesterase in the remaining blood in the tourniqueted extremity. If plasma cholinesterase activity is inhibited by hexaflurenium, the best local anesthetic in man is 2-chloroprocaine, which may provide the safest i.v. regional anesthesia (Zsigmond and Flynn, 1974). Nevertheless, a slight chance for toxic reactions still remains. Therefore, an agent free of central nervous system and cardiovascular toxicity may be the safest drug for i.v. regional anesthesia. The results of the studies of Dowdy *et al.* (1973) and Weber *et al.* (1975) indicate that ketamine possesses local anesthetic activity. If ketamine does provide local anesthesia sufficient for the conduction of surgical procedures, it would be the ideal agent for i.v. regional anesthesia since the worst reaction in a patient after accidental or intentional tourniquet release at the end of a procedure would be amnesia, analgesia, and anesthesia without the hazards of central nervous system or cardiovascular toxicity. Hence, the possible occurrence of cardiac arrest could be completely prevented.

In order to study this possible advantage of ketamine for i.v. regional anesthesia, our research team set out to study ketamine for this application in healthy human volunteers (Durrani *et al.*, 1989).

Methods and Materials

Healthy, young adult volunteers (N = 15) participated in these studies. Informed written consent was obtained after previous approval from the Institutional Review Board. The volunteers received either a 0.5% (Group A, N=5), or 0.3% (Group B, N=5), or 0.2% (Group C, N=5) solution of ketamine HCl. Since the volunteers in Group C found the tourniquet pain unbearable, the study in some of these volunteers was terminated early, although the initial onset of blocks was evaluated in all 5 volunteers in this group.

A heparinized plastic i.v. catheter was inserted into a vein in the arm to be studied. The arm was exsanguinated with an Esmarch bandage, a double cuffed tourniquet was applied, the proximal cuff of the tourniquet was inflated, and the Esmarch bandage removed. Ketamine, in a total volume of 30-50 ml (0.6 ml/kg) in 0.9% NaCl in the concentration scheduled for the volunteer, was then injected. For safety, another i.v. line was inserted in the contralateral arm vein and Ringer's lactate solution was slowly infused. Blood pressure was taken with an automatic recording oscillometer (Dinamap, Critikon Corp.) at 3 min intervals. The ECG was continuously monitored on a polygraph throughout and for 1 hr following the experiment.

The onset of sympathetic, sensory, and motor block was determined by psychogalvanometric recording on a polygraph, by pinprick and cold stimulation, and by recording the motor response to ulnar nerve stimulation via a hand held plethysmograph stimulator (Emerson Relaxaid Stimulator, Model 91-E2X). After maintenance of a successful block for 1 hr, the tourniquet was deflated by a cyclic deflation/inflation sequence with progressively increasing periods of deflation for 10-60 sec. The volunteers were observed for 2 hr after the end of tourniquet deflation for symptoms and signs of toxicity or adverse effects. An ANOVA computer program was used for statistical analysis. Differences were considered significant with $P<0.05$. All values are expressed as mean ± S.E.

Results

Groups A and B did not differ as to age, weight, height, and mean body surface area. The onset of sympathetic block was 6.0 ± 0.5 min in Group A and 7.2 ± 0.4 min in Group B (Fig. 1). Sensory blocks took longer in Group A than in Group B. There were no significant differences between the two groups in any of the onset times. However, the onset of sensory block took longer than sympathetic block, while that of motor

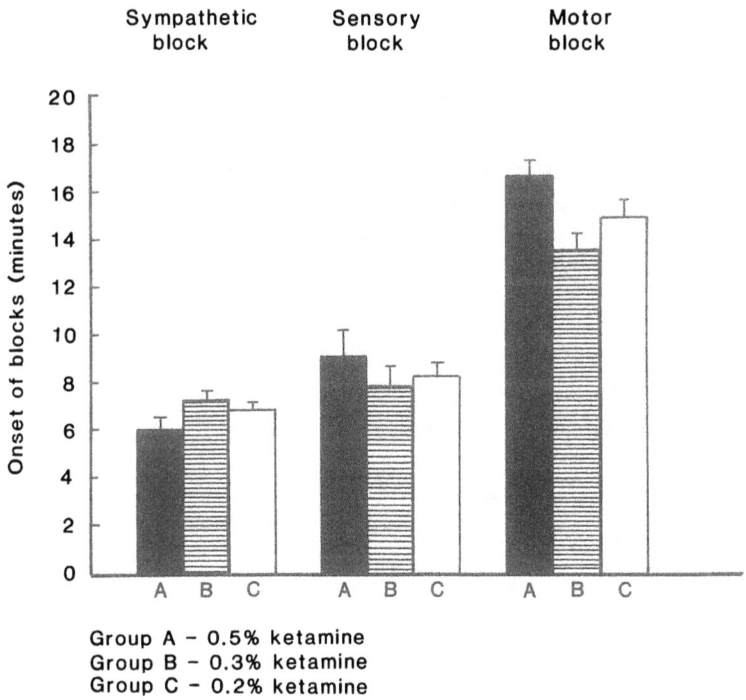

Fig. 1. Onset of i.v. regional anesthesia following different concentrations of ketamine.

block was the slowest in Group A. In Group B, the onset of motor block also took longer than that of either sensory or sympathetic block. No significant changes in heart rate or blood pressure occurred during the studies or during the deflation of the tourniquet (Fig. 2). During the 1 hr poststudy observation period, all of the volunteers had nystagmus or psychotomimetic sequelae. One volunteer in Group B lost consciousness. Hypersecretions (3/5) and nausea (2/5) occurred in Group A, while vomiting (2/5) occurred in Group B. Sweating was observed in all of the volunteers. Headache occurred in 2/5 and 1/5 in Group A and B, respectively. Diazepam (0.1-0.15 mg/kg i.v.) restored normal orientation in all volunteers within 20 min.

Discussion

The local anesthetic effect of ketamine was confirmed in this study. The sequential onset of sympathetic, sensory, and motor block is identical

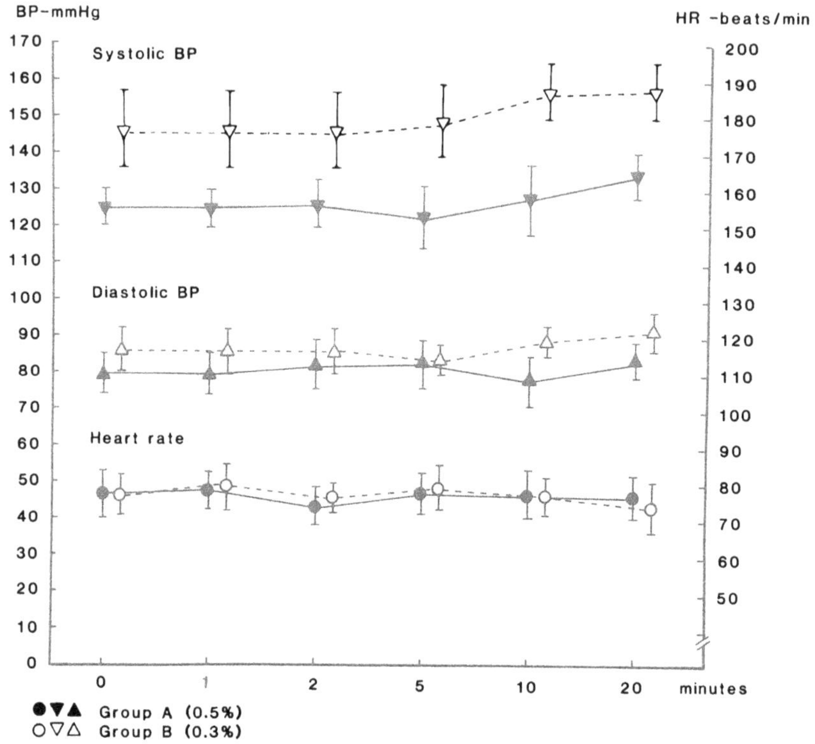

Fig. 2. No significant changes in heart rate or blood pressure are observed with i.v. regional ketamine anesthesia.

to that observed following administration of other local anesthetics. The potency of ketamine is slightly lower than that of procaine. In his classical experiment with i.v. regional anesthesia, Bier (1908) observed adequate analgesia with 0.25% procaine. Bion (1984) utilized intrathecal ketamine in war surgery. Recently, Tsai *et al.* (1988) confirmed the local anesthetic effects of intrathecal ketamine in monkeys.

Although ketamine may be suitable for i.v. regional anesthesia with the greatest safety margin, indeed without the fear of serious central nervous system or cardiovascular toxicity, its unpleasant and disturbing psychotomimetic effects and emetic sequelae prevent its use without diazepam premedication. Our pilot study was the first study to evaluate the effectiveness *vs* the safety of ketamine for i.v. regional anesthesia, so we intentionally avoided premedication. Diazepam, however, controlled the psychotomimetic effects promptly. Our earlier series of investigations showed that diazepam prevents not only the circulatory but also the psychotomimetic effects of ketamine (Kothary *et al.*, 1975). Hence, diazepam given prior to ketamine i.v. regional anesthesia might prevent all of the adverse sequelae of ketamine observed in this pilot study.

Conclusions

Ketamine may serve as an alternate, safer agent to currently used local anesthetics for i.v. regional anesthesia provided the patients receive benzodiazepine pretreatment. Ketamine used alone without diazepam premedication induces clinically unacceptable side effects following tourniquet removal. This possible clinical combination of diazepam and ketamine needs to be investigated.

Acknowledgement

We are grateful to all of the volunteers who participated in the study, conducted in 1981, to our secretaries, Natalka and Ellen Howard for their excellent work in typing the manuscript, and to Dr. Eva Barabas for the illustrations. The assistance of Dr. E.F. Domino with the review of this manuscript is acknowledged.

References

Bier, A.: Concerning a new method of local anesthesia of the extremities (German). Arch. Klin. Chir. 86: 1007-1016, 1908.

Bion, J.F.: Intrathecal ketamine for war surgery. A preliminary study under field conditions. Anaesthesia 39: 1023-1028, 1984.

Cox, J.M.R.: Intravenous regional analgesia. Can. Anaesth. Soc. J. 11: 503-508, 1964.

Dowdy, E.G., Kaya, K., and Gocho, Y.: Some pharmacologic similarities of ketamine, lidocaine, and procaine. Anesth. Analg. 52: 839-842, 1973.

Durrani, Z., Winnie, A.P., Zsigmond, E.K., and Burnett, M.L.: Ketamine for intravenous regional anesthesia. Anesth. Analg. 68: 328-332, 1989.

Heath, M.L.: Deaths after intravenous regional anesthesia. Br. Med. J. 285: 913-914, 1984.

Kennedy, B.R., Duthie, A.M., and Parbrook, G.D.: Intravenous regional analgesia: An appraisal. Br. Med. J. 1: 954-957, 1965.

Kothary, S.P., Zsigmond, E.K., and Matsuki, A.: Antagonism of the ketamine-induced rise in plasma-free norepinephrine, blood pressure and pulse rate by intravenous diazepam. Clin. Pharmacol. Ther. 17: 238, 1975.

Tsai, S.K., Mok, M.S., Hung, H.L., *et al.*: Analgesic effect of intrathecal ketamine in primates. Anesth. Analg. 67: S234, 1988.

Weber, W.V., Jawalekar, K.S., and Jawalekar, S.R.: The effect of ketamine on the nerve conduction in isolated sciatic nerves of the toad. Neurosci. Lett. 1: 115-120, 1975.

Zsigmond, E.K. and Flynn, K.: Intravenous regional anesthesia with hexafluoronium bromide and 2-chloroprocaine. Excerpta Med. Int. Cong. Series No. 330: 553, 1974.

Zsigmond, E.K., Durrani, Z., Burnett, M.L., and Winnie, A.P.: Ketamine for intravenous regional anesthesia. Reg. Anes. 7: 82-83, 1982.

Status of Ketamine in Anesthesiology,
edited by E.F. Domino©1990, NPP Books
P.O. Box 1491, Ann Arbor, MI 48106

Rectal Administration of Ketamine for Anesthesia Induction in Children: A Randomized, Controlled Clinical Study

J.-P. Jantzen, I. Tzanova, and A.M. Klein

Department of Anesthesiology
Johannes Gutenberg University Medical School
Mainz, F.R. Germany

Introduction

Rectal administration of barbiturates for preoperative sedation was introduced by Gwathmey in 1936 and is now widely used for premedication and induction of anesthesia (Kraus and Taeger, 1982; Kühn *et al.*, 1983; Liu *et al.*, 1980). Complications have been reported following the rectal administration of methohexital (Kaiser and Al Rafai, 1985; Liu *et al.*, 1984). The problems associated with rectal methohexital are lack of analgesic properties (Dundee, 1964) and irritation of the rectal mucosa (Hinkle and Weinlander, 1984, 1985). Ketamine is a potent analgesic which does not irritate mucous membranes, making ketamine an attractive alternative to barbiturates for rectal induction of anesthesia. The aim of this study was to clinically evaluate rectally administered ketamine *vs* methohexital for the induction of anesthesia in children.

Methods

The study was performed by three anesthesiologists and two nurse anesthetists according to a defined protocol. Fifty children presenting for minor surgery (ASA I, ≤ 12 months), with a maximum body weight of 20 kg, were randomly allocated to two groups (methohexital or ketamine). No premedication was given. Prior to induction, the mood of the children was evaluated by the anesthesiologist and rated either positive (cooperative, friendly, playful) or negative (introverted, fearful, aggressive). According to the degree of oro-tracheal secretion, the children were rated as wet or dry. Anesthesia was induced with either 10% methohexital (25 mg/

kg) or 5% ketamine (15 mg/kg) administered rectally in combination with 0.03 mg/kg of atropine.

The following were assessed at a 2 min sequence: visual contact, reaction to optical, acoustical, and tactile stimulation (blood pressure cuff), tolerance of vein puncture, and mask ventilation. Arterial oxygen saturation was monitored in 10 children by pulse oximetry. Hypoxygenation was assumed at $SaO_2<90\%$. Applications that did not produce tolerance of assisted mask ventilation within 20 min were rated as failures.

Anesthesia was maintained with halothane and nitrous oxide/ oxygen (1.3 MAC; $FiO_2 = 0.35$). After the termination of halothane exposure, the time intervals to onset of spontaneous movements and eye opening were noted. Further documentation included complications during emergence and recovery, and duration of postoperative analgesia and recovery room stay. The postoperative status was assessed by the ward nurse in the afternoon of the day of the operation and in the morning of the first postoperative day. Behavior was rated positive, normal or negative. The nurse was blinded to the induction agent used. Statistical analysis utilized the t-test; significance was assumed at $P \leq 0.01$.

Results

There were no differences among patients and procedures in the two groups (Table 1).

Rectal induction was rated successful in 12 of 20 children receiving methohexital and in 15 of 20 children receiving ketamine (Figs. 1 and 2). The course of induction and complications during induction is shown in Figs. 3 and 4. Defecation was seen in the methohexital group only (20%). Arterial oxygen desaturation was observed in 2 of 5 children in the methohexital group. The course of emergence and recovery is shown in Fig. 5. Complications are shown in Fig. 6. Respiratory complications were seen primarily in children receiving methohexital. Arterial hypoxygenation occurred in 2 methohexital children during recovery. Emergence, postoperative analgesia, and recovery lasted significantly longer in the ketamine children. The postoperative condition on the ward was rated more favorable in children receiving ketamine (Fig. 7).

Discussion

Ano-rectal induction is becoming increasingly popular in pediatric anesthesia. To go to sleep in the mother's arms is associated with a reduction of endocrine stress parameters (Birkhahn *et al.*, 1986). In a com-

TABLE 1. Comparison of methohexital and ketamine groups

Parameter	*Methohexital*	*Ketamine*
Number of subjects	25	25
Age (months)	39 ± 23 (12-89)	38 ± 18 (13-72)
Weight (kg)	15 ± 3 (10-20)	14 ± 3 (9-20)
Sex (M/F)	21/4 20/5	
Mask/Intubation	16/9	13/12
Surgery (min)	49 ± 28 (10-105)	54 ± 34 (6-135)
Anesthesia (min)	100 ± 38 (45-210)	105 ± 38 (45-210)
Preoperative condition (pos/neg)	7/18	10/15
Preoperative salivation (dry/wet)	15/10	19/6

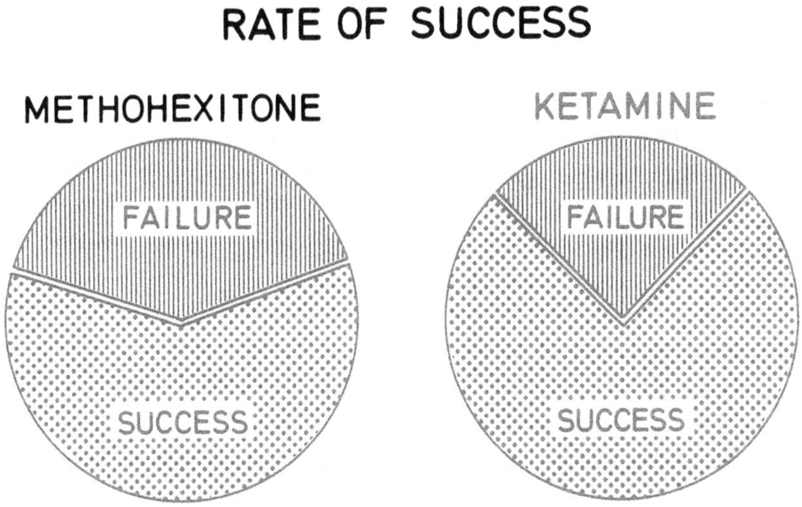

Fig. 1. Success rates of rectal induction with methohexital (N = 20) and ketamine (N = 20).

parative investigation, methohexital was shown to be a more suitable agent for rectal induction as compared to midazolam or etomidate (Kretz *et al.*, 1985). Reported complications associated with the rectal administration of methohexital include anaphylactoid reactions (Liu *et al.*, 1984), airway problems during induction (Kretz and Piepenbrock, 1983; Thülig *et al.*, 1985), emergence (Kühn *et al.*, 1983), and recovery (Kaiser and Al Rafai, 1985), as well as restlessness and agitation (Kretz and Piepenbrock, 1983; Kretz *et al.*, 1985). Ketamine could be a suitable alternative with regard to its analgesic properties, and lack of tissue irritation and histamine libera-

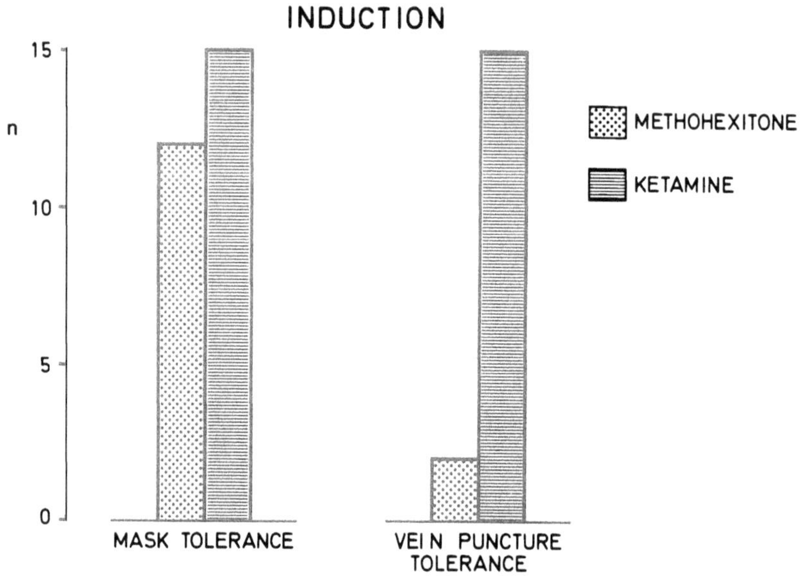

Fig. 2. Tolerance of vein puncture (N = 20) and face mask (N = 20).

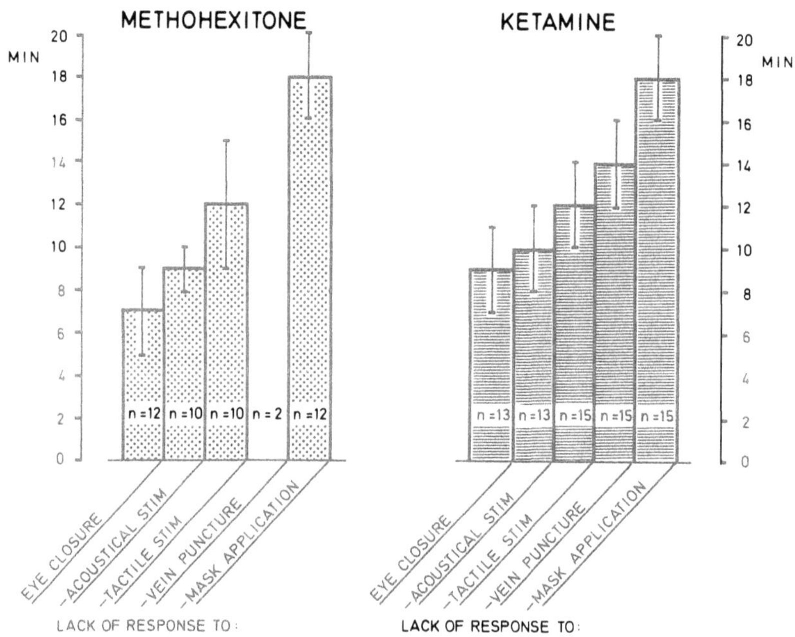

Fig. 3. Course of induction (N = 20) per group; x ± S.D.

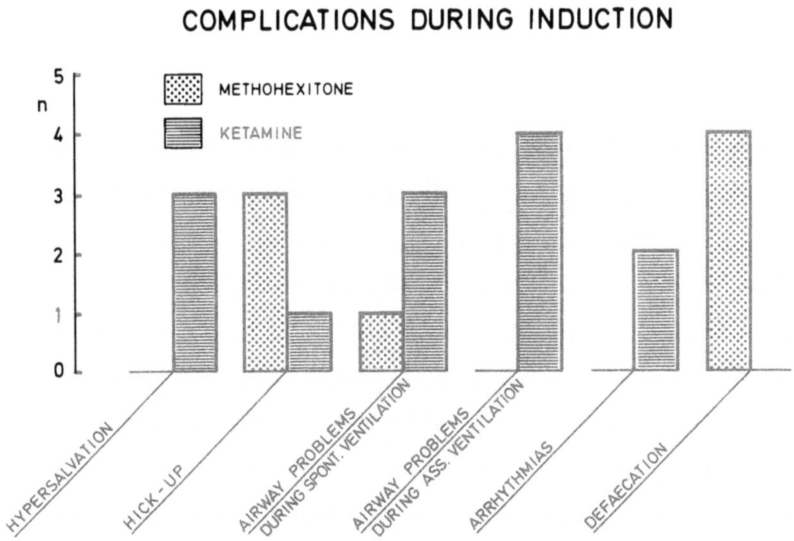

Fig. 4. Complications during induction.

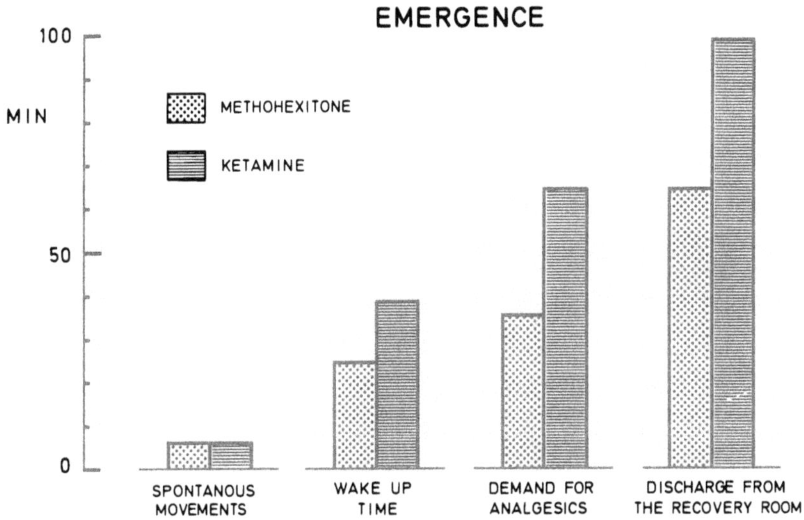

Fig. 5. Course of emergence (N = 50).

tion. We investigated the usefulness of methohexital and ketamine in the present randomized prospective clinical study.

Dosage recommendations for methohexital extend from 15 to 30 mg/kg as a 1%, 5%, or 10% solution (Engelhardt *et al.*, 1986; Liu *et al.*,

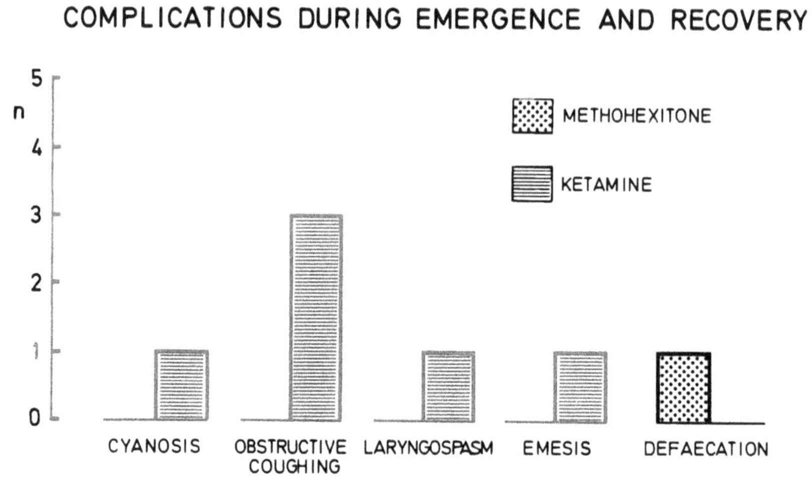

Fig. 6. Complications during emergence and recovery.

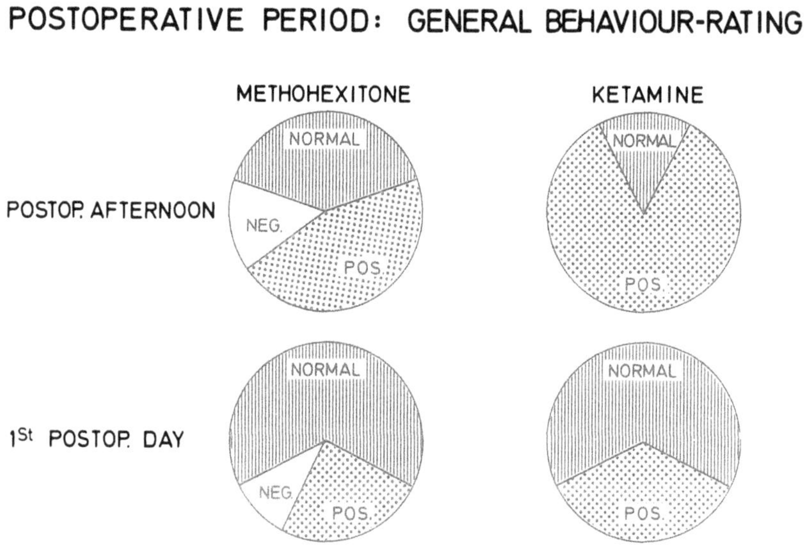

Fig. 7. Assessment of patient condition on the postoperative afternoon and the first postoperative day (N = 25 per group).

1980). We investigated the most frequently used dose of 25 mg/kg as a 10% solution (= 0.25 ml/kg). The recommended dosage for ketamine ranges from 8 to 15 mg/kg (Cetina, 1982; Idvall *et al.*, 1983; St. Maurice *et al.*, 1979). We chose to administer 15 mg/kg of the 5% preparation

(=0.3 ml/kg), following a pilot study using 10, 12.5, and 15 mg/kg in 3 children each. Because a mask ventilation was planned for the majority of the children, the administration of atropine was desirable in order to reduce oro-tracheal secretions. Because the main rationale of rectal induction is the avoidance of an i.m. injection, the atropine (0.03 mg/kg; Quaynor *et al.*, 1985) was administered rectally together with the induction agent. Successful induction, based on the criteria of this study, was accomplished in only 60% of the children receiving methohexital. This is considerably less than what has been reported by others using the same dosage (80%, Kretz and Piepenbrock, 1983; 82%, Liu *et al.*, 1980; 85%, Liu *et al.*, 1985; 100%, Thülig *et al.*, 1985). This discrepancy is likely due to different definitions of the term "induction". Probably for the same reason, induction with ketamine (75%) was also less successful than reported by others (92%, Kühn and Hausdörfer, 1983; 100%, Idvall *et al.*, 1983).

Both groups were comparable with respect to patient and procedure data (Table 1). The slightly higher percentage of tracheal intubations in ketamine children was due to the greater number of longer procedures in that group. The children's mood prior to induction was rated mostly negative, which was not unexpected because no premedication had been given.

An i.v. line could be established without resistance in only 2 of 20 methohexital treated children; the other children moved the arm in response to vein puncture. If more than one attempt was necessary for venous cannulation, the degree of resistance increased. Twelve of 20 methohexital children tolerated mask ventilation 18 ± 2 min after induction. The other 8 cases (40%) were, by definition, considered failures. It is possible that tolerance could have been accomplished if more time had been allowed. We believe, however, that an induction period of 20 min is the maximum that is acceptable for a clinical routine procedure.

In the ketamine group, 13 of 20 children displayed nystagmus and a characteristic "empty gaze" after 9 ± 2 min. An i.v. line could be started in 14 of 20 children after 14 min. Fifteen of 20 children (75%) tolerated mask ventilation 18 ± 2 min after rectal induction. Five cases were rated as failures.

Specific observations of the respective groups were nystagmus in the ketamine children (85%) and defecation in the methohexital group (20%). As almost identical volumes had been administered in both groups, defecation is most likely due to local tissue irritation and appears to be a specific effect associated with methohexital (Hinkle and Weinlander,

1984, 1985). Airway obstruction occurred in one methohexital child, a complication that had also been observed by others (Kretz and Piepenbrock, 1983). In the ketamine group, 3 children displayed laryngospasm. Both complications were immediately identified and corrected. Besides these apparent complications, subclinical compromise of gas exchange ($SaO_2 < 90\%$) was detected by means of pulse oximetry in 2 of 5 children receiving methohexital. This corresponds to observations made by others who found a decrease in capillary PO_2 10 min following rectal administration of methohexital (Kretz and Piepenbrock, 1983). Despite the rectal administration of atropine, hypersalivation, which required oral suctioning, was observed in 15% of ketamine children pre-, intra-, and postoperatively. The rectal administration of atropine (Olsson *et al.*, 1983) was reported to produce maximal plasma levels after 30 min (range of 5 to 60 min). In our study, the plasma levels were apparently insufficient to exert an antisialogogue effect. In 15% of the children in both groups, bradycardic and tachycardic arrhythmias were observed during mask ventilation. An additional 2 ketamine children displayed polytopic ventricular extrasystoles. At the termination of surgery, halothane and nitrous oxide were eliminated from the inspiratory gas mixture. Spontaneous movements commenced 6 ± 2 min later in both groups. Recovery was complete after about 24 min in the methohexital group, which agrees with reports by others (Kretz and Piepenbrock, 1983; Thülig *et al.*, 1985). Recovery in the ketamine group took significantly longer (39 ± 19 min). While emergence was uneventful in the methohexital children, serious complications were observed in the ketamine group. These included 3 instances of bronchospasm and one laryngospasm; one child became cyanotic, one vomited. These complications were limited, however, to those children whose tracheas had been intubated.

The methohexital children began to express discomfort or pain 32 ± 23 min after termination of anesthesia. This interval was considerably longer in children receiving ketamine (54 ± 21 min). Analgesics, administered at the discretion of the recovery room nurse, were given after 35 ± 19 min to 18 methohexital children and after 64 ± 28 min to 8 ketamine children. Children of the methohexital group were ready for discharge from the recovery room after 64 ± 39 min. This took 99 ± 37 min in the ketamine children (Fig. 5). We ascribe these differences in the course of recovery to the analgesic properties of ketamine, which appear to outlast the duration of surgery. The absence of the stress factor "postoperative pain" results, however, in a prolonged recovery. About 12.5% of the ketamine children vomited during recovery, which is in agreement with other reports (Idvall *et al.*, 1985; St. Maurice *et al.*,

1979). Vomiting after methohexital was not observed in this investigation nor reported in other studies; it seems to be a complication associated with ketamine.

Five children in each group were monitored by pulse oximetry. Arterial desaturation (SaO_2<90%) was observed in 2 children receiving methohexital; one of these had already displayed hypoxygenation during induction. As cyanosis is not visible unless $Sa0_2$ decreases to below 80% (Mertzlufft, 1986), a desaturation of SaO_2 > 80, < 90%, such as observed in this study, will not be diagnosed clinically. This finding might elucidate the current controversy regarding the safety of rectally administered methohexital with respect to possible respiratory compromise (Hausdörfer, 1986; Kaiser and Al Rafai, 1985; Kretz and Eyrich, 1986).

The childrens' postoperative condition was assessed by the same two ward nurses throughout the study. Based on the nurses' extensive clinical experience, the children were rated normal, positive, or negative. We believe that this means of assessment yields more informative results as compared to an assessment by the parents (Quaynor *et al.*, 1985) because of the range of parents' personalities and their individual reactions to their first exposure to a child in a postoperative state. Children receiving ketamine were rated more favorably on both the postoperative afternoon and the next day. The ketamine children also required less analgesics on the ward than the methohexital children. This is possibly due to the analgesic effect of ketamine extending into the recovery period.

Conclusions

Ketamine may be used for ano-rectal induction of anesthesia in children with success rates and onset times similar to those achieved with methohexital. Due to its analgesic properties, ketamine offers certain advantages during induction and recovery. On the other hand, the administration of ketamine was associated with a high incidence of complications, some of them severe.

An esthetic and hygienic problem of methohexital is defecation.

Further investigations are required to assess the significance of arterial oxygen desaturation, such as seen after methohexital in this study.

We conclude that the ideal drug for ano-rectal induction of anesthesia in children is still being sought.

References

Bejersten, A., Olsson, G.L., and Palmer, L.: The influence of body weight on plasma concentrations of atropine after rectal administration in children. Acta Anaesth. Scand. 29: 782, 1985.

Birkhahn, J., Tadmor, C., Bar-Maor, J.A., and Shoshany, G.: Effective psychological preparation in elective pediatric surgery can reduce stress. J. Israel Soc. Anesth. Suppl. 1: 133, 1986.

Cetina, J.: Schonende Narkoseeinleitung bei Kindern durch orale und rektale Ketamin-Dehydrobenzperidol-Applikation. Anaesthesist 31: 277, 1982.

Dundee, J.W.: Alterations in response to somatic pain associated with anaesthesia. XVI. Methohexitone. Brit. J. Anaesth. 36: 798, 1964.

Engelhardt, W., Ebert, W., Rietbrock, I., and Richter, E.: Dosis-Wirkungsbeziehung und Serumkonzentrationen von Methohexital und Hydroxymethohexital nach rektaler Anästhesieeinleitung mit 1 % iger und 2 % iger Methohexitallösung bei Kindern. Anaesthesist 35: 491, 1986.

Gwathmey, J.T.: Rectal administration of evipal soluble, a safe, reversible and controllable preanesthetic medication. A preliminary report. Am. J. Surg. 32: 411, 1936.

Hausdörfer, J.: Bemerkungen zur Arbeit von H. Kaiser und S. Al-Rafai. Anaesthesist 35: 389, 1986.

Hinkle, A.J. and Weinlander, C.M.: Rectal mucosal injury after rectal premedication with methohexital. Anesthesiol. 61: A436, 1984.

Hinkle, A.J. and Weinlander, C.M.: The rectal toxicology of 10% methohexital: Gross and histological mucosal effects in an animal model. Anesthesiol. 63: A461, 1985.

Idvall, I., Holasek, J., and Stenberg, P.: Rectal ketamine for induction of anaesthesia in children. Anaesthesia 38: 60, 1983.

Jantzen, J.P., Erdmann, K., Hilley, D.M., and Klein, A.M.: Vergleichende Untersuchung von Analgesie und Plasmaspiegeln nach rektaler, intramuskulärer und intravenöser Gabe von Ketamin. Anaesthesist 34: 346, 1985.

Kaiser, H. and Al Rafai, S.: Wie sicher ist die rektale Narkoseeinleitung mit Methohexital in der Kinderanästhesie?: Anaesthesist 34: 359, 1985.

Kraus, G. and Taeger, K.: Methohexital zur rektalen Narkoseeinleitung bei Kindern. Anästh. Intensivther. Notfallmed. 17: 285, 1982.

Kretz, F.J. and Eyrich, K.: Bermerkungen zur Arbeit von H. Kaiser und S. Al-Rafai. Anaesthesist 35: 390, 1986.

Kretz, F.J. and Piepenbrock, S.: Narkoseeinleitung bei Kleinkindern durch rektale Applikation von Methohexital. In: Prämedikation im Kindesalter/Kinderanästhesie, J. Hausdörfer, ed., Springer, Berlin, 1983.

Kretz, F.J., Heppe, M., and Gonzalez, J.: Die rektale Narkoseeinleitung im Kleinkindalter mit Methohexital, Midazolam und Etomidate sowie postoperative Analgesie mit Paracetamol oder Fentanyl-eine vergleichende randomisierte Doppelblindstudie bei 120 Kindern. Anaesthesist 34: Suppl., 189, 1985.

Kühn, K., Hausdörfer, J., Weiss, Ch., and Rothe, K.F.: Die rektale Prämedikation mit einem kurzwirkenden Barbiturat in der Kinderanästhesie. Anästh. Intensivmed. 24: 308, 1983.

Kühn, K. and Hausdörfer, J.: Rektale Narkoseeinleitung bei Kindern. In: Prämedikation im Kindesalter/Kinderanästhesie, J. Hausdörfer, ed., Springer, Berlin, 1983.

Liu, L.M.P., Gauderault, P., Friedmann, P., Goudsouzian, N.G., and Liu, P.:

Methohexital plasma concentrations in children following rectal administration. Anesthesiol. 62: 567, 1985.

Liu, L.M.P., Goudsouzian, N.G., and Liu, P.L.: Rectal methohexital premedication in children. A dose-comparison study. Anesthesiol. 53: 343, 1980.

Liu, L.M.P., Liu, P.L., and Moss, J.: Severe histamine-mediated reaction to rectally administered methohexital. Anesthesiol. 61: 95, 1984.

Mertzlufft, F.: Kriterien zur Beurteilung des postoperativen O_2-Status. Beitr. Anaesth. Intensivmed. 18: 221, 1986.

Olsson, G.L., Bejersten, A., Feychting, H., Palmer, L., and Petterson, B.M.: Plasma concentrations of atropine after rectal administration. Anaesthesia 38: 1179, 1983.

Quaynor, H., Corbey, M., and Björkmann, S.: Rectal induction of anaesthesia in children with methohexitone-patient acceptability and clinical pharmacokinetics. Br. J. Anaesth. 57: 573, 1985.

St. Maurice, C., Laguenie, G., Courturier, C., and Goutail-Flaud, F.: Rectal ketamine in paediatric anaesthesia. Br. J. Anaesth. 51: 573, 1979.

Thülig, B., Reinhold, P., Radig, C.H., Bohn, G., and Wedy, C.: Methohexital rektal-die Narkoseeinleitung der Wahl bei Kindern? Anästh. Intensivther. Notfallmed. 20: 316, 1985.

Status of Ketamine in Anesthesiology,
edited by E.F. Domino©1990, NPP Books
P.O. Box 1491, Ann Arbor, MI 48106

Ketamine Clinic: A Model Clinic for Sedation of Mentally Handicapped Patients Undergoing Routine Gynecologic Examinations

D.A. Rosen, K.R. Rosen, T.E. Elkins, S.G. McNeeley, C.J. Heaton, C. Sorg, and H.F. Andersen

Department of Anesthesia, Section of Pediatric Anesthesia,
C.S. Mott Children's Hospital
and
Department of Obstetrics and Gynecology
Women's Hospital
University of Michigan
Ann Arbor, MI

Introduction

The elective use of deep sedation in settings other than the operating room and intensive care is a controversial topic. Even in these areas there is little information available about the safety and/or efficacy of specific sedation regimens. Sedation of both inpatients and outpatients is a common issue in several specialty areas: pediatrics, dentistry, radiology, and emergency medicine. Guidelines for the safe practice of sedation have been established for some of these areas (Committee on Drugs, 1985; Anesthesia and Sedation—Consensus Conference, 1985).

The care of the mentally handicapped patient presents additional physical, medical, emotional, and ethical problems. Limitations in communication and understanding may prevent these patients from obtaining adequate preventative health care, such as a routine gynecologic examination. Examination under general anesthesia is often required. Minimal information is available about sedation of the mentally handicapped in any setting. It has been suggested that these patients may exhibit altered sensitivity to sedative agents.

The ideal sedative for mentally handicapped patients undergoing gynecologic examination should possess specific properties, in addition to being safe and effective with minimal side effects. Any agent utilized in an outpatient clinic needs to have rapid onset and limited duration. A noninvasive route of administration is preferred. Analgesic properties are also desirable. The objective of this study was to evaluate oral and intranasal ketamine in this context.

METHODS

This study was approved by The Institutional Human Use and Ethics Committee. Examination in the gynecology outpatient clinic under this sedation study protocol was offered to patients who were unable to cooperate in prior examinations. All patients were maintained NPO for 6 hr. Demographic variables were recorded for each patient: age, weight, medical, allergy and medication histories, prior ketamine clinic attendance and degree of mental handicap (see Table 1).

Baseline vital signs were obtained and recorded. Resuscitation equipment was available at the bedside including: ambu bag, mask, suction and oxygen. Oral ketamine (3.5-15 mg/kg) was administered by the anesthesiologist. Parenteral ketamine (100 mg/ml) was mixed with a flavor extract to disguise the bitter taste. To enhance mucosal absorption, the ketamine was delivered in as small a volume as possible. An alternative carrier solution was sought when the flavor extracts were noted to be associated with a high incidence of gastric distress. Chocolate syrup was found to provide the necessary flavoring in a minimal volume with fewer gastric side effects.

An anesthesiologist was present during the entire duration of the ketamine clinic to monitor vital signs (heart rate, blood pressure and respirations) and assess level of sedation every 15 min until discharge. Sedation was rated on a 5 point scale; a score of 1 indicated no change from the patient's baseline, and an asleep patient received a score of 5.

TABLE 1. Level of functional impairment

Score	*Description*	*Definition*
1	Normal	
2	Minimal	Able to understand procedure and instructions
3	Moderate	Able to answer simple questions
4	Severe	Able to follow simple direct instructions
5	Total	No communication or understanding

The gynecologic examination was attempted when a sedation score of 3 was attained. The occurrence of any side effects was recorded.

Additional sedatives were administered by either the oral or intranasal route if the patient's sedation score was only 1 or 2 after 45 min. Although clinic patients resisted intranasal administration of the initial sedative, the majority readily accepted an intranasal medication after receiving the oral ketamine. The intranasal route offers greater speed and reliability of absorption. Midazolam (0.04-0.25 mg/kg) was selected as the supplemental sedative instead of ketamine (3.5-10.0 mg/kg) if only a small increase in sedation was desired. The patients continued to be observed until they had returned to a sedation score of 1. The patients were then discharged from clinic and the time from examination to discharge noted. Families were contacted by phone within 24 hr of discharge from clinic to assess any delayed problems with the sedation protocol. Statistical analysis of the data was performed with ANOVA to determine differences between level of mental function and dose of ketamine required to achieve sedation.

Results

The ketamine clinic was attended by 42 different patients with mental handicaps, for a total of 68 clinic visits. The median patient age was 29, with a range of 18-55 yr. The mean patient weight was 52 kg. Approximately 2/3 of the patients rated an impairment score of 5. Impairment ratings of 3 or 4 were given to 15 and 19% of the patients, respectively. A successful gynecologic examination was performed for 88% of the patients (see Table 2).

Five patients were not able to be examined on one or more occasions for a variety of reasons. One patient became quite well sedated during 4 different appointments but excessive muscle tone impeded examination. One patient experienced severe and repeated vomiting after receiving the oral elixir. One patient refused supplemental medication by either the oral or intranasal route. Two patients simply failed to become sedated.

A single dose of oral ketamine produced sedation adequate for the

TABLE 2. Patients undergoing gynecologic examination

	N	*Successful Examination*	*Percent*
Patients	43	38	88
Visits	68	56	82

intended procedure in 50% of the sedation attempts. The remainder required 1-2 supplemental sedative doses. The sedative dose was found to be inversely related to the degree of functional impairment (see Table 3). Patients with moderate impairment required significantly less ketamine than those with a more severe handicap (P <0.01).

The most frequently observed side effect was vomiting, which occurred in 1/2 of patients receiving ketamine in the alcohol containing flavor extracts. The incidence of vomiting decreased to 1/3 when the switch to chocolate syrup was made. One patient complained of dizziness and 2 patients experienced prolonged lethargy. No respiratory depression was observed. The only patient with baseline hypertension (150/90 mm Hg) demonstrated a moderate (180/110 mm Hg) but self-limited increase in blood pressure following the administration of ketamine (10 mg/kg) which resolved without treatment within 45 min. No patient experienced excessive sedation. All patients were discharged within 90 min of examination (see Table 4).

Discussion

Thus far, utilization of the ketamine sedation protocol has enabled 38 patients to obtain medical care which had been previously unavailable on

TABLE 3. Impairment *vs* ketamine dose

Impairment Score	*Range*	*Ketamine Dose mg/kg* *Mean*	*SD*
3	3.5– 8.5	6.1	2.2
4	7.9–15	10.8*	3.5
5	3.7	9.6*	3.9

*Ketamine dose significantly different from group 3 (P<0.01)

TABLE 4. Side effects

	Frequency	*Percent*
Nausea alone	3	4.5
Vomiting:	26	38
Single episode	18	26.5
Two or more episodes	8	12
Prolonged lethargy	2	3
Respiratory	0	0
Cardiovascular	1	1.5
Dizziness	1	1.5
Total	33/68	49

56 visits. It is an important alternative to the unethical use of force or to the risk and expense of general anesthesia in this patient population. A single dose of oral ketamine was an adequate sedative in 50% of the patients. The dose that is required to produce sedation in this mentally handicapped population (10 mg/kg) is approximately 10 fold greater than the reported sedative dose of oral ketamine in a normal adult (0.5-1.0 mg/kg; Grant *et al.*, 1981). The dose necessary to produce sedation also appears to be inversely related to the degree of mental handicap. Ketamine does exhibit many desirable properties as a sedative in this milieu. It has a relatively rapid onset and short duration. It possesses analgesic properties which may also facilitate a gynecologic examination. It is reliably absorbed from mucosal surfaces, allowing nonparenteral routes of administration. Finally, it produces deep sedation without the loss of protective airway reflexes or impairment of ventilatory drive.

Ketamine, however, does fall short of the ideal in a number of areas. There is a potential for adverse central nervous system effects, including seizures and hallucinations. These were not observed in any of our patients. Hypertension may be a problem in patients with underlying cardiovascular disease. We observed no hypertension in patients with normal baseline blood pressure despite the use of up to 22 mg/kg of ketamine. The most prevalent difficulty of this regimen is the lack of available nonparenteral formulations for ketamine. The parenteral solution is quite bitter and unpalatable. Despite attempts to disguise the flavor, there was a significant incidence of gastric complaints. The inability to sedate 2/5 patients was related to this issue.

All patients who were successively examined were able to be examined again during subsequent clinic appointments. The 2/4 patients who were not adequately sedated during an initial clinic visit returned to ketamine clinic. None of these return patients were able to be examined despite increasing doses of ketamine. Sedation failures were noted to be more frequent in patients who were chronically taking thioridazine. The number of patients in this group was too small to allow determination of statistical significance. The 2/5 thioridazine patients were not able to be sedated during 5 clinic visits.

In conclusion, although ketamine is not the ideal outpatient sedation agent, it was effective in the great majority of our mentally handicapped patients. No serious or long lasting side effects were observed. The experience with this technique is still relatively small and we do not recommend omitting any of the precautions which we practiced, *i.e.*, NPO, monitoring, and resuscitation availability. Finally, our ketamine clinic was a very cost efficient alternative to the use of general anesthesia for performance of a gynecologic examination in the mentally handicapped.

Acknowledgements

We would like to thank Tina Foster for her help in preparation of this manuscript.

References

Committee on Drugs, Section of Anesthesiology: Guidelines for the Elective Use of Conscious Sedation, Deep Sedation, and General Anesthesia in Pediatric Patients. Pediatrics 76(2): 317-321, 1985.

Anesthesia and Sedation-Consensus Conference: Anesthesia and Sedation in the Dental Office. JAMA 254(8): 1073-1076, 1985.

Grant, T.S., Nimmo, W.S., and Clements, J.A.: Pharmacokinetics and analgesic effects of i.m. and oral ketamine. Br. J. Anaesth. 53: 805-810, 1981.

Status of Ketamine in Anesthesiology,
edited by E.F. Domino©1990, NPP Books
P.O. Box 1491, Ann Arbor, MI 48106

Ketamine Update: Its Clinical Uses in Anesthesia[1]

P.F. White

Department of Anesthesiology
Washington University School of Medicine
St. Louis, MO

INTRODUCTION

Interest in finding an i.v. anesthetic with sedative-hypnotic, amnestic, and analgesic properties prompted the investigation of phencyclidine (Sernyl, Parke-Davis) and its congener, cyclohexamine. These drugs produced an adequate anesthetic state, but the long-lasting psychotomimetic activity during the postanesthetic period precluded their widespread clinical use. Further research led to the clinical evaluation of ketamine (an arylcyclohexylamine) which provided adequate surgical anesthesia, more rapid recovery, and less prominent emergence reactions. Although approved for general clinical use in 1970, the clinical usefulness of ketamine has been limited because of its cardiovascular-stimulating properties and high incidence of psychotomimetic emergence reactions (White *et al.*, 1982). Because the ketamine molecule contains a chiral center, it exists as one of two optical isomers or enantiomers. In this article, recent clinical studies involving ketamine (Ketalar, Parke-Davis; Morris Plains, NJ or Ketaject, Bristol Laboratories; Evansville, IN) and its individual isomers will be discussed. Clinical applications of this unique sedative, analgesic and anesthetic drug will also be reviewed (Tables 1 and 2).

Pharmacological properties of the ketamine isomers

The commercially available ketamine solutions contain equal amounts of two isomers, S(+) ketamine and R(-) ketamine (Fig. 1).

Since the optical isomers of a number of psychoactive compounds (*e.g.*, hallucinogens, sedative-hypnotics, opiates) differ in their phar-

[1]Editor's note: This article, with slight alterations, is reprinted with permission of the publishers of the original, which appeared in Seminars in Anesthesia 8: 113-126, 1988.

TABLE 1. Clinical uses of ketamine in the practice of anesthesiology

- Induction of anesthesia in poor risk patients
  - Shock or cardiovascular instability
  - Severe dehydration
  - Bronchospasm secondary to asthma or chronic obstructive pulmonary disease
  - Severe anemia
  - Major thoracoabdominal procedures (*e.g.*, one lung anesthesia)
  - Cardiac tamponade or constrictive pericarditis
- Obstetrical patients
  - Induction of general anesthesia
    - Severe hypovolemia
    - Acute hemorrhage
    - Acute bronchospasm
  - Low dose for analgesia
    - To supplement regional anesthetic techniques
    - At the time of delivery or during the postpartum period
- Adjunct to local and regional anesthetic techniques
  - For sedation and analgesia during performance of nerve block procedures
  - To supplement an inadequate block
- Outpatient surgery
  - For brief diagnostic and therapeutic procedures (*e.g.*, cardiac catheterization; oral surgery; urologic surgery, head and neck surgery; orthopedic surgery; ophthalmology; radiotherapy)
  - To supplement local and regional block techniques
  - For diagnostic and therapeutic procedures (*e.g.*, endoscopy)
- Uses outside the operating room
  - In burn units (*e.g.*, debridement, dressing changes)
  - In emergency rooms (*e.g.*, closed reductions)
  - In intensive care units (*e.g.*, sedation, painful procedures)
  - In recovery rooms (*e.g.*, postoperative sedation and analgesia)

TABLE 2. Contraindications to the use of ketamine

- Cardiovascular disease
  - Poorly controlled hypertension
  - Intracranial, thoracic, or abdominal aneurysms
  - Unstable angina or recent myocardial infarction
  - Right or left heart failure*
- Central nervous system disorders
  - Cerebral trauma
  - Intracerebral mass or hemorrhage
- Open globe injury to eye or increased intraocular pressure*
- Thyrotoxin states*
- Otolaryngologic procedures involving pharynx, larynx, or trachea*
- Psychiatric disorders (*e.g.*, schizophrenia) or history of adverse reactions to ketamine or one of its congeners*

* Indicates a relative contraindication to the use of ketamine

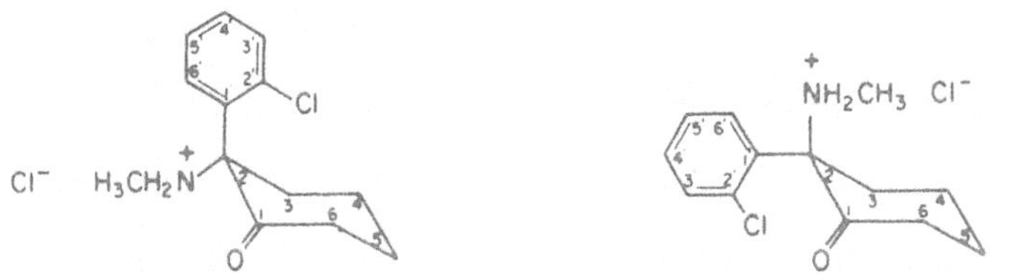

S,(+)-Ketamine hydrochloride R,(−)-Ketamine hydrochloride

Fig. 1. Structural configuration of the two optical isomers of ketamine. The commercial formulation consists of the 2 isomers. (Reprinted with permission, White *et al.*, 1980.).

macological properties, it was not surprising to learn that the ketamine isomers differed in their neuropharmacological effects. In animal studies, the S(+) ketamine isomer was shown to have a higher therapeutic index, produce more profound sedation and analgesia, and to cause less excitatory activity than the R(-) ketamine isomer.

In a randomized double blind clinical study, the S(+) isomer of ketamine was judged to produce more effective anesthesia than either the racemic mixture or the R(-) isomer (White *et al.*, 1980). Quantification of verbal responses in the postanesthetic period suggested that more agitation and psychic emergence reactions occurred after administration of R(-) ketamine than the racemic compound or S(+) ketamine. A more recent study in healthy young volunteers indicated that S(+) ketamine was three to five times more potent than the R(-) isomer in terms of its anesthetic effects (White *et al.*, 1985). However, both isomers produced similar degrees of cardiovascular stimulation and psychotomimetic activity. The pharmacokinetic variables for the ketamine isomers did not differ from those for the racemic mixture. Pharmacodynamic modeling of the EEG effects of ketamine and its enantiomers revealed that R(-) ketamine was not as effective as racemic or S(+) ketamine in causing EEG slowing (Fig. 2, Schuttler *et al.*, 1987). These data suggest that the R(-) isomer may function as a partial agonist (or an agonist-antagonist) with respect to its effects on the CNS.

Given the rather minor qualitative differences between the ketamine isomers with regard to their clinical effects, the pharmaceutical industry has been reluctant to pursue further studies with the S(+) ketamine. Thus, it would seem unlikely that the more potent S(+) isomer will ever be available for widespread clinical use. Nevertheless, it is possible that a derivative of S(+) ketamine could prove to be a valuable addition to our anesthetic armamentarium.

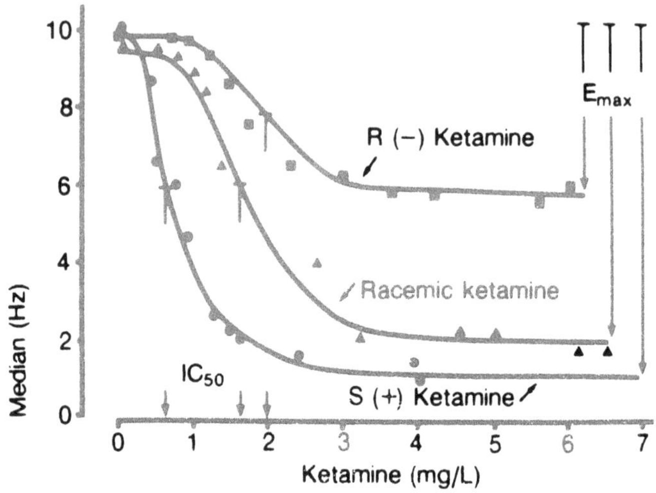

Fig. 2. Relationship between the changes in the EEG median frequency and serum ketamine concentrations in a volunteer receiving racemic ketamine, S(+), and R(-) ketamine on separate occasions. (Reprinted with permission, Schuttler *et al.*, 1987.).

Effects of ketamine on the central nervous system

Ketamine produces a "dissociative" anesthetic state that has been described as a functional and electrophysiological dissociation between the thalamo-neocortical and limbic systems. Early EEG studies reported that ketamine depressed thalamocortical pathways and concomitantly activated the limbic system. Subsequent studies demonstrated that ketamine produced excitatory activity in both the thalamus and limbic systems; however, there was no clinical evidence that this seizure like activity spread to cortical areas. In fact, ketamine has been used to successfully treat status epilepticus (Sybert and Kyff, 1983).

The EEG changes produced by racemic ketamine (and the S(+) isomer) can be described by three sequential phases (Fig. 3). The unique clinical anesthetic state, which is produced by ketamine and its isomers, has been characterized as a state of catalepsy, in which the eyes often remain open with a slow nystagmic gaze, while corneal and light reflexes remain intact. Reduced glucose utilization in the somatosensory and auditory systems suggests that a selective sensory deprivation occurs during ketamine anesthesia (Crosby *et al.*, 1982). Anesthesia is considered adequate when there is no purposeful response to noxious stimuli. However, varying degrees of hypertonus and occasional spontaneous movements,

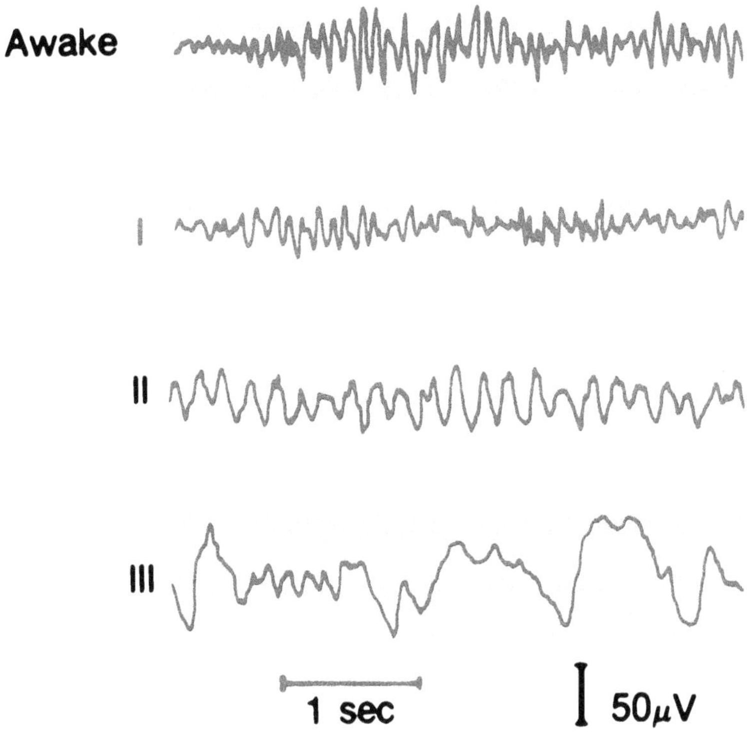

Fig. 3. Progressive changes in the EEG produced by ketamine. Phases I to III were seen with racemic ketamine and its S(-) isomer. With R(-) ketamine, the maximal EEG effect was Phase II. (Reprinted with permission, Schuttler *et al.*, 1987.).

seemingly unrelated to painful stimuli, may be noted when surgical anesthesia is adequate.

Clinical observations suggest that ketamine analgesia can outlast ketamine anesthesia and that this analgesic effect occurs even at subanesthetic doses. More recent studies indicate that ketamine's analgesic action is mediated in part through interactions with the opiate receptor system. Yet, the analgesic effects of subanesthetic doses of ketamine remain highly controversial. In volunteer studies, investigators have suggested that it was possible to provide effective analgesia without producing undesirable side effects by using a ketamine infusion (Clements *et al.*, 1982). However, Owen *et al.* (1987) reported that a ketamine infusion was ineffective in providing a postoperative analgesia. Compared to morphine, ketamine was significantly less effective for the relief of

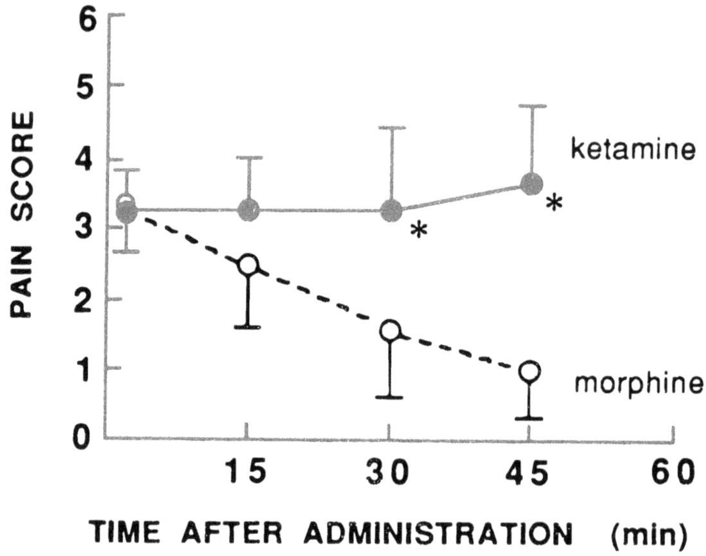

Fig. 4. Effects of epidural ketamine, 10-12 mg followed by infusion of 12 mg/hr, and morphine, 0.05-0.1 mg/kg, on postoperative pain scores, 0 = no pain to 5 = intolerable pain. (Reprinted with permission, Ravat *et al.*, 1987.).

postoperative pain. Epidural ketamine was similarly ineffective in relieving postoperative pain when compared to morphine (Fig. 4; Ravat *et al.*, 1987).

The psychotomimetic activity produced by ketamine can be disturbing to the physicians and nurses and may upset other patients in the recovery room. Typically, the psychic sensations during emergence from ketamine anesthesia are described as alterations in mood state and body image, extracorporeal (out-of-body) experiences, floating sensations, vivid dreams or illusions, "weird trips" and occasional frank delirium. The loss of skin and musculoskeletal sensations decreases the patient's ability to feel gravity, thereby producing a sensation of body detachment or "floating in space." The vivid dreams and visual illusions disappear on wakening, although recurrent illusions (flashbacks) have been reported several weeks after ketamine administration in adults and children.

The reported incidence of psychic disturbances following ketamine vary from <5% to >30%. Factors associated with a higher incidence of emergence reactions include: age (> 16 years old); sex (females>males); subjects who frequently dream during sleep; large doses of ketamine (>2 mg/kg i.v.); rapid i.v. administration (>40 mg/min); or a history of personality problems. When compared to thiopental, ketamine was found to be associated with a significantly greater incidence of psychological abnormalities in the immediate postoperative period (Moretti *et al.*, 1984). The ketamine induced changes were short lived (<24 hr) and no differences were found between the two groups with regard to long term changes in personality.

Despite many statements in the literature to the contrary, neither covering the eyes during the operative and postoperative periods, nor allowing patients to emerge in a quiet area alters the incidence of emergence reactions. In fact, it is important to discuss the common side effects of ketamine (*e.g.* dreaming, floating sensations, dizziness, and blurred vision) with the patient, both before and after the operation. Adverse reactions to ketamine can be minimized by informing the patient in advance of the likelihood of "vivid visual imagery" during the anesthetic experience.

Several premedicants and adjunctive agents have been evaluated in preventing emergence reactions caused by ketamine. Atropine premedication before ketamine administration may increase the frequency of unpleasant dreams. Although droperidol was first reported to reduce the incidence of adverse emergence reactions when used as a premedicant, others found that it could increase the occurrence of vivid dreams. Furthermore, patients receiving droperidol tend to be significantly less responsive and more disoriented during the recovery period. Several investigators have reported a decrease in posthypnotic emergence phenomenon when ketamine was used with thiobarbiturates or other general anesthetics. Concomitant use of nitrous oxide significantly decreased the ketamine dose required for surgical anesthesia, decreased the incidence of emergence reactions, and shortened the recovery period.

Benzodiazepines appear to be the most effective drugs for attenuating the psychic actions of ketamine during the emergence period. Diazepam (0.15 to 0.3 mg/kg, i.v.) has been reported to significantly decrease the incidence of dreams and to eliminate postoperative illusions when administered before induction of ketamine anesthesia. Others have reported diazepam to be equally effective in attenuating emergence sequelae, whether administered at the start or the end of the procedure. Although diazepam is highly effective in preventing vivid emergence reactions and delirium following ketamine, a high incidence of floating sensations, dizziness, and dreaming can be seen even in the presence of diazepam.

Of the currently available benzodiazepines, lorazepam (2 to 5 mg, p.o. or i.v.) is reported to be the most effective in preventing unpleasant dreams and emergence sequelae after ketamine. Lorazepam's enhanced effectiveness may be related to its ability to produce more effective and longer lasting amnesia than diazepam. Flunitrazepam (0.03 mg/kg i.v.) also attenuates the emergence sequelae associated with ketamine anesthesia. Freuchen *et al.* (1981) found that a combination of flunitrazepam and ketamine for induction, followed by a ketamine infusion and nitrous oxide for maintenance anesthesia compared favorably to an inhalational anesthetic technique. Similarly, diazepam-ketamine-nitrous oxide anesthesia was associated with fewer adverse sequelae than a droperidol-fentanyl-nitrous oxide combination (Klausen *et al.*, 1983).

Midazolam, a rapid and short acting water soluble benzodiazepine, also prevents unpleasant dreaming and emergence sequelae when used as an adjunct to ketamine for inducing general anesthesia (White, 1982). In a more recent comparative study, Cartwright and Pingel (1984) reported that midazolam was more effective than diazepam in preventing unpleasant dreams when used as an adjuvant to ketamine anesthesia.

Use of ketamine in cardiothoracic anesthesia

Prior to discussing the uses of ketamine in cardiothoracic surgery, the effects of ketamine on the cardiovascular system will be described. Ketamine produces a dose related rise in the rate-pressure product and a transient rise in the cardiac index, but does not significantly alter the stroke work index. When ketamine is injected directly into the cerebral circulation, it produces immediate increases in BP, heart rate, and cardiac output. The cardiovascular effects of intracerebral ketamine could be markedly attenuated by pretreatment with a barbiturate. The volatile anesthetics also block the cardiovascular stimulating properties of ketamine such that significant cardiovascular depression can be produced when ketamine is used during inhalational anesthesia.

Based on these studies and others, it is felt that ketamine produces its sympathomimetic actions primarily by directly stimulating CNS structures. In the absence of autonomic control, ketamine has direct myocardial depressant properties. Ketamine also directly dilates vascular smooth muscle, which tends to counteract its sympathetically mediated vasoconstriction. The net effect is that systemic vascular resistance is not significantly altered by ketamine. Even though ketamine increases coronary blood flow, the increase may not meet the increased metabolic demands produced by ketamine on the myocardium, which result from the rise in the rate-pressure product and cardiac work.

Extensive experience with the use of ketamine for pediatric cardiac catheterizations has shown it to be highly effective with fewer catheter associated arrhythmias than the volatile anesthetics. Yet, clinical evidence suggests that ketamine can sensitize the myocardium to circulating catecholamines, and thereby enhance epinephrine induced arrhythmic activity. Nevertheless, a combination of midazolam and low dose ketamine has been used successfully for sedation and analgesia during electrical cardioversions. Interestingly, when ketamine is used for adult cardiac catheterization, it can produce significant decreases in blood pressure.

The cardiostimulatory properties of ketamine can produce serious sequelae in patients with cardiac disease. Although labetalol (1 mg/kg, i.v.) is reportedly the most effective drug in attenuating the ketamine induced rise in heart rate and BP, the benzodiazepines are also utilized for this purpose. When a ketamine infusion was administered in combination with high dose diazepam and nitrous oxide for cardiac anesthesia, smooth anesthetic conditions are produced with minimal effect on the cardiorespiratory system, excellent anterograde amnesia, satisfactory analgesia, and no postoperative emergence reactions. Diazepam (0.3 to 0.5 mg/kg i.v.) effectively prevents the rise in the rate-pressure product following administration of ketamine. Thus, ketamine induced cardiovascular stimulation and the concomitant rise in plasma norepinephrine levels can be significantly decreased by premedication with diazepam. Flunitrazepam and midazolam also effectively attenuate the cardiostimulatory response produced by ketamine (White, 1982).

In a study comparing a morphine-diazepam-nitrous oxide combination with ketamine-nitrous oxide anesthesia for coronary bypass surgery, Reves *et al.* (1978) found that although the overall number of changes in the rate-pressure product were similar, the mean maximal increases in systolic blood pressure and the rate-pressure product were significantly higher in the ketamine group. The incidence of changes in the rate-pressure product might have been less if diazepam had also been incorporated into the ketamine regimen. Nevertheless, these investigators found no significant difference between the two treatment groups with respect to perioperative morbidity and mortality.

In a controlled study of the circulatory responses during induction and maintenance of anesthesia in patients undergoing heart valve replacement, Dhadphale *et al.* (1979) found no significant differences between the diazepam-ketamine-nitrous oxide and morphine-nitrous oxide techniques. These investigators felt that high dose diazepam (0.5 mg/kg, i.v.) combined with ketamine (1 to 2 mg/kg for induction and 15 to 30 μg/kg/min for maintenance) was a satisfactory alternative to morphine-nitrous oxide anesthesia for patients with coronary artery disease, as well as for those undergoing heart valve replacement. A potential advantage of the diazepam-ketamine technique is that the nitrous oxide concentration is not critical, and therefore, 100% oxygen can be used. However, there may be recall of intraoperative events during cardiac surgery with diazepam-ketamine anesthesia. Apart from its intrinsic anesthetic properties, ketamine produces minimal, if any, anterograde amnesia. The concomitant use of either lorazepam or midazolam would be expected to further decrease the possibility of intraoperative recall when ketamine is used without nitrous oxide.

When used to induce anesthesia in patients with valvular heart disease, ketamine produces dose related increases in pulmonary vascular resistance and increases the minute work of the heart. In patients without cardiopulmonary disease, ketamine produces a significant increase in pulmonary vascular resistance, a secondary increase in right heart work, and a transient increase in the intrapulmonary shunt. Yet, ketamine is frequently used to induce anesthesia in children with pulmonary hypertension and right to left shunts without apparently worsening of their clinical or hemodynamic conditions (Hickey *et al.*, 1984). Nevertheless, ketamine might be deleterious to patients with limited right ventricular reserve (*e.g.*, pulmonary emboli and primary pulmonary hypertension).

High dose narcotic techniques (*e.g.*, fentanyl 50 to 150 μg/kg, sufentanil 5 to 15 μg/kg) are extremely popular for anesthetic induction of hemodynamically unstable patients undergoing cardiac surgery. In a comparison of ketamine and sufentanil for induction of patients with severe cardiomyopathy undergoing cardiac transplantation, Gutzke *et al.* (1987) reported that ketamine maintained a stable cardiac index and heart rate at the expense of increased wall tension. On the other hand, narcotic inductions were characterized by similar hemodynamic stability without any changes in myocardial wall tension. In patients undergoing elective coronary bypass surgery, fentanyl (50 μg/kg) effectively obtunded the sympathomimetic actions of ketamine (1.5 mg/kg; Newsome *et al.*, 1985). In contrast to the commonly used sedative hypnotics (thiopental and etomidate), the use of ketamine to supplement fentanyl anesthesia was not associated with significant hemodynamic changes. Furthermore, when ketamine or fentanyl were administered as i.v. adjuncts during thoracic surgery, ketamine was associated with more prolonged postoperative analgesia than fentanyl (Benumof *et al.*, 1981).

Many cardiac anesthetists consider ketamine the drug of choice for inducing and maintaining anesthesia in patients with cardiac tamponade or constrictive pericarditis because ketamine maintains sympathetic nervous system activity, even though ketamine may further increase the pulmonary vascular resistance. In these patients, the hemodynamic response to ketamine varies considerably, especially if the pulmonary capillary wedge pressure exceeds 15 mm Hg. Further studies are needed in these surgical populations.

Use of ketamine in the critically ill

Ketamine has been used in critically ill patients where a period of hypotension or apnea could be life threatening. Park *et al.* (1987) described the use of a ketamine infusion as a sedative, inotrope, and bronchodilator in a critically ill patient. However, it is difficult to obtain meaningful data from uncontrolled clinical reports. When ketamine was used in critically ill patients, it has been reported to provide good surgical anesthesia with a greater margin of safety than "conventional" anesthesia.

Use of ketamine during major surgical procedures in elderly, high risk patients has been reported to be associated with hemodynamic stability and a rapid emergence, with a low incidence of unpleasant dreams. Stefansson *et al.* (1982) reported that using ketamine as the sole anesthetic for hip fracture surgery in the geriatric patient resulted in a survival rate that did not differ significantly from other common anesthetic techniques, including epidural and volatile anesthetics. Furthermore, Pedersen *et al.* (1982) reported that ketamine, in contrast to thiopental, did not decrease the cardiac output when used for induction of anesthesia in critically ill patients. The so called "slow-dose" ketamine technique, which consists of a benzodiazepine, (*e.g.*, diazepam 2 to 5 mg, i.v.) followed by an infusion of ketamine (2 to 4 mg/min) can also be extremely useful in aged and high risk patients (Sher, 1980).

Ketamine has been regarded by some as advantageous for patients in hemorrhagic shock, while others have disputed its usefulness in this situation. In contrast to the marked pressor response following ketamine administration to normovolemic subjects, induction of ketamine anesthesia in patients who are hypovolemic secondary to acute hemorrhage causes no significant change or even a slight decrease in blood pressure. Rather than clarifying the cardiovascular and metabolic actions of ketamine, animal studies have produced conflicting results.

In experimental hemorrhagic and septic shock, ketamine significantly increases both systolic and diastolic blood pressure. Compared to hypovolemic barbiturate anesthetized rats, hypovolemic rats anesthetized with ketamine had significantly greater perfusion to their vital organs. Using a dog model, ketamine was found to be more effective than either thiopental or diazepam in maintaining renal blood flow (Priano, 1982). Furthermore, a higher survival rate was reported in hypotensive rats anesthetized with ketamine compared to halothane. In contrast to the volatile anesthetics, Longnecker, Ross, and Silver (1982) demonstrated that ketamine diminished or abolished the arteriolar response to hemorrhage, and therefore, tissue hypoxia did not occur. On the other hand, Weiskopf *et al.* (1981) found that ketamine produced a greater base deficit and larger increases in arterial lactate concentration than the volatile agents. These investigators reported that in spite of its ability to increase catecholamines, use of ketamine was associated with cardiovascular depression and metabolic acidosis (Bogetz *et al.*, 1982).

Critically ill patients occasionally respond to ketamine with an unexpected drop in blood pressure, which may result from the inability of the sympathomimetic actions of ketamine to counterbalance its direct myocardial depressant and vasodilatory effects. Diminished catecholamine response to ketamine following prolonged stress could result in a maldistribution of systemic blood flow. Waxman *et al.* (1980) observed occasional decreases in cardiac and pulmonary performance when ketamine was used to induce anesthesia in critically ill and acutely traumatized patients.

Use of ketamine in patients with pulmonary disease

Most studies in humans indicate that ketamine does not produce significant respiratory depression. In fact, a recent study reported that low doses of ketamine were capable of producing mild ventilatory stimulation (Morel *et al.*, 1986). In early clinical studies, an increase in pulmonary and bronchospasm was noted when ketamine was given to patients with reactive airway disease. *In vitro* bronchial smooth muscle studies with ketamine demonstrated muscle relaxation, antagonism of the spasmogenic effects of carbachol and histamine, and a potentiation of the antispasmodic effects of epinephrine. Ketamine was found to be as effective as halothane or enflurane in preventing experimentally induced bronchospasm in dogs. The ability of ketamine to antagonize antigen induced bronchospasm is related in part to its vagolytic and direct smooth muscle relaxant effects. However, the major component *in vivo* appears to be related to ketamine's sympathomimetic properties, since the protective effect against antigen induced bronchospasm is lost in the presence of β-adrenergic blockade. Several case reports describe the use of ketamine to treat severe bronchospasm refractory to conventional bronchodilators. Ketamine increases pulmonary compliance and reduces airway resistance in patients with asthma. Investigators have also found ketamine to be effective in treating bronchospasm occurring during halothane anesthesia. As a result of its salutary effects on airway resistance, ketamine may be the agent of choice for rapid induction of anesthesia in patients with reactive airway disease. Furthermore, ketamine is an alternative to the volatile agents for maintenance of anesthesia in patients who are receiving parenteral bronchodilators. However, concurrent administration of ketamine and aminophylline may decrease the seizure threshold (Hirshman *et al.*, 1982).

Ketamine is an excellent alternative to the volatile agents for one lung anesthesia in patients with pre-existing lung disease and abnormal preoperative blood gas values. When one lung anesthesia was used during thoracic surgery, patients with impaired pulmonary function had improved oxygenation and decreased pulmonary shunt fractions when a diazepam-ketamine infusion-muscle relaxant anesthetic technique was used as an alternative to conventional inhalational techniques. The difference appeared to be a result of ketamine's ability to preserve the hypoxic vasoconstrictor reflex. Ketamine would also be advantageous in clinical situations where a high inspired oxygen concentration is required to maintain adequate tissue oxygenation (*e.g.*, severe anemia and cerebrovascular insufficiency).

Use of ketamine for obstetrical anesthesia and analgesia

Early studies using ketamine for anesthesia during routine vaginal deliveries reported an unacceptably high incidence of maternal complications and depressed infants with low Apgar scores. These problems were shown to be dose-related and when lower doses of ketamine (0.2 to 0.5 mg/kg, i.v.) were used, neonates were not depressed, and complications were minimal with high patient acceptance. Nevertheless, even when subanesthetic doses of ketamine are used to produce obstetrical analgesia, a majority of these patients will experience a pleasant, dream-like state.

Ketamine given in combination with nitrous oxide for obstetrical anesthesia produces virtually no recall of pain during delivery, and although dreaming occurs in many patients, a majority of the dreams are pleasant with excellent patient acceptance. Use of larger doses of ketamine ($\geq$ 1.5 mg/kg, i.v.) for inducing anesthesia in unpremedicated parturients produces good surgical anesthesia; however, recovery from anesthesia is often unpleasant. In a large obstetrical series comparing low dose ketamine (0.5 mg/kg, i.v.) with methoxyflurane (0.25 to 10 percent), ketamine produced a more rapid onset of action and proved to be the superior analgesic, while patient acceptance was similar for the two groups. The use of droperidol as an adjunct to ketamine prolonged the recovery period without decreasing the incidence of adverse emergence reactions.

When compared with thiopental for induction of anesthesia prior to cesarean section, ketamine provided for a rapid induction, greater analgesia and amnesia, with a similar incidence of unpleasant emergence reactions. However, the incidence of undesirable psychotomimetic responses was low following both induction agents. Using ketamine as the sole anesthetic for cesarean section in Third World countries has been reported to result in lower fetal mortality rates than other general anesthetic techniques. Some investigators have suggested that ketamine may be a useful analgesic for managing the hemodynamically unstable preeclamptic patient, because of its anticonvulsant properties; however, it should be used with caution in this situation because its cardiostimulatory properties could precipitate a hypertensive crisis.

There have been no clinical reports regarding fetal acid base changes following ketamine anesthesia; however, animal studies indicate that ketamine increases uterine blood flow without adversely affecting fetal cardiovascular or acid base status. Using a chronic sheep preparation with induced fetal acidosis, Pickering *et al.* (1982) found blood pressure and cerebral blood flow to be preserved better following administration of ketamine than thiopental. Arterial blood gas evaluations in mothers and infants receiving ketamine analgesia for vaginal delivery showed no significant differences when compared to regional anesthesia. In a comparative study of ketamine and thiopental for rapid i.v. induction prior to cesarean section, ketamine treated patients showed higher maternal umbilical artery and vein pH and base excess values (Dick-Nielsen and Holasek, 1982).

Neonatal arterial blood pressure has been reported to be less depressed after maternal ketamine anesthesia compared with a similar group receiving thiopental. Neonatal neurobehavioral agents following vaginal delivery with ketamine, 0.7 mg/kg i.v. and 50% nitrous oxide, thiopental, 4 mg/kg i.v. and 50% nitrous oxide, or 2% chloroprocaine epidural anesthesia revealed the greatest percentage of high scores in the epidural group, intermediate values following ketamine-nitrous oxide, and the lowest scores after thiopental-nitrous oxide.

The reduced blood loss that has been reported when ketamine is used as an induction agent for first trimester abortions may be related to its ability to increase both uterine tone and the intensity of uterine contractions. In parturients, ketamine has been reported to have variable effects on uterine tone and contractility. Ketamine can induce contractions equal to ergometrine when administered during the first trimester of pregnancy and produces dose related changes in uterine activity in the full term pregnant uterus. So called "analgesic" doses of ketamine (0.2 to 0.4 mg/kg, i.v.) produce no significant effects, while larger induction doses (1 mg/kg, i.v.) increase the intensity of uterine contractions. Similarly, ketamine increases both basal uterine tone and the intensity of contractions in the nonpregnant uterus.

Use of ketamine for induction of anesthesia

Children. Intramuscular ketamine (4 to 8 mg/kg) has proven extremely useful for induction of anesthesia prior to administering an inhalational agent, and for diagnostic and minor surgical procedures not requiring i.v. cannulae or endotracheal intubation. Ketamine has been used successfully for oral surgical procedures and diagnostic muscle biopsies lasting from 5 to 30 min using doses of 1 to 3 mg/kg i.m., or 0.5 to 1.0 mg/kg i.v.. However, side effects that have been reported include cardiovascular stimulation, partial airway obstruction and minor postanesthetic complications, including unpleasant dreams. Diazepam (5 to 10 mg, p.o.) combined with ketamine (3 mg/kg, i.m.) can provide excellent sedation with few side effects for children requiring oral surgical procedures lasting 45 to 60 min (Duperon and Jedrychowski, 1983).

In children undergoing minor otolaryngological procedures, i.v. ketamine (2 mg/kg) compared favorably with thiopental (4 mg/kg). Although operating conditions are similar, thiopental produces more cardiorespiratory depression and a greater need for postoperative analgesics, while ketamine is associated with a higher incidence of restlessness and a somewhat more prolonged recovery period. Ketamine (10 mg/kg, i.m.) has also been used for bronchoscopy in children without significant complications. However, ketamine stimulated production of copious amounts of upper airway secretions, necessitating concomitant use of an antisialagogue. Furthermore, anecdotal reports indicate that ketamine may produce "hyper-reactive" airway reflexes, especially when the upper respiratory tract is inflamed.

Finally, rectal ketamine (7.5 to 15 mg/kg) has been used successfully as an induction agent in pediatric anesthesia. Compared to rectal methohexital (25 mg/kg), use of ketamine (15 mg/kg, per rectum) for induction was associated with a higher incidence of airway complications during the perioperative period (Jantzen *et al.*, 1987). There is a high degree of acceptance of ketamine in children undergoing repeated anesthesias; however, CNS tolerance may develop.

Adults. In a large series comparing low-dose ketamine (0.5 mg/kg, i.v.) with barbiturate compounds when combined with nitrous oxide for minor gynecological procedures, investigators have reported that ketamine is associated with fewer intraoperative problems. However, in patients premedicated with droperidol, the ketamine induced dreams were more vivid and unpleasant than those associated with barbiturates. Although pentobarbital reduced the incidence of psychic emergence reactions after ketamine, it also prolonged the recovery period.

In evaluating the effectiveness of ketamine (1 to 3 mg/kg, i.v.) for induction and maintenance of general anesthesia for midtrimester abortions, side-effects included visual distortions (45%), dizziness/light-headedness (35%), and agitation/ disorientation (30%; White, 1983). Overall, 85% of the patients experienced dreams (70% of which were pleasant experiences), with 35% stating that they would prefer a different anesthetic in the future. Although recovery was occasionally prolonged, most patients were discharged within two hr of awakening from the anesthetic. Use of lower doses of ketamine (1 mg/kg, i.v.) as an i.v. adjuvant during brief gynecological procedures was associated with highly satisfactory operating conditions, few postanesthetic side effects, and a rapid recovery from anesthesia.

It appears that i.v. ketamine can be used for induction and maintenance for outpatient anesthesia if the minimal effective dose of ketamine (0.5 to 1.0 mg/kg for induction followed by continuous infusion of 15 to 30 μg/kg/min) is administered in combination with nitrous oxide and thiopental (1 to 3 mg/kg), or midazolam (0.07 to 0.15 mg/kg). To provide for a more rapid recovery following brief outpatient procedures, a combination of thiopental (3 to 5 mg/kg, i.v.) or methohexital (1 to 2 mg/kg, i.v.) for induction followed by a continuous infusion of ketamine (3 to 6 mg/min) and nitrous oxide (70% in oxygen) is recommended. Use of a continuous infusion of ketamine significantly decreases the drug dosage requirement, improves intraoperative conditions, and decreases recovery time compared with the traditional intermittent bolus technique (White, 1983). Although ketamine produced superior intraoperative conditions compared with fentanyl, recovery times were more prolonged and side effects were more frequent with ketamine (White *et al.*, 1983).

Use of ketamine in balanced anesthesia

In a study comparing intermittent bolus and continuous infusion of ketamine as adjuncts to nitrous oxide for maintenance of anesthesia during outpatient gynecologic procedures, the maintenance dosage requirement was decreased 30% to 40% in patients receiving ketamine by continuous infusion compared to the intermittent bolus group (White, 1982). Evaluation of the intraoperative conditions revealed fewer hypertensive episodes and less tachycardia with the infusion technique. Other investigators have found that ketamine is largely devoid of respiratory depressant effect when administered by continuous infusion (Morel *et al.*, 1986). In addition, superior intraoperative conditions can result from improved titration of ketamine dosage with the infusion technique.

During the recovery phase, a significant decrease in awakening time as well as less sedation and fatigue were seen with the ketamine infusion (*vs* intermittent bolus) technique (White, 1983). In addition, the incidence of emergence reactions was reduced significantly. Trieger test scores also indicated a significantly more rapid return of cognitive function. These advantages presumably are a result of the decreased dosage requirement during the maintenance period when a continuous ketamine infusion is used.

Pharmacokinetics of ketamine infusion

Titration of i.v. anesthetics like ketamine using small, incremental bolus doses has been performed by anesthesiologists for many years. Continuous infusion is a logical extension of this method of titration, minimizing the fluctuations in blood and brain ketamine concentrations that follow bolus injecttions. To achieve a therapeutic blood level more rapidly, it is necessary to administer a "loading" dose. To maintain a desired drug concentration, it is necessary to continuously infuse the drug. Although i.v. infusions are usually administered on an empirical basis, a knowledge of pharmacokinetic principles may allow the anesthetist to more accurately predict the dosage requirements. Pharmacokinetic data for ketamine can be used to calculate the loading dose (LD) and the initial maintenance infusion rate (MIR).

Two simple equations can be used to estimate the LD and MIR for ketamine: LD (μg/kg) = Cp (μg/mL) x Vd (mL/kg); and MIR (μg/kg/min) = Cp (μg/mL) x Cl (mL/kg/min) where Cp = plasma drug concentration; Vd = volume of distribution (the extent of drug uptake by the tissues) and Cl = clearance of drug (the rate of elimination). The range of pharmacokinetic values reported for ketamine are: Cp = 0.25 to 2.5 μg/mL, Vd = 0.6 to 3.0 mL/kg, and Cl = 15 to 20 mL/kg/min.

The LD can be administered as either a bolus or as a short "priming" infusion. Since side effects appear to be more common with rapid fluctuations in plasma drug concentrations, a loading infusion may be preferred to a loading bolus. The required plasma drug concentration will depend on the desired pharmacologic effect (*e.g.*, sedation and hypnosis), the presence of other centrally active drugs (*e.g.*, thiopental, midazolam, nitrous oxide, and opioid analgesics), the type of operation (*e.g.*, superficial, intra-abdominal), and the individual's sensitivity to the drug (*e.g.*, age, level of anxiety, and drug history). The influence of premedication, adjunctive drugs, nitrous oxide, and type of operation on the maintenance requirement for ketamine is shown in Table 3.

What clinical signs are most useful in deciding whether to increase or decrease the MIR of ketamine? Although the most sensitive clinical signs of depth of anesthesia appear to be changes in muscle tone and ventilatory pattern, one must rely on evidence of autonomic hyperactivity (*e.g.*, diaphoresis, lacrimation, tachycardia, and hypertension) if the patient has received muscle relaxants. While the blood pressure response to surgical stimulation may be a useful guide in judging the depth of anesthesia with volatile anesthetics, it is a less reliable index when i.v. drugs like ketamine are used. Table 4 summarizes an approach to using a ketamine infusion as part of a "balanced" anesthetic technique as well as for sedation and analgesia during local and regional anesthesia.

Use of ketamine for sedation and analgesia

During the performance of a painful nerve block, the ideal adjunctive drug would provide analgesia, sedation, and amnesia without cardiorespiratory depression. In comparing the clinical effectiveness and acceptability of diazepam, Innovar, and ketamine for sedation and analgesia prior to intercostal nerve blocks, ketamine was reported to produce more optimal conditions during the block procedure and higher patient acceptance (Thompson and Moore, 1971). Furthermore, the use of a diazepam (0.15 mg/kg)-ketamine (0.5 mg/kg) combination was not associated with any more side effects or a greater need for postoperative care than an unpremedicated group undergoing similar nerve block procedures. More importantly, patient acceptance was significantly higher in the diazepam-ketamine group. Low-dose ketamine combined with a benzodiazepine has become increasingly popular before injection of local anesthetics for outpatient cosmetic surgical procedures (White, 1985). Patients are reported

TABLE 3. Use of ketamine infusion as part of a balanced anesthetic technique

		Induction				
Investigator	*Premedication*	*Adjunct*	*(mg/kg)*	*Ketamine (mg/kg)*	*Nitrous Oxide (percent)*	*Maintenance Ketamine (μg/kg/min)*
Major abdominal surgery						
Martinez-Aguirre (1977)	Atropine	Diazepam	(0.5)	2.0	50	40
Hatano *et al.* (1979)	Diazepam	Diazepam	(0.2-0.3)	1.3-2.0	66	10-15
Houlton & Downing (1978)	Omnopon	Flunitrazepam	(0.3)	—	—	33
Idvall *et al.* (1979)	Atropine/meperidine, droperidol/fentanyl	—	2.0	50	41	
Cardiac surgery						
Hatano *et al.* (1976)	Diazepam		0.3-0.5	1.0	50	12
Jackson *et al.* (1978)	Morphine		0.4	2.0	—	90
Dhadphale *et al.* (1979)	Morphine		0.4	2.0	50	17
Gynecologic surgery						
El-Naggar *et al.* (1977)	Diazepam	Diazepam	(0.2)	0.5-1.0	66	17-34
Liburn *et al.* (1978)	Lorazepam		—	1.0	—	66-83
Barclay *et al.* (1980)	Papaveretum, atropine	Flunitrazepam, atropine	(0.3)	—	40-60	16-31
Freuchen *et al.* (1981)	Flunitrazepam, atropine	Flunitrazepam	(0.3)	1.0	60	18

TABLE 4. Using ketamine as a sedative, analgesic or anesthetic during the perioperative period

Premedication: A benzodiazepine administered either orally (*e.g.*, diazepam, 15-30 mg, lorazepam, 2-5 mg) 60-90 min before surgery or i.v. (*e.g.*, midazolam, 0.05-0.1 mg/kg) immediately prior to induction as an adjunct to ketamine. If preoperative sedation is contraindicated, a benzodiazepine can be administered i.v. prior to the termination of surgery. A noncentrally active antisialogogue (*e.g.*, glycopyrrolate, 0.005 mg/kg, i.v.) can decrease secretions if administered 5-10 min prior to induction.

Induction of anesthesia: Ketamine, 0.5-1.5 mg/kg, i.v., or 2-6 mg/kg, i.m. Lower doses of ketamine are used if thiopental (1-2 mg/kg, i.v.) or midazolam (0.1-0.2 mg/kg, i.v.) is used as an adjunct in place of the premedicant or if the patient is elderly or critically ill.

Maintenance of anesthesia: Ketamine 15-45 μg/kg/min (1-3 mg/min) via continuous i.v. infusion with supplemental nitrous oxide, 50-70% in oxygen. If ketamine is infused in combination with nitrous oxide, 70%, following a barbiturate induction, a higher maintenance infusion rate may be required (*e.g.*, 30-90 μg/kg/min).

Sedation and analgesia: Ketamine, 0.2-0.8 mg/kg, i.v. (over 2-3 min), or 2-4 mg/kg i.m., followed by continuous ketamine infusion (5-20 μg/kg/min) with or without supplemental oxygen.

to be comfortable, cooperative, and highly satisfied with this drug combination (White *et al.*, 1988).

In a randomized double blind study, midazolam was compared to diazepam for sedation when administered as an adjuvant to ketamine during local anesthesia (White *et al.*, 1988). Midazolam (0.05 to 0.15 mg/kg, i.v.) was found to produce a spectrum of CNS activity which was similar to diazepam (0.1 to 0.3 mg/kg, i.v.). However, the slope of midazolam's dose-response curve for sedation appeared to be steeper (*i.e.*, a narrower therapeutic dosage range). In a comparative evaluation, midazolam (0.1 mg/kg, i.v.) was found to produce more profound sedation and amnesia than diazepam (0.2 mg/kg, i.v.). Midazolam was associated with significantly less pain on injection and a lower incidence of postoperative venoirritation. Although recovery characteristics were similar for the two benzodiazepines when used as adjuvants to ketamine, overall patient acceptance was higher with midazolam compared to diazepam-ketamine.

Ketamine has also been used extensively in burn units for dressing changes, debridements, and skin grafting procedures in children and adults. Intramuscular ketamine (2 to 6 mg/kg) produces excellent surgical conditions for eschar excision. The rapid recovery from ketamine caused a minimal delay in resuming nutritional intake. Rare emergence reactions (mild excitement and/or illusions) were noted in these unpremedicated burn patients. In premedicated patients, even lower doses of ketamine (1 to 2 mg/kg, i.m.) can produce good operating conditions, amnesia and satisfactory analgesia with a rapid recovery and reestablishment of routine activities. However, an apparent tolerance to ketamine developed in all patients receiving more than two exposures, and the dose requirement increases progressively in patients receiving repeated administration of ketamine.

Ketamine infusions (1 to 1.5 mg/min) have been used during the early postoperative period for sedation and analgesia. To achieve adequate postoperative analgesia with ketamine, it is usually necessary to produce profound sedation. When used to sedate patients requiring postoperative ventilatory support, ketamine was reported to decrease agitation and the opiate analgesic requirement (Joachimsson *et al.*, 1986).

Use of ketamine in patients with uncommon diseases

Although ketamine can increase skeletal muscle tone and occasionally produces muscle spasms, it has been used safely in patients with a variety of myopathies, as well as those with a history compatible with malignant hyperthermia (Lees *et al.*, 1982). Even though ketamine increases ALA synthetase activity in animals, it has been used successfully to anesthetize patients with acute intermittent porphyria (Bancroft and Lauria, 1983) and hereditary coproporphyria (Capouet *et al.*, 1987). A diazepam and ketamine combination was used successfully to provide anesthesia for a patient with malignant carcinoid syndrome and associated tricuspid valvular disease (Eisenkraft *et al.*, 1981). Ketamine anesthesia was also used for a patient with Shy-Drager syndrome (Saarnivaara *et al.*, 1983).

Summary

Ketamine is a safe, rapid-acting parenteral anesthetic and analgesic agent. Ketamine alone markedly elevates BP and heart rate, produces profuse salivation, lacrimation, diaphoresis, skeletal muscle hypertonus, involuntary purposeless movements, and agitation or even frank delirium during emergence. Benzodiazepines are highly effective in preventing the marked cardiovascular responses and unpleasant emergence reactions associated with ketamine anesthesia. Furthermore, by using a continuous ketamine infusion technique the anesthetist can titrate the drug more closely, and thereby, reduce the amount of drug required.

A combination of ketamine and midazolam (a benzodiadepine with a pharmacokinetic profile similar to that of ketamine) has proven useful for rapid induction of anesthesia and can also be used for maintenance of anesthesia during total i.v. techniques.

Numerous clinical studies have appeared in the literature over the last 15 years using ketamine infusion techniques (Table 3). Clinical applications for ketamine in anesthesia include a role in total i.v. anesthesia for major surgery, in the management of acute trauma, and in outpatient anesthesia. Ketamine is widely used for sedation and analgesia during procedures under local anesthesia. In addition, ketamine can be used in intensive care units and emergency rooms for providing acute pain relief during brief procedures or painful manipulations. Although it is apparent that ketamine does not possess all the physicochemical and pharmacologic properties of an ideal i.v. anesthetic, its diverse pharmacological properties may provide important insights in the continuing search for i.v. drugs that will be closer to the ideal.

References

Bancroft, G.H. and Lauria, J.I.: Ketamine induction for Caesarian section in a patient with acute intermittent porphyria and achondroplastic dwarfism. Anesthesiol. 53: 143-144, 1983.

Benumof, J.L., Canada, E.D., and Scanlon, T.S.: Intravenous anesthesia and postoperative analgesia. Anesth. Analg. 60: 240-241, 1981.

Bogetz, M.S., Weiskopf, R.B., and Roizen, M.F.: Ketamine increases catechols but causes cardiovascular depression and acidosis in hypovolemic swine. Anesthesiol. 57: 29, 1982.

Capouet, V., Dernovoi, B., and Azagra, J.S.: Induction of anaesthesia with ketamine during an acute crisis of hereditary coproporphyria. Can. J. Anaesth. 34: 388-390, 1987.

Cartwright, P.D. and Pingel, S.M.: Midazolam and diazepam in ketamine anaesthesia. Anaesthesia 39: 439-442, 1984.

Clements, J.A., Nimmo, W.S., and Grant, I.S.: Bioavailability, pharmacokinetics, and analgesic activity of ketamine in humans. J. Pharm. Sci. 71: 539-542, 1982.

Crosby, G., Crane, A.M., and Sokoloff, L.: Local changes in cerebral glucose utilization during ketamine anesthesia. Anesthesiol. 56: 437-443, 1982.

Dich-Nielsen, J. and Holasek, J.: Ketamine as induction agent for Cesarean section. Acta Anaesthesiol. Scand. 26: 139-142, 1982.

Duperon, D.F. and Jedrychowski, J.R.: Preliminary report on the use of ketamine in pediatric dentistry. Pediat. Dentist. 5: 75-78, 1983.

Dhadphale, P.R., Jackson, A.P.F., and Alserti, S.: Comparison of anesthesia with diazepam and ketamine vs. morphine in patients undergoing heart valve replacement. Anesthesiol. 51: 200-203, 1979.

Eisenkraft, J.B., Dimich, I., and Miller, R.: Ketamine-diazepam anaesthesia in a patient with carcinoid syndrome. Anaesthesia 36: 881-885, 1981.

Freuchen, I., Ostergaard, J., and Mikkelsen, B.O.: Anaesthesia with flunitrazepam and ketamine. Br. J. Anaesth. 53: 827-830, 1981.

Gutzke, G.E., Shah, K., Glisson, S.N., *et al.*: Sufentanil or ketamine: Induction in cardiomyopathy patients. Anesthesiol. 67: 64, 1987.

Hickey, P.R., Hansen, D.D., Norwood, W.I., *et al.*: Anesthetic complications in surgery for congenital heart disease. Anesth. Analg. 63: 657-664, 1984.

Hirshman, C.A., Krieger, W., Littlejohn G., *et al.*: Ketamine aminophylline induced decrease in seizure threshold. Anesthesiol. 56: 464-467, 1982.

Jantzen, J.P., Tzanova, I., Klein, A.M., *et al.*: A clinical evaluation of methohexitone and ketamine for ano-rectal induction of anesthesia in children. Anasth. Intensivmed. 28: 56-61, 1987.

Joachimsson, P.O., Hedstrand, U., and Eklund, A.: Low dose ketamine infusion for analgesia during postoperative ventilator treatment. Acta Anaesthesiol. Scand. 30: 697-702, 1986.

Klausen, N.-O., Wiberg-Jorgensen, F., and Chraemmer-Jorgensen, B.: Psychotomimetic reactions after low dose ketamine infusion—Comparison with neuroleptanaesthesia. Br. J. Anaesth. 55: 297-301, 1983.

Lees, D.E., Kim, Y.D., and MacNamara, T.E.: The safety of ketamine in pediatric neuromuscular disease. Anesth. Rev. 9: 17-21, 1982.

Longnecker, D.E., Ross, D.C., and Silver, I.A.: Anesthetic influence on arteriolar diameters and tissue oxygen tension in hemorrhaged rats. Anesthesiol. 57: 177-182, 1982.

Morel, D.R., Forster, A., and Gemperie, M.: Noninvasive evaluation of breathing pattern and thoraco-abdominal motion following the infusion of ketamine or droperidol in humans. Anesthesiol. 65: 392-398, 1986.

Moretti, R.J., Hassan, S.Z., Goodman, L.I., *et al.*: Comparison of ketamine and thiopental in healthy volunteers: Effects on mental status, mood, and personality. Anesth. Analg. 63: 1087 1096, 1984.

Newsome, L.R., Moldenhauer, C.C., Hug, C.C., *et al.*: Hemodynamic interactions of moderate doses of fentanyl with etomidate and ketamine. Anesth. Analg. 64: 260, 1985.

Owen, H., Reekie, R.M., Clements, J.A., *et al.*: Analgesia from morphine and ketamine—a comparison of infusions of morphine and ketamine for postoperative analgesia. Anaesthesia 42: 1051-1056, 1987.

Park, G.R., Manara, A.R., Mendel, L., *et al.*: Ketamine infusion—Its use as a sedative, inotrope, and bronchodilator in a critically ill patient. Anaesthesia 42: 980-983, 1987.

Pedersen, T., Engback, J., Klausen, N.O., *et al.*: Effects of low-dose ketamine and thiopentone on cardiac performance and myocardial oxygen balance in high risk patients. Acta Anaesthesiol. Scand. 26: 235-239, 1982.

Pickering, B.G., Palahniuk, R.J., Cote, J., *et al.*: Cerebral vascular responses to ketamine and thiopentone during foetal acidosis. Can. Anaesth. Soc. J. 29: 463-467, 1982.

Priano, L.L.: Alterations of renal hemodynamics by thiopental, diazepam and ketamine in conscious dogs. Anesth. Analg. 61: 853-862, 1982.

Ravat, F., Dorne, R., Baechle, J.P., *et al.*: Epidural ketamine or morphine for postoperative analgesia. Anesthesiol. 66: 819-822, 1987.

Reves, J.G., Lell, W.A., McCraken, L.E., *et al.*: Comparison of morphine and ketamine. Anesthetic techniques for coronary surgery: a randomized study. South. Med. J. 71: 33-36, 1978.

Saarnivaara, L., Kautto, U.-M., and Teravainen, H.: Ketamine anesthesia for a patient with the Shy-Drager syndrome. Acta Anaesthesiol. Scand. 27: 123-125, 1983.

Schuttler, J., Stanski, D.R., White, P.F., *et al.*: Pharmacodynamic modeling of the EEG effects of ketamine and its enantiomers in man. J. Pharmacokinet. Biopharm. 15: 241-253, 1987.

Sher, M.H.: Slow dose ketamine—A new technique. Anaesth. Intensive Care J. 8: 359-361, 1980.

Stefansson, T., Wickstrom, I., and Haljamae, H.: Hemodynamic and metabolic effects of ketamine anesthesia in the geriatric patient. Acta Anaesthesiol. Scand. 26: 371-377, 1982.

Sybert, J.W. and Kyff, J.V.: Ketamine treatment of status epilepticus. Anesthesiol. 58: 203, 1983.

Thompson G.E. and Moore, D.C.: Ketamine, diazepam, and Innovar: a computerized comparative study. Anesth. Analg. 50: 458-463, 1971.

Waxman, K., Shoemaker, W.C., and Lippman, M.: Cardiovascular effects of anesthetic induction with ketamine. Anesth. Analg. 59: 355-358, 1980.

Weiskopf, R.B., Townsley, M.I., Riordan, K.K., *et al.*: Comparison of cardiopulmonary responses to graded hemorrhage during enflurane, halothane, isoflurane and ketamine anesthesia. Anesth. Analg. 60: 481-491, 1981.

White, P.F., Comparative evaluation of intravenous agents for rapid sequence induction-thiopental, ketamine, and midazolam. Anesthesiol. 57: 279-284, 1982.

White, P.F.: Use of continuous infusions versus intermittent bolus administration of fentanyl or ketamine during outpatient anesthesia. Anesthesiol. 59: 294-300, 1983.

White, P.F.: Use of ketamine for sedation and analgesia during injection of local anesthetics. Ann. Plast. Surg. 15: 53-56, 1985.

White, P.F., Dworsky, W.A., Horai, Y., *et al.*: Comparison of continuous infusion fentanyl or ketamine versus thiopentone—Determining the mean effective serum concentrations for outpatient surgery. Anesthesiol. 59: 564-569, 1983.

White, P.F., Ham, J., Way, W.L., *et al.*: Pharmacology of ketamine isomers in surgical patients. Anesthesiol. 52: 231-239, 1980.

White, P.F., Schuttler, J., Shafer, A., *et al.*: Comparative pharmacology of ketamine isomers. Studies in volunteers. Br. J. Anaesth. 57: 197-203, 1985.

White, P.F., Vasconez, L.E., Mathes, S., *et al.*: Comparison of midazolam and diazepam for sedation during plastic surgery. J. Plast. Reconstr. Surg. 81: 703-709, 1988.

White, P.F., Way, W.L., and Trevor, A.J.: Ketamine-Its pharmacology and therapeutic uses. Anesthesiol. 56: 119-136, 1982.

Status of Ketamine in Anesthesiology,
edited by E.F. Domino©1990, NPP Books
P.O. Box 1491, Ann Arbor, MI 48106

Induction of Anesthesia with Sufentanil and Ketamine

I. Davies, M.A.E. Marcus*, S.J. Sperring, N.J. Robson, N.J. Sinisi, M.S. Cohen, M.C.O. van den Nieuwenhuyzen*, and T.H. Stanley**

The Department of Anesthesiology
University of Texas Medical School
Houston, Texas

**State University of Leiden*
The Netherlands

***The Department of Anesthesiology*
University of Utah School of Medicine
Salt Lake City, Utah

Introduction

Ketamine is a rapid acting analgesic and anesthetic which has been available for more than 15 years but has not achieved great popularity as an anesthetic induction agent (Corssen and Domino, 1965; Traber *et al.*, 1968; White *et al.*, 1982). The most important reasons for this are that ketamine causes hypertension and tachycardia, and a high incidence of vivid, frightening dreams and related emergence side effects (Fine and Finestone, 1973; Traber *et al.*, 1968; White *et al.*, 1982). While numerous investigators have documented that benzodiazepines, other sedative/hypnotics, or potent inhaled agents, administered prior to ketamine, attenuate the hemodynamic responses and minimize the emergence phenomena associated with its use (Fine and Finestone, 1973; White *et al.*, 1982), no one approach has been found to be sufficiently reliable and/or practical to improve ketamine's popularity. Evaluation of analgesic doses of sufentanil (0.25-2.0 μg/kg, i.v.) administered 3 to 5 min prior to induction of anesthesia with sodium thiopental or ketamine, has suggested that pretreatment with a potent narcotic may be a simple method of reducing or eliminating virtually all of ketamine's detriments as an induction anesthetic. This study was undertaken to test that hypothesis.

Methods

Approval was received from the Human Institutional Review Board of the University of Texas Health Science Center at Houston and written informed consent was obtained from 60 ASA physical status I-II adults, 18 to 60 years of age, scheduled for elective gynecological, orthopedic, plastic, otolaryngologic, or general surgical operations. Following enrollment in the study, patients were randomly assigned to one of three groups of 10 patients each. Patients in group I were scheduled to receive sufentanil (1 $\mu g\ kg^{-1}$ diluted to 5 ml with 0.9% NaCl), those in group II sufentanil (0.5 $\mu g\ kg^{-1}$ diluted to 5 ml with 0.9% NaCl), and those in group III 5 ml of 0.9% NaCl prior to induction of anesthesia.

Each patient was bought to the preoperative holding area approximately one hr prior to operation and asked to grade their baseline (control) pain score on a standard 10 cm visual analog scale. Following this, i.v. access was obtained via a peripheral arm vein and 500 ml of lactated Ringer's solution were administered over 20 min followed by an infusion of 125 ml/hr. Five min after arrival in the operating room, baseline systolic (SBP) and diastolic (DBP) arterial blood pressures, heart rate (HR), oxygen saturation (O_2 Sat), and endtidal carbon dioxide concentration (${}_{ET}CO_2$) were measured by an investigator unaware of the patient's group allocation using a Dinamap noninvasive blood pressure monitor, a standard lead II electrocardiogram, an Ohmeda pulse oximeter and a Perkin-Elmer model M400A mass spectrometer, respectively. The patients then received their pretreatment (sufentanil or 0.9% NaCl) medication. Three min later, patients in groups I and II received ketamine (0.3 $mg\ kg^{-1}$ i.v.) and those in group III received sodium thiopental (4.5 $mg\ kg^{-1}$ i.v). The induction doses of ketamine and thiopental were repeated if patients were still able to respond to verbal commands one min after administration of the initial induction dose. When unconscious, patients were evaluated for the presence of rigidity using the following scoring system: no rigidity = 0; mild rigidity (some difficulty with mechanical ventilation) = 1; moderate rigidity (appreciable difficulty with mechanical ventilation but gas exchange adequate following insertion of an oral airway) = 2; severe rigidity (little or no gas exchange with mechanical ventilation in spite of insertion of an oral airway) = 3.

One min following loss of consciousness, patients' SBP, DBP, HR, O_2Sat and ${}_{ET}CO_2$ were remeasured and each received succinylcholine (1.5 $mg\ kg^{-1}$ i.v). One min later, hemodynamic and 0_2Sat data were recorded again, the patients' tracheas intubated and maintenance anesthesia begun with isoflurane (0.1-2.5%) in N_2O (60%) and oxygen in order to maintain

HR and SBP within ± 20% of baseline. Muscle relaxation was maintained with vecuronium (0.05 to 0.1 μg kg^{-1}) as needed. The duration of laryngoscopy (in sec) was measured. Hemodynamic data, $_{ET}CO_2$ and endtidal isoflurane concentrations were remeasured 1, 2, 4, 7, and 12 min after intubation and every 5 min thereafter.

At the conclusion of the operation, isoflurane and nitrous oxide were discontinued, residual neuromuscular paralysis was antagonized with atropine (0.2 mg kg^{-1}), and neostigmine (0.05 mg kg^{-1}) and the patients were extubated when able to respond to command. The duration of operation and anesthesia were measured and recorded. Arousal time, the time from discontinuation of the last anesthetic until the patient first responded to command, was also recorded.

The presence or absence of nausea (as solicited by a recovery room nurse every 30 min) and vomiting (as noted by another investigator) were recorded every 10 min for the first 90 min in the recovery room. Subjective (as determined by the patient) and objective (as determined by the recovery room nurse) 10 cm visual analogue pain scores were obtained 30, 60, and 90 min after arrival in the recovery room. I.V. morphine (2 mg) was requested by the recovery room nurse (who was unaware of the patient's group allocation) for control of moderate or severe postoperative pain (as determined by an anesthesiologist uninvolved with the study). All data were recorded by nurses and investigators unaware of the patient's group allocation. Twenty-four hr after the operation, all patients filled out a questionnaire addressing intraoperative awareness, dreams, and related intraoperative and emergence memories.

Continuous dependent variables (blood pressure, heart rate, endtidal carbon dioxide, and oxygen saturation) were analyzed for statistical significance using analyses of variance. Individual comparisons were analyzed by the Tukey's method. Nominal dependent variables (sex, ASA score, height, weight, incidence of nausea, vomiting, dreaming, awareness, and postoperative analgesic requirements) were analyzed with contingency tables and either the Chi square or Fisher's exact test, depending on cell size. $P < 0.05$ was considered statistically significant.

RESULTS

Patients in the 3 groups were similar with respect to gender distribution, the type of operation scheduled, ASA physical status distribution, age, weight, height, baseline vital signs, baseline oxygen saturation, endtidal carbon dioxide, baseline preoperative pain scores, and the duration of laryngoscopy, surgery, and anesthesia, as shown in Tables 1 to 3.

TABLE 1. Demographic data in 60 patients having anesthesia induced with sufentanil and ketamine or sodium thiopental, mean (± SD)

Induction Agents	*Group I Sufentanil (1.0 μgkg⁻¹) + ketamine*	*Group II Sufentanil (0.5 μgkg⁻¹) + ketamine*	*Group III Sodium Thiopental*
Gender M/F	3/17	6/14	5/15
Age (yr)	36.06 ± 9.89	34.70 ± 10.66	34.70 ± 11.88
Weight (kg)	68.00 ± 17.94	59.96 ± 15.17	73.85 ± 17.04
Height (cm)	165.65 ± 9.72	168.75 ± 7.27	168.10 ± 10.85
	Preoperative, Operative and Recovery Data		
End tidal CO_2 (%) 3 min after sufentanil or 0.9% NaCl	4.62 ± 0.98	4.14 ± 0.90	4.52 ± 0.57
Duration surgery/min	88.20 ± 47.90	97.60 ± 54.10	111.00 ± 82.80
Duration laryngoscopy/sec	22.65 ± 13.92	17.40 ± 8.20	26.55 ± 16.42
Arousal time (min)	5.65 ± 4.71	5.4 ± 4.19	7.95 ± 6.41

Pretreatment with sufentanil did not produce significant changes in endtidal carbon dioxide concentrations between the 3 groups just prior to anesthetic induction (Table 1). However, group I required significantly less ($P < 0.05$) ketamine (0.32 ± 0.07 *vs* 0.55 ± 0.11 mg kg^{-1}) than group II for induction of anesthesia. All patients in group III lost consciousness with their initial dose of thiopental. Rigidity following induction of anesthesia occurred in 45 and 30 percent of group I and II patients, respectively, and was also thought to have occurred in one patient in group III (Table 4). The difference in incidence of rigidity between groups I and III was statistically significant ($P < 0.007$) but that between groups I and II, and II and III was not.

Tables 2 and 3 display HR, SBP and DBP from baseline until 7 min after tracheal intubation. During that interval, HR remained unchanged in group I, but became significantly ($P < 0.01$) elevated in groups II and III, particularly 2 min after tracheal intubation. Similarly, SBP and DBP remained unchanged in group I but were significantly ($P < 0.01$) increased in groups II and III (except DBP remained unchanged in group II), particularly after tracheal intubation.

Arousal times (5.7 ± 4.7, 5.4 ± 4.2, and 8.0 ± 6.4 in groups I to III, respectively) were similar in the 3 groups but patients in group I had significantly lower objective pain scores upon arrival in the recovery room and 30 min later than those in group III (Table 5).

Patients in group I also required significantly ($P < 0.009$) less mor-

TABLE 2. Mean (± SD) heart rate (beats/min) in 60 patients receiving sufentanil and ketamine or sodium thiopental for induction of anesthesia

	Baseline	1 Min Following Loss of Consciousness	Prior to Intubation	Min After Intubation		
				2	4	7
Group I	72.4 ± 9.92	75.7 ± 16.4	83.9 ± 16.5	80.7 ± 20.0	67.5 ± 12.4	59 ± 9.1
Group II	74.4 ± 15.5	84.7 ± 16.8	90.0 ± 22.7	91.2 ± 26.7	79.6 ± 21.1	68.2 ± 16.0
Group III*	77.4 ± 15.7	81.5 ± 17.4	100.6 ± 16.1	100.5 ± 16.8	97.9 ± 21.0	89.9 ± 11.8

*P<0.01 ANOVA for linear regression

TABLE 3. Mean (± SD) systolic (SBP) and diastolic (DBP) in 60 patients receiving sufentanil and ketamine or sodium thiopental for induction of anesthesia

		Baseline	1 Min Following Loss of Consciousness	Prior to Intubation	Min After Intubation		
					2	4	7
Group I	SBP	122.8 ± 22.2	121.1 ± 30.7	130.1 ± 23.1	130.2 ± 23.1	1183 ± 23.0	108.3 ± 16.2
	DBP	70.2 ± 15.3	70.4 ± 13.6	74.4 ± 19.7	68.4 ± 14.8	62.4 ± 14.8	57.0 ± 9.7
Group II	SBP*	129.3 ± 19.7	137.5 ± 17.4	139.8 ± 22.3	146.7 ± 29.7	126.8 ± 20.6	112.3 ± 13.1
	DBP	73.8 ± 11.6	80.7 ± 14.6	78.9 ± 17.0	80.0 ± 19.9	67.4 ± 14.1	60.5 ± 14.9
Group III	SBP*	132.9 ± 14.0	127.3 ± 21.6	145.1 ± 25.0	161.8 ± 30.3	138.6 ± 29.4	119.2 ± 20.8
	DBP*	75.8 ± 7.7	74.3 ± 17.7	967.3 ± 15.4	97.65 ± 20.9	79.3 ± 23.3	63.5 ± 17.6

SBP = Systolic pressure mm Hg
DBP = Diastolic pressure mm Hg
*P<0.01 ANOVA for linear regression

TABLE 4. Frequency (%) of rigidity in 60 patients receiving sufentanil and ketamine or sodium thiopental for induction of anesthesia

	No rigidity	*Minimal Rigidity*	*Moderate Rigidity*	*Severe Rigidity*
Group I	55	25	5	15
Group II	70	15	10	5
Group III	95*	5	0	0

*P <0.007, Chi square test when compared to group I

TABLE 5. Objective postoperative pain scores in 60 patients receiving sufentanil and ketamine or sodium thiopental for induction of anesthesia, Mean ± S.D.

	Arrival in PACU	*30 min*	*60 min*	*90 min*
Group I	2.1 ± 1.1*	2.5 ± 1.4*	2.5 ± 1.6	2.1 ± 1.9
Group II	2.6 ± 1.9	3.1 ± 1.8	3.1 ± 1.9	1.8 ± 1.4
Group III	3.9 + 2.7	4.1 + 1.6	3.0 + 1.5	1.9 + 1.9

Results expressed as mean score on a visual analogue scale of 1 (no pain) to 10 (worst pain imaginable) as assessed by an investigator unaware of the patient's group allocation.
*P < 0.05, analysis of variance with Tukey's adjustment when compared to group III at the same interval.

phine in the recovery room (1.5 ± 2.6 mg) than group III (3.7 ± 2.5 mg). Difference in objective pain scores between groups I and II, and II and III, and in subjective pain scores between all 3 groups were not statistically significant.

The incidence of nausea and vomiting was similar among the 3 groups (Table 6). No patient in any of the groups was aware during the operation and none reported vivid, colorful, or frightening dreams, although two patients in each group thought they may have had a pleasant dream.

Discussion

The clinical usefulness of ketamine is limited because of its cardiovascular stimulating properties and high incidence of disturbing emergence reactions. Ketamine alone produces a dose related rise in the rate pressure product but without significant alternation of stroke index (Tweed *et al.*, 1972; Idvall *et al.*, 1979). In contrast, sufentanil can decrease arterial blood pressure and heart rate (Larsen *et al.*, 1980). This study demonstrates that a dose (1 $\mu g\ kg^{-1}$) of sufentanil, given before anesthetic induction with ketamine, prevents cardiovascular stimulation

TABLE 6. Frequency (%) of side effects in 60 patients having anesthesia induced with sufentanil and ketamine or sodium thiopental

	Awareness during operation	*Recovery Room*		*Frightening or colorful dreams*
		Nausea	*Vomiting*	
Group I	0	18	20	0
Group II	0	18	25	0
Group III	0	25	31	0

during the induction-tracheal intubation sequence in ASA physical status I-II patients. In the group of patients that received 1 μg kg^{-1} of sufentanil, HR, SBP and DBP remained unchanged, while in the other groups there was a significant rise in these variables.

The combination of ketamine with 1 μg kg^{-1} of sufentanil provided significant analgesia after the operation. This group required significantly less morphine during their recovery room stay than the other two groups. Sufentanil and ketamine have two different sites for analgesic action. Sufentanil binds to opiate receptors whereas ketamine produces a selective depressant effect on the medial thalamic nuclei and nuclei involved in the transmission of impulses within the medial medullary reticular formation, a presumed relay station for the transmission of the affective-emotional components of nociception from the spinal cord to higher brain centers (Massopust *et al.*, 1972; Ohtani *et al.*, 1979). Sufentanil and ketamine may be synergistic because of these different sites of analgesic action.

A variety of premedicants and adjunctive agents have been evaluated in an attempt to prevent the untoward emergence reactions following ketamine anesthesia. Benzodiazepines have been most efficacious in attenuating the psychic actions of ketamine during the emergence periods but do not obviate the incidence of floating sensations, dizziness, and dreaming (Mattila *et al.*, 1979). In our study, premedication with sufentanil completely prevented frightening or colorful dreams. The dose of 1 μg kg^{-1} of sufentanil may be more effective than lower doses because it decreases the need for ketamine and provides more analgesia.

Rapid injection of any potent opioid can produce truncal rigidity (Grell *et al.*, 1970; Freund *et al.*, 1973). In this study, the incidence of moderate and severe rigidity was directly related to the dose of sufentanil used. However, rigidity had no effect on intubation time or $ETCO_2$. Rigidity is controllable and does not usually create hazardous situations for the experienced anesthesiologist. There are data that suggest that chest wall rigidity and reduced ventilatory compliance after high doses of iv fentanyl, sufentanil, and similar opioids are related to the dose and speed with which the drugs are given and thus presumably the speed and concentration achieved in CNS tissue. The percentage of rigidity could perhaps be decreased by giving a smaller dose of sufentanil (0.4 μg kg^{-1}) or by administering the drug via a continuous i.v. infusion over 3 min.

In conclusion, a low or moderate dose of sufentanil followed by a low dose of ketamine appears superior to sodium thiopental for induction of anesthesia. The combination provides amnesia and unconsciousness, stable hemodynamics during intubation, and superior early postoperative analgesia without causing unpleasant emergence phenomena.

References

Corssen, G. and Domino, E.F.: Dissociative anesthesia: Further pharmacologic studies and the first clinical experience with the phencyclidine derivative CI-581. Anesth. Analg. 45: 29-40, 1965.

Fine, J. and Finestone, S.C.: Sensory disturbances following ketamine anesthesia-Recurrent hallucinations. Anesth. Analg. 52: 428-430, 1973.

Freund, F.G., Martin, W.E., Wong, K.C., and Hornbein, T.F.: Abdominal muscle rigidity induced by morphine and nitrous oxide. Anesthesiol. 38: 358, 1973.

Grell, F.L., Koons, D.A., and Denson, J.S.: Fentanyl in anesthesia: A report of 500 cases. Anesth. Analg. 49: 523, 1970.

Idvall, J., Ahlgren, I., Aronsen, K.F., *et al.*: Ketamine infusions: Pharmacokinetics and clinical effects. Br. J. Anaesth. 51: 1167-1172, 1979.

Larsen, R., Sonntag, H., Schenk, H.-D., Radke, J., and Hilfiker, O.: Die Wirkungen von sufentanil and fentanyl auf hämodynamik, coronardurchflutung and myocardialen metabolismus des menschen. Anaesthesist 29: 277-279, 1980.

Massopust, L.C., Jr., Wolin, L.R., Albin, M.S., *et al.*: Electrophysiologic and behavioral responses to ketamine hydrochloride in the rhesus monkey. Anesth. Analg. 51: 329-341, 1972.

Mattila, M.A.K., Larni, H.M., Nummi, S.E., *et al.*: Effect of diazepam on emergence from ketamine anesthesia: A double blind study. Anaesthesist 28: 20-23, 1979.

Ohtani, M., Kikuchi, H., Kitahata, L.M., *et al.*: Effects of ketamine on nociceptive cells in the medial medullary reticular formation of the cat. Anesthesiol. 51: 414-417, 1979.

Traber, D.L., Wilson, R.D., and Priano, L.L.: Differentiation of the cardiovascular effects of CI-581. Anesth. Analg. 47: 769-778, 1968.

Tweed, W.A., Minuck, M.S., and Mymin, D.: Circulatory responses to ketamine anesthesia. Anesthesiol. 37: 613-619, 1972.

White, P.F., Way, W.L., and Trevor, A.J.: Ketamine—Its pharmacology and therapeutic uses. Anesthesiol. 56: 119-136, 1982.

Status of Ketamine in Anesthesiology,
edited by E.F. Domino©1990, NPP Books
P.O. Box 1491, Ann Arbor, MI 48106

Ketamine in Obstetrical Anesthesia

A.-R.M. Yousef

Department of Anesthesia and Intensive Care
Shatby Maternity University Hospital
University of Alexandria
Alexandria, Egypt

INTRODUCTION

Ketamine is an arylcyclohexylamine that is structurally related to phencyclidine with which it shares certain neuropharmacological properties. Ketamine acts rapidly on the central nervous system (CNS), although a little slower than thiobarbiturates. Ketamine is effectively absorbed via the i.m. route with more than 90% bioavailability but with a 15 min delay in peak plasma levels (Grant *et al.*, 1981). The precise mechanisms of ketamine dissociative anesthesia are not completely known. Ketamine exerts multiple effects on the CNS. At the level of the spinal cord it is selective in reducing polysynaptic reflexes (Tang and Schroeder, 1975). Ketamine blocks NMDA receptor membrane ion channels in their open position. The dissociative state produced by ketamine is due to a functional and an electrophysiological dissociation between the neocortical and limbic systems. The nystagmus and myoclonic movements seen during ketamine anesthesia make it difficult to judge the depth of anesthesia. Ohtani *et al.* (1979) reported a selective depression of nuclei within the medical medullary reticular formation that are involved in the transmission of the affective emotional components of pain perception from the spinal cord to higher brain centers. They suggested that ketamine analgesia may be related to its ability to suppress lamina-specific spinal cord activity. Ketamine produces a dose related increase in arterial blood pressure and heart rate. This is due to stimulation of the CNS. Also, a dose related respiratory depression is noted during ketamine anesthesia. This depression leads to a slight decrease in PO_2 but CO_2 responsiveness is maintained quite well. In patients with reactive airway disease, ketamine decreases airway resistance and bronchospasm. In our experience, 4 min after the administration of ketamine there is a sharp momentary drop in uterine contractions which rapidly regains its preanalgesic level. A steady increase in uterine activity occurs which reaches its maximum by the beginning of the second stage (Figs. 1 and 2). Ketamine stimulates salivary secretions. Thus the prior administration of an anticholinergic agent is mandatory. Ketamine is unique in the fact that it is nonirritant to tissues (Way and Trevor, 1986).

The onset of sleep is rapid, occurring in 2 to 8 min. Recovery of consciousness is also rapid but complete recovery may take 3 hr. Postanesthetic emergence reactions vary between 5 to 30%. These reactions are more common in adults than in children (White *et al.* 1982, Meyers and Charles, 1978; Smith, 1984). Posthypnotic emergence reactions can be aborted by the use of small doses of thiobarbiturates, diazepam or opioids or by keeping the patient completely undisturbed (Way and Trevor, 1986).

Patients and Methods

Vaginal deliveries

One hundred parturients undergoing normal vaginal deliveries were chosen among those in Shatby Maternity University Hospital. Fifty parturients received ketamine i.m. (2-3 mg/kg). Ketamine was given i.v., in a dose of 0.2-0.3 mg/kg to the other 50 patients. These parturients were compared to a similar group receiving various other analgesic agents for alleviation of pain. The parturients were monitored for the efficacy and duration of analgesia by an objective questionnaire, cervical dilation

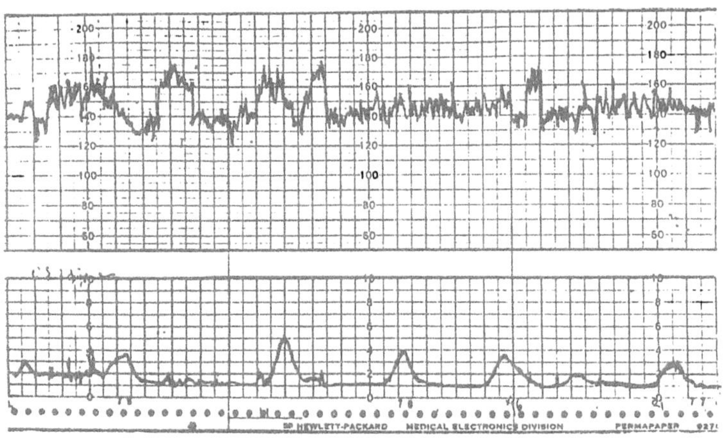

Fig. 1. Initial decrease in uterine contractions following i.m. ketamine. Upper tracing-fetal heart rate; lower tracing-uterine contractions in this and Fig. 2.

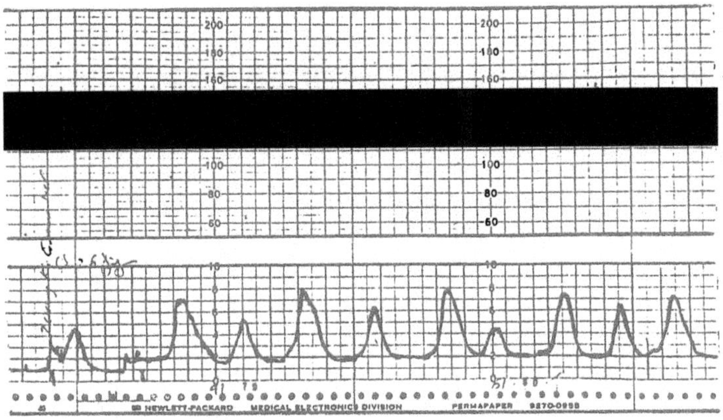

Fig. 2. A subsequent steady increase in uterine contractions following i.m. ketamine is observed (lower tracing).

score, uterine contractions, and fetal cardiac rate and rhythm by cardiotocography. The uterine activity was calculated in Alexandria Units (El-Sahwi *et al.*, 1976). The duration of the second stage was recorded. The newborn infants were assessed by Apgar scores at 1 and 5 min (Apgar 1953).

Cesarean section

Ketamine was administered i.v. in a dose of 1-2 mg/kg as an induction agent for cesarean section in 50 parturients to achieve analgesia and prevent the occurrence of awareness during the events of the procedure. These patients were compared to a similar group who received routine i.v. anesthesia for cesarean section not including ketamine.

RESULTS

The analgesia achieved by ketamine given either i.m. or i.v. was superior to other agents used to alleviate labor pains during spontaneous normal deliveries. The scores showed that ketamine produced excellent analgesia compared to good, fair, or poor analgesia in other groups of patients who received agents other than ketamine. Side effects in the form of posthypnotic emergence reactions were minimal. Patients who received other agents had a slow increase in uterine contractions preceeded by a gradual diminution of uterine activity to the preanalgesic level after a long time of 60 min. The pelvic and cervical scores were much improved after the administration of ketamine. The mean ± S.E. duration of the second stage of 32.0 ± 18.7 min lies within the normal physiological range. Parturients who received other analgesic agents had a prolonged second stage (41.3 ± 24.9, 44.5 ± 15.8 and 55.0 ± 15.8). The duration of analgesia following ketamine anesthesia was 82.0 min, in comparison with other agents where the duration was 68.0, 77.5, and 136.7 min.

Assessment of newborn infants

The fetuses were assessed during labor by continuous monitoring of cardiac rate and rhythm, and after delivery by Apgar scores at 1 and 5 min. Ketamine anesthesia produced no ominous signs in the rhythm or heart rate of the fetus (Figs. 1 and 2).

The fetal heart rate ranged between 120-160 beats/min with normal beat to beat variations. The changes in fetal heart rate during ketamine were nonsignificant despite the fact that few cases showed momentary early "cardiac dips". Other agents produced an increase in heart reactivity during uterine contractions or late cardiac dips or loss of beat to beat variations. After delivery, the newborn infants were assessed by Apgar scores at 1 and 5 min. All babies cried lustily and had good Apgar scores, 9/10 at 1 min and 10/10 at 5 min when their mothers were given ketamine.

Cesarean sections

Awareness was not experienced by any of the parturients who received ketamine in the induction period, as compared to a 9% incidence in those who did not receive ketamine.

Discussion

At the present time, there is no ideal pain relieving agent. In evaluating the ideal pain relieving agent, three aspects should be considered: efficacy to alleviate pain and lack of side effects, effect on uterine activity, and action on the fetus and newborn infant.

Ketamine given to parturients in labor produces CNS depression. Its analgesic effect is rapid and excellent. Analgesia began about 4 min after i.m. administration, a fact supported by Coppel *et al.* (1973) who stated that the onset of sleep occurred 2 to 8 min after i.m. injection. Unfortunately, this excellent analgesia in some patients is offset by a variable incidence of delirium and hallucinations posthypnotically. Ketamine produces a transient decrease in uterine activity for a few min after its administation, but normal physiological uterine contractions are achieved rapidly. Fifteen min after i.m. injection, ketamine produces a pronounced and sharp increase in uterine activity which is increased both in force and frequency. This ultimately shortens the duration of the second stage of labor.

The depression of uterine contractions encountered during the early phase of the administration of ketamine is transient in comparison to other agents used for pain relief in obstetrics. Some patients may show a state of uterine hypertonus, but without any ominous signs in the fetus or mother. This fact was noted by Bovill *et al.* (1971) and Moore *et al.* (1971).

The duration of the second stage was short. This is explained by the increased expulsion forces experienced by the mother together with a significant improvement in uterine activity. Ketamine also produces improvement in the cervical dilation score, and thus shortens the overall duration of delivery. Vaginal delivery need not be assisted as usually is the case with other analgesic agents.

Fetuses delivered under ketamine analgesia were in good cardiac status, as judged by monitoring the fetal cardiac rate and rhythm. No ominous signs were observed during ketamine anesthesia. Serious "cardiac dips" or decelerations of heart rate were not recorded. Infants showed good Apgar scores at 1 and 5 min.

Ketamine does not appear to pass through the placental membranes because it does not affect the overall state of the newborn. Akamatsu *et al.* (1974) found that there were no noticeable serious effects on neonates even if i.v. ketamine was administered immediately prior to delivery.

Ketamine administered as an induction agent in patients scheduled for cesarean section easily reduces awareness, which is a common finding in about 9% of patients not given ketamine. This experience may be remembered as unpleasant dreams. This is important because the increased stress of awareness may stimulate sympathetic tone resulting in decreased uteroplacental blood flow at a crucial time. The incidence of awareness in obstetrical anesthesia is usually marked because sedatives and depressant drugs are avoided and a high percentage of oxygen is given for the benefit of the fetus before delivery. Ketamine as an induction agent may be the answer to reducing the incidence of awareness during cesarean section (Tunstall, 1979).

ACKNOWLEDGEMENT

The author is deeply endebted to the staff of his anesthesia and obstetric department for their help. Thanks are extended to all of the patients with whom this research was accomplished. This research was supported by Parke Davis Scientific Department, Egypt.

References

Akamatsu, T.J., Bonica, J.J., Rehmey R., Eng, M., and Veland, K.: Experience with the use of ketamine for parturition. Anesth. Analg. 53: 2, 1974.

Apgar, V.: Proposal of a new method of evaluation of newborn infants. Anesth. Analg. 32: 260, 1953.

Bovill, J.G., Coppel, D.L., Dundee, J.W., and Moore, J.: Current status of ketamine anaesthesia. Lancet 1: 1285, 1971.

Coppel, D.L., Bovill, J.G., and Dundee J.W.: The taming of ketamine. Anaesthesia 28: 293, 1973.

El-Sahwi, S., Gaafar, A.A, and Toppozada, H.K.: A new unit for evaluation of uterine activity. Amer. J. Obstet. Gyn. 98: 900, 1967.

Grant, I.S., Nimmo, W.S., and Clements, J.A.: Pharmacokinetics and analgesic effects of i.m. and oral ketamine. Brit. J. Anaesth. 53: 805, 1981.

Meyers, S.F. and Charles, P.: Prolonged adverse reactions to ketamine in children. Anesthesiol. 49: 39, 1978.

Moore, J., McNobb, T.G., and Dundee, J.W.: Preliminary report on ketamine in obstetrics. Brit. J. Anaesth. 43: 779, 1971.

Ohtani, M., Kikuchi, H., Kitahata, L.M., Taub, A., Toyooka, H., Hanaoka, H., and Dohi, S.: Effects of ketamine on nociceptive cells in the medial medullary reticular formation of the cat. Anesthesiol. 51: 414,1979.

Smith, S.E.: Intravenous anaesthesia, In A Practice of Anaesthesia, Chapter 19, pp. 626, Wylie and Churchill-Davidson, 5th Ed., Lloyd. Lake Pub., 1984.

Tunstall, M.E.: The reduction of amnesic wakefulness during caesarean section. Anaesthesia 34: 316, 1979.

Tang, A.H. and Schroeder, L.A.: Spinal cord depressant effects of ketamine and etoxadrol in the cat and the rat. Anesthesiol. 39: 37, 1973.

Way, W.L. and Trevor, A.J.: Pharmacology of intravenous nonnarcotic anesthetics. Chap. 24, pp. 799. In Anesthesia, 2nd Ed., Miller, R.D., ed., Churchill-Livingstone, 1986.

White, P.F., Way, W.L., and Trevor A.J.: Ketamine: Its pharmacology and therapeutic uses. Anesthesiol. 56: 119, 1982.

Status of Ketamine in Anesthesiology,
edited by E.F. Domino©1990, NPP Books
P.O. Box 1491, Ann Arbor, MI 48106

Epidural Injection of Ketamine Hydrochloride: An Experimental Study in Rats

G. Guinto-Enriquez, R.Y. Enriquez** and L. Reyes de Castro***

**Division of Anesthesiology and*
***Neuropathology Research Laboratory*
Faculty of Medicine and Surgery
University of Santo Tomas
Manila, Philippines

Introduction

The spinal administration of opiates produces powerful modulation of the rostral processing of nociceptive impulses. These occur as a result of mediation by several recognized subpopulations of opiate receptors, notably the *mu*, *delta*, and *kappa* receptors (Yaksh *et al.*, 1986). Clinically, epidurally, and intrathecally administered opiates, particularly morphine, have gained popularity for relief of postoperative pain (Bromage *et al.*, 1980; Rutter *et al.*, 1981). Though intrathecal morphine may be effective in relieving postoperative pain, such administration is often associated with several side effects. These include respiratory depression, urinary retention, nausea, vomiting, and pruritus (Gustafsson *et al.*, 1982). Hence, the search for an alternative agent continues.

Ketamine, a phencyclidine derivative, is a potent analgesic. In a series of experiments done with subhypnotic doses, ketamine was proven to produce dose related analgesia that is significantly antagonized by administering the narcotic antagonist, naloxone. This led investigators to infer a similarity between ketamine induced analgesia and that produced by morphine (Finck and Ngai, 1982). This indicates that analgesia produced by ketamine is mediated by opiate receptors. Since ketamine administered systemically is unlikely to produce respiratory depression, it seems to offer an obvious advantage over opiates. Islas *et al.* (1985) evaluated the use of epidural ketamine for control of postoperative pain. They concluded that it produces potent analgesia without major respiratory depression and other side effects. Naguib *et al.* (1986) likewise concluded that 30 mg of ketamine epidurally was a safe and effective method for postoperative analgesia. Neither study, however, evaluated any of the possible neurotoxic effects that ketamine may exert on the spinal cord. Since intrathecal and epidural ketamine administration may prove to be of use for postoperative analgesia, we decided to do an experiment on rats with the following objectives:

1. To evaluate the efficacy of epidurally administered ketamine as an analgesic.
2. To describe the time course for the analgesic, motor function, and behavioral effects of epidural ketamine.
3. To examine if ketamine administered by the epidural route has any neuropathological effects on the spinal cord.
4. To determine if epidural ketamine has any systemic toxic effects.

Materials and Methods

I. Preparation of epidural catheters

Polyethylene tubing PE-10 with a 0.28 mm internal diameter and 0.61 mm outer diameter was cut into segments 15 cm long. Each catheter was sterilized with ethylene oxide gas and flushed with sterile 0.9% NaCl prior to implantation.

II. Animal preparation and surgical procedure of Durant and Yaksh (1986), with slight modifications.

Thirty male Sprague-Dawley rats, weighing 150-200 gm, obtained from the National Standard Testing Center, Bicutan, Metro Manila, were used in this study.

Anesthesia was induced and maintained with diethyl ether in air until the end of the procedure. The back was shaved from the neck to the tail and Povidone-iodine cleansing and antiseptic solutions were applied. A 50 ml syringe was placed transversely under the abdomen to obtain maximal flexion of the lumbar vertebrae during the procedure. The iliac crests were then palpated to locate the sixth lumbar vertebra which lies between them. A midline skin incision was made over the spinous processes of L5-L6. The fascia was opened and the interspinous ligament between L5-L6 and L6-L7 was cut. The superficial muscles around the spinous process of L6 were dissected and retracted. The L6 spinous process was removed to allow the insertion of the catheter parallel to the dura. A dissecting microscope was then used at 10x magnification. The area between the two posterior articular processes of L5 was cleared to reach the ligamentum flavum. Using a right angle hook made of a G22 hypodermic needle, the ligamentum flavum was pierced at the base of the L-5 spinous process.

The catheter was then gently introduced cephalad into the lumbar epidural space to a length of 2 cm. The catheter tip was located at L3 level, one segment above the caudal end of the spinal cord. The catheter was flushed with isotonic saline and it was noted that no solution leaked around the point of entry for volumes up to 100 μl.

The remainder of the catheter was tunneled s.c., emerging through the skin in the neck region. The catheter was anchored appropriately. An aseptic technique was used throughout the entire procedure. The catheter tip was then sealed with a sterile steel pin. Diethyl ether anesthesia was then discontinued. Only those animals which showed normal motor and sensory function after recovery from anesthesia were included. Immediately upon recovery from anesthesia, the location of the catheter was verified by injection of 0.8 mg 2% lidocaine through the epidural catheter. Hindlimb paralysis and lumbar analgesia indicated that the catheter was in the epidural space. Rats in which there was any doubt about the location of the catheter were not included in the experiment.

III. Drugs and schedule of injection

Twenty-four hr after surgery, each animal received an initial dose of the assigned drug. Drugs for epidural injection were mixed in such a way that all doses were administered in a 40 μl solution followed by a 10 μl 0.9% NaCl solution for flushing (dead space of catheter = 10 μl). The investigators observed that an epidural volume of 40 μl was adequate to produce sensory and motor blockade of the lower half of the body.

To assess the initial range of dosage, an "up and down" method was used. A dose of 2 mg/kg, shown by Ivankovich and McCarthy (1986) to have some effect after intrathecal injection in dogs, was administered epidurally. This failed to produce significant analgesia. A threefold increase in the dose was administered to the next rat. At 6 mg/kg, significant sensory and motor blockade were observed. This dosage was utilized in the experimental series. To determine at what dose a selective spinal analgesia would be produced, the significant dose of 6 mg/kg was decreased by 1/3, *i.e.*, a dose of 4 mg/kg was given.

Ketamine HCl was given to two study groups in the following schedule:

Group I. Ketamine HCl 40 μl, 6 mg/kg, once daily for 3 consecutive days, N = 6. Group II. Ketamine HCl 40 μl, 4 mg/kg, once daily for 3 consecutive days, N = 6.

Group III. (Control group) 0.9% NaCl 40 μl, once daily for 3 consecutive days, N = 6.

Each epidural injection was done at a specific period of time each day.

IV. Evaluation of clinical effects

A. Clinical effects in rats were observed prior to administration, immediately after administration, every 5 min for one hr, and every 30 min thereafter, if necessary.

B. The following tests were done:

1. Nociceptive tests.

Paw pinch:	The hindpaws were pinched with a pair of forceps. A withdrawal response was considered positive.
Tail flick:	A polysynaptic reflex, this response was elicited by placing the rat's tail through a slit over which the light of a 300 watt bulb was focused. Response latency was described as the time between presentation of the stimulus and the rapid removal of the tail from the slit. To avoid tissue damage, the test was terminated automatically after 6 sec.
Hot plate:	The animal was placed on top of a metal surface maintained at 56°C. Response latency was recorded as the time between placing the animal on the metal surface and the time the rat jumped or licked its hindpaws.

2. Non-nociceptive tests.

Motor function:	The ability to negotiate a 60° inclined plane was assessed. Dragging of both hindlegs was considered as a sign of motor dysfunction.
Behavioral observations:	The animals were observed carefully for untoward manifestations like abdominal breathing, confusion, catalepsy, etc. Catalepsy was defined as a lack of movement for 15 sec or more when the animal's forelimbs were placed on a bar 4 cm in height.

V. Morphology

A separate group of 6 rats was given benzethonium chloride (the preservative component of Ketalar), 40 μl, 0.01%, once daily for 3 consecutive days to serve as control in the morphologic studies. Twenty four hr after the last dose, all 24 animals were sacrificed with an overdose of diethyl ether. The chest was opened to expose the aorta. Ten percent buffered formalin solution was perfused. The vertebral column was removed en bloc, fixed in formalin and decalcified in a nitric acid-alcohol mixture. Different levels of the spinal column were blocked and processed for paraffin sections. Hematoxylin-Eosin stain and Luxol Fast Blue-Cresyl Violet stain were done on all sections. Slides were evaluated for morphologic changes.

VI. Statistical analysis

Response latencies were expressed as the mean ± S.E. These were eventually plotted against time in graphic format. Two factor analysis of variance was done to determine if the response latency is affected by the dose of ketamine and the time interval between administration and clinical testing.

Results

A total of 30 rats was used. Two rats died because of diethyl ether overdose during the operative procedure. One had the catheter inside the subarachnoid space, as manifested by leakage of CSF during the procedure. Three rats which showed signs of spinal cord injury (monoparesis and paraparesis) after surgery were excluded from the study. Twenty four (80%) rats found to have the catheter inside the epidural space were included in this study. None of these 24 rats showed signs of leakage when the catheters were flushed with 0.9% NaCl at the end of each necropsy.

Figs. 1 and 2 illustrate the time course of the effect of epidural ketamine and epidural 0.9% NaCl on the tail flick and hot plate responses 24 hr after catheterization. Two-factor analysis of variance revealed that the response latency in both tail flick and hot plate tests was significantly affected by the dose of epidural ketamine as well as the time interval between administration and clinical testing ($P < 0.001$).

Ketamine, in a dose of 6 mg/kg, produced a complete block of both the tail flick and hot plate responses. Peak effect was noted to occur within 5 min of administration. On the other hand, the tail flick and hot plate responses were not completely blocked in the animals given epidural

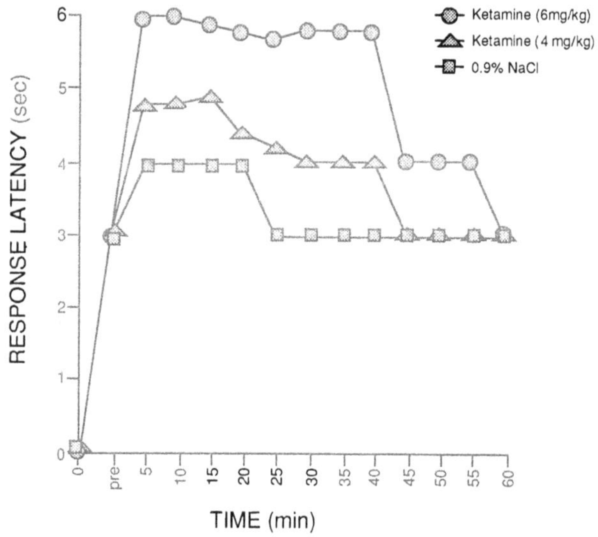

Fig. 1. Time course of the nociceptive response to tail flick after epidurally administered 0.9% NaCl, 4 and 6 mg/kg of ketamine.

ketamine at 4 mg/kg. This was manifested by a shorter latency period than in those animals to which 6 mg/kg was given. No significant effect was noted in the saline group.

Table 1 summarizes the behavioral signs observed one day after catheterization. Motor dysfunction was produced by ketamine in a dose of 6 mg/kg. Likewise, no withdrawal was noted during pinching of the hindpaws in all 6 rats. The onset of both motor and sensory blockade occurred within 30-60 sec. It took 5-15 min for motor function to return to normal. Sensory blockade, on the other hand, lasted for 25-45 min. Behavioral dysfunction in the form of confusion was observed in one animal. No respiratory depression was observed.

A selective analgesic effect was noted with 4 mg/kg of ketamine. There was absence of the withdrawal response to pinching of the hindpaws in 4 out of 6 animals. No motor blockade was observed. The time of onset for sensory blockade was within 45-60 sec. The duration of action, on the other hand, was noted to be 15-30 min. No behavioral dysfunction was observed.

Gross observation at necropsy revealed a brownish appearance in the levels of the spinal column surrounding the catheter. A fibrotic reaction was observed mainly at the site of entry of the catheter into the epidural space. Microscopic examination in ketamine treated rats revealed the

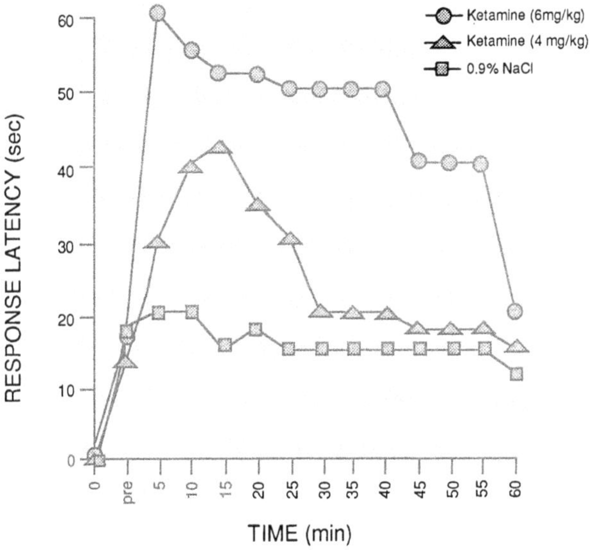

Fig. 2. Time course of the nociceptive response to a hot plate after epidurally administered 0.9% NaCl, 4 and 6 mg/kg ketamine.

following: 1. A few lymphocytes and occasional red blood cells and a connective tissue reaction were present around the catheter (see Fig. 3). 2. No granuloma, giant cells, nor fats were found in the epidural space near the catheter. 3. Thickening of the dura in areas between the catheter and the spinal cord. 4. Mild deformation of the spinal cord in areas where it lays with the catheter (see Fig. 4). 5. Minimal demyelination in these deformed areas.

Basically the same histologic findings were observed in rats treated with benzethonium chloride and isotonic saline.

Discussion

Recent studies have shown that narcotic drugs produce an unusually intense, prolonged, and segmental analgesic action when injected into the subarachnoid or extradural space of animals and man (Bahar *et al.*, 1979; Cousins *et al.*, 1979; Leslie *et al.*, 1979; Wang *et al.*, 1979). These observations stemmed from earlier laboratory investigations into the site of action of morphine and morphinomimetic substances in the spinal cord and brainstem. Several groups of investigators have shown that it exerts a profound and depressing action on the nociceptive pathways in the dorsal horn (Kitahata and Collins, 1981). Autoradiographic studies have con-

TABLE 1. Summary of behavioral effects observed after epidural injection of ketamine hydrochloride

		Absence of Withdrawal Response During Pinching		*Time of Onset*		*Time to Regain Normal Function*			
	Motor Dysfunction	***Hindpaw***	***Forepaw***	***Motor***	***Absence of Withdrawal***	***Motor***	***Withdrawal***	***Confusion***	***Catalepsy***
Ketamine HC1 (6 mg/kg)	6/6	6	0	<1 min	<1 min	5-15 min	25-45 min	1	0
Ketamine HC1 (4 mg/kg)	0/6	4	0	0	<1 min	0	15-30 min	0	0
Ketamine	0/3	0	0	0	0	0	0	0	0

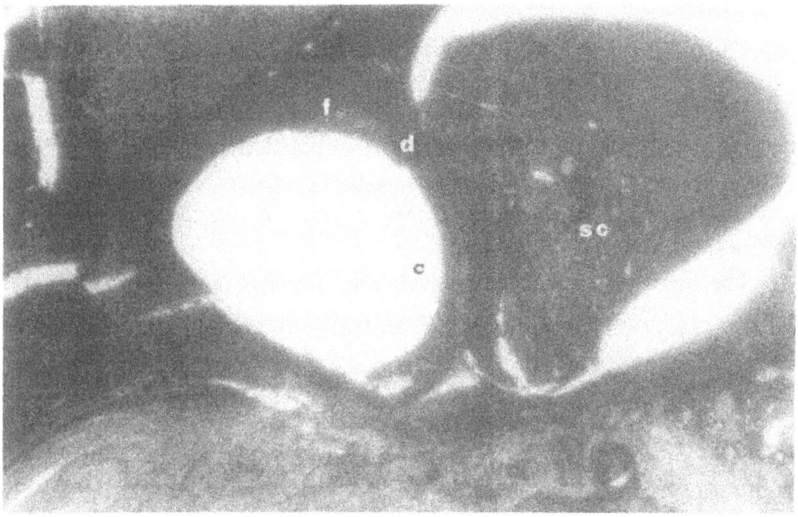

Fig. 3. Cross section of the caudal end of the spinal cord (sc) showing the relationship of the catheter (c) to the spinal cord. Note the fibrotic reaction (f) around the catheter (60x magnification).

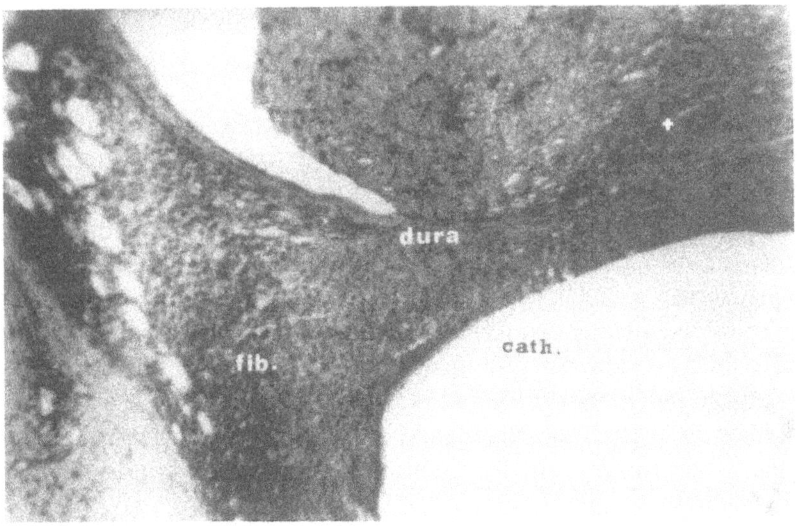

Fig. 4. A closer magnification (150x) of the catheter and the spinal cord showing mechanical compression of the spinal cord (+). Note the lymphocytic infiltration of the dura surrounding the catheter.

firmed that abundant opiate receptors exist in the substancia gelatinosa of the dorsal horn, especially in Lamina 1 and 2 (Kitahata and Collins, 1981; Nordberg *et al.*, 1984).

Following the identification of these opiate receptors in the spinal cord, the epidural and intrathecal use of opioids has increased. However, these methods of pain relief are not without side effects, the most serious of which is delayed respiratory depression (Cousins *et al.*, 1979; Gustafsson *et al.*, 1982).

There are two possible mechanisms for this untoward effect: 1) An unknown portion of the drug, after diffusion into the CSF and uptake into the substancia gelatinosa of the dorsal horn, gains access to the respiratory center by the blood stream after absorption through the epidural venous plexus. 2) Excessive diffusion into CSF may allow significant quantities of the narcotic to reach the fourth ventricle by cephalad subarachnoid spread, and then direct depression of the respiratory center may occur (Bromage *et al.*, 1980; Cousins and Bridenbaugh, 1980). These important studies have provided a new way to exploit analgesics by selective analgesia without the risk of appreciable respiratory or autonomic depression.

Ketamine has been used extensively in clinical practice for more than 10 years. Among the myriad of pharmacologic effects produced by this "dissociative" anesthetic is profound analgesia without respiratory depression (Pender, 1971). Experimentally, subhypnotic doses of ketamine produce a dose related analgesia in both animals and man (Finck and Ngai, 1982; Slogoff *et al.*, 1974). It would, therefore, seem to be a suitable drug for pain relief.

In an experimental study in mice, it was observed that the analgesia produced by ketamine was significantly antagonized by the administration of the narcotic antagonist, naloxone (Finck and Ngai, 1982). Ryder *et al.* (1978) further speculated that ketamine might produce analgesia by releasing or potentiating endogenous opioid peptides whose action was then antagonized by naloxone. Alternatively, ketamine might interact directly with opiate receptors (Finck and Ngai, 1982). These findings were corroborated by a study of Finck and Ngai (1982). They showed that ketamine at pharmacologically relevant concentrations binds to opiate receptors in two standard *in vitro* test systems and that ketamine displaces the radioactively labeled narcotic agonist, etrophine, from opiate receptors *in vivo*. They concluded that the mechanism for the analgesia produced by ketamine is mediated by opiate receptors. These theories led the investigators to infer a similarity between ketamine induced analgesia and the analgesia produced by narcotics when administered epidurally.

Consequently, we were able to demonstrate that the administration of ketamine in rats has produced a significant elevation in the behaviorally defined nociceptive threshold on a variety of tasks ranging from simple spinal nociceptive reflexes (tail flick and paw pinch) to a more complex operant task such as the hot plate.

Two factor analysis of variance revealed that the response latency in both tail flick and hot plate was significantly affected by the dose of epidural ketamine used as well as the time interval between administration and clinical testing ($P < 0.01$). This indicates that the analgesic effect of epidural ketamine is dose related and the increase in the response latency is statistically significant.

Epidurally, ketamine, in a dose of 6 mg/kg, produced a maximal response on hot plate and tail flick tests. There was a significant increase in the response latency period in both tests when compared to the baseline values. The paw pinch likewise showed a significant result. There was no normal withdrawal of hindpaws in any of the six animals given such a dose.

At a lower dose of 4 mg/kg, a selective spinal analgesia was observed. There was a shorter response latency period in the tail flick and hot plate responses than those in which 6 mg/kg was given. The withdrawal response to pinching of the hindpaws was absent in 4 of 6 animals injected. From these results, one can deduce that epidural ketamine exerts a desirable effect on the spinal cord. The significant analgesia produced can be presumed to be of the same mechanism as epidural morphine, *i.e.*, mediated by opiate receptors. Nevertheless, there are significant differences. The time of onset for epidural ketamine, as demonstrated in this study, was less than one min as compared to the established onset of action of epidural morphine which is 15 to 30 min (Durant and Yaksh, 1986). This rapid onset of action may be attributed to the lower molecular weight of ketamine (MW 238) as compared to morphine sulfate (MW 669). It is a known theory that molecular diffusion through the extracellular channels, as represented by the dura, varies inversely with the square root of the molecular weight (Moore *et al.*, 1982). This faster onset of action is of obvious significance since pain is more easily relieved at its onset than when it is already well pronounced.

The duration of action with regard to sensory blockade was 25 to 45 min in group 1 and 15 to 30 min in group II. Morphine, administered epidurally in rats, had a duration of action of 30 to 60 min (Durant and Yaksh, 1986). Islas *et al.* (1985) evaluated the efficacy of epidural ketamine for postoperative pain control in man. They established that the mean duration of action was 4.06 ± 1.34 hr. This relatively long duration of action can be attributed to its hydrophillic properties and relatively delayed clearance from the subarachnoid space.

A significant motor dysfunction was noted at the 6 mg/kg dose level. This implies that the drug appears to have a local anesthetic action in relatively higher concentrations. This motor blockade, however, lasted for only 5 to 15 min compared to sensory blockade of 25 to 45 min. Furthermore, at a dose of 4 mg/kg, where there is selective analgesia, no motor dysfunction was observed.

One animal, given a dose of 6 mg/kg, manifested confusion. Such an effect may be attributed to a rapid vascular absorption which eventually results in a functional and electrophysiological dissociation between the thalamo-neocortical and limbic systems (Corssen *et al.*, 1968). This did not pose a serious problem inasmuch as it only lasted for 5 min.

In this study, ketamine analgesia was not associated with any respiratory depression. Soliman *et al.* (1975) observed that ketamine did not produce any significant respiratory depression and the respiratory response to a carbon dioxide challenge was maintained during ketamine anesthesia. In contrast, respiratory depression after epidural narcotics has been described by many authors (Cousins *et al.*, 1979; Gustafsson *et al.*, 1982).

Naguib *et al.*, (1986) likewise conducted a study on epidural ketamine for postoperative pain relief in man. The analgesic doses of ketamine he used, given by epidural and i.m. routes, were not associated with any changes in cardiovascular parameters. In contrast, general anesthesia with ketamine produces a dose related rise in the heart rate systolic pressure product (often in excess of 100%), with a transient rise in the cardiac index but without altering the stroke index (Tweed *et al.*, 1972) through a central adrenergic stimulation (Chodoff, 1972). This cardiovascular stability may be an obvious advantage of epidural ketamine over epidural opiates which usually cause cardiovascular depression.

The morphologic changes observed in this study revealed no significant difference between the control and study groups. The reaction to the catheter appears to be an inflammatory response to the chronic presence of the tubing. Likewise, the minimal demyelination observed may be attributed to a mechanical compressive effect the catheter exerts on the spinal cord. These findings are consistent with the previous experimental studies using other drugs in animals chronically implanted with catheters (Durant and Yaksh, 1986). Based on these results, we may conclude that ketamine, even in combination with benzethonium chloride, does not produce significant changes attributable to ketamine itself.

The importance of investigating the potential spinal neurotoxicity before clinical experiments are started cannot be overemphasized. Remarkably, many agents have been used by clinical investigators without such preliminary screening. When spinal administration of morphine was introduced clinically (Bahar *et al.*, 1979), neurotoxicologic data were not available.

One may argue whether morphological investigation is adequate to detect neurotoxic effects of spinally administered drugs because such effects may be functional rather than structural. Clearly, the absence of morphological change alone is not sufficient to free a drug from possible neurotoxic effect. However, findings from morphological studies, *e.g.*, lesions in special cell types or location, are important because the morphological basis of functional changes may then be detected.

Summary

An experiment was performed to determine effects of epidural ketamine, as the HCl salt, on neuromuscular function. Ketamine was found to have local anesthetic effects (sensory and motor blockade) in doses of 6 mg/kg with a mean onset of < 1 min and a duration of action of 25-45 min and 5-15 min for sensory and motor blockade, respectively (ANOVA: $P < 0.01$). Epidural ketamine, in a dose of 4 mg/kg, was observed to have a selective analgesic property as manifested by the absence of motor dysfunction. The only undesirable effect observed was confusion in one rat. No respiratory depression was observed. Morphologic studies revealed that epdirually administered ketamine has no significant histotoxic effect on the spinal cord when compared with controls using light microscopy.

References

Bahar, M., Olshwang, D., Magora, F., *et al.*: Epidural morphine in treatment of pain. Lancet 1: 527-529, 1979.

Bromage, P.R., Camporesi, E., and Chestnut, D.: Epidural narcotics for postoperative analgesia. Anesth. Analg. 59: 473-480, 1980.

Chodoff, P.: Evidence for central adrenergic action of ketamine. Anesth. Analg. 51: 247-250, 1972.

Corssen, G., Miyasaka, M., and Domino, E.F.: Changing concepts in pain control during surgery: Dissociative anesthesia with CI-581. Anesth. Analg. 47: 746-759, 1968.

Cousins, M.J. and Bridenbaugh, P.O.: Neural Blockade in Clinical Anesthesia and Management in Pain. First Edition, p. 180, J.B. Lippincott Co., Philadelphia, 1980.
Cousins, M.J., Mather, L.E., Glynn, C.J., *et al.*: Selective spinal analgesia. Lancet 1: 1141-1142, 1979.
Durant, P.A. and Yaksh, T.L.: Epidural injection of bupivacaine, morphine, fentanyl, lofentanil, and DADL in chronically implanted rats: A pharmacologic and pathologic study. Anesth. 64: 43-53, 1986.
Finck, A.D. and Ngai, S.H.: Opiate receptor mediation of ketamine analgesia. Anesth. 56: 291-297, 1982.
Gustafsson, L.L., Schildt, B., and Jacobsen, K.J.: Adverse effects of extradural and intrathecal opiates: Report of a nationwide survey in Sweden. Br. J. Anesh. 54: 479-486, 1982.
Ivankovich, A.D. and McCarthy, R.J.: Epidural ketamine for control of postoperative pain. Letter to the Editor. Anesth. Analg. 65: 988-992, 1986.
Islas, J.A., Astorga, J., and Laredo, M.: Epidural ketamine for control of postoperative pain. Anesth. Analg. 64: 1161-1162, 1985.
Kitahata, L.M. and Collins, J.G.: Spinal action of narcotic analgesics. Anesth. 54: 153-163, 1981.
Leslie, J., Camporesi, E., Urban, B., *et al.*: Selective epidural analgesia. Lancet 1: 151, 1979.
Moore, R.A., Bullingham, R.E.S., *et al.*: Dural permeability to narcotics: *In vitro* determination and application to extradural administration. Br. J. Anaesth. 54: 1117-1128, 1982.
Naguib, M., Gyamfi, Y. *et al.*: Epidural ketamine for postoperative analgesia. Can. Anaesth. Soc. J. 33: 16-21, 1986.
Nordberg, G., Hedner, T., *et al.*: Pharmacokinetic aspects of intrathecal morphine analgesia. Anesth. 60: 448-454, 1984.
Pender, J.V.: Dissociative anesthesia. J.A.M.A. 215: 1126, 1971.
Rutter, D.V., Shewes, D.G., and Morgan, M.: Extradural opioids for postoperative analgesia. Br. J. Anes. 53: 915-920, 1981.
Ryder, S., Way, W.L., and Trevor, A.J.: Comparative pharmacology of the optical isomers of ketamine in mice. Eur. J. Pharm. 49: 15-23, 1978.
Slogoff, S., Allen, G.W., Wessels, J.V., *et al.*: Clinical experience with subanesthetic ketamine. Anesth. Analg. 53: 354-358, 1974.
Soliman, M.G. Brinale, G.F., and Kuster, G.: Response to hypercapnea under ketamine anesthesia. Can. Anaesth. Soc. J. 22: 486-494, 1975.
Tweed, W.A., Minuck, M.S., and Mymin, D.: Circulatory response to ketamine anesthesia. Anesth. 37: 613-619, 1972.
Wang, J.K., Naus, L.A., and Thomas, J.E.: Pain relief by intrathecally applied morphine in man. Anesth. 50: 149-151, 1979.
Yaksh, T.L., Noueihed, R.Y., and Durant, P.A.: Studies of the pharmacology and pathology of intrathecally administered 4-anilo-piperidine analogues and morphine in the rat and cat. Anesthesiol. 64: 54-66, 1986.

Status of Ketamine in Anesthesiology,
edited by E.F. Domino©1990, NPP Books
P.O. Box 1491, Ann Arbor, MI 48106

Studies with Epidural Ketamine and Local Anesthetic Combinations for Obstetrical Analgesia and Anesthesia

S.M. Shulman, A.T.C. Peng, L.S. Blancato, F. Cutrone, and K. Nyunt

Department of Anesthesiology
St. Lukes-Roosevelt Hospital Center
Columbia University, New York, NY 10025

INTRODUCTION

Ketamine given epidurally has interested medical researchers for its possible use to induce epidural analgesia or anesthesia without sympathetic blockade or the side effects of epidural narcotics. Reports about the analgesic effectiveness of epidural ketamine, however, yield conflicting results. Some researchers have reported prolonged analgesia (Mankowitz *et al.*, 1982; Islas *et al.*, 1985; Naguib *et al.*, 1986; Samaras *et al.*, 1988). Other researchers (Brock-Utne *et al.*, 1985; Auwera *et al.*, 1987; Ravat *et al.*, 1987; Mori and Shingu, 1988; Mok *et al.*, 1987; Kawana *et al.*, 1987; Ivankovich and McCarthy, 1986) have reported transient analgesia with a rapid onset and a duration less than 60 min. Similarly, intrathecal ketamine (Ahuja, 1983; Bion, 1984) causes motor blockade which lasts less than 30 min. It is unknown whether the short duration of epidural and intrathecal ketamine is caused by diffusion of the drug away from the spinal cord or caused by a biochemical alteration at the site of action. The possibility of a local anesthetic action of ketamine has also been proposed as a mechanism of analgesia (Kawana *et al.*, 1987).

It is important to note the site of surgery in reviewing the reports of epidural ketamine analgesia. Epidural ketamine is consistently reported to cause effective analgesia when the source of the pain is somatic (*e.g.* bone, muscle, skin). On the other hand, when a visceral component of the pain is present (*e.g.* pleura, peritoneum), epidural ketamine causes only poor analgesia. The first report of epidural ketamine was by Mankowitz *et al.*, (1982) who reported analgesia for up to 6 hr in chronic pain patients. These patients had back, lower abdominal, or leg pain. In a later report from this group, Brock-Utne *et al.*, (1985) reported that up to 50 mg of epidural ketamine provided only 30 min of analgesia in patients after upper abdominal surgery. Islas *et al.*, (1985) reported prolonged analgesia in postoperative patients. A dose of 4 mg of epidural ketamine provided pain relief for about 4 hr after lower abdominal, perineal, and lower extremity operations. We have also observed this (unpublished results). This analgesia is not surprising since those types of surgery mainly cause somatic pain postoperatively.

The doses of epidural ketamine should also be noted in reviewing reports (Naguib and Adu-Gyamfi, 1988; Kawana *et al.*, 1987). If a low dose is used and no analgesia occurs, then the only conclusion is that the dose was ineffective. Naguib *et al.* (1986) reported using up to 30 mg of epidural ketamine and found that 10 and 30 mg of epidural ketamine further decreased analgesic requirements for the first 24 hr after cholecystectomy. This is a complex study to interpret because (1) it was not double-blind, (2) cholecystectomy pain may be either predominantly somatic, visceral, or mixed, and (3) only further analgesic requirements were noted; the duration of action of the initial dose was not reported.

We sought to determine the efficacy of epidural ketamine in combination with either lidocaine or bupivacaine. We report double blind randomized studies on (1) the effect of 10 and 30 mg epidural ketamine, combined with 0.125% bupivacaine, in relieving patients' pain after cesarean section, (2) the effect of adding epidural ketamine 0.1% to epidural lidocaine anesthesia during cesarean section, and (3) the effect of adding epidural ketamine (0.1%) to epidural bupivacaine (0.125%) on labor analgesia.

Methods

Postcesarean study protocol

Following approval of the Institutional Review Board, all patients who were to receive a lumbar epidural catheter for anesthesia for elective cesarean section were asked to participate in this study provided they were not preeclamptic, eclamptic, and did not have other medical illness. Cesarean section anesthesia was achieved with epidural 3% chloroprocaine or 2% lidocaine and i.v. sedation. After cesarean section, the patients' pain was assessed by the Prince Henry pain score (PH) and the Visual Analog Scale (VAS). Once the PH score was 4 and no neurological deficit remained, they were randomly assigned to groups A, B, or C. Groups A, B, and C received 20 ml of 0.125% bupivacaine alone, 0.125% bupivacaine and 10 mg ketamine, or 0.125% bupivacaine and 30 mg ketamine, respectively, in double blind fashion. Subsequently, the PH, neurologic exam, and vital signs were determined at least every 30 min. Analgesia was defined as a PH decrease of 1. Excellent analgesia was defined as a PH of 0 or 1.

Cesarean study protocol

Following approval of the Institutional Review Board, 41 healthy patients who were to receive epidural anesthesia for elective repeat cesarean section consented to this study. Ketamine (20 mg) or 0.9% NaCl (0.4 ml) was added to 20 ml of 2% lidocaine with 1:200,000 epinephrine in a double blind fashion. A total of 15 to 20 ml of the mixture was administered. The sensory level, latency time of anesthesia, interval between induction and delivery (IDI), and Apgar scores were recorded. The discomfort during cesarean section was scored as follows: 0 = severe, 1 = moderate, 2 = mild, and 3 = none. Duration of the initial dose of anesthesia was measured from the end of the epidural injection to the time any supplementary analgesic or anesthetic was administered.

Labor study protocol

Following approval of the Institutional Review Board, 31 healthy laboring parturients who were to receive epidural analgesia consented to this study. Ketamine (10 mg) or 0.9% NaCl (0.2 ml) was added to 10 ml of 0.125% bupivacaine with 1:200,000 epinephrine in a double blind fashion. The linear analog scale (LAS) was assessed at 20 min intervals. The cervical dilations at the initial dose (CD-1) and at the return of pain (CD-2) were noted. Duration of analgesia, motor strength, and Apgar scores were also recorded.

Statistical analysis

The statistical significance of the differences between groups were determined by either Student's t test, Chi square test, or Rank Spearman non-parametric test, when appropriate. A P value less than 0.05 was considered significant.

Results

Postcesarean results

There was a statistically significant increase in duration of analgesia after cesarean section in the group of patients who received 30 mg of epidural ketamine (see Table 1). A good correlation between the PH and the VAS was noted. As both yielded similar results, only the PH will be

TABLE 1. Postcesarean study and results: The effect of epidural ketamine on the duration of analgesia

Group	*Epidural ketamine (mg)*	*Duration of analgesia (min)*	*Patients with excellent analgesia*
A	0 (N = 11)	81 ± 70	64 %
B	10 (N = 6)	112 ± 56 NS	83 %
C	30 (N = 6)	204 ± 96 *	100 %

NS = Not Significant * = Statistically significant

further mentioned. One patient in group C developed blurry vision. No hallucinations, burning, floating sensations, numbness, muscle weakness, hemodynamic changes, pruritus, respiratory depression, or other side effects were observed. Apparently, the addition of epidural bupivacaine eliminated the burning sensation reported to accompany 40% of epidural ketamine injections (Naguib *et al.*, 1986).

Cesarean study results

The addition of ketamine decreased the latency and the discomfort, and increased the duration of the anesthesia (see Table 2). One patient who received ketamine experienced blurred vision which resolved within 10 min without requiring treatment. No hallucinations or other side effects were observed. Sensory level, IDI, and Apgar scores between the two groups were not significantly different.

TABLE 2. Cesarean study: Demographic data and results

	Only epidural lidocaine (N = 21)	*Epidural ketamine (30mg) and lidocaine (N = 20)*
Age (years)	28.9 ± 5.2	32.5 ± 6.3
Sensory Level (T)	5.3 ± 1.4	4.6 ± 1.5 NS
Gravida	2.8 ± 1.0	2.4 ± 1.1 NS
Parity	1.5 ± 0.9	1.5 ± 1.0 NS
IDI (min)	31.9 ± 7.4	29.5 ± 11 NS
APGAR at 1 min	8.4 ± 1.2	8.5 ± 0.6 NS
APGAR at 5 min	9.0 ± 0.4	9.2 ± 0.4 NS
Latency (min)	18 ± 5.4	11 ± 4.7 *
Discomfort Score	2.1 ± 0.8	2.8 ± 0.4 *
Duration (min)	83 ± 52	142 ± 65 *

* = statistically significant
NS = not significant

Labor study results

The addition of ketamine increased the intensity and duration of analgesia during labor as measured by the linear analog scale (LAS, see Table 3). All Apgars were above 7. No hallucinations or other side effects were observed. Motor strength, cervical dilatation (CD), fetal heart tracing, cesarean section rate, and Apgar scores between the two groups were not significantly different. Epidural ketamine (0.1%) and bupivacaine (0.125%) analgesia is superior to bupivacaine alone.

Discussion

The efficacy of epidural ketamine as an analgesic is controversial because conflicting results have been reported. The negative results have led some investigators to conclude that ketamine has no effect on the spinal opiate receptors (Mori and Shingu, 1988), despite previous reports of ketamine affecting lamina V receptors (Kitahata *et al.*, 1973). In our 3 studies, epidural ketamine substantially increased or improved the analgesia of local anesthetics. One hypothesis is that the epidural ketamine relieves the pain in skin, muscle, and bone, whereas the local anesthetic relieves the visceral pain.

In reviewing the results of the bupivacaine control group in the postoperative pain study, there was a bimodal distribution of patients. One group had no analgesia while the other group had up to 2 hr of analgesia.

Postcesarean section pain is an interesting type of postoperative pain. Structures with somatic innervation include skin, subcutaneous tissue,

TABLE 3. Epidural ketamine for labor: Demographic data and results

	Only Epidural Bupivacaine (N = 12)	*Epidural Ketamine and Bupivacaine (N = 19)*
Age	25.8 ± 4.2	29.2 ± 5.1 NS
Gravida	2.7 ± 1.8	2.2 ± 1.0 NS
Para	1.0 ± 1.6	0.5 ± 0.7 NS
LAS Initial	9.6 ± 0.7	9.4 ± 1.0 NS
LAS at 20 min	4.4 ± 2.5	1.8 ± 2.1 *
Cervical dil. init (cm)	4.3 ± 1.3	5.1 ± 1.9 NS
Cervical dil. final (cm)	6.9 ± 2.2	6.8 ± 2.6 NS
Duration (min)	77.3 ± 2.2	119.7 ± 50 *

NS = not statistically significant
* = statistically significant

and muscle. Visceral innervation is present in the uterus which is incised but not removed during surgery. The basis for our argument is that some patients have principally somatic pain while others have principally visceral pain and a third group has both types of pain. Since the 0.125% bupivacaine blocks mainly the fibers from the uterus, the ketamine was useful in providing somatic analgesia.

Perhaps, the epidural ketamine is both an effective somatic and visceral analgesic for only 30 min due to the high levels of ketamine reached after epidural administration. Ahuja (1983) noted in catheterized rats that some demonstrated analgesia in the tail flick test while others did not. Little is known of the pharmacokinetics of epidurally administered ketamine.

In the postoperative study, we found that analysis with the Prince Henry Pain Scale (Torda and Pybus, 1984) was easier than with the Visual Analog Scale. The Prince Henry Pain Scale correlates pain with movement, deep breathing, and coughing. Although the statistical analysis requires a non-parametric analysis, the results can be correlated with the patient analgesia during different activities.

Epidural 0.1% ketamine and 2% lidocane anesthesia for cesarean section is superior to lidocaine alone. To the authors' knowledge, there are no reports of epidural ketamine being used intraoperatively to supplement local anesthetics. Epidural ketamine decreased the latency time and patient discomfort. Despite decreased anesthesia latency, surgical preparation and dissection resulted in no change in the IDI. Here, the improved patient comfort may be due to analgesia of the abdominal wall and perineal structures which may be pushed during surgery.

The question of epidural ketamine toxicity is a serious one. Ahuja (1983) noted no histopathological finding in rats after treatment with ketamine. He also noted epidural catheterization alone caused a 20% incidence of neurological damage. Saissy reported vacuolization with high doses of ketamine. Mok *et al.* (1987) did not observe microscopic pathology in two adult monkeys many weeks after intrathecal ketamine. Brock-Utne *et al.* (1982) observed no histological changes due to intrathecal ketamine. In fact, they noted edema of a few nerve roots whether 0.9% NaCl or ketamine was given. We considered these results to be consistent with no neurotoxicity of epidural ketamine. Recently, Enriquez *et al.* (1988) reported no changes in rat spinal cord histology due to ketamine. Since benzethonium chloride preservative is present, however, we designed the dilution of ketamine to minimize the concentration of the preservative.

Conclusion

Epidural ketamine has not proven to be better than epidural narcotics. The risks include the possibility of the neurotoxicity of ketamine and its preservative, the need for a spinal injection, and overdose causing motor blockade. The combination of a local anesthetic and ketamine avoids neither the risk of sympathetic blockade nor of inadvertent subdural injection. We did not succeed in improving safety over the use of local anesthetics used for labor analgesia. While the effect of ketamine in the epidural space is complex, the only clear advantage it may offer would be in the relief of pure somatic pain. This pain is present in patients after peripheral orthopedic or vascular surgery.

Note: The postcesarean study was presented at the Southern Society of Anesthesia meeting in Orlando, Florida, March, 1987. The cesarean study was presented at the ASA meeting in Atlanta, Georgia, October, 1987. The labor study was presented at the World Congress in Washington, D.C., May, 1988.

Acknowlegements

We would like to acknowledge the assistance of Ms. Edith Flaster, Irving Center for Clinical Research, Columbia University, with the statistical analysis.

References

Ahuja, B.R.: Analgesic effect of intrathecal ketamine in rats. Br. J. Anaesth. 55: 991-995, 1983.

Auwera, D.V., Verbsorgh, C., and Camu, F.: Epidural ketamine for postoperative analgesia. Anesth. Analg. 66: 1340, 1987.

Bion, J.F.: Intrathecal ketamine for war surgery. A preliminary study under field conditions. Anaesthesia 39: 1023-1028, 1984.

Brock-Utne, J.G., Rubin, J., and Mankowitz, E.: Epidural ketamine for control of postoperative pain. Anesth. Analg. 65: 990, 1985.

Brock-Utne, J.G., Kallichurum, S., Mankowitz, E., Maharaj, R.J., and Downing, J.W.: Intrathecal ketamine with preservative histological effects on spinal nerve roots of baboons. South Africa Med. J. 61: 440-441, 1982.

Enriquez, G.G., Enriquez, R.Y., and De Castro, L.R.: Epidural injection of ketamine hydrochloride: An experimental study in rats. World Congress A727, May 1988.

Islas, J.A., Astorga, J., and Laredo, M.: Epidural ketamine for control of postoperative pain. Anesth. Analg. 64: 1161-1162, 1985.

Ivankovich, A.D., and McCarthy, R.J.: Epidural ketamine for control of postoperative pain: Two comments. Anesth. Analg. 65: 989, 1986.

Kawana, Y., Sata, H., Shimade, H., Fujita, N., Ueda, Y., Hayashi, A., and Araki, Y.: Epidural ketamine for postoperative pain relief after gynecologic operations: A double-blind study and comparison with epidural morphine. Anesth. Analg. 66: 735-738, 1987.

Kawana, Y., and Sato, H.: Epidural ketamine for postoperative pain relief after gynecological operations: A double-blind study and comparison with epidural morphine. Anesth. Analg. 67: 798, 1988.

Kitahata, L.M., Taub, A., and Kosaka, Y.: Lamina-specific suppression of dorsal-horn unit activity by ketamine hydrochloride. Anesthesiol. 38: 4-11, 1973.

Mankowitz, E., Brock-Utne, J.G., Cosnett, J.E., and Green-Thompson, R.: Epidural ketamine: A preliminary report. South Africa Med. J. 61: 441-442, 1982.

Mok, M.S., Chan, K.H., Chung, S.K., Lee, T.Y., and Lippmann, M.: Evaluation of the analgesic effect of epidural ketamine. Anesth. Analg. 66: S121, 1987.

Mok, M.S. and Tsai, S.K.: Evaluation of intrathecal ketamine as an analgesic in primates. Reg. Anesth. 13: S10, 1988.

Mori, K., and Shingu, K.: Epidural ketamine does not produce analgesia. Anesthesiol. 68: 296-297, 1988.

Naguib, M., Adu-Gyamfi, Y., Gamil, H.A., Farag, H., and Gyasi, H.K.: Epidural ketamine for postoperative analgesia. Can. Anaesth. Soc. J. 33: 16-21, 1986.

Naguib, M., and Adu-Gyamfi, Y.: Epidural ketamine for postoperative analgesia. Anesth. Analg. 67: 798, 1988.

Ravat, F., Dorne, R., Baechle, J.P., Beaulaton, A., Lenoir, B., Leroy, P., and Palmier, B.: Epidural ketamine or morphine for postoperative analgesia. Anesthesiol. 66: 819-822, 1987.

Samaras, V.A., Gyftonicolou, A., Evagelssopoulou, E., Siafaca, J., and Sikiotis, C.: Postoperative analgesic effect of ketamine HCl administered epidurally in gynecological procedures. Reg. Anesth. 13: S76, 1988.

Torda, T.A., and Pybus, D.A.: Extradural administration of morphine and bupivacaine: A controlled comparison. Br. J. Anesth. 56: 141-145, 1984.

Status of Ketamine in Anesthesiology,
edited by E.F. Domino©1990, NPP Books
P.O. Box 1491, Ann Arbor, MI 48106

Assessment of Epidural Ketamine for Relief of Pain Following Vaginal and Lower Abdominal Surgery

O. E. El-Khateeb*, A. Ragab, M. Metwalli, and H. A. Hassan

Anesthesia Department, Faculty of Medicine
University of Alexandria
Alexandria, Egypt
*and *Anesthesia and ICU Department, Jahra Hospital*
Jahra, Kuwait

INTRODUCTION

In a significant percent of surgical patients, severe postoperative pain and abnormal responses, especially reflex skeletal muscle spasm which decreases chest wall compliance if unrelieved, cause a marked decrease in inspiratory capacity with consequent pulmonary dysfunction, which progresses to atelectasis and hypoxaemia (Craig, 1981). In addition, unrelieved severe spasm and associated responses often cause circulatory and metabolic dysfunctions, consisting of a marked increase in cardiac output, blood pressure, metabolism, and oxygen consumption (Bonica, 1987).

Many methods have been used to relieve postoperative pain, among them intrathecal and epidural opiates which have shown encouraging results. However, opiates have drawbacks, *e.g.*, delayed respiratory depression, urine retention, itching, nausea and vomiting, etc. (Torda *et al*, 1980; Bromage 1980; Rutter *et al.*, 1981).

Since respiratory depression, which is the chief disadvantage of epidural opiates, is unlikely to occur with ketamine when given through the i.v. or the i.m. route, the use of epidural ketamine for postoperative pain relief was suggested by Mankowitz, *et al.* (1982).

The aim of this work was to study the efficacy, advantages, and possible side effects of epidural ketamine as a method for postoperative pain relief in women undergoing vaginal or lower abdominal surgery.

Patients and Methods

Thirty adult female patients, who had to undergo vaginal or lower abdominal surgery, were chosen to participate in this study after receiving informed consent. The study was approved by the local ethical committee. All patients were free from any systemic or metabolic diseases, as judged by clinical examination and routine laboratory testing.

Method

I. Anesthesia—Surgery was done under epidural analgesia with 2% xylocaine (10-15 ml). When the intraoperative analgesia had worn off, as indicated by restoration of normal response to pin prick, and the patient began to experience pain, a dose of 8 mg ketamine HCl diluted in 10 ml sterile normal 0.9% NaCl was injected through a fixed epidural catheter. If an inadequate response was obtained, further incremental doses of 2 mg in 2 ml 0.9% NaCl were given at intervals of 15 min, with a maximum dose of 12 mg. If again no response occurred, it was considered a failure.

II. Measurements—Pulse rate, arterial blood pressure and respiratory frequency per min were recorded preoperatively, intraoperatively, and in the postoperative period until 24 hr after administration of the analgesic.

III. Assessment of pain.

A. Subjective methods (Parkhouse *et al.*, 1963).

Patients graded their pain using a questionnaire which was scored as follows:

No pain	___ 0
Mild pain	___ 1
Moderate pain	___ 2
Severe pain	___ 3

The score recorded before analgesia gave the total pain intensity score (T.P.I.S.), and that after analgesia gave the total pain relief score (T.P.R.S.).

B. Objective Assessment Scores (Steinhouse *et al.*, 1982, modified)

a) Facial expression		b) Body movements	
Relaxed	___ 0	Little movement	___ 0
Tense	___ 1	Moderate movement	___ 1
Very tense	___ 2	Excessive movement	___ 2
Extremely tense	___ 3	Very excessive movement	___ 3

c) Cooperation		d) Level of consciousness	
Complete cooperation	___ 0	Fully conscious	___ 0
Good cooperation	___ 1	Drowsy	___ 1
Fair cooperation	___ 2	Semiconscious	___ 2
Poor cooperation	___ 3	Unconscious	___ 3

IV. Side effects (immediate or late), *e.g.*, hypotension, sickness syndrome, itching, neurological complications, etc.

Statistical analysis of the data was done by Student's "t" test. The values were considered to be statistically significant if P was equal or <0.05.

Results

The physical characteristics of the patients and the dose of xylocaine used for operative anesthesia are shown in Table 1. The dose of ketamine ranged from 8-12 mg (0.1-0.25 mg kg^{-1}), with a mean value of 10.6 ± 1.59 mg (0.16 ± 0.03 mg kg^{-1}). The onset time of ketamine analgesia ranged from 15 to 30 min, with a mean of 20.0 ± 5.9 min. The duration of analgesia ranged from 2 to 24 hr, with a mean value of 5.73 ± 5.6 hr (Table 2).

Clinical assessment of pain (Tables 3, 4, 5 and 6). Excellent analgesia was obtained in 21 patients, whereas partial analgesia occurred in 4 patients, and 5 patients showed no response at all. The resultant analgesia lasted for 24 hr in 2 patients; in the others (23 patients) it lasted for 2-9 hr. All of the patients in whom analgesia was obtained showed full con-

TABLE 1. Physical characteristics of patients and amounts of 2% xylocaine used

	N	*Age (yr)*	*Wt (kg)*	*Dose of 2% xylocaine (ml)*
Mean ± S.D.	30	36.0 ± 5.8	67.9 ± 10.85	12.5 ± 2.54

TABLE 2. Dose, onset time and duration of epidural ketamine analgesia

	Total dose (mg)	*Dose/kg wt (mg kg^{-1})*	*Onset time (min)*	*Duration (hr)*
Range	8 – 12	0.10 – 0.22	15 – 30	2 – 24
Mean	10.6	0.16	20.8	5.73
S.D.	±1.59	±0.03	±5.89	±5.6

Table 3. Total pain scores before and after analgesia

Patients	*No Pain*	*Mild*	*Moderate*	*Severe*	*Mean Score TPIS*	*Mean Score TPRS*	*±S.D.*	*t*	*P*
Before analgesia	—	4	11	15	2.3666		0.718		
After analgesia	21	4	5	—		4.6666	0.776	14.636	<0.001

sciousness, better cooperation, fewer body movements, and fewer changes in facial expression towards relaxation after epidural ketamine administration.

No significant changes have been reported regarding the hemodynamic and respiratory effects of epidural ketamine analgesia. Neither immediate nor delayed side effects were observed after epidural ketamine as evidenced by follow-up of the patients for 4 days.

Discussion

Kitahata *et al.* (1974) showed in animals that abundant opiate receptors are present in the substantia gelatinosa of the dorsal horn of the spinal cord. This important finding opened up new possibilities in the treatment of pain.

Investigators all over the world have extensively studied the behavior of opiates intrathecally and epidurally. They have reported many side effects, of which respiratory depression (immediate and/or late) was the most common (Torda *et al.*, 1980; Bromage, 1980; Rutter *et al.*, 1981).

In the present study, 15 patients had severe pain, 11 had moderate, and 4 had mild pain after operative analgesia and prior to ketamine administration. Within 15-30 min of ketamine injection, a decrease in the intensity of pain was obtained in 25 patients, with 21 noting no pain and 4 reporting mild pain. At the same time, 5 patients gave no response (failed analgesia), although the catheter was still in the epidural space and patients were given the maximum dose of ketamine. All the patients in whom ketamine was effective (25 patients), showed better cooperation, fewer body movements, and fewer changes of facial expression towards relaxation.

The time of onset of epidural ketamine analgesia ranged from 15-30 min, with a mean of 20.8 ± 5.9 min. The same results were reported by Mankowitz *et al.* (1982). This relatively long onset may be attributed to

TABLE 4. Facial expression scores before and after analgesia

Patients	*Relaxed*	*Tense*	*V. Tense*	*Ext. Tense*	*Mean Score*	*±S.D.*	*t*	*P*
Before analgesia	1	11	13	5	1.733	0.785		
After analgesia	22	4	4	0	0.4	0.724	13.372	<0.001

t is significant if ≥ 2.045

TABLE 5. Body movement scores before and after analgesia

Patients	*Little*	*Moderate*	*Excessive*	*Very Excessive*	*Mean Score*	*±S.D.*	*t*	*P*
Before analgesia	1	15	10	4	1.567	0.774		
After analgesia	22	6	2	0	0.333	0.606	13.399	<0.001

TABLE 6. Co-operation scores before and after analgesia

Patients	*Complete*	*Good*	*Fair*	*Poor*	*Mean Score*	*±S.D.*	*t*	*P*
Before analgesia	2	10	12	6	1.7333	0.8683		
After analgesia	17	8	5	0	0.6	0.7701	12.24	<0.001

t is significant if ≥ 2.045

the time needed for the drug to reach the spinal cord and exert its analgesic action.

From the subjective and objective assessment of pain relief and the hourly follow-up of the patients, the duration of analgesia ranged from 2 to 24 hr. Although the duration of analgesia was longer in patients who received 12 mg ketamine, no linear relation could be obtained. Mankowitz *et al.* (1982) found that the duration of analgesia in patients given 4 mg ketamine epidurally varied from 30 min to 6 hr.

The effective dose of epidural ketamine ranged between 8 and 12 mg, although even the 12 mg dose failed to produce any effect in 5 patients. More importantly, we did not notice any correlation between the dose of ketamine and the body weight of the patients. However, in a similar study (Mankowitz *et al.*, 1982), a dose of 4 mg epidural ketamine was effective in alleviating pain. This difference could be explained by many factors: *e.g.*: indication for analgesia (postoperative *vs* chronic pain), wide variation in pain threshold, and unpredictability of ketamine action even when given i.v., i.m., or rectally (Bonica, 1977; Paul *et al.*, 1982).

The mechanism of action of epidural ketamine is not known. Mankowitz *et al.* (1982) have suggested that epidural ketamine relieves pain by an interaction with opiate receptors. Altura *et al.* (1980) showed that ketamine has a local anesthetic action. Against this proposal is evidence that ketamine analgesia is not associated with motor block, loss of sensitivity to temperature, touch or pin prick, or any signs of sympathetic block. The new concept of an *alpha*-adrenergic mechanism for analgesia which is antagonized by *alpha* blocking agents but not by naloxone could also explain ketamine analgesia (Gordh, 1987).

Conclusion

We have found that epidural ketamine induced analgesia is a simple and relatively safe method for relief of postoperative pain. However, this technique needs more study before it can be considered for recommendation as a standard method of postoperative analgesia.

References

Altura, B.M., Altura, B.T., and Corella, A.: Effects of ketamine on vascular smooth muscle function. Br. J. Pharmacol. 70: 257, 1980.

Bonica, J.J.: Importance of effective pain control. Acta Anaesthiol. Scand. 31: Supp 85: 1-16, 1987.

Bonica, J.J.: Neurophysiologic and pathologic aspects of acute and chronic pain. Arch. Surg. 112: 750, 1977.

Bromage, P.R.: Epidural narcotics for postoperative analgesia. Anesth. Analg. 59: 473, 1980.

Craig, D.G.: Postoperative recovery of pulmonary function. Anesth. Analg. 60: 46-52, 1981.

Gordh, T.J.: *Alpha*-adrenergic and cholinergic mechanisms of analgesia. Acta Anaesthesiol. Scand. 86: 31 Supp. 28, 1987.

Kitahata, L.M., Kosaka, Y., Taub, A., Bonikos, K., and Hoffert, M.: Lamina specific suppression of dorsal horn unit activity by morphine sulphate. Anesthesiol. 41: 39, 1974.

Mankowitz, E., Brock-Utne, J.G., Cosnett, J.E., and Green Thompson, R: Epidural ketamine, a preliminary report. S. Afr. Med. J. 61: 441, 1982.

Parkhouse, J., and Holmes, C.M.: Assessing post-operative pain relief. Proc. Roy. Soc. Med. 56: 579, 1963.

Rutter, D.W., Skewes, D.G., and Morgan, M.: Extradural opioids for postoperative analgesia. Br. J. Anaesth. 53: 915, 1981.

Steinhaus, J.E., Bevan, W., Webb, S.C., and Thompson, W.R.: Evaluation of analgesics by the rating of patient behavior. Anesthesiol. 25: 64, 1964.

Torda, T.A., Pybus, D.A., Liberman, H., and Clark, M.: Experimental comparison of extradural and i.m. morphine. Br. J. Anaesth. 52: 939, 1980.

White, P.F., Way, W.L., and Trevor, A.J.: Ketamine-Its pharmacology and therapeutic uses. Anesthesiol. 56: 119, 1982.

Status of Ketamine in Anesthesiology,
edited by E.F. Domino©1990, NPP Books
P.O. Box 1491, Ann Arbor, MI 48106

Caudal Ketamine for Relief of Pain Following Anorectal Surgery

O.E. El-Khateeb

Anesthesia and ICU Department
Jahra Hospital
Jahra, Kuwait

Introduction

Since the identification of opioid receptors in the spinal cord (Pert and Yaksh, 1979), intrathecal and epidural opiates have been widely used to relieve pain and provide postoperative analgesia (Cousins and Mather, 1984). However, their use has been limited by the potential danger of early or delayed respiratory depression (Gustafsson *et al.*, 1982). Therefore, to avoid the drawbacks of opiates, other substances have been tried.

Ketamine is a potent analgesic with minimal respiratory depressant effects (Pender, 1971) which seemed to offer an advantage over the opiates. The demonstration of the safety of intrathecal ketamine with its preservative in baboons by Brock-Utne *et al.* (1981) led Mankowitz *et al.* (1982) to administer ketamine, with the preservative benzethonium chloride, into the extradural space of humans suffering from chronic pain. This was followed by a few other studies with different results (Naguib *et al.*, 1986; Ravat *et al.*, 1987; El-Khateeb *et al.*, 1988). However, nothing is mentioned in the literature regarding the caudal use of ketamine. The purpose of this work was to study efficacy, advantages, and possible side effects of caudal ketamine as a method for postoperative pain relief in patients undergoing anorectal surgery.

Patients and Methods

A single blind, controlled study was performed on 50 ASA I patients who had to undergo a variety of anorectal surgeries (piles, chronic fissure and anorectal fistula). All patients gave their written consents, and the study was approved by the local Ethical Committee. Physical examination, as well as a complete biochemical profile, was done on all patients to exclude any cardiovascular, renal, hepatic or metabolic disorder.

All patients received diazepam (10 mg orally) 1 hr before being brought to the operating theater. Caudal epidural block was performed while the patient was lying down on his face with hips flexed (jack-knife position). Using a 19 gauge spinal needle, 25 ml of 2% xylocaine was injected in a single shot technique. Through the same needle, ketamine (20-50 mg diluted with xylocaine) was injected in 25 patients. In the control group, only 25 ml of 2% xylocaine was injected for operative intervention. Routine intraoperative monitoring included E.C.G., cardiac rate, blood pressure, and oxygen saturation using a pulse oximeter. In the postoperative period, pulse rate, blood pressure, and respiratory frequency per min were monitored.

The onset time of xylocaine block, as well as the duration of the block, were recorded. The time between the end of the xylocaine block (as evidenced by return of pin prick sensation) and the first dose of analgesic within the first 24 hr, was recorded as duration of postoperative analgesia. The dose and timing of the analgesic drug (only pentazocine was used in all patients) were recorded. Side effects noticed during the first 24 hr postoperatively were dealt with and recorded.

Assessment of pain relief was done by the author who had to visit patients every 2 hr during the period of postoperative analgesia, and on the next day after removal of the pack. Assessment was based on subjective (Parkhouse and Holmes, 1963) as well as objective means (Steinhaus *et al.*,1984). The results are shown in Table 1.

Statistical analysis of the data was done by the Student "t" test. The values were considered to be statistically significant at $P \leq 0.05$. A linear regression analysis was also done. The incidence of postoperative complications in both groups was compared using the "Z" test.

Results

The physical characteristics of patients studied and the surgical procedures done were comparable in the 2 groups, as shown in Table 2.

Table 3 shows the dose, onset time, and duration of caudal xylocaine block. The onset of block, as judged by loss of pin prick sensation, was 10.56 ± 4.4 min in the ketamine group, and 10.48 ± 3.9 min in the control group. The difference was statistically insignificant ($t = 0.068$). There was a statistically significant increase in the ketamine group ($t = 2.69$, $P < 0.02$) in the duration of surgical analgesia, which ended at the return of pin prick sensation.

TABLE 1. Modified pain assessment score (M.P.A.S.)

Subjective Parameters	*Objective Parameters*			*Score*
Patient Questionnaire	*Facial Expression*	*Body Movement*	*Cooperation*	
No pain	Relaxed	Little	Complete	0
Mild pain	Tense	Moderate	Good	1
Moderate pain	Very tense	Excessive	Fair	2
Severe pain	Extremely tense	Very excessive	Poor	3

TABLE 2. Age, sex, and type of surgery

			Surgical procedure		
Group	*Sex M/F ratio*	*Age (yr)*	*Piles*	*Fissure*	*Fistula*
Ketamine	19/6	37.88 ± 13.12	20	2	3
Control	14/11	40.32 ± 13.57	18	4	3

TABLE 3. Characteristics of the caudal "xylocaine" block

Group	*Dose ml (2%)*	*Onset (min)*	*Duration (min)*
Ketamine	25	10.56 ± 4.4	87.2 ± 8.9
Control	25	10.48 ± 3.9	79.2 ± 11.9
"t"		0.068	2.69
P		NS	< 0.02

Postoperative analgesia

A statistically significant improvement in all parameters of postoperative analgesia was observed. The duration of analgesia increased from 4.9 ± 4.9 hr in the control group to 10.3 ± 8.8 hr in patients who received ketamine. The total dose of pentazocine used was 57.6 ± 19.2 mg in the control group, while that used by the ketamine group was 37.2 ± 27.7 mg. The difference was statistically significant (t = 3.026, P <0.01). While the M.P.A.S. was 2.04 ± 0.7 in the control group, it reached 0.92 ± 0.99 in the ketamine group. The difference was highly significant (P < 0.001) as shown in Table 4.

The correlation study between the dose of ketamine used and the duration of postoperative analgesia proved to be statistically insignificant

TABLE 4. Characteristics of postoperative analgesia

Group	*Duration of analgesia (hr)*	*Total dose of pentazocine (mg)*	*M.P.A.S.*
Ketamine	10.3 ± 8.8	37.2 ± 27.7	0.92 ± 0.99
Control	4.9 ± 4.9	57.6 ± 19.2	2.04 ± 0.7
"t"	2.681	3.026	4.59
P	<0.02	<0.01	<0.001

TABLE 5. Correlation between dose of ketamine and duration of analgesia

Dose mg	*Number of patients*	*Duration of postoperative analgesia (hr)*
20	18	9.16 ± 8.28
30	2	14.25 ± 13.78
50	5	13.0 ± 10.23

r = + 0.185, "t" = 0.90

(r = 0.185, t = 0.903). Although there was an increase in the duration of postoperative analgesia in patients who received 50 mg of ketamine relative to those who received 20 mg only, the difference was statistically insignificant (t = 0.772; see data, Table 5).

Side Effects

No significant changes were observed in pulse rate, ECG, blood pressure, or respiratory rate in either group, neither during the operative time nor postoperatively for 24 hr. However, other side effects were reported, as listed in Table 6.

Discussion

In the last few years, a few studies have appeared in the literature discussing the analgesic effect of epidural ketamine. However, the results reported are very controversial. While Islas *et al.*, (1985), Naguib *et al.*, (1986), and Abdel Fattah *et al.*, (1988) found lumbar epidural ketamine (in doses of 4 to 120 mg) to be effective in postoperative pain control, other authors (using mostly a smaller range of doses) found that epidural ketamine was unable to relieve postoperative pain (Ivankovich and McCarthy, 1986, Kawana and Araki, 1987; Ravat *et al.*, 1987).

In our present study, there was a definite increase in the duration of postoperative analgesia from 4.9 ± 4.9 to 10.3 ± 8.8 hr. Also, the

TABLE 6. Reported side effects

Group	*Intraoperative*	*Postoperative*	
		Nausea/vomiting	*Urine retention*
Ketamine	Drowziness + involuntary movements (2 Pts)	3	3
Control	—	4	6
Computed			
Z		1.33	3.63
P		NS	<0.01

quality of the postoperative analgesic state was much better than that of the control group (M.P.A.S. of 0.92 ± 0.99 and 2.04 ± 0.7 in each group, respectively). However, the number of patients in the ketamine group who did not need any other form of analgesia in the 1st 24 hr was 7 (28%). In the study of Naguib *et al.* (1986), 54% of patients were completely free of pain after a single 30 mg epidural injection of ketamine. However, their patients were cholecystectomy cases and they used the lumbar epidural approach.

Although we could not find a statistically significant correlation between dose of ketamine and the duration of postoperative analgesia (r = 0.185), there was still a demonstrable increase in the duration of postoperative analgesia (13.0 ± 10.23 hr) in patients who received 50 mg ketamine relative to those who received only 20 mg (9.16 ± 8.28 hr). The same observation has been made by Mankowitz *et al.* (1982) and Naguib *et al.* (1986), who attributed it to the ketamine receptor affinity or the development of tachyphylaxis.

Although postoperative pain, especially that following anorectal surgery, is known to be multifactorial in origin, we can attribute pain relief in the ketamine group to the action of the drug rather than other factors. This is probably true because of the control group used, and as observed in the study by Goligher *et al.* (1984). In that study, 100 patients were operated upon using 5 different techniques for hemorrhoidectomy; there was no statistical difference in postoperative pain scores.

As regards side effects, we noticed involuntary movements in 2 patients in the ketamine group shortly after the block which were associated with drowziness and incoherent speech. Most relevant studies deny such ketamine side effects (Islas *et al.*, 1985; Naguib *et al.*, 1986). However, Ravat *et al.*, (1987), using a dose of 10 mg ketamine epidurally, have reported a sedative effect that could be explained by the vascular uptake from epidural space and a systemic action. Furthermore, psychic disturbances following ketamine anesthesia are well known and vary between 3 and 30 percent (Krestow, 1974; Oduntan and Gool, 1975).

Other side effects (nausea, vomiting, and urine retention) have been reported in the postoperative period. However, their incidence was less in the ketamine group than in the control group. Anorectal surgery, especially hemorrhoidectomy, is known to be associated with a high incidence of urine retention, which is mostly reflex in origin due to the severe pain commonly present (Goligher *et al.*, 1985; Davis, 1987). No cardiovascular or respiratory complications were reported in any of our patients, an observation which is in agreement with almost all related studies.

The mechanism of the analgesic action of epidural ketamine is not clear. While some authors suggest an opioid agonist effect (Smith *et al.*, 1980, Finck and Ngai, 1982), other investigators have failed to demonstrate such interaction with specific opioid receptors (Fratta *et al*, 1980). Ketamine's ability to produce lamina selective suppression of dorsal horn unit activity has been reported by Kitahata *et al.* (1973). The most recent explanation is ketamine's *alpha*-adrenergic effect acting on the noradrenergic pathway (Kawana *et al.*, 1987). Systemic or spinal administration of an $alpha_2$-adrenoreceptor agonist in animals produces an antinociceptive effect antagonized by *alpha*-blocking agents but not by naloxone (Yaksh and Reddy, 1981).

Summary

Caudal epidural ketamine in doses of 20 to 50 mg, although not very predictable, can be considered a simple and quite safe method of postoperative pain relief following anorectal and allied surgical procedures.

References

Abdel Fattah, M.M., Sayed, A.A., Abdel Salem, M.W., Omar, N.S., and Younis, M.M.: Epidural ketamine *vs* morphine for postoperative analgesia. Egypt. J. Anaesth. 4: 65-76, 1988.

Brock-Utne, J.G., Kallichurum, S., Mankowitz, E., Maharaj, R.J., and Dowing, J.W.: Intrathecal ketamine with preservative: Histological effects on spinal nerve root of baboons. S. Afr. Med. J. 61: 440-441, 1981.

Cousins, M.J. and Mather, L.E.: Intrathecal and epidural administration of opioids. Anesthesiol. 61: 276-310, 1984.

Davis, J.E.: Major ambulatory surgery of the general surgical patients, management of anorectal conditions, peripheral vascular problems, and gastrointestinal endoscopy. Surg. Clin. N. Am. 67(4): 761-778, 1987.

El-Khateeb, O.E., Ragab, A., Metwalli, M., and Hassan, H.A.: Assessment of epidural ketamine for relief of pain following vaginal and lower abdominal surgery. 9th World Congress of Anesthesiology, II: A0728, 1988.

Fink A.D. and Ngai, S.H.: Opiate receptor mediation of ketamine anesthesia. Anesthesiol. 56: 291-297, 1982.

Fratta, A.D., Casu, M., Loviselli, A., Biggio, G., and Gessa, G.L.: Failure of ketamine to interact with opiate receptor. Eur. J. Pharmacol. 61: 389-391, 1980.

Goligher, J., Outhie, H. and Nixon, H.: Haemorroids or piles. In Surgery of the Anus, Rectum and Colon, 5th Ed. pp. 129-138, Bailliere Tindall, London, 1984.

Gustafsson, L.L., Schildt, B., and Jacobsen, K.J.: Adverse effects of extradural and intrathecal opiates: Report of a nationwide survey in Sweden. Br. J. Anaesth. 54: 479-486, 1982.

Islas, J., Astorga, J., and Laredo, M.: Epidural ketamine for postoperative pain. Anesth. Analg. 64: 1161-1162, 1985.

Ivankovich, A.D. amd McCarthy, R.J.: Epidural ketamine for control of postoperative pain: Two comments. Anesth. Analg. 65: 989, 1986.

Kawana, A. and Araki, Y.: Epidural ketamine for postoperative pain relief after gynecological operations. A double-blind study and comparison with epidural morphine. Anesth. Analg. 66: 735-738, 1987.

Kitahata, L. M., Taub, A., and Koseka, Y.: Lamina-specific suppression of dorsal-horn unit activity by ketamine hydrochloride. Anesthesiol. 38: 4-11, 1973.

Krestow, M.: The effect of post-anaesthetic dreaming on patients acceptance of ketamine anaesthesia. A comparison with thiopentone-nitrous oxide anaesthesia. Can. Anesth. Soc. J. 21 : 385-389, 1974.

Mankowitz, E., Brock-Utne, J.G., Cosnett, J.E., and Green Thompson, R.: Epidural ketamine—A preliminary report. S. Afr. Med. J. 61: 441-442, 1982.

Naguib, M., Abu-Gyamfi, Y., Absood, G.H., Farag, H., and Gyasi, H.K.: Epidural ketamine for postoperative analgesia. Can. Anesth. Soc. J. 33 : 16-21, 1986.

Oduntan, S.A. and Gool, R.Y.: Clinical trial of ketamine (Cl-581). Can. Anesth. Soc. J. 22: 100-105, 1975.

Parkhouse, J. and Holmes, G.M.: Assessing postoperative pain relief. Proc. Roy. Soc. Med. 56: 579-582, 1963.

Pender, J.W.: Dissociative anaesthesia. JAMA. 215: 1126, 1971.

Pert, A. and Yaksh, T.L.: Site of morphine induced analgesia in primate brain: Relation to pain pathway. Pharmacol. Biochem. Behav. 3: 133-138, 1975.

Ravat, F., Dorne, R., Baechle, J.P., Beaulaton, A., Lenair, B., Leroy, P., and Palmier, B.: Epidural ketamine or morphine for postoperative analgesia. Anesthesiol. 66: 819-822, 1987.

Smith, D.J., Pekoe, G.M., Martin, L.L., and Coalgate, B.: The interaction of ketamine with the opiate receptor. Life Sci. 26: 789-795, 1980.

Steinhaus, J.E., Bevan, W., Webb, S.C., and Thompson, W.R.: Evaluation of analgesics by the rating of patient behavior. Anesthesiol. 25: 64-66, 1964.

Yaksh, T. and Reddy, S.V.T.: Studies in the primate on the analgesic effects associated with intrathecal actions of opiates, alpha-adrenergic agonists and baclofen. Anesthesiol. 54: 451-457, 1981.

Status of Ketamine in Anesthesiology,
edited by E.F. Domino©1990, NPP Books
P.O. Box 1491, Ann Arbor, MI 48106

Anesthesia Requirements for the Severely Burned Patient

I. Feller

Department of Surgery
University of Michigan
Ann Arbor, MI

Anesthesia is a hazard for the severely burned patient. It is important that the anesthesiologist and surgeon cooperate to decrease the morbidity and mortality that can follow operative procedures since the severely burned patient often requires operations while he or she has one or more systemic complications. The anesthesiologist decreases the operative risks by selecting the anesthetic agent which has the least depressive effect on the specific systems. The surgeon contributes by organizing the operating room team so that the length of time anesthesia is needed is reduced to safe limits.

The important factors in determining the severity of a burn are: area of body involved, depth of tissue injury and destruction, age, past medical history, part of body burned, and concurrent injuries that occurred at the time of the accident. The patients at highest operative risk are those with full thickness burns over greater than 40% of the body surface, less than 4 years of age or over 40, having a past medical history involving one or more of the organ systems, and pulmonary injury during the burn accident. These factors, singly or in combination, affect the patient's morbidity and mortality.

The severely burned patient has organ system complications as the rule rather than the exception. The skin is the largest organ of the body. The loss of skin function in burns over 20% full thickness results in a loss of fluids with its electrolytes and allows the invasion of bacteria. The resulting septicemia, dehydration, electrolyte imbalance, and stress lead to organ system complications. The most common complications are septicemia, pneumonia, congestive heart failure, and renal insufficiency. Unfortunately, each patient may have more than one complication at the time an operation is necessary.

It is important to close the burn wound as quickly as possible by supporting the healing of partial thickness burns, debriding, and grafting of the full thickness loss areas. The number of operative procedures required to close a full thickness burn depends on the size of the full thickness injury. For example, full thickness burns involving 50% of the body surface may require five or more autografts. The anesthesiologist and the surgeon must work together to plan each procedure while simultaneously considering the total number of procedures that will have to be carried out. The duration of anesthesia for each procedure can be decreased by preparing the graft donor site and draping the patient before the anesthesia is given. Tranquilizers and hypnotics should be used to decrease the patient's apprehension. This cooperative event requires a team approach by all operating room personnel under the direction of the anesthesiologist and the surgeon. The anesthesia time can be shortened by an average of 30 min or more for each procedure.

The surgeon and his assistants should be at the operating table, gowned and prepared to start the painful part of the operation, as soon as the anesthesia is effective. The number of surgeons should be adequate to carry out all procedures requiring anesthesia for a period not to exceed 30 min. This is possible since the cutting of an autograft is painful but applying the graft is not. Therefore, the graft can be applied to the patient on the day following the operation. The added advantage of this technique is that hemorrhage is controlled, resulting in a higher percent of graft take.

Ketamine is one of the anesthetics of choice for these patients. The period of time necessary for induction is very short, intubation is not necessary, recovery following the cessation of administration of the i.v. dose is rapid, and the patient can resume normal oral alimentation within an hour after the operation.

We have used ketamine as the agent of choice since 1965 in over 2,000 procedures for more than 400 patients with excellent results and minimal complications. The only complication that we have encountered is an erythematous rash on the head, neck, and chest. This appeared in less than 5% of the cases. The duration of this reaction was usually less than one hour.

Psychologic aberrations following ketamine can be avoided by administering diazepam or an equivalent agent before the procedure and just prior to the last dose. We have also found that the dose of ketamine can be titrated to each individual patient. Most patients require less than the recommended dose. When multiple procedures are required, the titration method allows for the corrections needed when tolerance to the drug is noted. We have used ketamine in patients who required as many as 12 procedures to close their wounds.

The use of a nasal cannula for oxygen administration is advised when administering ketamine. Some patients have shallow respirations during the procedures and all benefit from the oxygen because of their basic pathophysiologic conditions.

Summary

The severely burned patient often requires operative procedures with general anesthesia when he or she has one or more organ system complications. This hazard can be lessened by coordinating the anesthesiologist's and surgeon's performance in the operating room. Ketamine is an anesthetic of choice because it has a minimum depressive effect on the organ systems. The surgeon should plan the operation so that the time for anesthesia is limited to 30 min.

Status of Ketamine in Anesthesiology,
edited by E.F. Domino©1990, NPP Books
P.O. Box 1491, Ann Arbor, MI 48106

Ketamine Anesthesia in the I.C.U.– Pros and Cons

J.V. Kyff and J.W. Sybert*

Department of Anesthesia
University of Michigan
Ann Arbor, MI
*and *Department of Anesthesiology*
Botsford General Hospital
Farmington Hills, MI

Introduction

Many uses have been found for ketamine (a "dissociative" anesthetic and derivative of phencyclidine) over the past 25 years. As a general anesthetic agent it has many desirable characteristics that make it easy to use, even in untrained hands. Ketamine leaves airway reflexes intact, and maintains respiration. In addition, it supports blood pressure due to the release of catecholamines. Ketamine also induces intense analgesia and amnesia and suppresses seizures. It has a large toxic to therapeutic dosage ratio, and it may be administered via i.v., i.m., intranasal, sublingual, buccal and epidural routes. On the other hand, protection against aspiration is not guaranteed with ketamine, and respirations may not be maintained. Also, airway reactivity is enhanced, increasing the likelihood of laryngospasm. Blood pressure may not be supported due to direct myocardial depression. In addition, seizures may be induced, and amnesia and analgesia are not guaranteed due to the difficulty in determining the depth of anesthesia (and therefore the timing of subsequent doses). Vivid dreams and hallucinations may occur, resulting in restless, even combative patients. Despite the concomitant administration of amnestic agents, patients often refuse further procedures under ketamine due to recall of these dreams. The ready availability and ease of ketamine administration have resulted in many patients being placed at risk by well meaning, but untrained personnel, both in the I.C.U. and in inappropriate locations, such as the general medical floor.

Early reports of induced seizure activity and cortical stimulation by ketamine in animals and humans, both epileptic and nonepileptic, have led to controversy regarding its use (Manohar *et al.*, 1972; Winters, 1972; Ferrer-Allado *et al.*, 1973; Bennett *et al.*, 1973; Rosen and Hagerdal, 1976; Nelson *et al.*, 1980; Black *et al.*, 1980). Ketamine's epileptogenicity, however, has been refuted by others (Corssen *et al.*, 1974; Celesia *et al.*, 1975; Callaghan and Schwark, 1980; Reder *et al.*, 1980; Myslobodsky *et al.*, 1981) and indeed it has been reported by some to suppress seizure activity (Corssen *et al.*, 1974; Reder *et al.*, 1980; Myslobodsky *et al.*, 1981). To date, no clinical trials of ketamine administration in the treatment of status epilepticus in humans have been reported. The following are three case reports in which status epilepticus, after proving refractory to the usual therapeutic regimen, was responsive to ketamine administration.

Case I

An estimated 70 kg, 55 year old white male was admitted to the Emergency Department after suffering cardiopulmonary arrest while shovelling snow. The patient had no significant past medical history and was taking no medications. Cardiopulmonary resuscitation had been initiated at the scene by Emergency Medical Services and was continued until a normal sinus rhythm was obtained in the Emergency Department following electrical defibrillation. The electrocardiogram demonstrated an acute anterior wall myocardial infarction. Twelve hours after admission, the patient developed status epilepticus which was felt to be due to massive post anoxic encephalopathy, secondary to cardiac arrest. The Neurology Department was asked to consult. An initial electroencephalogram demonstrated "continuous paroxysms of generalized high voltage spike and slow wave activity." The physical examination at this time revealed fixed and dilated pupils, no response to painful stimuli, and no spontaneous respirations (the patient was intubated and placed on controlled ventilation upon admission). Laboratory values were essentially unremarkable. In an attempt to control the status epilepticus, diazepam (40 mg), phenytoin sodium (700 mg), phenobarbital (390 mg), and amobarbital (60 mg) were administered i.v. without effect.

At this point, a member of the Anesthesia Department was asked to consult regarding the use of a general anesthetic agent for seizure control (Brain, 1974). Blood pressure at this time was 90/60 mm Hg, pulse 100 beats per min. Due to the patient's severely debilitated state the risk of hemodynamic depression resulting from a general anesthetic was felt to present too great a risk. Therefore, ketamine (125 mg) was administered i.v. as a bolus and seizure activity terminated immediately. A post ketamine electroencephalogram demonstrated "low voltage with poorly organized background activity . . . generalized depression of cortical function more severe in the left hemisphere."

Breakthrough seizures occurred 90 min following the initial dose of ketamine. These were suppressed following an additional i.v. bolus of 50 mg ketamine. Forty-five min following the second dose facial seizures began, but once again were suppressed following an additional 100 mg i.v. bolus of ketamine. No further seizure activity occurred.

On the third hospital day, the patient developed an apparent pneumonia. This progressed to generalized septicemia and cardiopulmonary arrest on hospital day 5, from which the patient could not be resuscitated. At no time did the patient regain consciousness, respond to painful stimuli, or the pupils constrict and react.

Case II

An estimated 59 kg, 23 year old white female presented to the Emergency Department with sudden onset of flu-like symptoms including fever, nausea, emesis, sore throat, progressing to myalgias, arthralgias, pallor, petachiae and ecchymosis. Her blood pressure was 90/60 mm Hg, heart rate 110 beats/min, temperature 104°F orally, and respirations 24 breaths per/min, with 7 ml per hr of urine output. The patient was admitted to the Intensive Care Unit, begun on triple antibiotic therapy, and closely monitored with a pulmonary artery catheter.

Despite intense monitoring and aggressive therapy, the patient's clinical course continued to deteriorate. She suffered meningoccemia, myocarditis, cardiac dysrhythmia, and ventricular tachycardia, necessitating resuscitation on two occasions. Progressive gangrene of both lower extremities required bilateral below the knee amputations. A toxic megacolon necessitated laparotomy, decompression and colostomy.

On the twelfth hospital day, the patient developed status epilepticus uncontrollable with phenytoin sodium (1.0 g), and phenobarbital (390 mg i.v). Her past medical history was positive for seizure disorder during the preceding three years, which was well controlled on phenytoin sodium (400 mg/day). One day prior to the development of status epilepticus, her serum phenytoin sodium and phenobarbital levels were 8.8 and 20.1 μg/ml, respectively. A serum lactate level of 3.4 was also recorded. We saw this patient in consultation regarding control of seizures (Brain, 1974).

An i.v. drip of 300 mg of ketamine in 50 ml of 5% dextrose in water D5W was established, along with maintenance administration of phenytoin, phenobarbital, and amobarbital. The patient also was cooled with little effect on body temperature. The seizure activity abated and did not reappear. Multiple electroencephalographic recordings obtained during and after ketamine therapy indicated "severe depression of cortical activity." None reported seizure activity.

On the 15th hospital day, the patient expired. Her final diagnosis included acute meningococcemia and Waterhouse-Friderichsen Syndrome.

Case III

An obese, estimated 80 kg, 23 year old white female was found unconscious and unresponsive to painful stimuli in a parked automobile during subfreezing weather. Approximately 4 hr earlier, she had ingested an estimated one-half liter of rum, thirty 50 mg amitriptyline HCl tablets, and 120 Triavil 2-25 (2 mg perphenazine and 25 mg amitriptyline HCl). Her serum ethanol level was 28.8 mg% and her pupils were fixed and dilated. She suffered tachy-brady arrhythmias, hypotension to 80 mm Hg systolic, respiratory insufficiency, and cardiopulmonary arrest, requiring intubation and controlled mechanical ventilation. She also showed generalized seizures of 15 to 30 sec duration at 2 to 3 min intervals, followed by decorticate posturing beginning upon admission to the Emergency Department.

At the time we were asked to see the patient regarding seizure control (Brain, 1974), her condition was as follows: blood pressure 85/49 mm Hg, apical rate of 70 to 80 beats/min with frequent ventricular ectopies, pulmonary artery pressure 19/6, wedge pressure 8, blood gases pH 7.38, PO_2 111, PCO_2 39, on an FIO_2 of 40%, and urine output of 230 ml over 5 hr. Her pupils remained fixed and dilated. The following i.v. medications had been administered: naloxone HCl 0.4 mg, physostigmine sulfate 10 mg, propanolol HCl 3 mg, lidocaine HCl in multiple boluses with a drip running at 4 mg per min, a bretylium tosylate drip at 2 mg per min, dexamethasone sodium phosphate 20 mg, a norepinephrine bitartrate drip at variable rates titrated to blood pressure, phenytoin sodium 700 mg, and phenobarbital 740 mg. In view of the depressed nature of the cardiovascular system, hypotension, irritability of the myocardium and our previous success with the use of ketamine in the treatment of status epilepticus, we once again chose this agent.

Ketamine HCl 125 mg (1.6 mg/kg) in incremental doses was administered i.v. with prompt control of seizure motor activity. A drip was established with 500 mg of ketamine in 100 ml of 0.9% NaCl and titrated to prevent breakthrough seizure activity, approximately 6.25 mg/kg/hr. Phenytoin and phenobarbital were continued every 6 hr. On our recommendation, the patient's arterial pH was adjusted upward toward the 7.5 range to improve cardiac stability and excretion of the tricyclic (Brown *et al.*, 1973; Brown, 1976; Callahan, 1979).

The electroencephalogram recorded 3 hr after the initial dose of ketamine, while on a decreased administration rate of 4.69 mg/kg/hr, showed no seizure activity during the initial 30 min of the tracing. Then, 4 episodes of 6 to 11 sec duration each, with spike and wave activity of central cephalic origin appeared, followed by a return to nonseizure activity. Approximately 12 hr after admission, the ketamine was discontinued by weaning. The remaining cardiovascular support medications, as well as ventilatory support, were removed gradually over the ensuing 3 days.

Subsequent electroencephalograms recorded on hospital days 3 and 7 indicated "moderately severe generalized nonspecific abnormality with suppression of electrocerebral activity" and "mild disturbance of brain function . . . abnormal electroencephalogram", respectively. The patient was discharged to her own care on hospital day 13 and displayed no gross neurologic or cardiovascular abnormalities at that time.

Discussion

Admittedly, a great deal of patient data is missing from the above cases. These data include exact weights, serum phenytoin and phenobarbital levels, mg/kg/min dosages, pre-, intra-, and postketamine administration electroencephalograms, plus additional items normally found in carefully controlled studies. However, the critical nature of these patients, and the urgency of establishing seizure control, led to the omission of much of these data.

While we do not claim to have solved the mystery of ketamine's central nervous system excitation and suppression, we have supplied clinical experience with three specific cases of status epilepticus and the use of ketamine. The catastrophic condition of these patients, and the extensive suppression therapy already utilized, led us to try an unconventional approach only hinted at in the current literature (White *et al.*, 1982).

The authors hope this information may be of value to clinicians called upon to consult when first line therapies for "breaking" status epilepticus have failed or offer risks significantly greater than benefits in specific clinical situations such as those presented here.

REFERENCES

Bennett, D.R., Madsen, J.A., Jordan, W.S., and Wiser, W.C.: Ketamine anesthesia in brain-damaged epileptics. Neurol. 23: 449-460, 1973.

Black, J.A., Golden, G.T., and Fariello, R.G.: Ketamine activation of experimental corticoreticular epilepsy. Neurol. 30: 315-318, 1980.

Brain, W.R.B.: Brain's Diseases of the Nervous System, 4th ed. edited by J.N. Walton, p. 1124, Oxford University Press, 1974.

Brown, T.C.K.: Sodium bicarbonate treatment for tricyclic antidepressant arythmias in children. The Med. J. Australia, 2: 380-382, 1976.

Brown, T.C.K., Barker, G.A., Dunlop, M.E., and Loughnan, P.M.: The use of sodium bicarbonate in the treatment of tricyclic antidepressant-induced arythmias. Anesth. Intens. Care, 1: 203-210, 1973.

Callahan, M.: Tricyclic antidepressant overdose. J. Am. Crit. Emer. Phys. 8: 413-425, 1979.

Callaghan, D.A. and Schwark, W.S.: Pharmacological modification of amygdaloid-kindled seizures. Neuropharmacol. 19: 1131-1136, 1980.

Celesia, G.G., Chen, R.C., and Bamforth, B.J.: Effects of ketamine in epilepsy. Neurol. 25: 169-172, 1975.

Corssen, G., Little, S.C., and Tavakoli, M.: Ketamine and epilepsy. Anesth. Analg. Cur. Res. 53: 319-333, 1974.

Ferrer-Allado, T., Brechner, V., Dymond, A., Cozen, H., and Crandall, P.: Ketamine-induced electroconvulsive phenomena in the human limbic and thalamic regions. Anesthesiol. 38: 333-344, 1973.

Manohar, S., Maxwell, D., and Winters, W.D.: Development of EEG seizure activity during and after chronic ketamine administration in the rat. Neuropharmacol. 11: 819-826, 1972.

Myslobodsky, M.S., Golovchinsky, V., and Mintz, M.: Ketamine: Convulsant or anti-convulsant. Pharmacol. Biochem. Behav. 14: 27-33, 1981.

Nelson, S.R., Howard, R.B., Cross, R.S., and Samson, F.: Ketamine induced changes in regional glucose utilization in the rat brain. Anesthesiol. 52: 330-334, 1980.

Reder, B.S., Trapp, L.D., and Troutman, K.C.: Ketamine suppression of chemically induced convulsions in the two-day-old White Leghorn cockerel. Anesth. Analg. 59: 406-409, 1980.

Rosen, I., and Hagerdal, M.: Electroencephalographic study of children during ketamine anesthesia. Acta Anesth. Scand 20:32-39, 1976.

White, P.F., Way, W.L., and Trevor, A.J.: Ketamine-its pharmacology and therapeutic uses. Anesthesiol. 56: 119-136, 1982.

Winters, W.D.: Epilepsy of anesthesia with ketamine. Anesthesiol. 36: 309-312, 1972.

Status of Ketamine in Anesthesiology,
edited by E.F. Domino©1990, NPP Books
P.O. Box 1491, Ann Arbor, MI 48106

Anesthesia with Propofol and Ketamine

A. Doenicke, H. Suttmann, G. Juhl, J. Kugler, O. Ochmann, and M. Laub

Institute for Anesthesiology
Ludwig-Maximilians University
Munich, F.R. Germany

INTRODUCTION

In the past 30 years there have been many efforts to replace thiopental as an induction agent with non-barbiturate compounds. Trials were undertaken with estil, propanidid, althesin, etomidate and, most recently, with propofol. The first three drugs are not on the market because they cause anaphylactoid reactions or vein irritation, resulting in s.c. necrosis of the forearm. Etomidate provides hemodynamic stability but causes depression of cortisol synthesis, especially when administered over a long period. The most recent development is propofol (a diisopropylphenol), a pure hypnotic with an extremely short half life. It produces some cardiocirculatory depression and reduces cardiac output. Its hemodynamic effects are dose dependent and can be modified by the concomitant administration of benzodiazepines and opioids.

We have shown that propofol reduces blood pressure, which recovers to baseline following tracheal intubation. Clinical experience indicates that the combination with opioids potentiates the decrease in blood pressure caused by propofol. The use of propofol as a continuous i.v. infusion for maintenance of anesthesia has recently become popular. Its extremely short half life results in rapid emergence and postoperative well being. However, as it is a pure hypnotic, clinical usage requires combination with an analgesic. In our investigation of a combination of propofol with ketamine, we have found that propofol abolishes the psychotomimetic effects of ketamine and that the hemodynamic effects of ketamine are opposite to those of propofol. The arterial hypotension associated with the administration of propofol is due partly to a decrease in cardiac output and partly to peripheral vasodilation. Following prolonged administration, especially if combined with fentanyl, propofol will reduce heart rate. In contrast, ketamine produces an increase in cardiac output, blood pressure, and heart rate.

Methods

A randomized, comparative study was conducted with 20 patients of ASA groups I and II undergoing general and orthopedic surgery. Ten patients received a combination of propofol and fentanyl, and 10 patients received a combination of propofol and ketamine. All patients were supplied with air. The depth of anesthesia was controlled via an automatic infusion pump in accordance with continuous EEG analysis. In the event of a decrease in anesthesia, a propofol bolus (0.5 mg/kg) was supplied by the pump in addition to the basal infusion (120 μg/kg/min). When anesthesia deepened below a predetermined level (E0 to E2 defined by EEG analysis), the basic infusion was interrupted. Increases in blood pressure and heart rate of more than 20% were interpreted as a reaction to pain. This was treated with the administration of an additional ketamine bolus of 0.5 mg/kg.

Results

An average of 2.9 mg/kg i.v. of propofol was required in both groups of patients for induction of anesthesia. Continuous EEG analysis made it possible to keep anesthesia at a predetermined level (anesthesia states E0 to E2). In the fentanyl group, the propofol maintenance rate was 124 μg/kg/ min. In the ketamine group it was 149 μg/kg/min. Analgesia was induced by infusion with an average of 4.2 μg/kg of fentanyl (fentanyl group), or 22 μg/kg/min of ketamine.

Blood pressure increased moderately during induction of anesthesia (intubation) and intraoperative blood pressure was stable. Neither hypertension (as observed with ketamine alone) nor hypotension (occasionally observed with propofol) occurred. Severe bradycardia was seen in a few patients but this was successfully treated with atropine. Maintenance of the vegetative and motor reflexes in the ketamine group led to restlessness of the patient during anesthesia. This had to be countered by increased doses of skeletal muscle relaxants.

Postoperative recovery was rapid in both groups. The patients in the ketamine group needed no or only a small dose of analgesics. In addition, they breathed spontaneously and deeply. A few patients reported pleasant dreams. There were no reports of unpleasant dreams, as has occasionally been reported after administration of ketamine alone. A few patients complained postoperatively about distorted and double vision (diplopia).

The combination of propofol and ketamine for the induction and maintenance of anesthesia is an interesting alternative to conventional anesthesia. This kind of anesthesia is a true form of total i.v. anesthesia (TIVA) inasmuch as the patients are supplied with air. Unfortunately, a certain amount of restlessness during the intraoperative phase has to be accepted or sufficient skeletal muscle relaxant has to be administered. In the postoperative phase, stable, satisfactory respiration, and long lasting analgesia can be expected. Our patients reported this anesthetic combination to be pleasant.

Conclusions

Based upon our experience with the combination of propofol and ketamine, the following advantages are apparent:

1. No hemodynamic side effects of propofol are seen during the induction of anesthesia.
2. No respiratory depression occurs postoperatively as opioids are not employed for anesthesia.
3. The psychotomimetic side effects of ketamine are abolished by propofol.

Status of Ketamine in Anesthesiology,
edited by E.F. Domino©1990, NPP Books
P.O. Box 1491, Ann Arbor, MI 48106

Present Position of Ketamine Infusions: A Study of 100 Cases and a Comparison with Propofol

D.L. Coppel and J.W. Dundee

Royal Victoria Hospital
Belfast, Northern Ireland

Continuous infusion of intravenous anesthesia is nothing new, being fairly widely practiced in the early days of thiopental, although not well documented at the time. In 1950 O'Donel Browne described the successful treatment of eclamptic convulsions with infusions of thiopental; however he found a high mortality resulting from "barbiturate overdosage". Clearly thiopental had neither the pharmacokinetic profile (too long lasting) nor the safety required for continuous infusion. The shorter acting methohexital had a satisfactory pharmacokinetics profile, but caused too high an incidence of muscle movement to make it acceptable in this field (McMurray *et al.*, 1986). Over the years it became obvious that one needed a drug with no "antanalgesic" action. For this reason the British steroid "Althesin" was very popular in this field, and its removal for toxicologic reasons left a vacuum in the anesthesiologist's armamentarium. We describe here attempts to fill this vacuum by ketamine, and compare it with more recent studies with propofol.

Uses

Before discussing our findings it is helpful to review the reason for using such techniques and other forms of total i.v. anesthesia. An increasing awareness of the danger of chronic exposure to low concentrations of gaseous or volatile anesthetic agents and their adverse effects on health has been the main stimulus for the development of total i.v. anesthesia (TIVA). This is coupled with the fact that in certain operations, for example neurosurgical procedures, the volatile and gaseous anesthetics do not provide the best or safest operating conditions. Another possible reason for this interest is that, on theoretical grounds, the apparatus used for TIVA should be much simpler and also much less expensive than that used for inhalation agents as one could possibly dispose of bulky cylinders or pipe line gases. (Dundee and Wyant, 1988).

If high frequency jet ventilation had achieved wider acceptance, this would have provided another field for TIVA. It is in this field that the experience reported in this paper has been gained.

The Ideal Drug

The requirement of the ideal drug for TIVA will vary with the circumstances of usage. As an example a long acting drug will be of use in the intensive therapy unit, while fulfilling no place in outpatient (day case) anesthesia. In addition to these pharmacokinetic factors, one should consider the analgetic properties of the agent. Perhaps more correctly, one should consider the absence of antanalgetic action (Dundee and Wyant, 1988). This is a major problem with the barbiturates and otherwise pharmacokinetically suitable agents, such as methohexital, which cause a clinically unacceptably high incidence of extraneous muscle movement when used as an infusion. To some extent, this disadvantage can be overcome by the simultaneous use of a short acting opioid such as alfentanil. However, a drug with some analgetic action would be more valuable (Table 1).

Cardiovascular depression can be a problem with large doses of some drugs or with prolonged infusions, but this also can be minimized by judicious use of opioids. Respiratory depression is more of a theoretical rather than a practical problem, as anesthesiologists are well equipped to deal with this and often induce it deliberately. Apart from problems with long term use of etomidate (Sear *et al.*, 1983), organ toxicity is not a major problem with TIVA and it does not influence the choice of agent.

Water solubility is one of the great advantages of ketamine as is its stability in solution. Drugs which used solubilizing agents, such as cremophor, have now been abandoned, including Althesin, the loss of which prompted the present studies. To date propofol given by continuous rate infusion pumps has caused no administration problems, although it is not suitable for infusion in diluted solutions.

TABLE 1. The ideal drug for total intravenous anesthesia

1. Satisfactory pharmacokinetic profile: not too long lasting, not too cumulative
2. Smooth anesthesia: analgetic action desirable
3. Acceptable degree of toxicity

Present Study

The present study involved 200 patients having major thoracic operations (Table 2). These were all sick subjects with 70+% in both series falling into ASA grades 3 or 4 of physical fitness. Operations lasted 120-135 min and were carried out by staff surgeons in one hospital. All anesthesia was given by senior staff. Infused drugs were administered by constant rate infusion syringes. The two studies were carried out consecutively, with propofol becoming available as the ketamine series was completed.

Preanesthetic medications. Except in very sick patients, 8-10 mg of morphine was given with atropine.

Induction. This varied with the two drugs. In the propofol series, induction was with 1-2 mg kg^{-1} given over 20-30 sec and varying with the fitness of the patient. It was preceded by a small dose of fentanyl or alfentanil. The infusion was started immediately after consciousness was lost. Initially, 2 mg kg^{-1} of ketamine was given for induction (also preceded by a short acting opioid), followed by either diazepam or midazolam. In order to see if thiopental would minimize the hypertension and reduce ketamine dosage, the initial ketamine was replaced in 40 patients by 5 mg kg^{-1} thiopental. Myoneural blockade was with pancuronium or vecuronium.

Infusion

a. The rate varied with the fitness of the patient.

b. The rate was reduced as the operation proceeded.

c. Infusion started at 3 mg kg^{-1} hr^{-1} ketamine or 3-10 mg kg^{-1} hr^{-1} propofol.

d. Infusion stopped on closure of the muscle layer.

With propofol, it soon became apparent that the age of the patient was an important factor. Elderly patients required very small amounts of the drug (Robinson *et al.*, 1985, Dundee *et al.*, 1986).

Ventilation and use of nitrous oxide-oxygen. This was similar in

TABLE 2. Types of operations

Infusion	*Ketamine*	*Propofol*
Lung resection	51	47
Oesophagogastrectomy	18	14
Pleurodesis	14	17
Fundoplication	9	10
Miscellaneous	8	12

both series. Sixty percent of patients received jet ventilation (Acutronic) with oxygen enriched air, while the remainder had double lumen tracheal tubes inserted, and were ventilated (Engstrom) with nitrous oxide and oxygen. Ventilation was adjusted to maintain normality of blood oxygen and CO_2 tensions.

Monitoring. This was standard throughout and included continuous EKG, arterial pressure, expired carbon dioxide, and ventilatory parameters with periodic blood gas analysis.

RESULTS

Clinical anesthesia was satisfactory in all 200 patients, apart from the cardiovascular changes, which will be discussed in detail. There was no evidence of light anesthesia with ketamine, but this was suspected (sweating, lacrimation, or movement) in 20 of the propofol cases (15 without nitrous oxide, 5 with; $P<0.01$). This responded to an increased infusion rate or supplementary opioid. There was no incidence of awareness during anesthesia.

Cardiovascular effects. These differed greatly with the two drugs. The predominantly stimulating action of ketamine contrasted with the depressive effect of propofol.

Table 3 lists the mean recorded rises in systolic blood pressure (SBP) on three occasions during surgery. Thiopental had no significant effect on the degree of hypertension except at the time of retraction of the lung ($P<0.015$). However, these changes were so small as to be of no clinical significance.

Overall, 40% of the patients induced with thiopental and 66% of those with ketamine had a sustained increase in SBP of over 30%. Although these differ significantly ($P <0.05$) even with a thiopental induction, this is clinically unacceptable as the maximum recorded rise in blood pressure was 62.5% after thiopental and 100% after ketamine induction. In one patient, a 60 year old man with a history of alcoholism, despite the use of adrenoreceptor blockers the technique had to be aban-

TABLE 3. Mean increase in systolic blood pressure (mm Hg) at fixed times of observation

Induction agent	*Ketamine*	*Thiopental*
Tracheal intubation	34 ± 3	27 ± 3
Opening of chest	34 ± 3	27 ± 2
Lung retraction	8 ± 2	1 ± 3

doned after 45 min. There were no significant changes in heart rate with ketamine and no significant arrhythmias.

Table 4 shows the degree of hypotension induced by propofol. The fall was was significant ($P<0.02$) immediately postinduction. One should note the attenuation of the hypertensive response to tracheal intubation and the ability of this manoeuvre to restore pressures to acceptable levels. The findings of previous studies (Hendricksson *et al.*, 1985; Coates *et al.*, 1985) were helpful in minimizing the degree of hypotension. Most marked was the benefit of preloading with crystolloid fluids (Verneyum *et al.*, 1987) and slow injection of the induction dose (Dundee *et al.*, 1986). In no cases was the anesthesia stopped or the anesthetic changed because of hypotension. Neither tachycardia nor arrythmias were a problem with propofol.

Propofol dosage. By using accepted criteria as evidence of too light anesthesia and adjusting dosage accordingly it was noted that nitrous oxide markedly reduced the requirement of this agent (Table 5).

Recovery

There were no problems of re-establishing spontaneous ventilation in any patient. Recovery was much more rapid after propofol than following

TABLE 4. Mean blood pressure (MBP) ± S.E. in mm Hg and heart rate (HR) in beats per min associated with propofol anesthesia

	–		+	
Use of nitrous oxide	*MBP*	*HR*	*MBP*	*HR*
Preinduction	92 ± 15	90 ± 18	100 ± 13	89 ± 18
Postinduction	*63 ± 13	87 ± 15	*70 ± 16	84 ± 16
Postintubation	97 ± 20	95 ± 17	104 ± 21	93 ± 19
Intraoperative				
High	92 ± 21	91 ± 16	97 ± 16	88 ± 13
Low	70 ± 16	81 ± 16	70 ± 15	76 ± 14

* Statistically significant fall

TABLE 5. Influence of nitrous oxide on dosage of propofol

Supplement	*Nil*	*Nitrous Oxide*
Mean (± SD) duration of infusion (min)	122 ± 56	121 ± 46
Average total dosage		
mg	915 ± 518	743 ± 37
mg kg^{-1} hr^{-1}	7.2 ± 2.7	5.7 ± 2.0

ketamine. Patients usually opened their eyes on request within 15 min of discontinuation of propofol compared with 20-40 min with ketamine. However the latter delay did not cause any problems.

The time to first postoperative analgesia (given on demand) was 60-70 min with propofol and 200-350 min after ketamine. This latter was significantly shorter ($P < 0.01$) when thiopental was used for induction; 204 ± 28 (SE) min compared with 341 ± 25 min. Unpleasant sequelae were noted only in 6 patients after ketamine (2 hallucinations, 4 unpleasant dreams) and did not constitute a clinical problem. Thiopental appeared to offer some protection (Table 6).

Discussion

It is interesting to note that in 1977-78 workers from our medical school carried out a study of infusions of ketamine in gynecology patients, with operations lasting from 60-90 min. In these studies, they infused a diluted ketamine solution (1 mg/ml) and adjusted the infusion rate manually as required (Lilburn *et al.*, 1978). This technique was abandoned because of excessive bleeding, tachycardia and hypertension, rather than because of the expected emergence delirium. Premedication with lorazepam 4 mg had eliminated this entirely.

Unpleasant postoperative sequelae were again not a problem with ketamine in this study. However, cardiovascular stimulation still caused concern. The attempt to minimize these concerns by using thiopental for induction was only partly successful (Table 6), and was paid for by less prolonged post operative analgesia.

Table 7 summarizes the main differences between ketamine and

TABLE 6. Ketamine infusions: Comparison of findings with ketamine and thiopental induction

Induction	*Ketamine*	*Thiopental*
N	60	40
Mean duration of		
infusion (min)	108	116
dose mg (± S.E.)	506 ± 27	385 ± 28
mg/kg	7.7 ± 0.3	5.9 ± 0.4
SBP rise of 30%	66%	40%
time to first postop analgesia (min)	341 ± 25	204 ± 28
Sequelae		
Hallucinations	1	1
Unpleasant dreams	4	0

TABLE 7. Comparison of the relative merits of ketamine and propofol for total intravenous anesthesia

	Ketamine	*Propofol*
Onset of action	Slow	Rapid
Analgesic action	+ +	+
Controlability	+	+ +
Cardiovascular effects	Stimulation	Depression
Recovery	Slow	Prompt
Postoperative analgesia	Good	Adequate

propofol which have emerged from this study. The slower onset of action of ketamine is only important when one has to suddenly increase the depth of anesthesia; this is unlikely with this agent. The more rapid onset of action of propofol also means greater danger of inadvertently producing too deep anesthesia with its accompanying hypotension; on the other hand, this is accompanied by an ability to rapidly lighten anesthesia. This all points out the need for extra vigilance with propofol, which also has the problem of lower dosage requirements in the elderly. Based on the experience of Robinson and her colleagues (1985), "elderly" could mean anyone over the age of 55 years. One should never underestimate the need for experience in anesthesiologists for TIVA. However, it would appear that this is more important with propofol than with ketamine.

One must not underestimate the dangers of cardiovascular depression with propofol but, as in the previous Belfast study (Lilburn *et al.*, 1978), the hypertensive response to ketamine produced problems and limits its use in certain patients. There are many patients who could not tolerate even temporary hypotension and for them ketamine could be the drug of choice.

Up to the moment we have not commented on the cost and availability of these two agents. Ketamine is inexpensive and available world wide. It can be administered in dilute solution without any special equipment. By contrast, propofol is expensive and available only in certain countries. It needs power driven syringes for continuous infusion.

The propofol data reported here, are described in more detail by Milligan *et al.* (1990).

Acknowledgements

These studies required great cooperation from the thoracic surgeons and nursing/technical staff in our hospital, to whom we are grateful. Thanks are also due to the many anesthetists who assisted in this work.

References

Coates, D.P., Prys-Roberts C., Spelina K.R., Monk, C.R., and Norley, I.: Propofol (Diprivan) by intravenous infusion with nitrous oxide: dose requirements and haemodynamic effects. Postgrad. Med. J. 61 (Suppl 3): 76-79. 1985.

Dundee, J.W., Robinson F.P., McCollum J.S.C., and Patterson C.C.: Sensitivity to propofol in the elderly: Anaesthesia 41: 482-485. 1986.

Dundee, J.W. and Wyant, G.M.: Intravenous Anaesthesia 2nd Ed., Churchill, Livingstone, 1988.

Henriksson, B.A., Carlsson, P., Hallen, B., Hagerdal M., Lundberg, D., and Ponten, J.: Propofol (Diprivan) versus thiopentone in nitrous oxide/oxygen anaesthesia for short gynaecological procedures (Abstract). Postgrad. Med. J. 61 (suppl 3): 102. 1985.

Lilburn, J.K., Dundee J.W., and Moore, J.: Ketamine infusions—observations on technique and dosage and cardiovascular effects. Anaesthesia 32,315-321, 1978.

Milligan, K.R., Coppel, D.L., Johnston, J.R., and Cosgrove, J.: Propofol as a total intravenous anaesthetic agent for major thoracic surgery. J. of Cardiothoracic Surg. In press, 1990.

McMurray, T.J., Robinson F.P., Dundee J.W., Riddell J.G., and McClean, E.: A new method for producing constant plasma drug levels: Application to methohexitone. Br. J. Anaes. 57: 1085-1090. 1986.

O'Donel Browne: The treatment of eclampsia. J. Obst. Gyn. of the British Empire 57: 773-582. 1980.

Robinson, F.P.: Propofol (Diprivan) by intermittent bolus with nitrous oxide in oxygen for body surface operations. Postgrad. Med. J. 61 (suppl 3): 116-19. 1985.

Sear, J.W., Allen, M.C., Gales, M., McQuay, H.J., Kay, N.H, McKenzie, P.J., and Moore, R.A.: Suppression by etomidate of normal cortisone response to anaesthesia and surgery. Lancet ii: 1028. 1983.

Vermeyen, K.M., Erpels, F.A., Jansen, L.A., Beeckman, C.P., and Hanegreefs, G.A.: Propofol-fentanyl anaesthesia for coronary bypass surgery in patients with good left ventricular function. Br. J. Anaes. 59 1115-1120. 1987.

Status of Ketamine in Anesthesiology,
edited by E.F. Domino©1990, NPP Books
P.O. Box 1491, Ann Arbor, MI 48106

The Role of Ketamine in Cardiac Anesthesia

K.J. Tuman and A.D. Ivankovich

Department of Anesthesiology
Rush-Presbyterian-St. Luke's Medical Center
Chicago, IL

INTRODUCTION

Anesthesia for cardiovascular surgery in patients with debilitating cardiac disease remains a significant challenge for anesthesiologists. The lack of cardiodepression and an anti-arrhythmic action make ketamine a useful agent for anesthetic induction and maintenance in patients at risk for hemodynamic instability. When ketamine became available as an i.v. anesthetic in 1970, these properties promised to lessen the dangers of severe hypotension and dysrhythmias which were associated with most other anesthetics available at that time. In addition, the intense analgesia and amnesia associated with ketamine were further desirable features. Despite these attributes, however, ketamine did not gain widespread acceptance in cardiovascular surgery during the 1970s. As clinical experience with ketamine increased, it was recognized that its use was occasionally associated with cardiostimulatory effects which could be deleterious in patients with coronary artery disease or certain types of valvular heart disease. As ketamine's pharmacokinetic and pharmacodynamic properties became better understood, it was recognized that continuous infusions of ketamine as the main component of balanced anesthesia provided not only profound analgesia-amnesia, but also remarkable cardiorespiratory stability.

Over the years, it has become apparent that any single-agent anesthetic approach is unlikely to provide optimal anesthesia in open heart surgery. The realization that anesthetic agents must be supplemented with other drugs in order to achieve hemodynamic stability and avoid wide swings in blood pressure or heart rate led to interest in "balanced" anesthetic techniques. For example, high dose morphine anesthesia was initially introduced as an alternative to inhalational agents for the management of patients undergoing cardiovascular surgery (Stanley *et al.*, 1973). With experience, however, it became apparent that morphine was associated with a significant incidence of breakthrough hypertension, as well as increased fluid requirements secondary to histamine release and increased vascular capacitance. The newer narcotic agonists, fentanyl and sufentanil, act more specifically at the *mu* opiate receptor and are associated with fewer side effects, such as histamine release and direct venodilation. As such, hypotension related to the latter mechanisms is not commonly seen intraoperatively when these narcotics are used as a single-agent anesthetic approach, but hypotension as well as breakthrough hypertension still occur in a significant proportion of patients when these drugs are used alone for cardiac anesthesia (Benthuysen *et al.*, 1988). Because of this, all available anesthetics usually require supplementation with drugs to maintain hemodynamic stability. Avoidance of a rigid approach by choosing the combination of drugs (anesthetic and non-anesthetic) to achieve this goal is probably more important than the individual drugs chosen. Thus, the other components of the balanced anesthetic technique may include benzodiazepines, barbiturates, nitrous oxide, inhalational agents, or non-anesthetic drugs which act on the cardiovascular system (*e.g.*, anticholinergics, *alpha*-adrenergic blockers, *beta*-adrenergic blockers, calcium entry blockers, etc.). It is well known that diazepam premedication predictably blocks not only the cardiostimulatory (Kothary *et al.*, 1975; Hatano *et al.*, 1976a,b; Jackson *et al.*, 1978; Dhadphale *et al.*, 1979; Zsigmond *et al.*, 1980; Idvall *et al.*, 1983), but also the neuropsychiatric (Kothary *et al.*, 1975; Idvall *et al.*, 1979; Zsigmond *et al.*, 1980) effects of ketamine while preserving its beneficial effects. As such, diazepam has been combined with ketamine in a balanced anesthetic technique since the early 1970s, and has proven to be a remarkably safe and well tolerated anesthetic for patients undergoing open heart surgery. The following discussion reviews the clinical experience with ketamine in open heart surgery, plus additional information about the drug's cardiovascular effects which is essential to understanding the role of ketamine in this setting.

Cardiovascular Effects of Ketamine

Ketamine is the only i.v. anesthetic that routinely stimulates the cardiovascular system. Early clinical researchers recognized this unique trait and proposed the use of ketamine for cardiac and poor risk patients because of its remarkable intraoperative cardiovascular stability (Corssen *et al.*, 1970; Nettle *et al.*, 1973; Rodney *et al.*, 1974; Reves *et al.*, 1978). The hemodynamic effects of ketamine have since been extensively studied in animals, human volunteers, and patients with a variety of cardiac diseases. Many studies have noted that when ketamine is used alone, there are significant increases in heart rate, mean arterial blood pressure, cardiac output, systemic and pulmonary artery pressures, and peripheral vascular resistance (Virtue *et al.*, 1967; Tweed *et al.*, 1972; Tweed and Mymin, 1974). These changes may cause an increase in both the minute work of the heart as well as myocardial oxygen consumption. Patients with severe coronary artery or myocardial disease have a limited ability to increase myocardial oxygen supply, and in this setting ketamine, as the sole agent, might be deleterious. Similarly, in patients with stenotic valvular lesions, tachycardia may severely limit diastolic filling, resulting in decreased preload and loss of cardiac output. On the other hand, the cardiac stimulatory effects of ketamine alone are invaluable in patients with cardiac tamponade, constrictive pericarditis, cardiogenic shock and severe terminal cardiomyopathy, as in heart transplant patients (Gutzke *et al.*, 1987). Indeed, these latter conditions are perhaps the only indications for the use of ketamine as the sole anesthetic agent for cardiac surgery.

The cardiostimulatory effects of ketamine were initially thought to arise from increased sympathetic nervous system activity and norepinephrine release secondary to depression of baroreceptor reflex activity (Dowdy and Kaya, 1968; Slogoff and Allen, 1974). Further investigations, however, revealed that the cardiostimulatory effects result primarily from the direct action of ketamine on the central nervous system structures (Chodoff, 1972). Experimental studies have found that ketamine cardiostimulation occurs only in the absence of significant central nervous system depression (Ivankovich *et al.*, 1974a,b). When central nervous system depressants such as thiopental or halothane are administered first, there is minimal cardiovascular stimulation. It has also been demonstrated that ketamine cardiostimulation is accompanied by a simultaneous increase in serum catecholamine levels, which occurs as early as 2 min after an i.v. dose and returns to control levels within 15 min (Kothary *et al.*, 1975; Zsigmond *et al.*, 1980). Thus, although direct central nervous system stimulation seems to be the primary mechanism of ketamine's cardiostimulatory effects, there may also be stimulatory effects on the peripheral sympathetic nervous system at the level of the sympathetic ganglia (Slogoff and Allen, 1974). Analogous to cocaine, ketamine is a potent inhibitor of neuronal norepinephrine reuptake, although this peripheral effect does not appear to play a significant role in cardiovascular stimulation (Miletich *et al.*, 1973). Some investigators have also reported a dose dependent inhibition of extraneuronal norepinephrine uptake (Nedergaard, 1973).

Experimental studies have shown that, in addition to indirect cardiostimulatory actions, high doses of ketamine may have a direct negative inotropic effect (Traver *et al.*, 1968). However, at the low doses used clinically, this depressant effect of ketamine is overridden by the central stimulatory effect, except in the presence of catecholamine depletion (such as might occur in severe, prolonged shock states).

As shown in Table 1, many different drugs can block or attenuate the cardiostimulatory effects of ketamine. Because ketamine's cardiovascular actions are primarily centrally mediated, *alpha*-and *beta*-adrenergic blocking drugs, cholinergic blocking drugs, and calcium entry blocking drugs provide only a partial blockade. The administration of central nervous system depressants is a more logical and effective method of attenuating the cardiostimulatory effects of ketamine. General anesthetics and barbiturates are both effective, but the most consistently effective and clinically practical drugs for this use are the benzodiazepines (Kothary *et al.*, 1975; Hatano *et al.*, 1976a,b; Jackson *et al.*, 1978; Dhadphale *et al.*, 1979; Zsigmond *et al.*, 1980; Idvall *et al.*, 1983).

Diazepam is the benzodiazepine which has been most commonly combined with ketamine for use in patients undergoing open heart surgery. Diazepam not only prevents the cardiostimulatory effects of ketamine but also greatly diminishes the risk of postoperative emergence reactions, such as nightmares, hallucinations, and disorientation (Kothary *et al.*, 1975; Zsigmond *et al.*, 1980). Moreover, diazepam pretreatment does not interfere with the desirable features of ketamine, which include amnesia, analgesia, maintenance of protective laryngeal and cough reflexes, and lack of organ system toxicity. The cardiostimulatory effects and the incidence of emergence reactions are further lessened when ketamine is administered as a continuous i.v. infusion rather than as bolus injections (Idvall *et al.*, 1979).

TABLE 1. Drugs that block or attenuate the cardiostimulatory effects of ketamine

Atropine	Barbiturates
Alpha-adrenergic blockers	Benzodiazepines
Beta-adrenergic blockers	High spinal or epidural anesthesia
Calcium entry blockers	Inhalational anesthetics
Chlorpromazine	
Droperidol	

Clinical Experience With Diazepam-Ketamine in Cardiac Surgery

Several studies have evaluated the effects of diazepam pretreatment on the cardiostimulatory action of ketamine in patients undergoing open heart surgery (Hatano *et al.*, 1976a,b; Jackson *et al.*, 1978; Dhadphale *et al.*, 1979; Idvall *et al.*, 1983). The induction and maintenance of anesthesia using this technique has been reported to produce satisfactory anesthesia with little or no increase in heart rate, mean arterial pressure, rate pressure product, cardiac index, or systemic vascular resistance (Hatano *et al.*, 1976a,b; Jackson *et al.*, 1978; Dhadphale *et al.*, 1979; Idvall *et al.*, 1983; Tuman *et al.*, 1988; see Table 2). The stability of circulatory parameters is enhanced when ketamine is administered by continuous infusion rather than bolus injection because rapid changes in plasma drug levels are avoided and the total ketamine dose is reduced (Idvall *et al.*, 1979).

Clinical experience at our institution using diazepam-ketamine anesthesia for open heart surgery was reported in a 1976 study of 200 patients. This study demonstrated that a continous "micro-mini" ketamine infusion, combined with intermittent i.v. doses of diazepam, resulted in minimal effects on the cardiovascular and respiratory systems, excellent amnesia, and a very low incidence of postoperative emergence reactions (Hatano *et al.*, 1976a,b). The results of this early work were so impressive that ketamine-diazepam became the most popular choice of anesthetic in

TABLE 2. Hemodynamic Parameters During Diazepam-Ketamine (DK) Anesthesia for Aortocoronary Revascularization

	Control	*After DK*	*Intubation*	*Sternotomy*
HR	75	76	75	78
MAP	101	91	94	90
MPAP	23	21	21	21
PAOP	14	14	14	13
CI	2.5	2.4	2.4	2.4
SI	34	33	33	31
SVR	1582	1460	1516	1581
PVR	123	126	134	131
LVSWI	41	34	37	34

HR = heart rate (beats/min); MAP = mean arterial pressure (torr); MPAP = mean pulmonary artery pressure (torr); PAOP = pulmonary artery occlusion pressure (torr); CI = cardiac index ($l/min/m^2$); SI = stroke index ($ml/beat/m^2$); SVR = systemic vascular resistance ($dyne\text{-}sec\text{-}cm^{-5}$); PVR = pulmonary vascular resistance ($dyne\text{-}sec\text{-}cm^{-5}$); LVSWI = left ventricular stroke work index ($gm\text{-}m/m^2$). (Adapted from Tuman *et al*: J. Cardiothorac. Anesth. 2:419, 1988.)

patients undergoing heart valve and aortocoronary bypass surgery at our institution. To date, diazepam-ketamine has been used in over 3000 heart valve and 8000 coronary artery bypass operations. Recent work has compared the outcomes of patients undergoing cardiac surgery under a variety of anesthetic techniques and has demonstrated that diazepam-ketamine was associated with excellent results (Tuman *et al.*, 1989). In addition to its well known intraoperative hemodynamic stability, this technique has also been demonstrated to have significant advantages in the postoperative period as well (Tuman *et al.*, 1988).

The current methods of administering diazepam-ketamine anesthesia are similar to that originally described by Hatano *et al.* (1976a,b). Patients are premedicated with oral diazepam (10-15 mg) 90 min before anesthesia is started. Sixty min before anesthesia, atropine (0.4 mg) is given i.m. as an antisialogogue to reduce excessive salivary secretions occasionally associated with ketamine administration. Following preoxygenation, induction of anesthesia is usually started with 5 mg increments of diazepam administered sequentially, while an infusion of 0.1% ketamine is simultaneously administered i.v. Blood pressure and other circulatory parameters are carefully monitored during this period, and total ketamine induction doses range from 1.5 to 2 mg/kg, while the total diazepam dose ranges from 0.4 to 0.8 mg/kg. In elderly and debilitated patients, the lower dosage is usually sufficient, while in younger, more robust patients, the higher doses are usually required. After the patient is unresponsive, a neuromuscular blocker is administered and the trachea is intubated. The ketamine infusion is continued at the rate of approximately 1 mg/kg/hr and is usually supplemented with approximately 5 mg of diazepam every 60-90 min.

Using this technique, blood pressure and heart rate usually remain close to preoperative values (Fig. 1), and there is usually little change, even with surgical stimulation. However, a hypertensive response to intubation and surgical stimulation may occur in the younger, more robust patients undergoing aortocoronary bypass procedures. To prevent this response, small doses of i.v. anesthetics, such as thiopental, or narcotics, as well as low doses of inhalational anesthetic agents, or vasodilators, such as nitroprusside or nitroglycerine, may need to be administered.

Comparison of Diazepam-Ketamine and Narcotic Anesthesia Techniques

The primary alternatives to diazepam-ketamine anesthesia for cardiac surgery are the narcotic based techniques. High dose morphine anes-

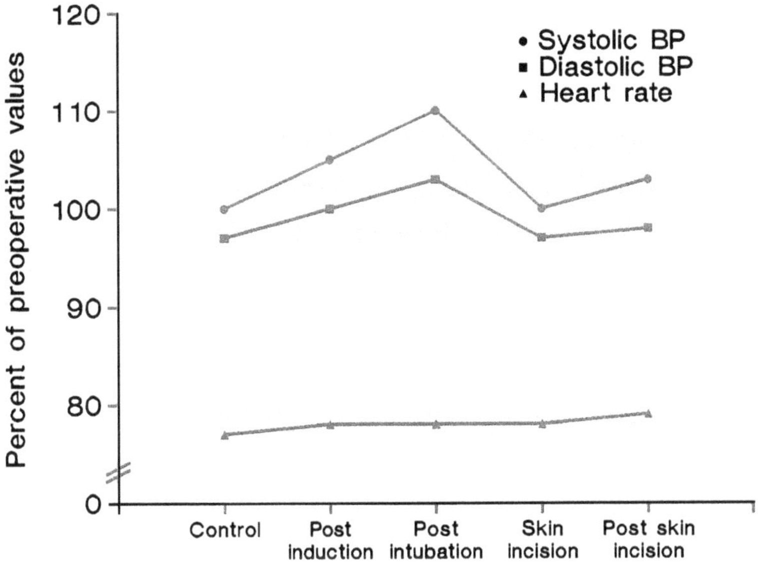

Fig. 1. Effect of diazepam-ketamine on blood pressure and heart rate. (Adapted from Anaesthesist, Hatano *et al.*, 1976b.)

thesia is no longer employed, primarily because of the cardiovascular difficulties entailed, most notably profound hypotension during induction. A sudden and profound drop in blood pressure following induction is one of the most hazardous intraoperative events in open heart surgical patients. It is very likely that the low morbidity and mortality rates reported with the use of diazepam-ketamine have in large part been due to the avoidance of hypotension with the latter technique. Another problem during high dose morphine anesthesia is the enormous increase in blood and fluid requirements, presumably due to histamine release. Moreover, intraoperative awareness has occurred with morphine "anesthesia", and significant cardiovascular depression often complicates attempts to increase doses above 1-3 mg/kg or to use various adjuvants to enhance anesthesia.

While less frequent, profound hypotension and other problems of morphine anesthesia may also occur with more potent opiate narcotics, such as fentanyl and sufentanil (Spiess *et al.*, 1986). Sufentanil and fentanyl are also associated with a high incidence of bradycardia, truncal rigidity, and breakthrough hypertension (Benthuysen *et al.*, 1988). Attempts to enhance anesthesia with diazepam or other agents increase the risk of significant cardiovascular depression (Tomicheck *et al.*, 1983).

Most high dose narcotic techniques that have been shown to produce intraoperative stability during cardiac surgery do so at the expense of significant amounts of residual anesthetic at the end of surgery. These residual plasma and tissue levels of narcotics may be unbalanced by noxious stimulation in the early postoperative period and are often responsible for lower blood pressures due to lower sympathetic and vascular tone. This is most profound when high dose morphine anesthesia is used, but occurs even when high-dose fentanyl is used for cardiac anesthesia. In one study, comparing diazepam-ketamine to high dose fentanyl anesthesia for open heart surgery, patients receiving high dose fentanyl had lower systemic arterial pressures and vascular resistances and required more vasopressors during the first 12 hr postoperatively. They also had a more positive cumulative fluid balance at 24 and 48 hr postoperatively, despite a higher incidence of postoperative diuretic use in patients receiving high-dose fentanyl (Tuman *et al.*, 1988). The decreased postoperative fluid and vasopressor requirements of diazepam-ketamine, compared to high dose fentanyl, may be related to its ability to preserve vascular tone, venous capacitance, and venous return (Hoka *et al.*, 1985). In addition, time until awakening from anesthesia and length of ICU stay were significantly greater with high dose fentanyl than with diazepam-ketamine. The diminished need for postoperative fluids and vasopressors, and a more rapid awakening time, suggest that diazepam-ketamine may provide a less complicated and less costly postoperative course than other types of anesthesia for cardiac surgery. The decrease in vasopressor requirements in patients receiving diazepam-ketamine compared to other primary narcotic or inhalational anesthetic techniques has also been demonstrated in a series of over 1000 consecutive aortocoronary bypass graft patients (Tuman *et al.*, 1989). Information on the postoperative effects of long acting anesthetic agents is sparse, and more studies of these effects and their mechanisms are necessary because they may affect patient management after cardiac surgery.

Conclusion

Compared with other techniques, the advantages of balanced diazepam-ketamine anesthesia far outweigh any potential drawbacks. While some patients experience hypertensive responses to intubation and surgical stimulation, such responses also occur with narcotic based anesthetic techniques. Moreover, hypertensive responses to ketamine can be safely and efficaciously overcome by administering small doses of other i.v. anesthetics, inhalational anesthetics, or vasodilators. The incidence of postoperative delirium does not appear to be significantly higher than it is following other anesthetic techniques used in open heart surgical patients.

The use of balanced anesthetic techniques, such as the diazepam-ketamine technique, offers greater intraoperative safety, a more stable postoperative course, and more complete anesthesia than "pure" anesthetic techniques, such as high-dose fentanyl. Recent studies suggest that moderate (rather than high) doses of fentanyl, combined with low doses of ketamine, not only provide more adequate anesthesia than fentanyl alone but also result in minimal hemodynamic changes, no recall of intraoperative events, and low risk of postoperative emergent phenomena (Newsome *et al.*, 1984). Such findings emphasize the value of a balanced approach to anesthesia administration in open heart surgery.

References

Benthuysen, J.L., Foltz, B.D., Smith, N.T., *et al.*: Prebypass hemodynamic stability of sufentanil, fentanyl and morphine-O_2 anesthesia during cardiac surgery. J. Cardiothorac. Anesth. 2: 749-757, 1988.

Chodoff, P.: Evidence for central adrenergic action of ketamine: Report of a case. Anesth. Analg. 51: 247-250, 1972.

Corssen, G., Allarde, R., Brosch, F., *et al.*: Ketamine as the sole anesthetic in open-heart surgery: A preliminary report. Anesth. Analg. 49: 1025-1031, 1970.

Dhadphale, P.R., Jackson, A.P.F., and Alseri, S.: Comparison of anesthesia with diazepam and ketamine *vs* morphine in patients undergoing heart-valve replacement. Anesthesiol. 51: 200-203, 1979.

Dowdy, E.G. and Kaya, K.: Studies of the mechanism of cardiovascular responses to CI-581. Anesthesiol. 29: 931-943, 1968.

Gutzke, G.E., Shah, K., Glisson, S.N., *et al.*: Sufentanil or ketamine: Induction in cardiomyopathy patients. Anesthesiol. 63: 64, 1987.

Hatano, S., Keane, D.M., Boggs, R.E., *et al.*: Diazepam-ketamine anaesthesia for open heart surgery—a micro-mini drip administration technique. Can. Anaesth. Soc. J. 23: 648-656, 1976a.

Hatano, S., Sadove, M.S., Keane, D.M., *et al.*: Diazepam-ketamine anaesthesia for open heart surgery: "Micro-mini" drip administration technique. Anaesthesist 25: 457-463, 1976b.

Hoka, S., Takeshita, A., Yamamoto, K., *et al.*: The effects of ketamine on venous capacitance in rats. Anesthesiol. 62: 145-148, 1985.

Idvall, J., Aronsen, K.F., Stenberg, P., *et al.*: Pharmacodynamic and pharmacokinetic interactions between ketamine and diazepam. Eur. J. Clin. Pharmacol. 24: 337-343, 1983.

Idvall, J., Ahlgren, I., Aronsen, K.F., *et al.*: Ketamine infusions: Pharmacokinetics and clinical effects. Br. J. Anaesth. 51: 1167-1173, 1979.

Ivankovich, A.D., Miletich, D.J., Reimann, C., *et al.*: Cardiovascular effects of centrally administered ketamine in goats. Anesth. Analg. 53: 924-933, 1974a.

Ivankovich, A.D., Miletich, D.J., and Albrecht, R.F.: Effect of ketamine on cerebral blood flow in goats. MAC XI: Anesthesia and the neuromuscular system. ISA Bulletin 7: 26-30, 1974b.

Jackson, A.P.F., Dhadphale, P.R., Callaghan, M.L., and Alseri, S.: Haemodynamic studies during induction of anaesthesia for open-heart surgery using diazepam and ketamine. Br. J. Anaesth. 59: 375-377, 1978.

Kothary, S.P., Zsigmond, E.K., and Matsuki, A.: Antagonism of the ketamine-induced rise in plasma free-norepinephrine, blood pressure and pulse rate by intravenous diazepam. Clin. Pharmacol. Ther. 17: 238, 1975.

Miletich, D.J., Ivankovich, A.D., Albrecht, R.F., *et al.*: The effect of ketamine on catecholamine metabolism in the isolated perfused rat heart. Anesthesiol. 39: 271-277, 1973.

Nedergaard, O.A.: Cocaine-like effect of ketamine on vascular adrenergic neurones. Eur. J. Pharmacol. 23: 153-161, 1973.

Nettle, D.C., Herrin, T.J., and Mullen, J.G.: Ketamine induction in poor-risk patients. Anesth. Analg. 52: 59-64, 1973.

Newsome, L.R., Moldenhauer, C.C., Hug, C.C., *et al.*: Hemodynamic interactions of moderate doses of fentanyl with etomidate and ketamine. Abstracts 6th Annual Society of Cardiothoracic Anesthesia Meeting, Boston, MA, pp 190-191, 1984.

Reves, J.G., Lell, W.A., McCracken, L.E., *et al.*: Comparison of morphine and ketamine anesthetic techniques for coronary surgery: A randomized study. South. Med. J. 71: 33-36, 1978.

Rodney, P.A., Arai, T., and Nagashima, H.: Ketamine-gallamine anaesthetic for great vessel operation in infant. Anesth. Analg. 53: 365-369, 1974.

Slogoff, S. and Allen, G.W.: The role of baroreceptors in the cardiovascular response to ketamine. Anesth. Analg. 53: 704-707, 1974.

Spiess, B.D., Sathoff, R., El-Ganzouri A., *et al.*: High dose sufentanil: Four cases of sudden hypotension on induction. Anesth. Analg. 65: 703-705, 1986.

Stanley, T.H., Gray, N.H., Stanford, W., *et al.*: The effect of high-dose morphine on fluid and blood requirements in open heart operations. Anesthesiol. 38: 536-541, 1973.

Tomicheck, R.C., Rosow, C.E., Philbin, D.M., *et al.*: Diazepam-fentanyl interaction-hemodynamic and hormonal effects in coronary artery surgery. Anesth. Analg. 62: 881-884, 1983.

Traver, D.K., Wilson, R.D., and Priano, L.L.: Differentiation of the cardiovascular effects of CI-581. Anesth. Analg. 47: 769-778, 1968.

Tuman, K.J., Keane, D.M., Spiess, B.D., *et al.*: effects of high-dose fentanyl on fluid and vasopressor requirements after cardiac surgery. J. Cardiothorac. Anesth. 2: 419-429, 1988.

Tuman, K.J., McCarthy, R.J., Spiess, B.D., *et al.*: Does choice of anesthetic agent significantly affect outcome after coronary artery surgery? Anesthesiol. 70: 189-198, 1989.

Tweed, W.A., Minuck, M., and Mymin, D.: Circulatory responses to ketamine anesthesia. Anesthesiol. 37: 613-619, 1972.

Tweed, W.A. and Mymin, D.: Myocardial force-velocity relations during ketamine anesthesia at constant heart rate. Anesthesiol. 41: 49-52, 1974.

Virtue, R.W., Alanis, J.M., Mori, M., *et al.*: An anesthetic agent: 2-orthochlorophenyl, 2-methylaminocyclohexanone HCI (CI-581). Anesthesiol. 47: 823-833, 1967.

Zsigmond, E.K., Kothary, S.P., Kumar, S.M., *et al.*: Counteraction of circulatory side effects of ketamine by pretreatment with diazepam. Clin. Ther. 3: 28-32, 1980.

Status of Ketamine in Anesthesiology,
edited by E.F. Domino©1990, NPP Books
P.O. Box 1491, Ann Arbor, MI 48106

The Use of a Ketamine-Midazolam Combination for Sedation and Analgesia in Intensive Care Patients

H.A. Adams, J. Biscoping, W. Russ, and G. Hempelmann

Department of Anesthesiology and Intensive Care Medicine
Justus-Liebig University
D-6300 Giessen, F.R. Germany

Introduction

Analgo-sedation in intensive care patients is one of the still unsolved problems in anesthesiology. One "standard regimen" follows the other at close intervals. In the early days of intensive care medicine, sedation and analgesia for respirator treatment were simply interpreted as a continuation of general anesthesia by other means. Today, emphasis is placed on the individual situation of the patients and toward maintaining their cooperation as far as possible.

Evaluation and comparability of clinical investigations in intensive care patients are difficult due to different basic diseases, heterogeneous groups of patients, and use of numerous potent drugs. The present investigation was undertaken with the same restrictions.

It was not the aim of this study to create a new "standard regimen", but to consider the following:

1. Assessment of sedation and analgesia in intensive care patients using reliable clinical, endocrine, and neurological data.
2. Comparison of two different regimens for sedation and analgesia, focusing on specific indications for a combination of ketamine and midazolam.

Methods

Patients and groups

A total of 16 patients in an operative intensive care unit was investigated. Due to their clinical situation, all patients needed controlled ventilatory support for at least 48 hours. Exclusion criteria consisted of:

Age under 18 years
Cranio-cerebral trauma
Myocardial infarction within the last 6 months
Stenocardia
Excessive hypertension (SAP > 180 mm Hg)

All patients received "routine" treatment with fentanyl and midazolam with the first measuring point being 8:00 a.m. of the first day. After evaluation of baseline values, patients were randomly allocated to the following groups:

1. Fentanyl group—approximately 0.2 mg/hr fentanyl, 2.5 mg/hr midazolam, and 2 mg/hr pancuronium in intermittent doses (continuation of routine treatment).
2. Ketamine group—about 50 mg/hr ketamine and 2.5 mg/hr midazolam by infusion pump; in addition, 2 mg/hr pancuronium in intermittent doses.

Parameters and measuring points

The following were observed:

Plasma epinephrine, norepinephrine, antidiuretic hormone (ADH), adrenocorticotrophic hormone (ACTH), cortisol, glucose, lactate and free glycerol (so-called stress metabolites)
Routine laboratory data
Compressed spectral EEG array and power bands
Hemodynamic parameters via pulmonary artery catheter and arterial line
Clinical observation (vigilance, adaptation to the respirator)
Ketamine plasma concentration

Epinephrine and norepinephrine in plasma were detected by high pressure liquid chromatography with electrochemical detection, HPLC/ECD (Bouloux *et al.*, 1985). ADH, ACTH, and cortisol were detected by radioimmunoassay (RIA), ketamine in plasma by gas chromatography. For detailed information see Adams *et al.* (1988) and Russ *et al.* (1985).

The observation period lasted 48 hr. Endocrine parameters, stress metabolites, and ketamine in plasma were determined in intervals of 6 hr. Hemodynamic parameters were analyzed in intervals of 12 hr, and EEG parameters in intervals of 24 hr. Clinical observation was documented in intervals of 2 hr. Routine laboratory data were compared once at the end of the investigation period.

Statistical analysis

Due to their non-normal distribution, the endocrine and EEG parameters, as well as shunt volume, were log transformed and analyzed using geometric mean values. For all other parameters arithmetic means and S.D. were used. Statistical evaluation was undertaken by analysis of variance with repeated measures on one factor. $P \leq 0.05$ was considered significant.

Results

Groups were comparable with regard to distribution of sex, age, height, and weight. Most patients suffered from septic disorders and/or polytrauma.

Endocrine parameters and stress metabolites

Infusions of epinephrine and norepinephrine were necessary in 3 patients for stabilization of their cardiovascular functions. All were randomly allocated to the ketamine group. After the onset of ketamine administration, cardiovascular stability allowed reduction and discontinuation of these infusions in all patients. No patient with exogenous application of catecholamines was investigated in the fentanyl group.

Norepinephrine (Table 1 and Fig. 1) levels were markedly increased in both groups. Group levels were comparable, and concentrations became largely similar after discontinuation of exogenous catecholamine application.

Epinephrine levels (Table 1 and Fig. 1) remained within the normal range in the fentanyl group. In the ketamine group, plasma epinephrine was initially higher due to exogenous administration. During the course of the investigation, the concentrations of epinephrine became comparable. No statistical differences between the groups became obvious with both catecholamines.

Levels of ADH, ACTH, and cortisol generally remained within the normal range (Table 2 and Fig. 2). ADH decreased significantly during the investigation period. No statistical differences between the groups were found.

No statistical differences were noted in the stress metabolites. Glucose concentrations were markedly elevated, and lactate values increased in both groups. Free glycerol was within the normal range. A comparison of routine laboratory data at the end of the observation period showed no statistical differences.

Neuromonitoring

EEG parameters were analyzed in 6 patients from the fentanyl and 5 patients from the ketamine group (Table 3 and Fig. 3). Compressed spec-

TABLE 1. Geometric mean and range of norepinephrine and epinephrine concentrations in plasma

Time (hr)	*Group*	*Norepinephrine (pg/ml)*	*Epinephrine (pg/ml)*
0	Fentanyl	588 211-1542	99 4-739
	Ketamine	899 379-1957	539 251-1150
6	Fentanyl	447 127-1263	67 4-533
	Ketamine	729 269-1163	289 49-835
12	Fentanyl	531 144-2467	101 34-512
	Ketamine	630 385-1269	219 40-1343
18	Fentanyl	528 72-2391	127 8-980
	Ketamine	727 223-1331	183 43-1869
24	Fentanyl	573 326-1674	143 19-491
	Ketamine	674 332-1158	192 18-1045
30	Fentanyl	529 297-1759	60 9-625
	Ketamine	685 261-1596	176 29-1148
36	Fentanyl	651 294-2738	87 22-307
	Ketamine	673 238-1487	252 24-3125
42	Fentanyl	678 421-271	107 21-676
	Ketamine	699 259-1723	164 39-3413
48	Fentanyl	568 355-2178	72 5-893
	Ketamine	624 267-1193	138 31-964

tral arrays of both groups showed reduced *alpha* (8-12 Hz) and *beta* (13-30 Hz), and a significant increase in *delta* (1-3 Hz) and *theta* (4-7 Hz) activities. Statistical evaluation of the data revealed a significantly higher *beta* activity in the ketamine group.

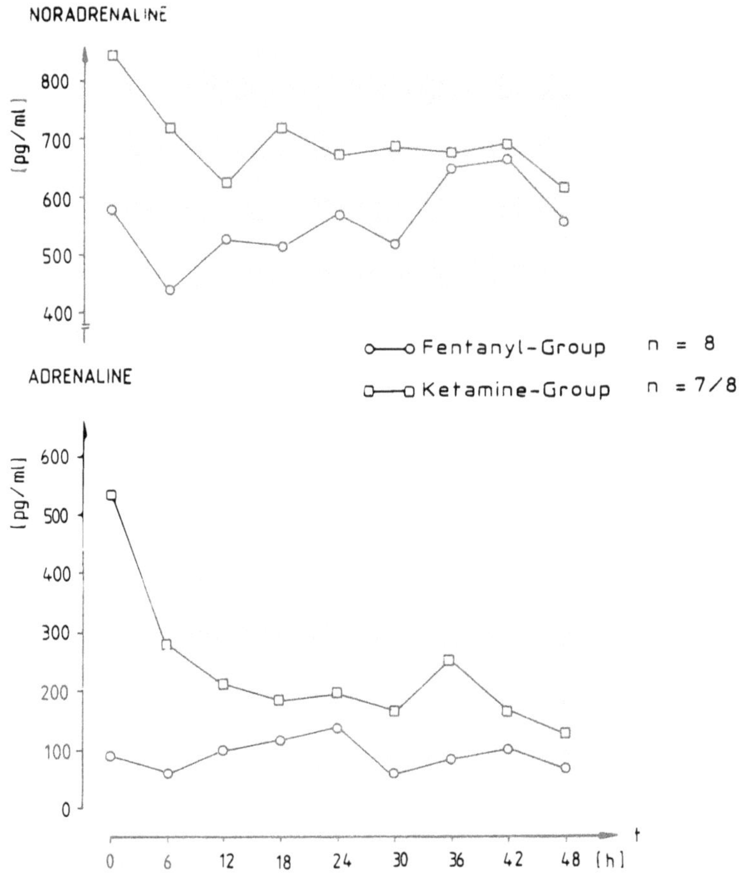

Fig. 1. Geometric mean values for plasma norepinephrine and epinephrine. The N for epinephrine is 7 in the ketamine group.

Plasma levels of ketamine

Plasma levels of ketamine indicated that there was no accumulation of the substance at the end of the investigation period after 48 hr (Fig. 4).

Hemodynamic data

In both groups, an increase in the cardiac index (CI) was significant over time (Table 4). The mean level of the CI in the ketamine group was about 0.7 l/min/m^2 higher than in the fentanyl group. Mean arterial pressure (MAP) and heart rate (HR) were comparable between the groups; ketamine caused no increase in HR. Right atrial pressure (RAP) was slightly increased in the fentanyl group. Mean pulmonary arterial pres-

TABLE 2. Geometric mean and range of ADH, ACTH, and cortisol concentrations in plasma

Time (hr)	*Group*	*ADH (pg/ml)*	*ACTH (pg/ml)*	*Cortisol (ng/ml)*
0	Fentanyl	3.2	16.7	228
		2.0-8.9	12.0-27.9	76-11
	Ketamine	3.7	25.4	323
		2.0-8.4	15.2-47.3	233-462
6	Fentanyl	2.9	19.5	185
		2.0-7.0	13.4-34.0	57-332
	Ketamine	3.1	19.3	254
		2.0-7.6	11.9-47.7	150-392
12	Fentanyl	2.8	23.8	176
		2.0-5.8	13.6-134.4	93-302
	Ketamine	4.3	21.1	254
		1.0-10.7	12.0-41.7	192-309
18	Fentanyl	2.2	23.9	217
		2.0-2.9	14.5-113.7	117-399
	Ketamine	2.9	22.1	234
		1.0-6.8	15.0-43.8	150-376
24	Fentanyl	2.7	21.4	160
		2.0-6.9	12.0-106.3	82-334
	Ketamine	3.0	20.2	227
		2.0-6.3	14.2-57.7	148-371
30	Fentanyl	2.6	20.0	181
		2.0-4.8	12.0-84.4	88-362
	Ketamine	2.7	22.2	250
		2.0-3.7	14.6-49.8	167-346
36	Fentanyl	2.7	22.9	181
		2.0-4.1	14.1-70.4	98-303
	Ketamine	2.2	22.6	249
		1.0-3.1	14.1-46.2	138-494
42	Fentanyl	2.8	20.1	189
		2.0-4.8	12.0-77.2	90-380
	Ketamine	2.2	19.9	264
		1.0-4.0	12.9-50.8	139-407
48	Fentanyl	2.3	21.9	176
		2.0-3.6	13.9-72.8	104-287
	Ketamine	1.9	22.4	273
		1.0-2.2	13.6-48.0	188-429

sure (PAP) and pulmonary capillary wedge pressure (PCWP) were nearly identical in both groups. In the ketamine group, systemic vascular resistance (SVR) and pulmonary vascular resistance (PVR) were generally lower. The reduction of shunt volume at the end of the investigation period reached statistical significance.

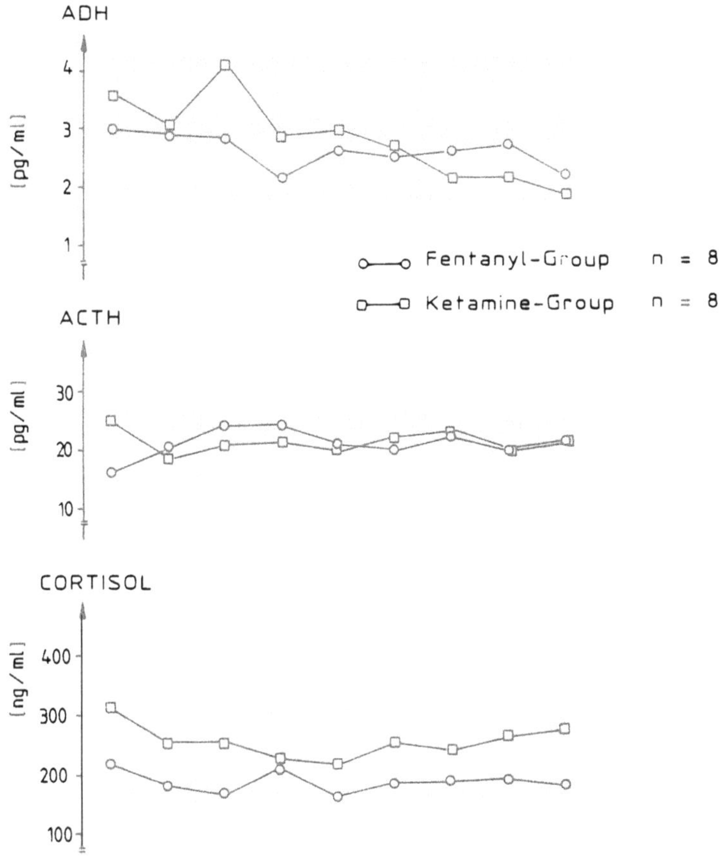

Fig. 2. Geometric mean values of ADH, ACTH, and cortisol concentrations in plasma.

Clinical observations

There was excellent adaptation to the respirator in both groups. Patients in the ketamine group reached higher vigilance levels, but without statistical significance (P=0.08). Sedation of one patient in each group was not sufficient. The data are summarized below:

Adaptation to respirator		*Vigilance*
4 Excellent		4 Full cooperation
3 Coughing		3 Limited cooperation
2 "Fighting"		2 Reaction to pain
1 Self-extubation		1 No pain reaction
3.98 ± 0.05	Fentanyl group	1.10 ± 0.09
3.96 ± 0.07	Ketamine group	1.31 ± 0.3

TABLE 3. Total EEG activity, power bands and compressed spectral array of 6 patients given fentanyl and 5 patients given ketamine. Geometric means and ranges are given.

Activity Parameter	*Group*	*0 hr*	*24 hr*	*48 hr*
Total (pW)	Fentanyl	67	67	52
		27-162	39-175	231-31
	Ketamine	105	95	119
		36-167	41-304	47-296
Alpha (pW)	Fentanyl	8	9	8
		3-18	3-30	3-51
	Ketamine	12	19	16
		6-26	6-51	11-40
Beta (pW)	Fentanyl	6	5	4
		2-33	3-13	3-10
	Ketamine	28	22	25
		9-89	7-88	8-110
Delta (pW)	Fentanyl	33	34	20
		8-116	12-161	9-120
	Ketamine	44	36	58
		14-109	17-136	14-103
Theta (pW)	Fentanyl	11	10	10
		5-46	7-23	4-30
	Ketamine	14	11	13
		7-28	4-29	7-43

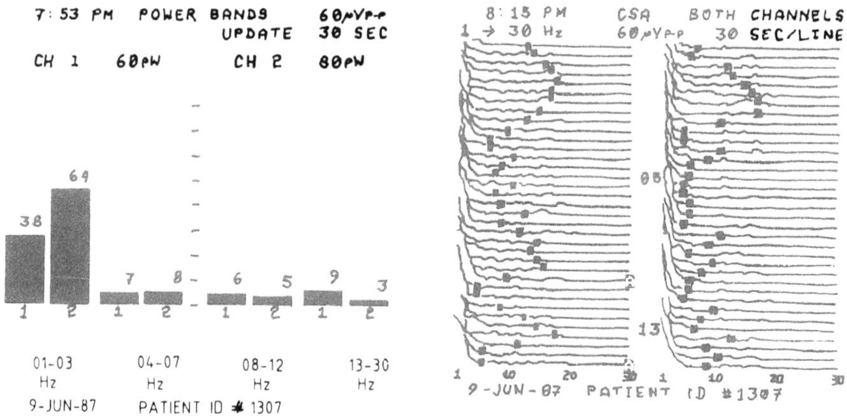

Fig. 3. Compressed spectral array and power bands of a patient in the ketamine group.

TABLE 4. Comparative hemodynamic data of the fentanyl and ketamine treated groups. Arithmetic means ± S.E. are given (for shunt volume, geometric means are given.)

Parameter Units	*Group*	*0 hr*	*12 hr*	*24 hr*	*36 hr*	*48 hr*
MAP	Fentanyl	95 ± 16	94 ± 10	100 ± 23	92 ± 18	87 ± 11
mm Hg	Ketamine	86 ± 11	89 ± 22	85 ± 14	90 ± 17	96 ± 24
HR	Fentanyl	107 ± 11	105 ± 16	103 ± 14	112 ± 8	109 ± 16
1/bpm	Ketamine	118 ± 11	114 ± 10	112 ± 16	118 ± 14	114 ± 17
CI	Fentanyl	3.2 ± 0.9	39 ± 0.9	4.0 ± 1.2	4.2 ± 1.4	3.8 ± 1.4
$1/min/m^2$	Ketamine	4.0 ± 1.2	4.9 ± 1.5	4.4 ± 1.3	48. ± 2.0	4.3 ± 1.2
RAP	Fentanyl	7 ± 3	10 ± 4	11 ± 3	12 ± 4	10 ± 3
mm Hg	Ketamine	8 ± 3	9 ± 5	8 ± 2	9 ± 4	10 ± 5
PAP	Fentanyl	22 ± 11	26 ± 9	23 ± 6	23 ± 6	23 ± 10
mm Hg	Ketamine	22 ± 6	25 ± 6	24 ± 5	26 ± 9	24 ± 5
PCWP	Fentanyl	16 ± 8	17 ± 7	14 ± 5	19 ± 8	15 ± 5
mm Hg	Ketamine	15 ± 7	19 ± 6	14 ± 4	19 ± 10	15 ± 4
SVR	Fentanyl	1206 ± 338	948 ± 291	1007 ± 289	872 ± 349	933 ± 331
$dynxsxcm^{-5}$	Ketamine	890 ± 495	745 ± 339	818 ± 286	831 ± 373	835 ± 236
PVR	Fentanyl	136 ± 63	108 ± 71	99 ± 38	108 ± 58	104 ± 58
$dynxsxcm^{-5}$	Ketamine	82 ± 42	64 ± 15	94 ± 37	73 ± 59	93 ± 32
Shunt	Fentanyl	13	14	12	12	12
Percent	Ketamine	13	14	13	14	7

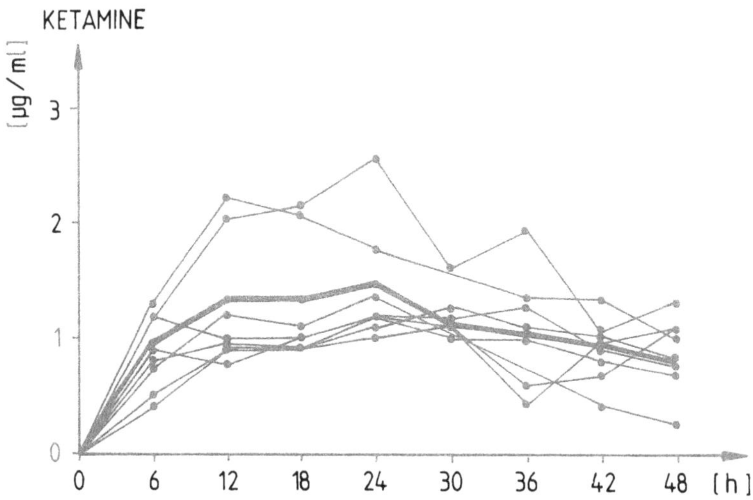

Fig. 4. Individual concentrations and arithmetic mean of plasma levels of ketamine.

Discussion

A careful interpretation of these results is necessary because of the methodological limitations mentioned in the Introduction. Epinephrine, ADH, ACTH, and cortisol, which are reliable stress parameters, demonstrated in both groups the absence of external systemic stress (Henry, 1980). This unexpected result was clearly supported by the analyses of the EEG parameters. In contrast, norepinephrine values were high in both groups throughout the whole period of investigation. This might be due to respirator therapy, positive endexpiratory pressure, or circulatory problems, and can be interpreted as the response of the organism to severe internal dysregulations.

The benefits of ketamine in patients with cardiovascular instability were demonstrated by a slightly increased cardiac index and a lower shunt volume. This might be due to the central stimulating sympathomimetic effect of ketamine (Ivankovich *et al.*, 1974; White *et al.*, 1982). Discontinuation of exogenous catecholamine administration in 3 of 8 patients supported this result.

Conclusions

1. Sedation and analgesia of intensive care patients with a combination of ketamine and midazolam is practicable.

2. Fentanyl/midazolam and ketamine/midazolam are comparable with regard to endocrine stress response and EEG monitoring.
3. Ketamine/midazolam is of special interest in intensive care patients with circulatory instability and can help to reduce the need for exogenous catecholamines.

References

Adams, H.A., Biscoping, J., Russ, W., Bachmann, B., Ratthey, K. and Hempelmann, G.: Untersuchungen zur sedativ-analgetischen Medikation beatmungspflichtiger Intensivpatienten. Anaesthesist 37: 268-276, 1988.

Bouloux, P., Perret, D., Besser, G.M.: Methodological considerations in the determination of plasma catecholamines by high performance liquid chromatography with electrochemical detection. Ann. Clin. Biochem. 22: 194-203, 1985.

Henry, J.P.: Present concept of stress theory. In Catecholamines and Stress: Recent Advances, pp 557-571, Elsevier/North Holland, New York-Amsterdam-Oxford, 1980.

Ivankovich, A.D., Miletich, D.J., Reimann, C. Albrecht, R.F. and Zahed, B.: Cardiovascular effects of centrally administered ketamine in goats. Anesth. Analg. 53: 924-933, 1974.

Russ, W., Kling, D., Krumholz, W., Fraedrich, G. and Hempelmann, G.: Erfahrungen mit einem neuen EEG-Spektralanalysator in der Karotischirurgie. Anaesthesist 34: 85-90, 1985.

White, P.F., Way, W.L., Trevor, A.J.: Ketamine—its pharmacology and therapeutic uses. Anesthesiol. 56: 119-136, 1982.

Status of Ketamine in Anesthesiology,
edited by E.F. Domino©1990, NPP Books
P.O. Box 1491, Ann Arbor, MI 48106

Analgosedation of Intensive Care Patients with a Low Dose Long Term Ketamine/Midazolam Combination

R. Klose, U. Hoppe, and P. Wresch

Department of Anesthesiology and Intensive Care Medicine
BG—Unfallklinik
Ludwigshafen, F.R. Germany

Introduction

Physical and psychological stress, *i.e.*, pain and emotional suffering, are well known factors that can lead to a complete breakdown of vegetative functions. A high sympathetic tone with subsequent high oxygen consumption and hemodynamic instability are possible consequences. It must be the goal of effective analgosedation to keep the severely ill patient free of pain and sufficiently sedated. The important anabolic contribution of deep levels of sleep to health and tissue restoration after trauma or surgery has been frequently stressed (Adam and Oswald, 1984). There are situations, such as physical therapy and positioning, where analgosedation is necessary only intermittently as it is advantageous if the patient can be somewhat awake.

From a clinical point of view, we believe ideal analgosedation must involve "dissociative anesthesia" with ketamine (Domino *et al.*, 1965). The ventilated patient is easy to waken, cooperative and, for the most part, pain free. He is capable of following instructions and does not remember the therapy because of simultaneous amnesia.

From the various possible analgosedation strategies, we chose a combination of ketamine and midazolam three years ago. Ketamine was considered optimal because of its wide therapeutic range and low toxicity. The benzodiazepine, midazolam, was chosen because of its controllability and few side effects. The combination seemed particularly beneficial because the elimination half lives of the medications are the same, about 2.5-3 hr (Clements and Nimmo, 1981).

METHODS

We are primarily responsible for the intensive care of the seriously burned and polytraumatized patients in our hospital. For their analgosedation we use a standard mixture of ketamine and midazolam in the weight ratio of 10:1, which has been empirically proven usable. We decided to use this fixed combination because of easy clinical handling of the medications. To prevent a possible fluctuation of therapeutic effectiveness, we prefer a continuous infusion of the medication to intermittent boluses.

We begin with a 3 ml bolus of the ketamine/midazolam mixture (60 mg ketamine and 6 mg midazolam). The infusion pump is set to administer 10 ml/hr of 200 mg ketamine and 20 mg midazolam. This setting must be corrected up or down according to the degree of analgosedation needed (see Table 1). An infusion setting of 15 ml/hr is the maximum dose. The average dose after the initial bolus is about 2.9 mg/kg/hr of ketamine. This dosage seems to be rather high when compared to the results of other authors (see Table 2).

TABLE 1. Details of infusion technique

Filling of the infusion pump
50 ml = 1000 mg ketamine + 100 mg midazolam
1. Bolus 3 ml = 60 mg ketamine + 6 mg midazolam
2. Initial setting 10 ml/hr (200 mg ketamine + 20 mg midazolam)
3. Adjust to desired effect - max. 15 ml/hr - 300 mg ketamine + 30 mg midazolam

TABLE 2. Investigations using analgosedation in intensive care

	Ketamine mg/kg/hr	*Benzodiazepine mg/kg/hr*
Kurth (1983)	0.3-0.5	Flunitrazepam 0.002-0.006
Nimmo and MacRae (1983)	0.18	—
Shetty *et al.* (1986)	0.2-0.8	—
Joachimsson *et al.* (1986)	0.7-1.4	Diazepam
Langrehr *et al.* (1986)	0.1-0.5	Flunitrazepam 0.002-0.005
Brost and Tzanova (1986)	0.3-0.5	Flunitrazepam 0.004-0.006
Emrich *et al.* (1987)	1.7	Midazolam 0.17
Adams *et al.* (1988)	0.7	Midazolam 0.04
Klose *et al.* (1989)[1]	2.9	Midazolam 0.3
Present study (1989)[2]	1.7	Midazolam 0.17

[1] Burn patients
[2] Polytraumatized patients

Thus, our method is not low dose analgosedation. It is definitely long term analgosedation. Large amounts of ketamine and midazolam are often used for weeks at a time. One patient was treated and ventilated for about 5 months. We must, therefore, critically evaluate the long term side effects of ketamine/midazolam.

From our everyday clinical observations we have determined that our present analgosedation technique performs effectively. Fig. 1 shows the plasma cortisol levels of 9 seriously burned, mechanically ventilated patients. The levels of cortisol were measured intermittently over a period of 6 weeks. Most of the plasma cortisol levels, as simple stress parameters, are in the normal range. This long term use of ketamine and midazolam can, nevertheless, only be considered harmless when several important clinical demands have been met. The demands of an analgosedation concept are summarized in Table 3.

TABLE 3. Demands of clinically useful analgosedation

No adverse cardiovascular effects
No respiratory depression
No accumulation with long term usage
No organ toxicity
Wide therapeutic margin of safety

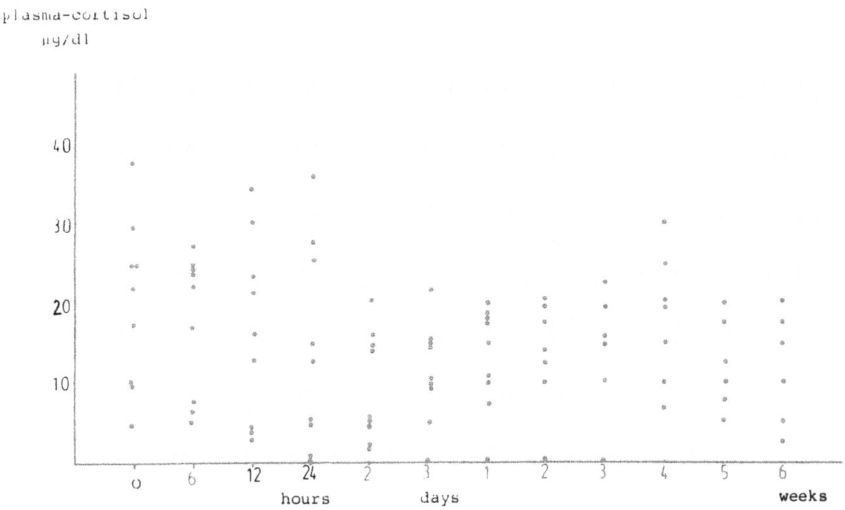

Fig. 1. Plasma cortisol levels in 9 severely burned patients during analgosedation with ketamine/midazolam.

The sympathomimetic side effects of ketamine are reduced by the addition of midazolam and this drug combination results in stabilization of the circulation. The majority of our patients showed no signs of hypertension. No conclusive correlation of hypertensive episodes and ketamine could be made. Many clinical causes could account for any hypertensive episodes in the burn patients.

Many investigators have described pulmonary hypertension caused by ketamine. We also noticed pulmonary hypertension, especially in burn patients. However, this could not be directly related to an action of ketamine. Burn patients often suffer from serious pulmonary insufficiencies, *e.g.*, due to inhalation trauma. In our observations, the hemodynamic effect of ketamine/midazolam does not seem to be detrimental. It is well known that ketamine produces bronchodilation and lowers airway resistance (White *et al.*, 1982). There is little central respiratory depression. The laryngopharyngeal reflexes remain intact, depending on the dosage. For this reason, our analgosedation technique with ketamine/midazolam uses small doses such as 5 ml/hr. It is possible to maintain a satisfactory level of analgosedation in the spontaneously breathing, well supervised patient. In addition, we feel that minimal respiratory depression helps in weaning from the respirator since the ability to cough up secretions is a positive feature in bronchial clearance. In 3 years of clinical observation of about 150 ventilator dependent patients we have seen only one patient with excessive secretion and a flooding of the bronchial system. On the other hand, approximately 15% of the patients with severe respiratory insufficiency and obvious pulmonary changes needed additional skeletal muscle relaxants. This was the only way to overcome the technical problems of mechanical ventilation.

The well known psychotomimetic side effects of ketamine were noted in about 10% of our long term ventilated patients. It is possible that their disorientation, unrest, and insomnia during the weaning period can be explained by a too drastic reduction or too abrupt cessation of the analgosedation. In these patients, an additional dose of midazolam led to clearcut psychological stabilization. All psychotomimetic side effects, of course, cannot be directly related to ketamine/midazolam. There are patients with pre-existing psychoses, especially alcohol and drug dependent burn patients. In addition, many other medications used in intensive care medicine can lead to central nervous system problems. There is no doubt that long term intensive care patients can acquire mental problems independent of medication.

Ketamine is biotransformed enzymatically by the liver. The metabolites are excreted by the kidney and the intestine. The main metabolite is norketamine (Chang and Glazko, 1974; Clements and Nimmo, 1981; Domino, 1981; Idvall *et al.*, 1979). We measured plasma ketamine and norketamine levels in some of our burn patients. The patient whose plasma levels of ketamine and norketamine are shown in Fig. 2 had a 48% thickness burn and third degree inhalation trauma.

Although a continuous increase in the ketamine/midazolam infusion rate from 1.7 to 2.9 mg/kg/hr was clinically necessary, the ketamine levels remained at a relatively steady state between 1000 and 1500 ng/ml. The norketamine level showed a marked initial increase and then fell below the ketamine level. The mechanism of P450 enzyme induction is a possible explanation for this lack of accumulation of ketamine despite the large ketamine doses given over a long period of time. In contradiction of this hypothesis, however, is the terminal fall of the norketamine level. Possibly, norketamine was even more efficiently biotransformed over a period of many days.

It is noteworthy that our burn patients seemed to need an increase in the dose of ketamine/midazolam mainly in the first week of treatment. A

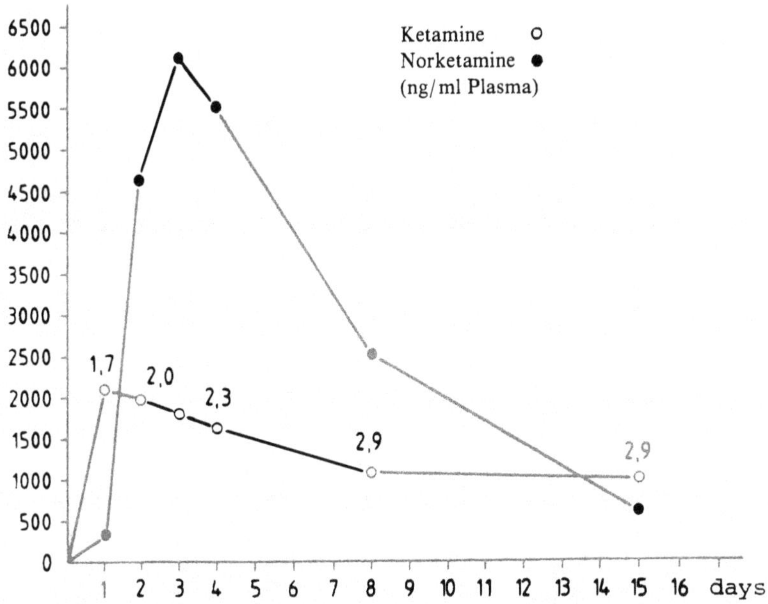

Fig. 2. Plasma levels of ketamine and norketamine. The numbers 1.7, 2.0, 2.3, and 2.9 indicate the infusion pump setting; mg ketamine/kg body weight/hr.

possible explanation for this could be the loss of plasma and drugs through the open body surface. Such burn patients often suffer from septic complications during which there is a well known catabolic glucose and protein need (Wilmore *et al.*, 1980). A faster hepatic metabolism and real drug elimination is the best possible explanation. Our observations agree with this hypothesis. The polytraumatized, nonseptic patients need only about half the amount of ketamine/ midazolam compared to the burn patients described in the literature (see Table 2). There were also burn patients who were not sufficiently sedated despite the maximum dose of 300 mg of ketamine and 30 mg of midazolam/hr. The ketamine/midazolam analgosedation was completely unsuccessful in about half of such patients and we had to choose a totally different regimen. We also administered opioids, other benzodiazepines, and neuroleptics in about 20% of the burn patients. A possible explanation for this lack of regularity between the ketamine dose, ketamine plasma level, and degree of analgesia is the fact that only free ketamine is responsible for its analgesic effect. A larger portion of plasma ketamine is bound to *alpha*-1-acid-glycoprotein and the remaining is bound to albumin. The concentration of *alpha*-1-acid-glycoprotein can be increased by stress and trauma. Thus, the amount of free ketamine is reduced (Martyn *et al.*, 1984).

We did not observe any side effects of ketamine in relation to acid base balance, glucose metabolism, or kidney function. We had the impression that there is no adverse effect on the intestine as there is, for example, with opioids. It is important to note that for clinical use the water soluble midazolam component almost always leads to phlebitis when peripheral veins are used. Therefore, a continuous dose should be given only through a central venous line. In addition, we noted pH dependent incompatibilities of midazolam, especially with amino acid solutions. As a result, ketamine/midazolam should be administered separately. Although the primary side effects of ketamine are reduced by midazolam, we do not use the combination in patients with excessive hypertension, *i.e.*, a systolic blood pressure higher than 180 mm Hg. We also do not use the combination in patients with recent myocardial infarction, a history of coronary heart disease, or an increased intracranial pressure (ICP). However, with continual ICP monitoring and controlled hyperventilation the use of ketamine may be less dangerous.

The analgosedation with ketamine/midazolam failed to work well in alcoholic patients because of tolerance development. In patients with a recognized psychosis we chose another form of analgosedation because the effect of ketamine is not predictable and the origin of possible psychotomimetic phenomena is not clear.

Conclusion

Long term analgosedation with ketamine/midazolam provides well controlled, nonaccumulative, and nonorganotoxic analgesia. It can be given by continuous infusion. The dosage is regulated by need. An easy weaning from the respirator is possible in long term mechanically ventilated patients because of minimal respiratory depression. During "dissociative analgesia" the ventilated patient is easily awakened and cooperative. Its use is possible even in high risk burn and polytraumatized patients because of the stable hemodynamic parameters. Even though this method of analgosedation is not suitable for all patients, it is accepted by our doctors and other health care workers because of ease in handling and effectiveness.

References

Adam, K. and Oswald, J.: Sleep helps healing, Brit. Med. J. 289: 1400-1401, 1984.

Adams, H.A., Biscoping, J., Russ, W., Bachmann, B., Ratthey, K., and Hempelmann, G.: Untersuchungen zur sedativ-analgetischen Medikation beatmungspflichtiger Intensivpatienten. Anaesthesist 37: 268, 1988.

Brost, F. and Tzanova, I.: Postoperative Langzeitanalgosedierung. Intensivbehandlung 12, 1987.

Chang, T. and Glazko, A.J.: Biotransformation and disposition of ketamine. Int. Anesthesiol. Clin. 12: 157-177, 1974.

Clements, J.A. and Nimmo, W.S.: The pharmacokinetics and analgesic effect of ketamine in man. Brit. J. Anaesth. 53: 27, 1981.

Domino, E.F.: Ketamine: Isomers and metabolites. In Anaesthesiology: Proceedings of the 7th Congress of Anaesthesiologists, Rügheimer, E. and Zindler, M., eds., pp. 696-699, Excerpta Medica, Amsterdam, 1981.

Domino, E.F., Chodoff, P., and Corssen, G.: Pharmacologic effects of CI-581, a new dissociative anesthetic in man. Clin. Pharmacol. Ther. 6: 279-291, 1965.

Emrich, O., Klose, R., Steen, M., and Büttner, J.: Ketamin in der Intensivtherapie—Analgosedierung mit der low-dose-long term-Ketamin/Midazolam-Kombination in kontinuierlicher Infusion. In Neue Aspekte zu Ketamin in der Anesthesie, Intensivu. Notfallmedizin Anaesthesiologie u Intensivmedizin, Bd 198, Tolksdorf, W., ed., p. 75, Springer, New York, 1988.

Idvall, J., Ahlgren, J., Aronsen, K.F., and Stenberg, P.: Ketamine infusions: Pharmacokinetics and clinical effects. Br. J. Anaesth. 51: 1167-1173, 1979.

Joachimsson, P.D., Hedsteand, U., and Eklung, A.: Low dose ketamine infusion for analgesia during postoperative ventilator treatment. Acta Anaesthesiol. Scand 30: 697, 1986.

Kurth, M.: Anästhesie und Analgosedierung mit Ketamin bei Patienten einer Intensivstation. Anaesth. Intensivmed. 24: 270, 1983.

Langrehr, D., Miranda, D.R., Stoutenbeck, C.P., Zandstra, D.F., and van

Saene, H.K.F.: Ketamin-Benzodiazepin-Kombination zur Sedierung von Intensivpatienten. In Langzeitsedierung des Intensivpatienten, Schulte am Esch, J., ed., Zuckschwerdt, Munich, 1986.

Martyn, J.A.J., Abernethy, D.R., and Greenblatt, D.J.: Plasma protein bindings of drugs after severe burn injury. Clin. Pharmacol. Ther. 35: 534-536, 1984.

Nimmo, W.S. and MacRae, W.A.: Sedation and analgesia. In Recent Advances in Critical Care Medicine 2, Ledingham, I. McA., and Hanning, C.D., eds., Churchill Livingstone, London, 1983.

Shetty, G.K., Kelsall, P.G., and Pyan, D.W.: Long term ketamine infusion. Anaesthesia 41: 1262, 1986.

White, P.F., Way, W.L., and Trevor, A.J.: Ketamine-Its pharmacology and therapeutic uses. Anesthesiol. 56: 119-136, 1982.

Wilmore, D.W., Goodwin, C.W., Aulick, L.H., Powand, M.C., Mason, A.D., and Pruitt, B.A.: Effect of injury and infection on visceral metabolism and circulation. Ann. Surg. 192: 491-504, 1980.

Status of Ketamine in Anesthesiology,
edited by E.F. Domino©1990, NPP Books
P.O. Box 1491, Ann Arbor, MI 48106

Ketamine in Induction of General Anesthesia and Regional Anesthesia

O. Schulte-Steinberg

Starnberg, Germany

Induction of General Anesthesia

We have had success in using ketamine as an induction agent for general anesthesia for several reasons. After one circulation time, the patient is analgesic and amnesic, an advantage in extremely urgent surgery (Langrehr and Stolp, 1969). For routine induction, ketamine is very attractive because it maintains stable blood pressure levels despite a high concentration of inhalational agents during this period. Ketamine anesthesia is at its peak between 3 and 5 min and remains active for approximately 10 to 20 min. When ketamine is used, analgesia lasts 2 to 3 min longer than barbiturates (Langrehr *et al.*, 1967, Fig. 1). This leaves enough time for difficult intubations as well as for fixation of the tracheal tube, positioning the patient, setting up the respirator, and performing other tasks which may take away the anesthetist's attention.

Inhalation anesthetics, in general, are taken up smoothly (Stephen *et al.*, 1970). Hypotension frequently occurs during induction of neurolept anesthesia (NLA). This drop in blood pressure will not be seen when ketamine is used at the start of NLA (Schumacher *et al.*, 1974; Holzrichter, 1974).

An induction agent like ketamine which maintains blood pressure (as shown in Figs. 2 and 3) can be used for the patient in shock (Peter *et al.*, 1970; Schlag, 1972; Nettles *et al.*, 1973).

On the other hand, the cardiovascular stimulation, so welcomed in the previously discussed situation, is unwarranted in hypertensive and cardiac risk patients with minimal coronary reserve in which cardiac stimulation results in elevated myocardial work and oxygen consumption. According to Langrehr *et al.* (1984), cardiovascular stimulation can safely be eliminated by the administration of a benzodiazepine before the ketamine. The dosages are: diazepam 0.25 mg/kg, flunitrazepam 0.015 mg/kg, or midazolam 0.15 mg/kg. This will produce a stable cardiovascular system and is thus an advantage of ketamine (White, 1982). Only the

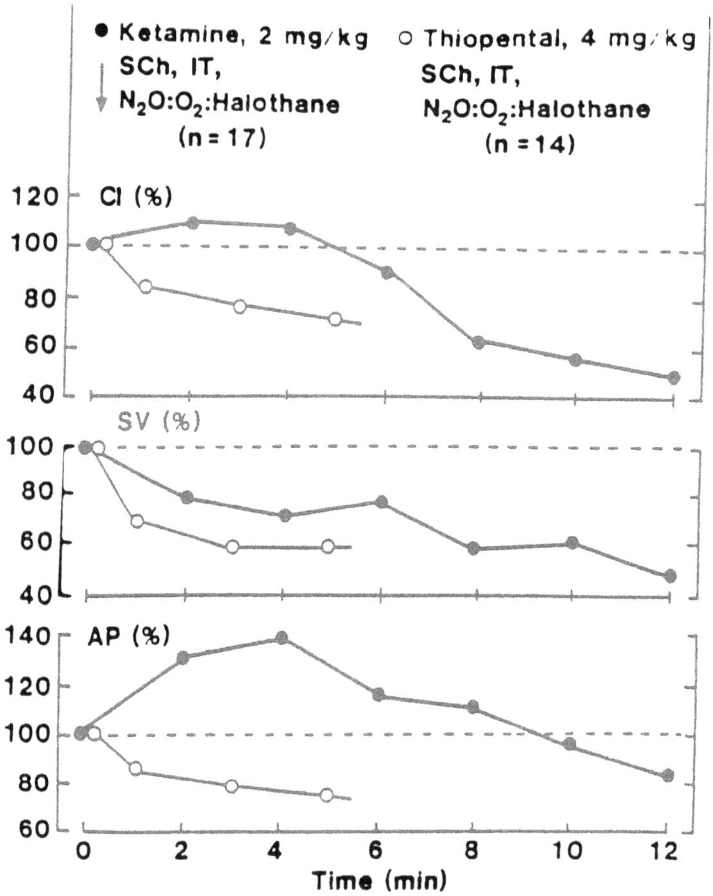

Fig. 1. Difference between ketamine and barbiturate induction. There was identical follow up maintenance regarding cardiac index (CI), stroke volume (SV), and blood pressure (AP). (Modified from Langrehr *et al.*, 1984.)

tendency to increase blood pressure is to be avoided. Respiration is only insignificantly depressed if the benzodiazepine is given alone in clinical dosages. Nevertheless, Langrehr *et al.* (1984) found a tendency for mild respiratory depression even during the short induction time when the combination of diazepam or flunitrazepam with ketamine was used. However, this did not occur when midazolam was combined with ketamine. Because diazepam also tends to cause hypotension (Kingston *et al.*, 1978), midazolam is preferable. When an appropriate dose of benzodiazepine is given before ketamine, or when ketamine is used solely as an induction agent and followed by a regular general anesthetic tech-

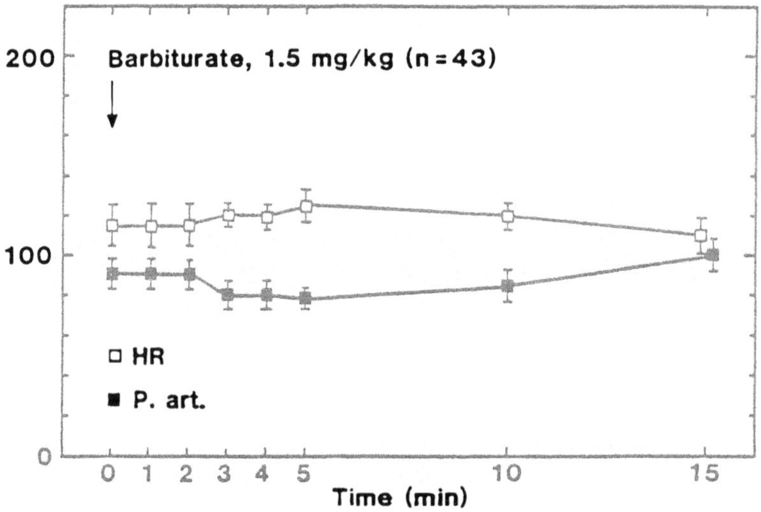

Fig. 2. Mean arterial blood pressure and heart rate after i.v. injection of a barbiturate (1.5 mg/kg) in patients with shock (Peter *et al.*, 1970).

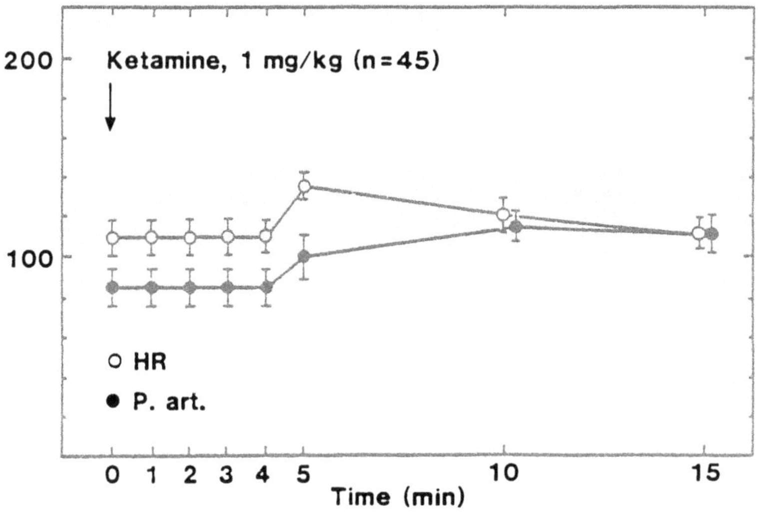

Fig. 3. Mean arterial blood pressure and heart rate after i.v. injection of ketamine (1 mg/kg) in patients with shock (Peter *et al.*, 1970).

nique, arousal reactions do not occur (Langrehr *et al.*, 1984; Kortilla and Levänen, 1978; Matilla *et al.*, 1979).

The signs of anesthesia with ketamine are completely different from those of other agents. Mild nystagmus, a slight flutter of the eyelid followed by wide opening of the eyes, and an inability to respond to verbal commands are sure indicators of anesthesia. It is important that the i.v. injection be given very slowly and stopped immediately when the above mentioned signs become apparent, regardless of the lid reflex. By doing this, the dose is limited. The induction dose varies from 0.7 to 1.5 mg/kg, rarely exceeding 2 mg/kg (Vontin *et al.*, 1976). Shock patients can be induced satisfactorily with 0.5 to 0.7 mg/kg. Patients with intestinal obstruction (full stomach), usually associated with hypotension induced in the anti-Trendelenburg position, particularly benefit from the cardiovascular stimulation when ketamine is used (Schmidt, 1977, Fig. 4). The agent also allows time for replacement of deficits in fluid volume.

Ketamine offers a number of special advantages for the induction of patients for cesarean section (Langrehr and Stolp, 1969). Besides the retained spontaneous respiration and the stable cardiovascular state of the mother, the lack of detrimental effects on the fetal cardiovascular system and the absence of respiratory depression of the child are of great importance (Langrehr and Neuhaus, 1973; Holzrichter, 1974; Marx, 1976). Consequently, as Marx and others have clearly shown, the Apgar rating is decidedly better when ketamine has been used in comparison to barbiturates for induction. After a hemorrhage from a placenta previa, hypovolemic patients, for example, can be induced safely with ketamine (Holzrichter, 1974). For urgent sections, the patient is ready for the inci-

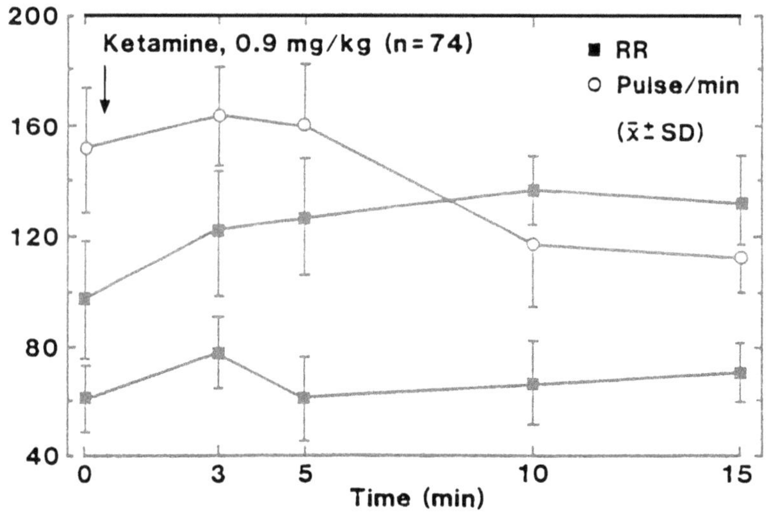

Fig. 4. Mean pulse rate and arterial blood pressure in 74 patients in shock following induction with ketamine (0.9 mg/kg). (Schmidt, 1977.)

sion about 1 min after injection. The only contraindications in these patients are preeclampsia and eclampsia.

The advantages of a sequence of ketamine followed by topical anesthesia via the nostril and pharynx and subsequent transtracheal block for patients with difficult airways have been described by Defalque (1971). We have frequently and successfully used this technique for years. Spontaneous maintenance of the airway is the real advantage of this technique.

In children, i.m. ketamine (4 to 7 mg/kg) is very practical for induction of general anesthesia, for the establishment of an i.v. access, and for the performance of a regional block (Schulte-Steinberg, 1989).

The only remaining contraindication to the induction of anesthesia with ketamine are patients with distinct hypertension. Even here, the blood pressure increase can be eliminated by the use of sufficient benzodiazepines (Langrehr and Stolp, 1969).

Regional anesthesia

Until the appearance of ketamine, other i.v. and inhalation agents were used as a supplement to regional anesthesia and, in particular, to central blocks. This combination has been blamed for the occurrence of respiratory failure and cardiovascular collapse in many cases (Szappanyos *et al.*, 1969). A drop in blood pressure is clearly observed when an inhalation anesthetic containing a halogenated agent is started in a patient with a central block. Ketamine offers a welcome alternative because of its analgesic properties, cardiovascular stimulation, lack of respiratory depression, and maintenance of protective reflexes. Piroelle (1980) showed that 1 mg/kg of ketamine during an epidural block leads to a small increase in heart rate (+12%) and systolic blood pressure (+15%). Langrehr *et al.* (1967) found a 20% increase in pressure with the same dose in unblocked patients. Boegl *et al.* (1973) showed similar findings for spinal anesthesia (Fig. 5).

Discomfort from tourniquets, exotic positions, and unsatisfactory analgesia can be avoided by the use of low dose ketamine and a benzodiazepine. A dose of 0.3 to 0.5 mg/kg of ketamine is sufficient for the positioning of patients with fractures for spinal or epidural anesthesia (Neumark and Halbgebauer, 1973; Austin, 1980). Blocks requiring multiple needle pricks, like intercostal blocks, can be performed without the patient feeling or remembering them (Schulte-Steinberg, 1978). These patients are not under general anesthesia and they will still respond to verbal commands. Again, to avoid cardiovascular stimulation and arousal reactions, midazolam is added to ketamine in a ratio of 1:10.

For several years we administered minute increments of ketamine

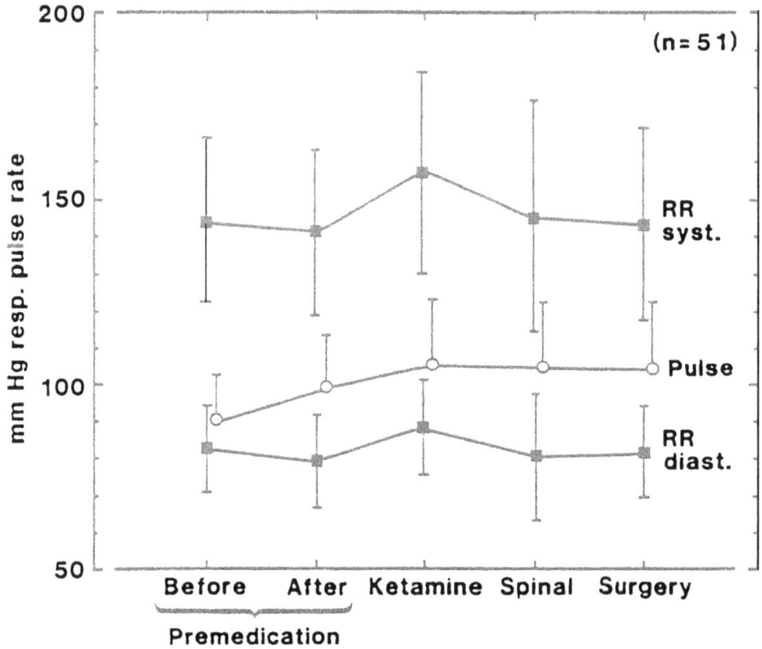

Fig. 5. Cardiovascular stability following combinations of ketamine with spinal anesthesia. (Modified from Boegl *et al.*, 1973.)

during surgical procedures in blocked patients. However, progress has been made with the use of infusion pumps. For peripheral nerve blocks, 0.5 mg/kg/hr of ketamine and 0.05 mg/kg/ hr of midazolam are sufficient.

Intubated patients with a spinal or epidural block require 0.6-0.9 mg/kg/hr of ketamine and 0.06-0.09 mg/kg/hr of midazolam during more extensive (*i.e.*, abdominal) surgery. This assures a stable cardiovascular situation in contrast to an inhalational method with halogenated agents (Wagner, 1989). The need to wait for a block to become effective can be avoided with ketamine; the surgeon can begin and the dose can be subsequently reduced as analgesia develops. In children, this method is practically routine. Surgery can begin immediately after the block has been performed under ketamine (4-7 mg/kg i.m.). Further increments of 0.5 mg/kg may be given until about 15 min after the block is initiated. Thereafter, N_2O/O_2 or small increments of midazolam is all that is needed. For more extensive surgery, intubated children, similar to adults, may require 0.6-0.9 mg/kg/hr of ketamine and one tenth of this dose of midazolam. At times, the benzodiazepine alone is sufficient at this stage.

Ketamine has added considerably to the safety and comfort of regional anesthesia. It should, however, always be combined with a benzodiazepine, preferably midazolam, because of its shorter duration and the absence of respiratory depression.

References

Austin, T.R.: Low dose ketamine and diazepam during spinal analgesia. Anaesthesia 35: 391-392, 1980.

Boegl, P. and Hutschenreuter, K.: Die Kombination der Ketamin—Narkose mit einer Leitungsanaesthesie. Anaesthesiology and Resuscitation, 69: 364-367. In Ketamin, Neue Ergebnisse in Forschung and Klinik, ed. by M. Gemperle, H. Kreuscher, D. Langrehr, Springer Verlag, Berlin-Heidelberg-New York, 1973.

Defalque, R.J.: Ketamine for blind nasal intubation. Anesth. Analg. 50: 984-986, 1971.

Holzrichter, P.L.: Ketanest als Einleitungsanaesthetikum bei der Sectio caesarea unter der NLA. Ketanest-Symposium Parke-Davis, Dortmund, 1974.

Kingston, H.G.G., Bretherton, K.W., Holloway, A.M. and Downing, J.W.: A comparison between ketamine and diazepam as induction agents for pericardiectomy. Anaesth. Intens. Care 6: 66-70, 1978.

Kortilla, K. and Levänen, J.: Untoward effects of ketamine combined with diazepam for supplementing conduction anesthesia in young and middle aged adults. Acta Anaesth. Scand. 22: 640-648, 1978.

Langrehr, D. and Stolp, W.: Der influss von Ketamin auf Verschiedene Vitalfunktionen des Menschen (Experimentelle Untersuchungen und klinische Erfahrungen bei 1300 Fällen). In Anaesthesiology and Resuscitation 40: 25-51, Ketamin, ed. by K. Kreuscher, Springer Verlag, Berlin-Heidelberg-New York, 1969.

Langrehr, D., Alai, P., Andjelkovic, J. and Kluge, I.: Zur Narkose mit Ketamine (CI 581): Bericht über erste Erfahrungen in 500 Fällen. Anaesthesist 16: 308-318, 1967.

Langrehr, D., Agoston, S. and Sia, R.: Ataranalgesia, a review. Acta Anaesth. Belg. 35: 165-187, 1984.

Langrehr, D. and Neuhaus, R.: Ketamin in der Geburtshilflichen-Anaesthesie, In Anaesthesiology and Resuscitation 69:277-284, Ketamin, Neue Ergebnisse in Forschung und Klinik, ed. by M. Gemperle, H. Kreuscher, D. Langrehr, Springer Verlag, Berlin-Heidelberg-New York, 1973.

Marx, G.F.: Ketamine in obstetrics and gynecology. 6th World Congress of Anaesthesiology, Mexico, International Congress Series No. 387, Excerpta Medica, Amsterdam-Oxford, 1976.

Matilla, M.A.K., Lavin, H.M., Nummi, S.E. and Pekkola, P.O.: Effect of diazepam on emergence from ketamine anaesthesia, a double-blind study. Anaesthesist 28: 20-23, 1979.

Nettles, D.C., Herrin, T.J. and Mullen, J.G.: Ketamine induction in poor risk patients. Anaesth. Analg. 52: 59-64, 1973.

Neumark, J. and Halbgebauer, I.: Ketamin-Halothan-Kombinations-narkose in der Alters-Unfallchirurgie. Wien. Med. Wschr. 31: 495-498, 1973.

Peter, K., Klose, R. and Lutz, H.: Ketanest zur Narkose-einleitung beim Schock. Zschr. F. Prakt. Anaesth. U. Wiederbelebung 5: 396-401, 1970.

Piroelle, Y., Samii, K. and Viars, P.: Association de l'anesthesie peridurale et de la ketamine. Anaesth. Analg. Reanim. (France) 37: 13-15, 1980.

Schlag, G.: Technik und Probleme der Anaesthesie beim Hypovolämisch-traumatischen Schock. Die Bedeutung des Ketamins. Anästh. Prax. 7: 23-29, 1972.

Schmidt, H.: Besondere Indikationen für die Verwendung von Ketamin. Erlanger Anaesthesie Seminare I. Medizin Media Analyse, Bubenreuth, 1977.

Schulte-Steinberg, O.: In Regional Anaesthesia in Children, ed. by C. Saint Maurice and O. Schulte-Steinberg. In press, 1989.

Schulte-Steinberg, O.: Anwendung und Dosierung von Flunitrazepam in Kombination mit der Regionalanaesthesie, In Klinische Anaesthesiolgie und Intensivetherapie, Rohypnol (Flunitrazepam), 179-181, Springer Verlag, Berlin-Heidelberg-New York, 1978.

Schumacher, W., Ilgaz, E., Muntasser, H. and Fadika, G.: Ketanest als Einleitungsanaesthetikum zur Neuroleptanaesthesie. Anaesthesist 23: 1-6, 1974.

Stephen, C.R., Johnson, E. and Burleson, J.: Induction of anaesthesia with ketamine in adults. Amer. Anesthesiol. Assn. Meeting, Oct. 21, New York, N.Y., 1970.

Szappanyos, G., Gemperle, M. and Gemperle, G.: The utilization of ketamine as an adjunct with spinal and epidural analgesia, In Anaesthesiology and Resuscitation 40:188-192, Ketamin, ed. by K. Kreuscher, Springer Verlag, Berlin-Heidelberg-New York, 1969.

Vontin, H., Heller, W. and Schorer, R.: Analgosedierung und Ataranalgesie: Rohypnol und Kombination mit Analgetika, 149, Editiones Roche: Erfahrungen mit Rohypnol, 1976.

Wagner, F.: Personal communication, 1989.

White, P.F.: Comparative evaluation of intravenous agents for rapid sequence induction. Thiopental, ketamine and midazolam. Anaesthesiol. 57: 279-284, 1982.

Status of Ketamine in Anesthesiology,
edited by E.F. Domino©1990, NPP Books
P.O. Box 1491, Ann Arbor, MI 48106

Comparative Study of the Effects of Midazolam-Ketamine Anesthesia and Thiopental Sodium Induced Enflurane-Nitrous Oxide Anesthesia for Minor Gynecological Operations

W. Tolksdorf, F. Reinhard, M. Hartung, and S. Bauman

Clinic for Anesthesiology
Medical Faculty
University of Technology
Aachen, F.R. Germany

INTRODUCTION

The principal reasons for the relatively rare use of ketamine in general anesthesia are its well known cardiovascular effects and psychotomimetic emergence reactions. The small number of comparative studies between ketamine combination anesthesia and other anesthetic methods is astonishing.

A critical view of the literature indicates that ketamine combination anesthesia shows no disadvantages in its acceptance by patients. The studies which ascertained this parameter indicate that the minimum percent acceptance for neuroleptic anesthesia is 70%. Ketamine combination anesthesia was judged positively by 85-93% of patients. About 92-100% of patients were satisfied with inhalational or barbiturate induced inhalational anesthesia. Considering these figures, it is necessary to elucidate the relative importance of the side effects of ketamine combination anesthesia. These side effects are primarily nightmares or bad dreams and are reported to be characteristic of the emergence period. Not all dreams were considered as bad; some patients recalled dreams as being pleasant. Other essential aspects become important in comparing different anesthetic methods, *e.g.*, pain sensations, shivering, etc.

The acceptance of an anesthetic method depends primarily on the totality of the experience of which the patient is aware. The sleeping patient is not conscious of alterations in blood pressure and heartrate; these are insignificant for his or her evaluation. Of course, the secondary cardiovascular and respiratory effects, among others, have to be taken seriously. On the other hand, it is necessary to view the larger picture and to pay attention to all of the patient's needs. The image of ketamine today is still influenced by reports from the days of ketamine monoanesthesia. Probably because of the euphoria over the discovery of an apparently ideal monoanesthetic, the side effects of ketamine were initially not considered to be very serious. Because of the emphasis on the use of ketamine monoanesthesia, it became difficult to show the importance of combining ketamine with other drugs, especially benzodiazepines, in order to reduce its side effects, which later were shown to be very objectionable.

After a very extensive study of the literature, it seemed convenient to compare the effects and side effects of a modern ketamine combination anesthesia, midazolam-ketamine, to a conventional thiopental sodium induced enflurane-nitrous oxide anesthesia.

Materials and Methods

From July to December 1986, we investigated 90 patients at the gynecological hospital, Medical Faculty Mannheim of the University of Heidelberg, who had to undergo minor gynecological procedures under a general anesthetic.

The women were randomly distributed into 3 groups of 30 patients each.

Sequence of examination

On the day before the operation, the following were conducted by the anesthesiologist:

- Medical history
- Clinical examination
- Information on anesthesia and inherent risks
- Prescription of a benzodiazepine in the evening (flunitrazepam) and/or morning (midazolam, 5 mg i.m.)

On the day of surgery the following were done:

a) In the ward:

Administration of the prescribed medication by a nurse 30-40 min before anesthesia

Transferring the patient to the operating room

b) In the preparatory room:
Measurement of blood pressure and heart rate by the anesthesiologist
Insertion of an i.v. indwelling cannula
Infusion of Ringer's solution

c) In the operating theater:
Induction of anesthesia

Anesthesia

Group 1 received 5 mg/kg body weight of thiopental sodium; by mask enflurane 2-3% and remainder oxygen, then maintenance with 1.5-2% in nitrous oxide/oxygen in a ratio of 2:1.

Group 2 received 5 mg of midazolam i.v. and 0.5-1 mg/kg body weight of ketamine i.v. If required, reinjection of 0.5-1 mg/kg body weight of ketamine i.v.

Group 3 received 7.5 mg/kg body weight of midazolam i.v. then 2-3 mg/kg body weight of ketamine i.v. If required, reinjection of 0.5-1 mg/kg body weight of ketamine i.v.

If required, patients in groups 2 and 3 were given oxygen by mask and assisted ventilation.

Monitoring. Continuous EKG lead, blood pressure and heart rate measurements were made at least every 5 min. Intraoperative complications were recorded.

Postoperative phase. All patients were observed during the emergence period. Recordings were made with regard to recovery of consciousness, stabilization of respiration, heart rate, and blood pressure, as well as of the time of transfer to the ward.

In the ward. Routine measurements were made of blood pressure and pulse rate, as well as supervising the physical and psychological state of the patient. About 180 min after the end of anesthesia, a final inquiry was made on the postoperative condition of each patient.

Documentation. All relevant measurements and patient statements were recorded.

Statistics. The relative and absolute frequencies in nominal and ordinal variables were determined. The minimum and maximum values of each measurement were retained. Extremely deviating values in a series were included. The arithmetical mean, median, standard deviation, and variance were calculated. The data from patients with no documentation of values at a given time of examination were excluded. The H-test of Kruskal-Wallis was used to check group variances. Statistical significance was accepted at the 5% level ($P < 0.05$).

RESULTS

The anthropometric data of the 3 groups of patients were comparable as shown in Table 1.

Preoperative anxiety. Preoperative anxiety was evaluated after arrival of the patients in the preparatory room. Three degrees of anxiety were noted: high, low and none. The degree of anxiety was estimated subjectively by the patients. The greatest degree of anxiety was caused by the unusual surroundings and equipment, as well as the busy operating team. The patients were anxious about the venipuncture, the infusion, and the anesthesia. The degree of preoperative anxiety was comparable in all 3 groups: 40% of the patients had high, 40% had low, and 20% had no preoperative anxiety.

Intraoperative assisted or controlled ventilation. All of the patients in group 1 had assisted ventilation. In groups 2 and 3, clinical criteria made it necessary to use an oxygen mask. This occurred in 12 patients in the 5 mg and 18 patients in the 7.5 mg midazolam group.

Length of surgery. The mean length of surgery was 20 min in all 3 groups. The shortest operation lasted 7-9 min and the longest 40-60 min, for an average of 30-34 min. The shortest anesthesia in all 3 groups lasted 15 min and the longest 57-70 min.

Circulatory parameters. Increases in blood pressure and tachycardia were observed in all 3 groups. The reason for this may be the sympathomimetic effects in the ketamine groups, and insufficient anesthesia or analgesia in the enflurane group. In groups 1 and 2, two patients showed increases in blood pressure which needed medical treatment. In one patient in the enflurane group ventricular extrasystoles were recorded, which disappeared after administration of 100% oxygen and cessation of the enflurane. There were no alarming decreases in blood pressure in any of the patients.

Time of recovery. The time of recovery was recorded when the patients were able to carry out simple orders such as lifting their head and

TABLE 1. Anthropometric data (minimum, median, and maximum values, and percent)

	Age (yr)	*Body weight (kg)*	*Percent anesthetic risk (Lutz)* 1	2	3
Group 1	19-40-84	47-64-83	48	38	14
Group 2	20-42-84	41-63-90	42	42	10
Group 3	19-41-84	39-63-92	40	42	18

stating their name and their ward. Patients given enflurane anesthesia had the shortest recovery times.

Movements. There were no marked differences between the 3 groups. In group 1, there were 5 patients who had uncoordinated movements of a low degree and 1 patient who had uncoordinated agitation. In both ketamine groups, there were 3 patients with uncoordinated, moderately marked movements but no cases of uncoordinated agitation. The patients in group 3 were relaxed with no noticeable movements.

Postoperative sedation. The patients in the ketamine groups were significantly ($P \leq 0.05$) more sedated (up to 30 min postoperatively) than the patients in the enflurane group. Later, there were no differences between any of the groups.

Nausea and vomiting. These side effects occurred very rarely (group 1–1 patient; group 2–5 patients; group 3–none).

Observations after completion of anesthesia (see Table 2). It is interesting that the typical side effects of ketamine monoanesthesia can be extensively suppressed depending upon the dose of midazolam given.

Dream sensations. The percentages of reports of dreaming in the 3 groups are shown in Table 3. Only 1 patient in group 2 had unpleasant dreams. The incidence of bad dreams or nightmares was reduced to 0 by giving 7.5 mg midazolam i.v.

Acceptance of anesthesia by the patients. As shown in Fig. 1, patient acceptance in groups 1 and 3 was identical and mainly positive; in group 2 it was a little less positive. The differences were not significant. The anesthesiologists judged ketamine anesthesia to be better than enflurane mask anesthesia because of ease of administration and the frequent problems of ventilation by mask.

Unpleasant emergence reactions. As shown in Fig. 2, unpleasant emergence reactions, such as motor restlessness, were identical in groups 1 and 2 (20%). Pain and shivering occurred only in the enflurane group (group 1).

DISCUSSION

The purpose of this study was to compare midazolam-ketamine anesthesia with spontaneous respiration to thiopental sodium induced enflurane anesthesia by mask with assisted ventilation. Special attention was paid to secondary psychotomimetic and circulatory effects as well as patient acceptance of each anesthetic method.

Preoperative anxiety had no influence on the course of anesthesia, particularly not on unpleasant experiences which seldom occurred. Ob-

TABLE 2. Frequency of adverse effects

Effect	*Group 1*		*Group 2*		*Group 3*	
	N	*Percent*	*N*	*Percent*	*N*	*Percent*
Rapid eye movements	0	0	4	13	2	7
Nystagmus	0	0	9	30	13	43
Diplopia and triplopia	0	0	18	60	13	43
Blurred vision	3	10	2	7	2	7
Blocked nostrils	0	0	2	7	0	0
Coughing	0	0	1	3	0	0
Respiratory problems	0	0	2	7	2	7
Sensation of pressure on the heart	0	0	1	3	0	0
Reddening	0	0	2	7	0	0
Moist hands	0	0	1	3	0	0
Fatigue, excessive sleep requirement	16	53	16	53	16	53
Heaviness of the limbs	0	0	3	10	0	0
Dizziness	2	7	16	53	20	67
Vertigo	10	33	16	53	1	3
Restlessness	6	20	3	10	1	3
Tremor	2	7	0	0	0	0
Continual logomania	0	0	5	17	1	3
Perseveration	0	0	8	27	1	3
Lamentation and moaning	1	3	6	20	1	3
Sudden emotional changes smiling/weeping	0	0	2	7	0	0
Smiling/giggling	0	0	4	13	0	0
Motor difficulties including speech	0	0	3	10	6	20
Panting, puffing	0	0	4	13	0	0
Strange sentiment	0	0	8	27	2	7

TABLE 3. Incidence of dreaming

Recall of dreams	*Group 1*		*Group 2*		*Group 3*	
	N	*Percent*	*N*	*Percent*	*N*	*Percent*
No recall	0	0	2	6.7	9	30
Pleasant	0	0	9	30	0	0
Indifferent	0	0	2	6.7	6	20
Unpleasant	0	0	1	3.3	0	0
None	30	100	16	53.3	24	80

servations of other authors (Sklar *et al.*, 1981; Tolksdorf *et al.*, 1982) for these anesthetic methods are not in agreement.

In group 1, no patient could remember any dreams. The incidence of dreaming was 40% in group 2 and 20% in group 3. The incidence of

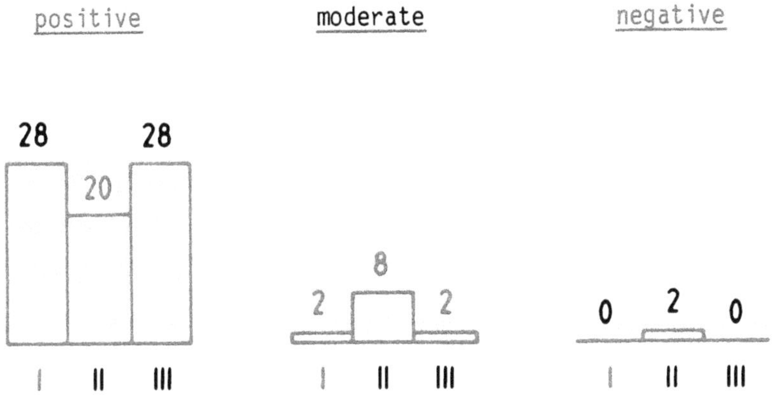

Fig. 1. Degree of acceptance of the different forms of anesthesia. N=30 in each group.

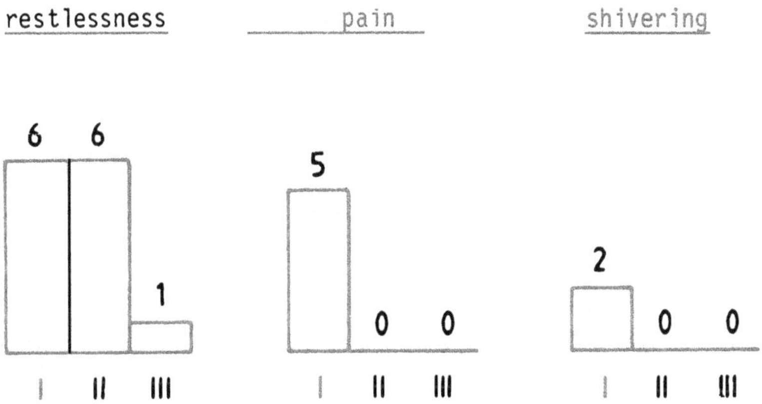

Fig. 2. Number of unpleasant emergence reactions in the 3 different groups of patients.

dreaming did not differ from that of ketamine monoanesthesia but there were clear distinctions. Unpleasant dream like experiences, as well as unreal imaginations and color impressions (Doenicke *et al.*, 1969; Schneider, 1980), and hallucinations (Meyers *et al.*, 1987; Pedersen, 1981; Sadove *et al.*, 1971), which are typical of ketamine monoanesthesia, were suppressed by its combination with midazolam with one exception. Studies concerning midazolam-ketamine anesthesia (Cartwright and Pingel, 1984; Funtan and Hetzel, 1986; Reinhold and Pfistere, 1986) report prevention or reduction of nightmares, hallucinations, and other psychological derangements. An analysis of the literature (Tolksdorf *et al.*, 1988) indicates a frequency of 5.1% of unpleasant dreams and hallucinations with benzodiazepine-ketamine anesthesia. Most of these studies were carried out with diazepam as the benzodiazepine used. According to Funtan and Hetzel (1986), neither ketamine nor midazolam dosage had any influence on dreaming. Unpleasant emergence reactions like nystagmus, rapid eye movements, diplopia and triplopia, which occurred exclusively in groups 2 and 3, have been observed by other investigators (Benke and Unger, 1969; Ghoneim *et al.*, 1985; Hagelin and Lundberg, 1981; Langrehr *et al.*, 1967; White, 1983). Harris *et al.* (1975) showed that the main reason for postoperative side effects was the preoperative condition of the patients. Obiaya *et al.* (1981) observed more postoperative side effects among introverted than extroverted patients.

We could not confirm any relationship between preoperative anxiety and unpleasant side effects. Intro- and extroversion were not determined. Other unpleasant emergence reactions, such as restlessness, were observed more frequently in the enflurane group (20%) than in the midazolam-ketamine group (3%). White (1982) observed only insignificant restlessness with midazolam-ketamine.

It should be stressed that the combination of midazolam and ketamine can eliminate the unpleasant side effects of ketamine monoanesthesia with increasing doses of midazolam. There is not much change in reports of dreaming, but the content of the dreams is indifferent. Probably the anterograde amnestic efficacy of midazolam is responsible for this.

Patient acceptance of the anesthetic method was comparable in groups 1 and 3 (more than 90%). Patients with the lower dose of midazolam (group 2) were less satisfied. Podlesch and Dähn (1986) found an acceptance rate of midazolam-ketamine anesthesia of 87%. This percentage is quite satisfactory.

Cardiovascular parameters were stable in all 3 groups. Circulatory complications did not occur. Typically, blood pressure and heart rate were higher in group 2 than in group 3, and lowest in group 1. There were no significant differences between groups. This result agrees with the experiences of others in the literature (Tolksdorf, 1988). Inherent to the method, all group 1 patients needed assisted ventilation by oxygen mask. This was seldom necessary in the patients in group 2.

The advantages of stable, spontaneous respiration are lost with increasing midazolam dosage. In group 3, 18 patients (60%) needed assisted ventilation.

The time of recovery was the same in all 3 groups. However, the patients in the ketamine groups were more sedated for up to 30 min more postoperatively than the patients in the enflurane group. This emphasizes the fact that ketamine is not a short but a middle lasting anesthetic. The analgesic effect of ketamine is useful after painful operative procedures. Far more patients in the enflurane group experienced postoperative pain than in the ketamine groups.

Conclusions

Midazolam-ketamine anesthesia is an easy and reliable anesthetic method which is accepted by anesthesiologists as well as patients. Patient acceptance is greater with larger doses of midazolam. However, the larger doses of midazolam eliminate some of the advantages of ketamine mono-anesthesia, *e.g.*, maintenance of pharyngeal and laryngeal reflexes. It is necessary to carefully supervise the patients, especially monitoring their cardiovascular and respiratory status.

Some undesirable side effects of ketamine are partly, and others completely, eliminated by midazolam. Reduction of the sympathomimetic effects of ketamine, as well as suppression of unpleasant dreams, should be stressed as the major advantages of a midazolam-ketamine combination.

References

Benke, A. and Unger, W.: Psychische und vestibuläre Effekte von Ketamine. Anaesthesiologie und Wiederbelebung 40: 167-169, 1969.

Cartwright, P.D. and Pingel, S.M.: Midazolam and diazepam in ketamine anesthesia. Anaesthesia 39: 439-442, 1984.

Doenicke, A., Kugler, J., Emmert, M., Laub, M., and Kleiner, H.: Ein Leistungsvergleich nach Ketamine und Methohexital. Anaesthesiologie und Wiederbelebung 40: 146-155, 1969.

Funtan, E. and Hetzel, W.: Kombination Midazolam/Ketamin zur Einleitung und Aufrechterhaltung von Narkosen bei kurzen, schmerzhaften Eingriffen. In: VII European Congress of Anaesthesiology, ed. by H. Bergmann, H. Kramar, and K. Steinbereithner, Anaesthesiologie und Intensivmedizin 17: 64, 1986.

Ghoneim, M.M., Hinrichs, J.V., Mewaldt, S.P., and Peterson, R.C.: Ketamine: Behavioral effects of subanesthetic doses. J. Clin. Psychopharmacol. 5: 70-76, 1985.

Hagelin, A. and Lundberg, D.: Ketamine for postoperative analgesia after upper abdominal surgery. Clin. Ther. 4: 229-233, 1981.

Harris, J.A., Beiersner, R.J., Edwards, D., and Bailey, L.W.: Attention, learning and personality during ketamine emergence. A pilot study. Anesth. Analg. 54: 169-172, 1975.

Langrehr, D., Alai, P., Andjelković, J., and Lluge, I.: Zur Narkose mit Ketamine (CI-591) Bericht über erste Erfahrungen in 500 Fällen. Anaesthesist 16: 308-318, 1967.

Meyers, E.F. and Charles, P.: Prolonged adverse reactions to ketamine in children. Anesthesiol. 49: 39-40, 1987.

Obiaya, M.D., Dakaraju, P., and Binitie, A.O.: Ketamine emergence and personality. East Afr. Med. J. 58: 489-493, 1981.

Pedersen, T.: Ketamine as continuous intravenous infusion combined with diazepam in non-abdominal surgery. A randomized double blind study. Anaesthesist 30: 111-114, 1981.

Podlesch, J. and Dähn, H.: Ataranalgetische Kombination mit Ketamin und Midazolam—eine multizentrische Studie. Fortschr. Anaest. 1: 1-8, 1986.

Reinhold, P., Pfisterer, T.: Ketamin-Midazolam-Stickoxydul-Intubationsnarkosen bei Kindern. In Ketamine. VII European Congress of Anaesthesiology, ed. by H. Bergmann, H. Kramar, and K. Steinbereither, Anaesthesiologie und Intensivemedizin 18: 93, 1986.

Sadove, M.S., Hatano, S., Zahed, B., Arastounejad, P., and Roman, V.: Clinical study of droperidol in the prevention of the side effects of ketamine anesthesia. A preliminary report. Anesth. Analg. 50: 388-393, 1971.

Schneider, D.: Kieferchirurgische Erfahrungen mit der Wirkung von Faustan (Diazepam) auf unerwunschte Aufwachreaktionen nach Ketamin-Kurznarkose. Zahn-Mund-Kieferheilkd. 68: 769-772, 1980.

Sklar, G.S., Zukin, S.R., and Reilly, T.A.: Adverse reactions to ketamine anesthesia. Anaesthesia 36: 183-187, 1981.

Tolksdorf, W. *et al.*: Das präoperative psychische Befinden. Med. Habil. Universitätsklinik Mannheim 18-26, 88-90, 1982.

Tolksdorf, W. *et al.*: Neue Aspekte zu Ketamin in der Anaesthesie, Intensiv- und Notfallmedizin. Springer Verlag Heidelberg, Anaesthesiologie und Intensivmedizin 198, 1988.

White, P.F.: Comparative evaluation of intravenous agents for rapid sequence induction—thiopental, ketamine and midazolam. Anesthesiol. 57: 279-284, 1982.

White, P.F., Dworsky, W.A., Horai, Y., and Trevor, A.J.: Comparison of continuous infusion fentanyl or ketamine versus thopental—determining the mean effective serum concentration for outpatient surgery. Anesthesiol. 59: 564-569, 1983.

Status of Ketamine in Anesthesiology,
edited by E.F. Domino©1990, NPP Books
P.O. Box 1491, Ann Arbor, MI 48106

I.M. Ketamine in Trauma Patients

M.F. Brandt, W. Dick, and H.W. Gervais

Department of Anesthesiology
Johannes Gutenberg University
Mainz, F.R. Germany

INTRODUCTION

Treatment of the injured patient is being progressively improved by providing good prehospital care (Shires, 1985). Pain relief for out of hospital trauma care is a difficult task for the staff of the emergency medical system. Analgesia is one of the stress reducing measures used to improve impairments of vital functions. In addition to unnecessary suffering, unrelieved acute pain is often associated with abnormal reflex responses that can exacerbate the underlying disease process leading to serious complications, even to the death, in some patients (Bonica, 1988). Moreover, some technical procedures, like the immediate management of fractures by traction, can only be carried out with sufficient pain relief. During the initial care of patients with multiple injuries in the field, there is a disproportion between theoretical requirements and practicability of pain control (Kreuscher, 1986). For example, it is almost never possible to perform regional blocks in the field. That means, pain management as part of initial care is limited mostly to the use of systemic analgesics or anesthetics.

Only drugs which do not adversely affect hemodynamics or ventilation can be used in prehospital treatment of trauma patients, because even short periods of hypotension or apnea could be life threatening in this class of high risk patients. In order that ambulance personnel with no or only limited experience in i.v. injections may be able to provide medication, a simple route of drug application, such as i.m. injection, must be possible. On the other hand, i.m. injection is only feasible if systemic absorption takes place even under limited peripheral blood flow conditions such as shock states in traumatized patients. Ketamine seems to be one of the few drugs which fulfill these requirements.

Previous investigations have proven the efficacy of subanesthetic doses of i.v. or i.m. ketamine in injured patients (Hirlinger and Dick,

1984; Hirlinger and Pfenninger, 1987). The present study was done to investigate the effects of low dose i.m. ketamine on consciousness, pain, peripheral microcirculation and hemodynamics in traumatized patients in shock. In addition, ketamine plasma levels were determined.

Methods

A randomized prospective experimental design was used. Low dose i.m. ketamine for analgesia was assessed in the field in 20 out of hospital trauma patients with clinical signs of shock. Shock was defined as a systolic blood pressure of 100 mm Hg or less, a heart rate of more than 100 beats/min, and visible signs of impaired microcirculation (pale skin or cyanosis). Patients with head injuries, impaired consciousness, known coronary artery disease or hypertension were excluded. Patients with prior administration of analgesics or after intake of alcoholic beverages were also excluded from the study.

Ten patients received ketamine in a dose of 0.5 mg/kg, and 10 other patients received ketamine in a dose of 1.0 mg/kg by deep injection into the deltoid muscle. Immediately before and at 5, 10 and 30 min after ketamine, heart rate, blood pressure, color of skin (normal = 1, pale = 2, or cyanotic = 3), level of consciousness (fully alert = 1, arousable = 2, or severely disoriented = 3), and degree of pain (no pain = 1, slight = 2, moderate = 3, or intensive pain = 4) were assessed.

Ketamine plasma levels (venous blood) were determined at the same time points in 5 patients of each group. Plasma levels were analyzed by gas chromatography, according to the method described by Hengy *et al.* (1978).

Clinical assessment of patients and ketamine injection in the field was done by a trained emergency physician who was a staff member of a physician equipped ambulance car. This so called "Notarztwagen" is part of the German emergency medical system which provides high level medical care in the field and during transportation to the hospital by means of a very well equipped special ambulance.

Results

Consciousness

Ten min after ketamine injection, maximum sedation was achieved in both groups. The level of consciousness, however, was still 1.6 ± 0.84 in the 0.5 mg/kg group and 1.5 ± 0.53 in the 1.0 mg/kg group (Fig. 1).

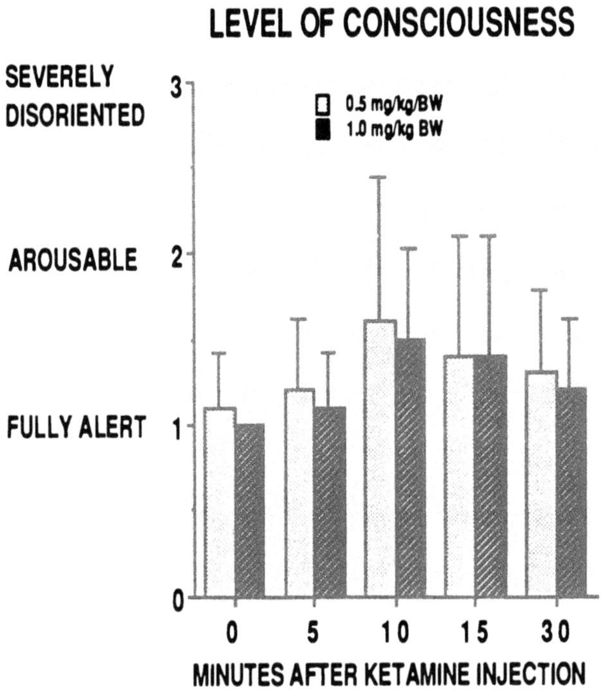

Fig. 1. Level of consciousness (mean ± S.D.).

Pain Relief

In the 0.5 mg/kg group, maximum pain relief occurred 10 min after ketamine. The pain score, which was 3.9 ± 0.32 before drug injection, decreased to 2.2 ± 0.79 at 10 min and slowly increased to a level of 2.9 ± 0.88 at the end of the observation period.

In the 1.0 mg/kg ketamine group, maximum relief of pain occurred after 15 min. Before drug injection, the pain score reached 3.5 ± 0.53. It decrementally decreased to a level of 1.5 ± 0.71 15 min after ketamine. At the end of the observation period, the pain score was 1.9 ± 1.1 (Fig. 2).

Microcirculation

Peripheral microcirculation, as assessed by the color of the skin, did not change in the 0.5 mg/kg group throughout the observation period (1.9 ± 0.57 before ketamine: 1.7 ± 0.48 at 30 min after ketamine.) In the 1.0 mg/kg group, a slight improvement could be seen 15 min after drug

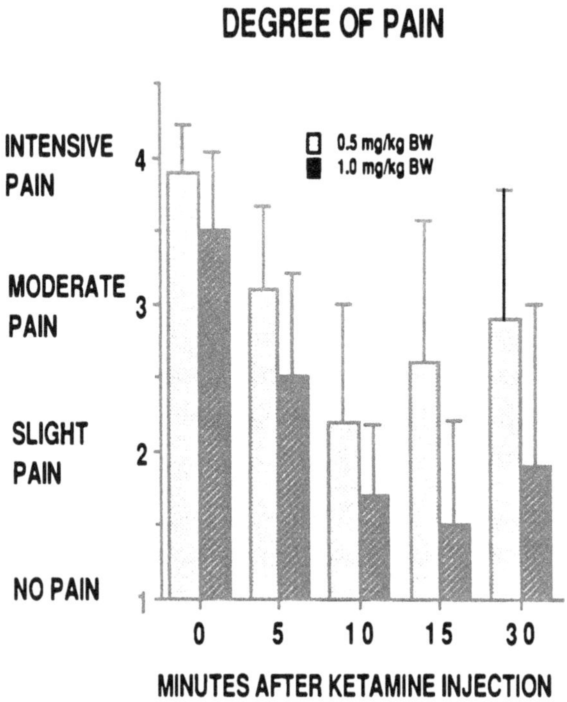

Fig. 2. Pain score (mean ± S.D.).

injection (from 1.8 ± 0.42 before to 1.2 ± 0.42 15 min after ketamine, Fig. 3).

Hemodynamics

There were only minor changes in heart rate or blood pressure throughout the 30 min period of the study (Figs. 4 and 5).

Plasma Levels

In the 0.5 mg/kg group, a maximum ketamine plasma level of 57.25 ± 62.73 ng/ml was achieved 30 min after injection. In the 1.0 mg/kg group, a peak plasma level of 181.5 ± 34.67 ng/ml was achieved 10 min after ketamine.

Plasma levels stayed in the respective range of their peaks throughout the entire observation period (Fig. 6).

Side Effects

There were no adverse effects in either of the two groups during the entire 30 min after ketamine injection.

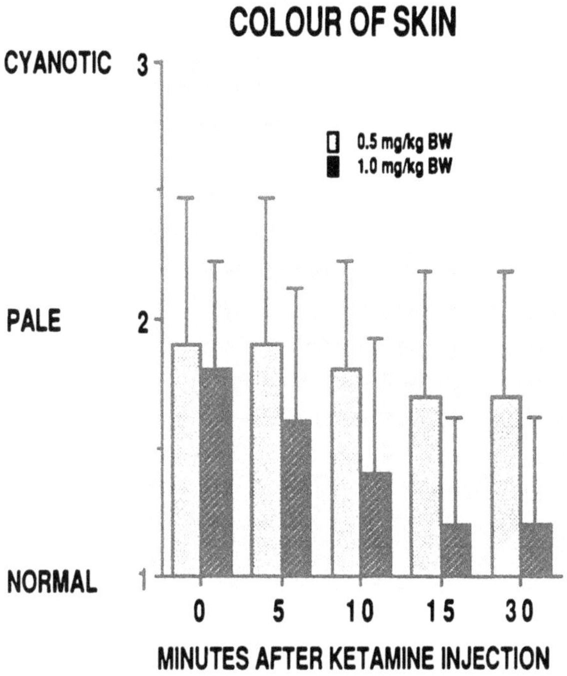

Fig. 3. Peripheral microcirculation (mean ± S.D.).

Discussion

In this study, ketamine proved to be a suitable agent to provide adequate pain relief in out of hospital trauma patients with clinical signs of shock.

It is noteworthy that there was no clinically important deterioration in the level of consciousness after ketamine injection. At the same time, analgesia could be achieved rapidly. Surprisingly, pain relief was sufficient even in the 0.5 mg/kg group though plasma concentrations were far below the commonly accepted effective range of between 100-150 ng/ml (Clements and Nimmo, 1981; Benet and Sheiner, 1985). In the 1.0 mg/kg group, plasma levels were within this therapeutic range. However, our plasma level data have to be interpreted with caution because of the great variability of the plasma concentrations, especially in the 0.5 mg/kg group, and the small number of patients.

The pain score used was deliberately simply structured. This 4-level pain score had been used successfully by other investigators under similar experimental conditions (Knoche *et al.*, 1981; Hirlinger and Dick, 1984;

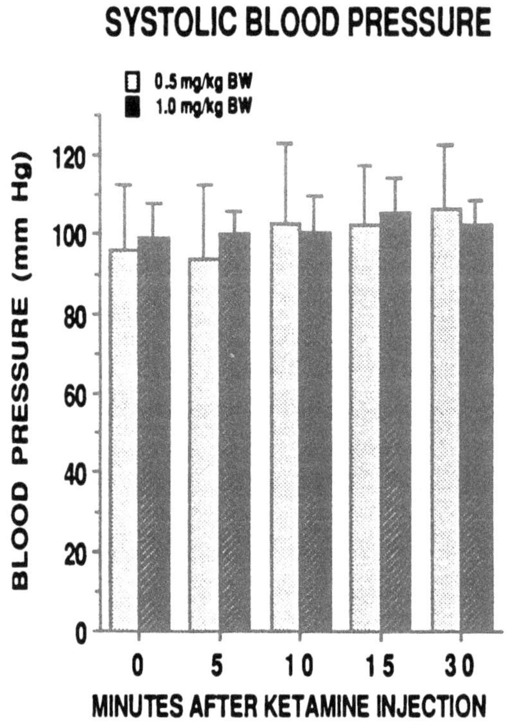

Fig. 4. Systolic blood pressure (mean ± S.D.).

Hirlinger and Pfenninger, 1987). Pilot studies had shown that this score was the maximum mental effort which could be obtained from patients under the conditions of trauma and stress.

With respect to hemodynamics, blood pressure and heart rate did not change. Theoretical considerations, from animal and isolated heart experiments that ketamine may lower blood pressure and decrease cardiac output because of its negative inotropic actions, especially under conditions of depleted catecholamine stores, must be kept in mind (Reves *et al.*, 1987; Goldberg *et al.*, 1970; Valicenti *et al.*, 1973; Tweed and Mymin, 1974; Urthaler *et al.*, 1976). A vasodilating effect of ketamine, which generally is overcome by sympathetic stimulation, also has to be considered (Fukuda *et al.*, 1983). Cardiac depression apparently did not occur in the subanesthetic dosage range we used. In order to avoid the interfering effects of ketamine and injury related impairments of mental status, head injured patients were excluded from the present study. There is a great deal of contradictory clinical and experimental data on the

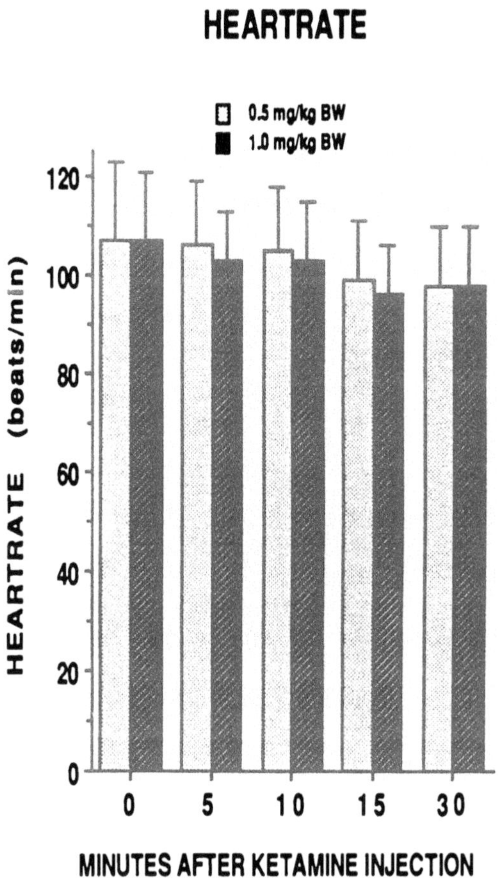

Fig. 5. Heart rate (mean ± S.D.).

subject of ketamine, cerebral blood flow, intracranial pressure, and patients with intracranial pathology. Most authors agree that, at least in man, ketamine increases cerebral blood flow and intracranial pressure, both in normal and abnormal brain (Takeshita *et al.*, 1972; Shapiro *et al.*, 1972; Sari *et al.*, 1972; List *et al.*, 1972; Hougaard *et al.*, 1974; Schwedler *et al.*, 1982). The same is true for many animal species, especially for the commonly used dog model (Dawson *et al.*, 1971). However, recently there seems to be evidence that the increase in intracranial pressure due to ketamine depends mainly on the ventilatory status of the patient (see report by Pfenninger *et al.* in this volume).

In several well controlled studies there was no increase in intracranial

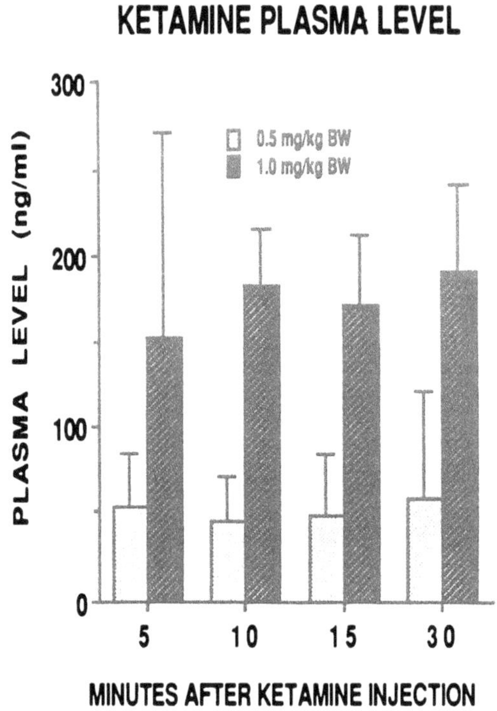

Fig. 6. Ketamine plasma level (mean ± S.D.).

pressure after ketamine if arterial PCO_2 was maintained, or if patients or experimental animals were hyperventilated (Schwedler *et al.*, 1982; Pfenninger *et al.*, 1985). Ketamine (0.5 mg/kg or 2.0 mg/kg) decreased cerebral perfusion pressure (Pfenninger *et al.*, 1985), especially in situations with impaired cerebral autoregulation like hypovolemic shock and simultaneously elevated intracranial pressure. The drop in cerebral perfusion pressure occurred because of reduced arterial blood pressure. This was caused by the combined negative inotropic effects of ketamine and excessive blood loss (approximately 30% of the total volume) under extreme shock conditions. In our study, the extent of shock was markedly less than in Pfenninger's study. This may explain why we failed to see any cardiovascular depression.

Pfenninger's results are in contrast to a recently published study of Artru and Katz (1989; see also this volume). These authors confirmed previous assumptions that ketamine elevates intracranial pressure because it increases cerebral blood volume, even when arterial PCO_2 is kept constant in mechanically ventilated dogs without intracranial pathology. The ketamine induced change in intracranial pressure could be reversed by pre- or postketamine hypocapnia or diazepam.

Summary

In summary, we conclude that the i.m. injection of a subanesthetic dose of ketamine in trauma patients provides fast and effective analgesia without serious side effects. The question of whether or not ketamine is an appropriate pharmacological agent for polytraumatized patients with concomitant head injuries still remains open and should be addressed in further clinical studies with well controlled ventilation of the patients.

References

Artru, A.A. and Katz, R.A.: Cerebral blood volume and CSF pressure following administration of ketamine in dogs: Modification by pre- or posttreatment with hypocapnia or diazepam. J. Neurosurg. Anesthesiol. 1: 8-15, 1989.

Benet, L.Z. and Sheiner, L.B.: Appendix II. Design and optimization of dosage regimens: Pharmacokinetic data. In The Pharmacological Basis of Therapeutics, 7th Edition, ed. by A. Goodman Gilman, L.S. Goodman, T.W. Rall, and F. Murad, pp. 1663-1733, Macmillan Publ. Co., New York, 1985.

Bonica, J.J.: Foreword. In Pain Management in Emergency Medicine, ed. by P.M. Paris and R.D. Stewart, Appleton & Lange, Norwalk, 1988.

Clements, J.A. and Nimmo, W.S.: Pharmacokinetics and analgesic effect of ketamine in man. Br. J. Anaesth. 53: 27-30, 1981.

Dawson, B., Michenfelder, J.D., and Theye, R.A.: Effects of ketamine on canine cerebral blood flow and metabolism: Modification by prior administration of thiopental. Anesth. Analg. 50: 443-447, 1971.

Fukuda, S., Murakawa, T., Takeshita, H., and Toda, N.: Direct effects of ketamine on isolated canine cerebral mesenteric arteries. Anesth. Analg. 62: 553-558, 1983.

Goldberg, A.H., Keane, P.W., and Phear, W.P.: Effects of ketamine on contractile performance and excitability of isolated heart muscle. J. Pharmacol. Exp. Ther. 175: 388-394, 1970.

Hengy, H., Vollmer, K.O., and Gladigau, V.: GLC-determination of tilidine, nortilidine and bisnortilidine in biological fluids with a nitrogen sensitive detector. J. Pharm. Sci. 67: 1765-1768, 1978.

Hirlinger, W.K. and Dick, W.: Untersuchungen zur intramuskulären Ketaminanalgesie bei Notfallpatienten. II. Klinische Studie an traumatisierten Patienten. Anaesthesist. 33: 272-275, 1984.

Hirlinger, W.K. and Pfenninger, E.: Intravenöse Analgesie mit Ketamin beim Notfallpatienten. Anaesthesist 36:140-142, 1987.

Hougaard, K., Hansen, A., and Brodersen, P.: The effect of ketamine on regional cerebral blood flow in man. Anesthesiol. 41: 562-567, 1974.

Knoche, E., Traub, E., and Dick, W.: Analgesie mit Ketamin bei Notfallpatienten und im Katastrophenfall. In Ketamin (Ketanest[R]) in Notfallund Katastrophenmedizin, ed. by W. Dick, perimed Fachbuch, Erlangen, 1981.

Kreuscher, H.: Schmerzbekämpfung am Katastrophenort. In Katastrophenmedizin-Probleme des Massenanfalls Kranker und Verletzter, ed. by E. Ungeheuer, pp. 71-75, Deutscher. Ärzte-Verlag, Köln, 1986.

List, W.F., Crumrine, R.S., and Cascorbi, H.F., *et al.*: Increased cerebrospinal fluid pressure after ketamine. Anesthesiol. 36: 98-99, 1972.

Pfenninger, E., Dick, W., and Ahnefeld, F.W.: The influence of ketamine on both normal and raised intracranial pressure of artificially ventilated animals. Eur. J. Anaesthesiol. 2: 297-307, 1985.

Pfenninger, E. and Reith, A.: Ketamine and intracranial pressure. This volume, 1990.

Reves, J.G., Flezzani, P., and Kissin, I.: Pharmacology of intravenous induction agents. In Cardiac Anesthesia, 2nd Ed., ed. by J.A. Kaplan, pp. 125-150, W.B. Saunders Co., Philadelphia, 1987.

Sari, A., Okuda, Y., and Takeshita, H.: The effect of ketamine on cerebral spinal fluid pressure. Anesth. Analg. 51: 560-565, 1972.

Schwedler, M., Miletich, D.J., and Albrecht, R.F.: Cerebral blood flow and metabolism following ketamine administration. Can. Anaesth. Soc. J. 29: 222-225, 1982.

Shapiro, H.M., Wyte, S.R., Harris, A.B. *et al.*: Ketamine anesthesia in patients with intracranial pathology. Br. J. Anaesth. 44: 1200-1204, 1972.

Shires, G.T.: Initial care of the injured patient. In Principles of Trauma Care, 3rd Ed., ed. by G.T. Shires, pp. 105-110, McGraw-Hill, New York, 1985.

Takeshita, H., Okuda, Y., and Sari, A.: The effects of ketamine on cerebral circulation and metabolism in man. Anesthesiol. 36: 69-75, 1972.

Tweed, W.A. and Mymin, D.: Myocardial force-velocity relations during ketamine anesthesia at constant heart rate. Anesthesiol. 41: 49-52, 1974.

Urthaler, F., Walker, A.A., and James, T.N.: Comparison of the inotropic action of morphine and ketamine studied in canine cardiac muscles. J. Thorac. Cardiovasc. Surg. 72: 142-149, 1976.

Valicenti, J.F., Newman, W.H., Bagwell, E.E., *et al.*: Myocardial contractility during induction and steady-state ketamine anesthesia. Anesth. Analg. 52: 190-194, 1973.

Status of Ketamine in Anesthesiology,
edited by E.F. Domino©1990, NPP Books
P.O. Box 1491, Ann Arbor, MI 48106

N-Methyl-D-Aspartate (NMDA) Antagonism is Central to the Actions of Ketamine and Other Phencyclidine Receptor Ligands

J. Church[1] and D. Lodge[2]

[1]*Department of Physiology*
University of British Columbia
Vancouver, Canada V6T 1W5

[2]*Department of Veterinary Basic Sciences*
Royal Veterinary College
London, United Kingdom

Ketamine and other anesthetic arylcyclohexylamines such as phencyclidine (PCP) and tiletamine share a wide range of behavioral effects. As well as being able to induce anesthesia, they also possess amnesic, analgesic, anticonvulsant, and psychotomimetic actions. This unique spectrum of activity, together with the fact that some members of this group of compounds have become important drugs of abuse which can elicit a schizophreniform psychosis (Domino and Luby, 1981), has prompted much research into the mechanism(s) which may underlie these complex actions. In this chapter we shall briefly review some of the behavioral effects of the dissociative anesthetics and related drugs. We shall then examine some of the many effects of these compounds on central transmitter systems and address the question of which of these effects might account for the major behavioral actions of these drugs. In particular, we shall detail the modulation by these drugs of neuronal excitation mediated by the N-methyl-D-aspartate (NMDA) subclass of postsynaptic excitatory amino acid (EAA) receptor, as much evidence now suggests that NMDA antagonism may be of fundamental importance to many of the central effects of ketamine and other PCP like drugs.

Behavioral Effects of Ketamine and Other PCP Like Compounds

With the obvious and single exception of anesthesia, each of the shared behavioral effects of the arylcyclohexylamines mentioned above has been reported to occur following the administration of subanesthetic doses of these compounds. As regards the general anesthetic state produced by these drugs, this is sufficiently different to that seen with other agents that a separate term, dissociative anesthesia, has been applied to it (see Corssen and Domino, 1966). Dissociative anesthesia is clinically a state of light hypnosis and analgesia in combination with the relative maintenance of pharyngeal/laryngeal and other protective reflexes with dissociation of limbic and cortical EEG patterns (Chen *et al.*, 1959, 1966; Domino, 1964; Corssen and Domino, 1966; White *et al.*, 1982). In contrast, the "triad of anesthesia" associated with the use of conventional general anesthetics combines deep hypnosis with obtunded reflex activity, analgesia being provided either by deepening the level of hypnosis with the general anesthetic agent or by a selective analgesic drug.

Initial reports suggested that ketamine was able to produce analgesia in humans when administered in subanesthetic doses, although after a single bolus injection the analgesia was of short duration (Sadove *et al.*, 1971; Clements *et al.*, 1982). More recently, however, doubt has been expressed regarding the ability of ketamine to provide significant analgesia following surgery unless near anesthetic doses of the drug are used (Owen *et al.*, 1987). Nor have initial reports of the analgesic efficacy of intrathecal or epidural ketamine been confirmed (Ravat *et al.*, 1987). Studies in laboratory animals, where ketamine is able to elicit antinociception only when anesthetic doses are given (Smith *et al.*, 1985), support the more recent human data.

In contrast to the uncertainty surrounding the analgesic potency of the arylcyclohexylamines, little doubt exists as to the psychotomimetic efficacy of these drugs (White *et al.*, 1982). Subjects emerging from dissociative anesthesia or who have abused low doses of arylcyclohexylamines may experience dysphoric and hallucinogenic effects which are qualitatively different from those produced by other psychoactive drugs. These effects are clearly dose related although even subanesthetic doses of ketamine (0.25 mg/kg) are able to produce psychotomimetic effects (Liang and Liang, 1975; White *et al.*, 1982; Ghoneim *et al.*, 1984).

Similarly, although there was at one time much debate over the profile of anticonvulsant/convulsant activity shown by the arylcyclohexylamines, there is now little doubt that at low doses anticonvulsant actions predominate. Thus, ketamine exerts dose related anticonvulsant activity, not only in a wide variety of experimental animal models of epilepsy, but also in convulsions associated with a variety of disease states in humans (see Church, this volume).

Finally, the amnesic effects of ketamine and PCP require comment. Both drugs disrupt learned behavior in animals (Balster, 1987) and, in subanesthetic doses, produce a retrograde amnesia in humans (Petersen and Stillman, 1978; Ghoneim *et al.*, 1984). Chronic PCP abuse results in memory loss and impairment of learning (Lerner and Burns, 1978; Siegel, 1978).

Neurotransmitter Interactions

The neuropharmacological and neurophysiological basis for the many shared behavioral effects of the anesthetic arylcyclohexylamines has been investigated extensively (see Kamenka *et al.*, 1983; Domino and Kamenka, 1988). Interactions with monoaminergic, cholinergic and *gamma*-aminobutyric acid (GABA) mediated systems have all been documented, as have effects on opioid receptors and neuromodulatory peptides such as cholecystokinin and substance P (Fratta *et al.*, 1981; Snell *et al.*, 1984; Johnson and Snell, 1985; Johnson, 1987; Pongdhana *et al.*, 1987). In turn, each of these interactions has been invoked either individually or in combination to explain the effects of these drugs. The large literature on this subject precludes an exhaustive review, but examination of the available evidence suggests that most of the actions of the arylcyclohexylamines on neurotransmitter systems so far described are insufficient in themselves to fully account for the shared behavioral effects of these compounds.

As an example, the hypothesis that many of the behavioral effects of PCP might be due to its indirect dopamine agonist activity has received much support. *In vitro*, PCP has been shown to stimulate tyrosine hydroxylase activity, facilitate dopamine release, and inhibit dopamine re-uptake; *in vivo*, it affects dopamine synthesis and metabolism (Johnson, 1987). Nevertheless, although the IC_{50} values for PCP and 8 arylcyclohexylamine analogues as inhibitors of dopamine re-uptake are highly correlated with the IC_{50} values for inhibition of specific binding to the PCP receptor (which is in turn highly correlated with some of the behavioral effects of dissociative anesthetics; see below), this correlation does not extend to dissociative anesthetics from different chemical classes which have similar behavioral properties to the arylcyclohexylamines (Snell *et al.*, 1984; Vignon and Lazdunski, 1984; Johnson and Snell, 1985).

Blockade of voltage-gated K^+ channels has also been proposed to explain the behavioral effects of dissociative anesthetics and related compounds (Bartschat and Blaustein, 1988). Nevertheless, it is apparent that the potency of a series of PCP like drugs for this effect is not well correlated with their potency in eliciting their common behavioral actions (Lodge *et al.*, 1988). Furthermore, the concentrations of the compounds required to block K^+ channels are higher than those found after the administration of subanesthetic doses of the drugs (Lacey and Henderson, 1986; Rothman, 1988), again suggesting that this property does not directly account for the behavioral effects of the drugs which are seen at subanesthetic doses. On the other hand, K^+ channel blockade by PCP like drugs may make a contribution to acute PCP toxicity (Lacey and Henderson, 1986).

In a similar manner, effects on serotonergic (Smith *et al.*, 1977), noradrenergic (Smith *et al.*, 1981), anticholinergic (Cohen *et al.*, 1974; Maayani *et al.*, 1974) and GABAergic (Dye and Taberner, 1975; Wood and Hertz, 1980) systems are not able to fully account for the behavioral properties listed earlier, although such effects are of obvious importance in determining the overall spectrum of activity of individual dissociative anesthetics. Johnson (1978), having reviewed the pharmacological actions of PCP on a number of transmitter systems, concluded: "Previous studies have suggested that the central biogenic amines, 5-hydroxytryptamine, dopamine, and norepinephrine, as well as acetylcholine (ACh) and GABA may be involved either directly or indirectly with the mechanism(s) underlying the behavioral effects of PCP. . .almost all of these studies neglected to establish a basic dose-response relationship for the observed effect . . . In summary, these studies have only suggested that 5-hydroxytryptamine, dopamine, norepinephrine, ACh and GABA may be involved in some way in the mediation of the behavioral effects produced by PCP." In a subsequent review eight years later, the same author concluded that further investigation of the effects of dissociative anesthetics on these transmitter systems had still not demonstrated their clear involvement in the causation of many of the behavioral effects of these drugs (Johnson and Snell, 1986). In the interim, however, a central binding site selective for dissociative anesthetics and drugs with similar behavioral properties had been described. A large body of evidence from animal behavioral discrimination and receptor binding studies indicates that some of the behavioral responses elicited by these groups of compounds might be mediated by their interaction with this receptor, one consequence of which is a reduction in the excitatory effects of NMDA on central neurons. In the remainder of this chapter we shall review the evidence which indicates that reduced excitatory transmission at central synapses utilizing NMDA receptors, a direct consequence of the binding of PCP like compounds to the PCP receptor, underlies at least some of the behavioral properties common to the dissociative anesthetics and related compounds.

Excitatory Amino Acids and PCP Like Drugs

Our knowledge of the mechanisms underlying the behavioral effects of dissociative anesthetics and related compounds advanced dramatically after the description of a central binding site in 1979 (Vincent *et al.*, 1979: Zukin and Zukin, 1979). The pharmacologic specificity of this site is unique in that only other dissociative anesthetics (including those from different chemical classes to the arylcyclohexylamines, *e.g.*, etoxadrol, dexoxadrol and (-)-2-methyl-3,3-diphenyl-3-propanolamine ((-)-2-MDP) and drugs which are known from animal behavioral discrimination studies to possess PCP like activity are able to displace [^{3}H]-PCP from its binding site. Included in this latter group are compounds such as N-allylnormetazocine (NANM), cyclazocine and pentazocine (benzomorphans); dextrorphan and dextromethorphan (morphinans); LY 154045 (a benz(f)isoquinoline); and MK-801 (a dibenzocycloalkenimine). Other classes of psychoactive drugs share neither the discriminative stimulus effects of PCP like drugs nor their affinity for the PCP receptor (Balster and Willetts, 1988; Lodge *et al.*, 1988).

The apparent affinities of these drugs for the PCP receptor are highly correlated, not only with their ability to act as PCP like interoceptive cues, but also with their ability to inhibit rotarod performance (Vincent *et al.*, 1979), suggesting that the binding site is a physiologically relevant receptor. In addition, other lines of evidence suggest commonalities between these groups of compounds. Thus, where the relevant studies have been performed, all of these drugs have been found to possess anticonvulsant, psychotomimetic, and amnesic effects and are able to disrupt learning (Balster, 1987; Lodge *et al.*, 1988; Church *et al.*, 1989). Cyclazocine, for example, has potent anticonvulsant activity in a variety of animal models of epilepsy (Church, this volume), is potently psychotomimetic in humans (Haertzen, 1970), and can disrupt associative learning (Tang and Franklin, 1983). Finally, members of these groups of drugs have similar neurophysiological profiles. Thus, in the chronic spinal dog they reduce certain reflexes (Vaupel, 1983), whereas in the intact animal polysynaptic reflexes are reduced with little concurrent effect on monosynaptic reflexes (Harris and Pierson, 1964).

The observation that ketamine selectively reduced polysynaptic rather than monosynaptic reflexes (Tang and Schroeder, 1973) was subsequently confirmed by Lodge and Anis (1984), who also found that this action was not accompanied by any marked effects on short duration glycinergic or long duration GABA-ergic inhibitions or dorsal root potentials at the subanesthetic doses employed (*i.e.*, 2.5-10.0 mg/kg i.v. in the cat). Nor did ketamine produce a barbiturate like enhancement of the effect of microelectrophoretic GABA on single spinal neurons in cats (Lodge and Curtis, 1978). These observations suggested not only that it was unlikely that enhancement of GABA mediated inhibitions makes a major contribution to the behavioral effects of ketamine (cf. the barbiturates), but also that ketamine might in some way be antagonizing the action of these neurotransmitters because polysynaptic excitations were already known to be mediated by EAAs (Watkins and Evans, 1981). Since ketamine does not interfere with the release of EAA transmitters (Minchin, 1981), subsequent investigations focussed on the effects of ketamine on the excitation of neurons by putative EAA neurotransmitters and their analogues.

Acidic amino acids such as L-glutamate and L-aspartate are likely to be major excitatory transmitters throughout the CNS (Watkins and Evans, 1981; Mayer and Westbrook, 1987). At present, there is a consensus that there are three major subtypes of postsynaptic receptors for the EAAs; these are named after their selective agonists, *i.e.* NMDA, quisqualic acid and kainic acid. Using the technique of microelectrophoresis, the effects of ketamine and PCP on neuronal excitations evoked by NMDA, quisqualate, kainate, and ACh were investigated. Whether administered locally or i.v., they were found to be selective NMDA antagonists (Fig. 1; Lodge *et al.*, 1982; Anis *et al.*, 1983). As expected from agonists capable of acting at all 3 postsynaptic receptor subtypes (Mayer and Westbrook, 1987), responses to L-glutamate and L-aspartate were reduced to an intermediate extent. The effects of ketamine and PCP on NMDA evoked excitations were seen at subanesthetic doses and, in the case of ketamine, showed a weak stereoselectivity with the (+) isomer being about 3 times as potent as the (-) isomer as an NMDA antagonist (Lodge *et al.*, 1982).

This NMDA blocking effect was soon found to be shared not only by other arylcyclohexylamines (*e.g.* tiletamine; Lodge *et al.*, 1983), but also by dissociative anesthetics from different chemical classes, such as etoxadrol and (-)-2-MDP (Berry *et al.*, 1984a; Blake *et al.*, 1986). In addition, all of those compounds which had a known affinity for the PCP receptor and exerted PCP like behavioral effects in animal discrimination studies were subsequently also found to be selective NMDA antagonists (Fig. 2). Their relative NMDA blocking potency closely paralleled their relative affinity for the PCP receptor and their relative ability to act as PCP like interoceptive cues (Lodge *et al.*, 1988). Opioid ligands, such as morphine and ethylketocyclazocine, had no selective action on responses of neurons to NMDA nor did naloxone reverse the NMDA antagonist effects of these

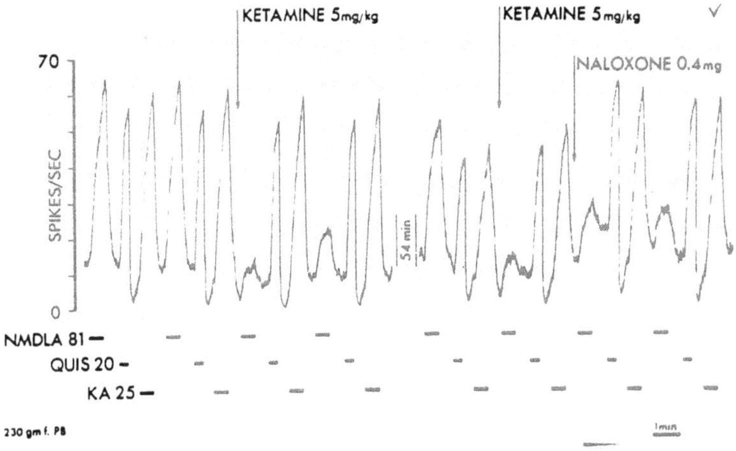

Fig. 1. Effect of i.v. ketamine 5 mg/kg on responses of a rat spinal neuron to electrophoretic administration of NMDA, quisqualate and kainate. Selective reduction of NMDA responses by ketamine recovers over a period of about one hr, and a subsequent dose produces a similar block of NMDA which is not reversed by naloxone (equivalent to 1.7 mg/kg i.v.).

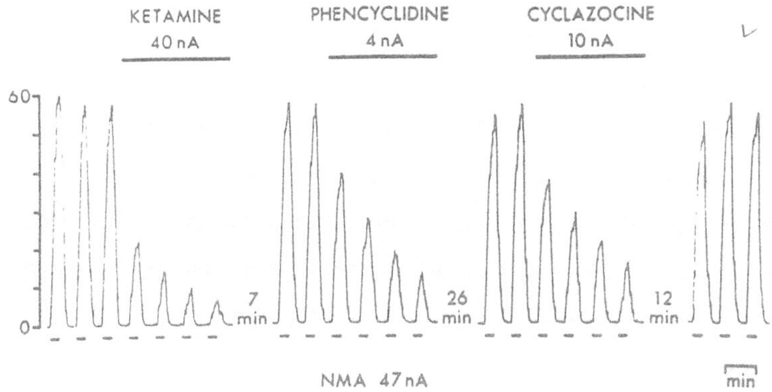

Fig. 2. Comparison of the potencies of ketamine, phencyclidine and cyclazocine as NMDA antagonists on a rat spinal neuron. Using the same protocol of electrophoretic administration, phencyclidine is approximately 10 and 2.5 times as potent as ketamine and cyclazocine, respectively. Ordinate: spikes/sec. Abscissa: time in min.

drugs (Fig. 1; Berry *et al.*, 1984b). Similarly, although many PCP like drugs show affinity for the *sigma* receptor as well as the PCP receptor (Quirion *et al.*, 1987), selective *sigma* receptor ligands show no selective antagonism of NMDA or other transmitter amino acids (Lodge *et al.*, 1988).

These observations, originally made *in vivo*, have now been confirmed in a variety of *in vitro* paradigms (see Domino and Kamenka, 1988). For example, PCP like drugs reduce the depolarizations evoked by NMDA application on frog spinal cords and slices of rat neocortex without affecting the actions of K^+, kainate or quisqualate (Harrison and Simmonds, 1985; Martin and Lodge, 1985). Relative NMDA antagonist potencies obtained using such quantitative *in vitro* techniques faithfully reflect those obtained in *in vivo* studies and, in turn, are consistent with binding at the PCP receptor and with PCP-like behaviors.

The use of *in vitro* electrophysiological and binding techniques has enabled a detailed investigation of the mechanism by which PCP like compounds exert their NMDA antagonist effects. Evidence now suggests that they act as noncompetitive antagonists by blocking the NMDA receptor operated ionophore. Ketamine, for example, displaces the dose response curve for NMDA to the left in a non-parallel fashion whether NMDA induced transmitter release or depolarization of cortical slices is the measured parameter and does not displace competitive NMDA receptor antagonists from the NMDA receptor (Harrison and Simmonds, 1985; Lodge and Johnston, 1985; Martin and Lodge, 1985; Johnson and Snell, 1986). Rather, excitatory amino acids enhance the binding of PCP like drugs to their receptor, indicating the agonist dependent nature of their antagonist actions (Loo *et al.*, 1986; Fagg, 1987). Finally, under voltage clamp, the block by ketamine of NMDA evoked currents is highly voltage and use dependent (MacDonald *et al.*, 1987). All of these data are consistent with the idea that PCP like compounds act as non-competitive NMDA antagonists by binding to a site (*i.e.* the PCP receptor) within the lumen of the NMDA receptor operated channel. That ketamine and PCP are able to attenuate the increase in intracellular Ca^{2+} levels evoked by NMDA (Fig. 3; O'Shaughnessy and Lodge, 1988) is also consistent with a channel blocking effect, the NMDA receptor operated ionophore being permeable not only to monovalent cations, but also to Ca^{2+}(Mayer and Westbrook, 1987).

It is now apparent that the PCP binding site within the NMDA receptor operated ionophore is but one of a number of modulatory sites which regulate the activity of the NMDA receptor complex. Included among these sites are the NMDA recognition site itself; a strychnine insensitive glycine binding site; a site also within the lumen of the receptor-linked channel, but distinct from the PCP binding site, which binds Mg^{2+} and other divalent cations in a voltage-dependent manner; and possible binding sites for Zn^{2+}, polyamines and tricyclic antidepressants

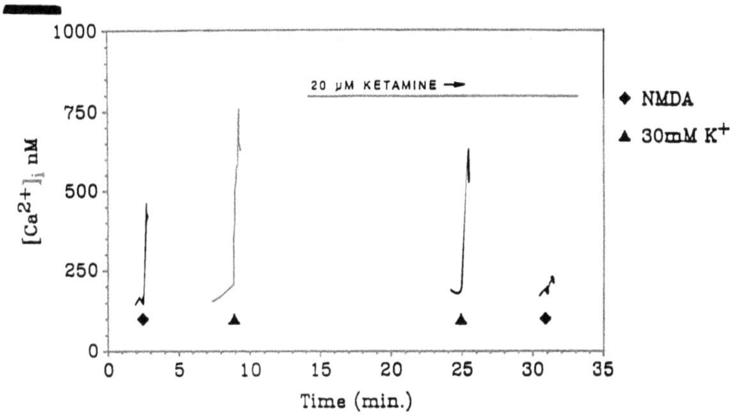

Fig. 3. Rise in intracellular $[Ca^{2+}]$ evoked in a cultured hippocampal pyramidal cell loaded with the Ca^{2+}sensitive dye FURA-2 AM. Responses to 200 μM NMDA (filled diamonds) and 30 mM K^+ (filled triangles) are shown. Ketamine (20 μM) blocked the rise in $[Ca^{2+}]$ evoked by NMDA with only a minor effect on that evoked by K^+. (Unpublished observations, J. Church.)

which are seemingly distinct from the others (Lodge, 1988). The multiplicity of regulatory sites on the NMDA receptor complex, together with its widespread distribution in the CNS, suggests that NMDA receptor mediated events are profoundly important for normal CNS function. The corollary of this, of course, is that any disruption of the normal functioning of this receptor complex might profoundly disrupt CNS function.

Behavioral Implications

The excellent correlations observed between the relative potencies of PCP like drugs to produce PCP-like discriminative stimuli, to displace tritiated ligands bound to the PCP receptor and selectively and noncompetitively to reduce neuronal excitations mediated by the NMDA receptor (Lodge *et al.*, 1988) suggests the possibility that reduced excitatory transmission at central synapses utilizing NMDA receptors underlies at least some of the behavioral properties common to these groups of compounds. A prerequisite for this suggestion is that activation of NMDA receptors occurs during synaptic transmission and that this can be blocked by ketamine (and other PCP receptor ligands). Many reports have now provided evidence for NMDA receptor involvement in excitatory synaptic transmission in many regions of the CNS, including neocortex (Thomson *et al.*, 1985), thalamus (Salt *et al.*, 1988), hippocampus (Coan and Collingridge, 1987) and spinal cord (Headley *et al.*, 1987). In each of the cited studies, ketamine (as well as some other PCP like compounds) has been shown to be capable of reducing a component of the synaptic response elicited either by electrical (Thomson *et al.*, 1985) or peripheral sensory (Headley *et al.*, 1987) stimuli.

Given the widespread distribution and importance of NMDA receptors in central synaptic transmission (Mayer and Westbrook, 1987), it is of interest to ask which of the behavioral effects of ketamine and other PCP like compounds might reflect their potent and selective NMDA blocking activity. As mentioned earlier, many PCP like compounds share amnesic, anesthetic, anticonvulsant, analgesic and psychotomimetic actions. To this list, at least in experimental animals, should also be added neuroprotective activity. Evidence for a causal relationship between NMDA antagonism and the neuroprotective and anticonvulsant properties of PCP like drugs is now extensive and is reviewed by Choi and Church, respectively (this volume). We shall therefore confine our remarks to an examination of whether NMDA antagonism might underlie the shared anesthetic, analgesic, amnesic or psychotomimetic actions of PCP like compounds.

Anesthesia

The fact that subanesthetic doses of ketamine are able to substantially reduce the excitatory actions of NMDA suggests that this action does not directly underlie its anesthetic efficacy. Thus, in the rat 2-5 mg/kg ketamine markedly attenuates responses to NMDA (Fig. 1; Anis *et al.*, 1983), whereas at least 50 mg/kg is required for surgical anesthesia (Flecknell, 1987). In addition, in the rat the range of concentrations of ketamine required for anesthesia lies between about 100 and 300 μM (Cohen *et al.*, 1973). Although such concentrations depress excitatory synaptic transmission (Oshima and Richards, 1988), this effect, in turn, is unlikely to be a specific consequence of NMDA antagonism. The IC_{50} for ketamine for reducing NMDA-induced depolarizations in slices of rat neocortex *in vitro* is 5.5 μM (Aram *et al.*, 1989). Concentrations of ketamine 20 to 50 times higher than this would have effects on numerous neurotransmitter systems and membrane ionic conductances which would better account for the reduction in synaptic transmission than NMDA antagonism (see Domino and Kamenka, 1988; Oshima and Richards, 1988).

Nevertheless, given the importance of NMDA receptors in mediating information transfer throughout many regions of the CNS, it seems likely that the NMDA blocking effects of dissociative anesthetics will, at least in part, determine the qualitative nature of the anesthesia induced by these drugs. Salt *et al.* (1988) have, for example, suggested that the ability of ketamine to reduce somatosensory input to the thalamus may account partly for the anesthetic action of the drug. In addition, competitive as well as noncompetitive NMDA antagonists are able to induce an anesthetic state in pigeons, rats and rhesus monkeys (Koek and Woods, 1988), although the relevance of these observations to anesthetic activity in humans awaits determination.

Analgesia/Antinociception

As referred to above, controversy now surrounds previous reports of the analgesic activity of subanesthetic doses of ketamine. Nevertheless, analgesia has also been documented following administration of PCP, dexoxadrol, etoxadrol and (-)-2-MDP (Chen and Weston, 1960; Lasagna and Pearson, 1965; Tang et *al.*, 1984), although in all cases the basis of this analgesic activity is ill understood. There is even conflicting evidence about the extent to which ketamine, for example, interacts with opioid receptors and whether or not naloxone is able to reverse ketamine induced analgesia (Fratta *et al.*, 1980; Smith *et al.*, 1985). In contrast to the dissociative anesthetics, the analgesic actions of PCP like NMDA antagonists, such as cyclazocine and pentazocine, appear largely to reflect activity at *mu* and *kappa* opioid receptors, although it is of interest that high doses of naloxone are required to reverse their analgesic effects (see Yaksh and Noueihed, 1985).

Evidence is available which supports the involvement of both NMDA receptors in nociceptive pathways within the CNS and NMDA antagonism in the genesis of ketamine's (weak) analgesic activity. Cahusac *et al.* (1984) reported that an intrathecally administered competitive NMDA antagonist elicited weak antinociception, although this was accompanied by clear motor weakness (an effect that does appear to reflect functional NMDA antagonism; see Polc, 1985; Turski *et al.*, 1985). Similarly, Headley *et al.* (1987) described the ability of ketamine, administered i.v. in doses which selectively reduce responses to NMDA, to reduce nociceptive responses of motoneurons. On the other hand, some PCP like compounds with potent NMDA antagonist actions (*e.g.*, dextrorphan; Church *et al.*, 1989) appear devoid of analgesic activity, even when administered intrathecally (Yaksh and Noueihed, 1985). At present, therefore, evidence tends to suggest that the NMDA blocking activity of PCP receptor ligands does not, in a simple or direct way, mediate their analgesic or antinociceptive activity.

Learning and Memory

Competitive and noncompetitive NMDA antagonists are able to impair learning and memory when administered in NMDA selective doses (*e.g.*, Morris *et al.*, 1986; Balster, 1987). Long term potentiation (LTP), a phenomenon often studied as an electrophysiological model of memory, is mediated, at least in part, by postsynaptic receptors of the NMDA type (Collingridge and Bliss, 1987) and can be blocked *in vivo* and *in vitro* by PCP receptor ligands, again administered in NMDA selective doses (Stringer *et al.*, 1983). Further, it has been demonstrated that blockade of LTP by a competitive NMDA antagonist is associated with learning impairment produced by the same compound (Morris *et al.*, 1986). Although the latter observation does not prove that these phenomena are causally related, it does support the possibility that the effects of PCP like compounds on learning and memory may reflect NMDA antagonism.

NMDA receptors have also been implicated in experience dependent changes in visual cortex (Rauschecker and Hahn, 1987) and in the storage of information during learning (McCabe and Horn, 1988). These observations suggest that NMDA receptor activation may be an important variable for the expression of activity dependent synaptic modifications. The possibility that PCP like compounds may be able to modulate neuronal plasticity in both the developing and mature CNS requires further investigation before these compounds can be safely administered in the long term (*e.g.*, as anticonvulsant agents).

Psychotomimesis

As described above, there is an excellent correlation for PCP like drugs between NMDA antagonist potency and the ability to produce PCP appropriate responding in animal behavioral discrimination studies (Lodge *et al.*, 1988). If such studies are predictive of the possibility of psychotomimetic activity in humans (Herling *et al.*, 1983), then this correlation would argue for the proposal that NMDA antagonism may mediate the psychotomimetic effects of PCP like drugs. However, there is obviously no guarantee that animal discrimination studies are predictive in this way and so it becomes necessary to examine the human data available. Such an examination reveals that there is a reasonably good relationship between the psychotomimetic potency of PCP like compounds in humans with their potency as NMDA antagonists in experimental animals (Lodge *et al.*, 1988; Church *et al.*, 1989). For example, ingestion of 5 mg of PCP by recreational users produces a similar frequency of psychotomimetic effects to 50-100 mg ketamine (Siegel, 1978), a relative potency ratio also seen for NMDA antagonism (Anis *et al.*,

1983). Indeed, it is apparent that of the PCP like NMDA antagonists so far used in humans, few have ever been or remain in clinical use. It would appear that this is largely because of their propensity to induce psychotomimetic effects. Thus, PCP, etoxadrol, dexoxadrol, tiletamine, N-allylnormetazocine, cyclazocine and bremazocine, although all potent NMDA antagonists (Lodge *et al.*, 1988), have never been widely used despite their useful anesthetic, analgesic or anticonvulsant properties. Of those PCP like NMDA antagonist compounds so far examined, only pentazocine, dextromethorphan, levorphanol and ketamine have found a place in routine clinical use. Pentazocine, dextromethorphan and levorphanol are very weak NMDA antagonists whose clinically useful activity (*e.g.* antitussive activity in the case of dextromethorphan) is found at doses lower than those which produce NMDA antagonism or elicit psychotomimetic effects. Ketamine, on the other hand, does induce dysphoria at normal therapeutic doses but is used only in the acute situation where this effect is outweighed by its spectrum of other (useful) effects.

There are obvious dangers in attempting to ascribe a causal link between a single neurophysiological parameter (*i.e.*, NMDA antagonism) and complex behaviors such as anesthesia, analgesia and psychotomimesis. Indeed, the hypotheses and correlations presented in the last part of this chapter must be regarded as very tentative. The evidence, although circumstantial, is nevertheless considerable that NMDA antagonism may contribute to the amnesic and psychotomimetic, as well as anticonvulsant and neuroprotective, actions of PCP like drugs. NMDA antagonism may, therefore, not only be central to some of the advantageous actions of PCP like compounds, but also may underlie some of their disadvantageous behavioral effects. This possibility may limit the clinical utility of all PCP-like drugs with NMDA antagonist activity to acute therapy in intensive care units where adverse reactions can be limited and managed.

Acknowledgements

We are indebted to Mrs. A.M. Forsyth for the preparation of the manuscript. Supported by the Wellcome Trust and the Medical Research Council (U.K.).

References

Anis, N.A., Berry, S.C., Burton, N.R., and Lodge, D.: The dissociative anaesthetics, ketamine and phencyclidine, selectively reduce excitation of central mammalian neurones by N-methyl-D-aspartate. Br. J. Pharmacol. 79: 565-575, 1983.

Aram, J.A., Martin, D., Tomczyk, M., Zeman, S., Millar, J., Pohler, G., and Lodge, D.: Neocortical epileptogenesis *in vitro*: Studies with N-methyl-D-aspartate, phencyclidine, *sigma* and dextromethorphan receptor ligands. J. Pharmacol. Exp. Ther. 248: 320-328, 1989.

Balster, R.L.: The behavioral pharmacology of phencyclidine. In Psychopharmacology: The Third Generation of Progress, H.Y. Meltzer, ed., pp. 1573-1579, Raven Press, New York, 1987.

Balster, R.L. and Willetts, J.: Receptor mediation of the discriminative stimulus properties of phencyclidine and *sigma* opioid agonists. In Transduction Mechanisms of Drug Stimuli, F.C. Colpaert and R.L. Balster, eds., pp. 122-135, Springer-Verlag, Berlin, 1988.

Bartschat, D.K. and Blaustein, M.P.: Psychotomimetic *sigma*-ligands, dexoxadrol and phencyclidine block the same presynaptic potassium channel in rat brain. J. Physiol. 403: 341-353, 1988.

Berry, S.C., Anis, N.A. and Lodge, D.: The effect of the dioxolanes on amino acid induced excitation in the mammalian spinal cord. Brain Res. 307: 85-90, 1984a.

Berry, S.C., Dawkins, S.L. and Lodge, D.: Comparison of σ- and κ-opiate receptor ligands as excitatory amino acid antagonists. Br. J. Pharmacol. 83: 179-185, 1984b.

Blake, J.C., Davies, S.N., Church, J., Martin, D. and Lodge, D.: 2-methyl-3,3-diphenyl-3-propanolamine (2-MDP) selectively antagonizes N-methylaspartate (NMA). Pharmacol. Biochem. Behav. 24: 23-25, 1986.

Cahusac, P.M.B., Evans, R.H., Hill, R.G., Rodriguez, R.E. and Smith, D.A.S.: The behavioral effects of an N-methylaspartate receptor antagonist following application to the lumbar spinal cord of conscious rats. Neuropharmacol. 23: 719-724, 1984.

Chen, G., Ensor, C.R., and Bohner, B.: The pharmacology of 1-(1-phenylcyclohexyl)piperidine HCl. J. Pharmacol. Exp. Ther. 127: 241-250, 1959.

Chen, G., Ensor, C.R., and Bohner, B.: The neuropharmacology of 2-(*o*-chlorophenyl)-2-(methylamino)cyclohexanone hydrochloride. J. Pharmacol. Exp. Ther. 152: 332-339, 1966.

Chen, G. and Weston, J.K.: The analgesic and anesthetic effect of 1-(1-phenylcyclohexyl)piperidine HCl in the monkey. Anesth. Analg. 39: 132-137, 1960.

Church, J., Jones, M.G., Davies, S.N., and Lodge, D.: Antitussive agents as N-methylaspartate antagonists: Further studies. Can. J. Physiol. Pharmacol., 67: 561-567, 1989.

Clements, J.A., Nimmo, W.S. and Grant, I.S.: Bioavailability, pharmacokinetics and analgesic activity of ketamine in humans. J. Pharm. Sci. 71: 539-542, 1982.

Coan, E.J. and Collingridge, G.L.: Effects of phencyclidine, SKF 10,047 and related psychotomimetic agents on N-methyl-D-aspartate receptor mediated synaptic responses in rat hippocampal slices. Br. J. Pharmacol. 91: 547-556, 1987.

Cohen, M.L., Chan, S.-L., Bhargava, H.N. and Trevor, A.J.: Inhibition of mammalian brain acetylcholinesterase by ketamine. Biochem. Pharmacol. 23: 1647-1652, 1974.

Cohen, M.L., Chan, S.-L., Way, W.L. and Trevor, A.J.: Distribution in the brain and metabolism of ketamine in the rat after intravenous administration. Anesthesiol. 39: 370-376, 1973.

Collingridge, G.L. and Bliss, T.V.P.: NMDA receptors—their role in long-term potentiation. Trends Neurosci. 10: 288-293, 1987.

Corssen, G. and Domino, E.F.: Dissociative anesthesia: Further pharmacologic studies and first clinical experience with the phencyclidine derivative CI-581. Anesth. Analg. 45: 29-40, 1966.

Domino, E.F.: Neurobiology of phencyclidine (Sernyl)—a drug with an unusual spectrum of pharmacological activity. Int. Rev. Neurobiol. 6: 303-347, 1964.

Domino, E.F. and Kamenka, J.-M., Eds.: *Sigma* and Phencyclidine-Like Compounds as Molecular Probes in Biology, NPP Books, Ann Arbor, MI, 1988.

Domino, E.F. and Luby, E.D.: Abnormal mental states induced by phencyclidine as a model of schizophrenia. In PCP (Phencyclidine): Historical and Current Perspectives, E.F. Domino, ed., pp. 401-413, NPP Books, Ann Arbor, MI, 1981.

Dye, D.J. and Taberner, P.V.: The effects of some new anaesthetics on the *in vitro* activity of glutamate decarboxylase and GABA transaminase in crude brain extracts and on the levels of amino acids *in vivo*. J. Neurochem. 24: 997-1001, 1975.

Fagg, G.E.: Phencyclidine and related drugs bind to the activated N-methyl-D-aspartate receptor channel complex in rat brain membranes. Neurosci. Lett. 76: 221-227, 1987.

Flecknell, P.A.: Laboratory Animal Anaesthesia, Academic Press, London, 1987.

Fratta, W., Casu, M., Balestrieri, A., Loviselli, A., Biggio, G., and Gessa, G.L.: Failure of ketamine to interact with opiate receptors. Eur. J. Pharmacol. 61: 389-391, 1980.

Fratta, W., Rossetti, Z., and Gessa, G.L.: Rapid depletion and restoration of striatal met-enkephalin after ketamine. Life Sci. 29: 93-97, 1981.

Ghoneim, M.M., Hinrichs, J.V., Mewaldt, S.P., and Petersen, R.C.: Ketamine: Behavioral effects at subanesthetic doses. Anesthesiol. 61: A390, 1984.

Haertzen, C.A.: Subjective effects of narcotic antagonists cyclazocine and nalorphine on the Addiction Research Center Inventory (ARCI). Psychopharmacol. 18: 366-377, 1970.

Harris, L.S. and Pierson, A.K.: Some narcotic antagonists in the benzomorphan series. J. Pharmacol. Exp. Ther. 143: 141-148, 1964.

Harrison, N.L. and Simmonds, M.A.: Quantitative studies on some antagonists of N-methyl-D-aspartate in slices of rat cerebral cortex. Br. J. Pharmacol. 84: 381-391, 1985.

Headley, P.M., Parsons, C.G. and West, D.C.: The role of N-methylaspartate receptors in mediating responses of rat and cat spinal neurones to defined sensory stimuli. J. Physiol. 385: 169-188, 1987.

Herling, S., Solomon, R.E. and Woods, J.H.: Discriminative stimulus effects of dextrorphan in pigeons. J. Pharmacol. Exp. Ther. 227: 723-731, 1983.

Johnson, K.M.: Neurochemical pharmacology of phencyclidine. NIDA Res. Monogr. 21: 44-52, 1978.

Johnson, K.M.: Neurochemistry and neurophysiology of phencyclidine. In Psychopharmacology: The Third Generation of Progress, H.Y. Meltzer, ed., pp. 1581-1588, Raven Press, New York, 1987.

Johnson, K.M. and Snell, L.D.: Effects of phencycldine (PCP)-like drugs on turning behavior, ^{3}H-dopamine uptake, and ^{3}H-PCP binding. Pharmacol. Biochem. Behav. 22: 731-735, 1985.

Johnson, K.M. and Snell, L.D.: Involvement of dopaminergic, cholinergic and glutamatergic mechanisms in the actions of phencyclidine-like drugs. NIDA Res. Monogr. 64: 52-66, 1986.

Kamenka, J.-M., Domino, E.F. and Geneste, P., Eds.: Phencyclidine and Related Arylcyclohexylamines: Present and Future Applications, NPP Books, Ann Arbor, MI, 1983.

Koek, W. and Woods, J.H.: Assessing directly observable behavioral effects of phencyclidine (PCP)-like drugs in pigeons, in rats, and in rhesus monkeys. In *Sigma* and Phencyclidine-Like Compounds as Molecular Probes in Biology, E.F. Domino and J.-M. Kamenka, eds., pp. 493-509, NPP Books, Ann Arbor, MI, 1988.

Lacey, M.G. and Henderson, G.: Actions of phencyclidine on rat locus coeruleus neurones *in vitro*. Neurosci. 17: 485-494, 1986.

Lasagna, L. and Pearson, J.W.: Analgesic and psychotomimetic properties of dexoxadrol. Proc. Soc. Exp. Biol. 118: 352-354, 1965.

Lerner, S.E. and Burns, R.S.: Phencyclidine use among youth: History, epidemiology and acute and chronic intoxication. NIDA Res. Monogr. 21: 66-118, 1978.

Liang, H.S. and Liang, H.G.: Minimizing emergence phenomena: subdissociative dosage of ketamine in balanced surgical anesthesia. Anesth. Analg. 54: 312-316, 1975.

Lodge, D., Ed.: Excitatory Amino Acids in Health and Disease, John Wiley and Sons, Chichester, 1988.

Lodge, D. and Anis, N.A.: Effects of ketamine and three other short acting anaesthetics on spinal reflexes and inhibitions in the cat. Br. J. Anaesth. 56: 1143-1151, 1984.

Lodge, D., Anis, N.A., Berry, S.C. and Burton, N.R.: Arylcyclohexylamines selectively reduce excitation of mammalian neurons by aspartate like amino acids. In Phencyclidine and Related Arylcyclohexylamines: Present and Future Applications, J.-M. Kamenka, E.F. Domino and P. Geneste, eds., pp. 595-616, NPP Books, Ann Arbor, MI, 1983.

Lodge, D., Anis, N.A., and Burton, N.R.: Effects of optical isomers of ketamine on excitation of cat and rat spinal neurons by amino acids and acetylcholine. Neurosci. Lett. 29: 282-286, 1982.

Lodge, D., Aram, J.A., Church, J., Davies, S.N., Martin, D., Millar, J., and Zeman, S.: *Sigma* opiates and excitatory amino acids. In Excitatory Amino Acids in Health and Disease, D. Lodge, eds., pp. 237-259, John Wiley and Sons, Chichester, 1988.

Lodge, D. and Curtis, D.R.: Time course of GABA and glycine actions on cat spinal neurones: Effect of pentobarbitone. Neurosci. Lett. 8: 125-129, 1978.

Lodge, D. and Johnston, G.A.R.: Effect of ketamine on amino acid-evoked release of acetylcholine from rat cerebral cortex *in vitro*. Neurosci. Lett. 56: 371-375, 1985.

Loo, P., Braunwalder, A., Lehmann, J. and Williams, M.: Radioligand binding to central phencyclidine recognition sites is dependent on excitatory amino acid receptor agonists. Eur. J. Pharmacol. 123: 467-468, 1986.

Maayani, S., Weinstein, H., Ben-Zvi, S., Cohen, S., and Sokolovsky, M.: Psychotomimetics as anticholinergic agents. I. l-cyclohexylpiperidine derivatives. Biochem. Pharmacol. 26: 1435-1439, 1974.

MacDonald, J.F., Miljkovic, Z., and Pennefather, P.: Use-dependent block of excitatory amino acid currents in cultured neurons by ketamine. J. Neurophysiol. 58: 251-266, 1987.

Martin, D. and Lodge, D.: Ketamine acts as a non-competitive N-methyl-D-aspartate antagonist on frog spinal cord *in vitro*. Neuropharmacol. 24: 999-1003, 1985.

Mayer, M.L. and Westbrook, G.L.: The physiology of excitatory amino acids in the vertebrate central nervous system. Prog. Neurobiol. 28: 197-276, 1987.

McCabe, B.J. and Horn, G.: Learning and memory: Regional changes in N-methyl-D-aspartate receptors in the chick brain after imprinting. Proc. Natl. Acad. Sci. USA 85: 2849-2853, 1988.

Minchin, M.C.W.: The effect of anaesthetics on the uptake and release of γ-aminobutyrate and D-aspartate in rat brain slices. Br. J. Pharmacol. 73: 681-689, 1981.

Morris, R.G.M., Anderson, E., Lynch, G.S., and Baudry, M.: Selective impairment of learning and blockade of long-term potentiation by an N-methyl-D-aspartate receptor antagonist, AP5. Nature 319: 774-776, 1986.

O'Shaughnessy, C.T. and Lodge, D.: N-methyl-D-aspartate receptor mediated increase in intracellular calcium is reduced by ketamine and phencyclidine. Eur. J. Pharmacol. 153: 201-209, 1988.

Oshima, E. and Richards, C.D.: An *in vitro* investigation of the action of ketamine on excitatory synaptic transmission in the hippocampus of the guinea pig. Eur. J. Pharmacol. 148: 25-33, 1988.

Owen, H., Reekie, R.M., Clements, J.A., Watson, R., and Nimmo, W.S.: Analgesia from morphine and ketamine. Anaesthesia 42: 1051-1056, 1987.

Petersen, R.C. and Stillman, R.C.: Phencyclidine: An overview. NIDA Res. Monogr. 21: 1-17, 1978.

Polc, P.: 2-amino-7-phosphonoheptanoic acid depresses *gamma* moto-neurons and polysynaptic reflexes in the cat spinal cord. Eur. J. Pharmacol. 117: 387-389, 1985.

Pongdhana, K., Ogawa, N., Hirose, Y., Ono, T., Kosaka, F. and Mori, A.: Effects of ketamine on the cholecystokinin, somatostatin, substance P, and thyrotropin releasing hormone in discrete regions of rat brain. Neurochem. Res. 12: 73-77, 1987.

Quirion, R., Chicheportiche, R., Contreras, P.C., Johnson, K.M., Lodge, D., Tam, S.W., Woods, J.H., and Zukin, S.R.: Classification and nomenclature of phencyclidine and *sigma* receptor sites. Trends Neurosci. 10: 444-446, 1987.

Rauschecker, J.P. and Hahn, S.: Ketamine-xylazine anaesthesia blocks consolidation of ocular dominance changes in kitten visual cortex. Nature 326: 183-185, 1987.

Ravat, F., Dorne, R., Baechle, J.P., Beaulaton, A., Lenoir, B., Leroy, P. and Palmier, B.: Epidural ketamine or morphine for postoperative analgesia. Anesthesiol. 66: 819-822, 1987.

Rothman, S.: Noncompetitive N-methyl-D-aspartate antagonists affect multiple ionic currents. J. Pharmacol. Exp. Ther. 246: 137-142, 1988.

Sadove, M.S., Shulman, M., Hatano, S. and Fevold, N.: Analgesic effects of ketamine administered in subdissociative doses. Anesth. Analg. 50: 452-457, 1971.

Salt, T.E., Wilson, D.G. and Prasad, S.K.: Antagonism of N-methylaspartate and synaptic responses of neurones in the rat ventrobasal thalamus by ketamine and MK-801. Br. J. Pharmacol. 94: 443-448, 1988.

Siegel, R.K.: Phencyclidine and ketamine intoxication. NIDA Res. Monogr. 21: 119-147, 1978.

Smith, D.J., Azzaro, A.J., Zaldivar, S.B., Palmer, S., and Lee, H.S.: Properties of the optical isomers and metabolites of ketamine on the high affinity transport and catabolism of monoamines. Neuropharmacol. 20: 391-396, 1981.

Smith, D.J., Perrotti, J.M., Mansell, A.L., and Monroe, P.J.: Ketamine analgesia is not related to an opiate action in the periaqueductal gray region of the rat brain. Pain 21: 253-265, 1985.

Smith, R.C., Meltzer, H.Y., Arora, R.C., and Davis, J.M.: Effects of phencyclidine on ^{3}H-catecholamines and ^{3}H-serotonin uptake in synaptosomal preparations from rat brain. Biochem. Pharmacol. 26: 1435-1439, 1977.

Snell, L.D., Mueller, Z.L., Gannon, R.L., Silverman, P.B. and Johnson, K.M.: A comparison between classes of drugs having phencyclidine-like behavioral properties on dopamine efflux *in vitro* and dopamine metabolism *in vivo*. J. Pharmacol. Exp. Ther. 231: 261-269, 1984.

Stringer, J.L., Greenfield, L.J., Hackett, J.T., and Guyenet, P.G.: Blockade of long-term potentiation by phencyclidine and opiates in the hippocampus *in vivo* and *in vitro*. Brain Res. 280: 127-138, 1983.

Tang, A.H., Cangelosi, A.A., Code, R.A., and Franklin, S.R.: Phencyclidine-like behavioral effects of 2-methyl-3,3-diphenyl-3-propanolamine (MDP). Pharmacol. Biochem. Behav. 20: 209-213, 1984.

Tang, A.H. and Franklin, S.R.: Acquisition of brightness discrimination in the rat is impaired by opiates with psychotomimetic properties. Pharmacol. Biochem. Behav. 18: 873-877, 1983.

Tang, A.H. and Schroeder, L.A.: Spinal cord depressant effects of ketamine and etoxadrol in the cat and the rat. Anesthesiol. 39: 37-43, 1973.

Thomson, A.M., West, D.C., and Lodge, D.: An N-methylaspartate receptor-mediated synapse in rat cerebral cortex: A site of action of ketamine? Nature 313: 479-481, 1985.

Turski, L., Schwarz, M., Turski, W.A., Klockgether, T., Sontag, K.-H., and Collins, J.F.: Muscle relaxant action of excitatory amino acid antagonists. Neurosci. Lett. 53: 321-326, 1985.

Vaupel, D.B.: Naltrexone fails to antagonize the effects of PCP and SKF 10,047 in the dog. Eur. J. Pharmacol. 92: 269-274, 1983.

Vignon, J. and Lazdunski, M.: Structure-function relationships in the inhibition of synaptosomal dopamine uptake by phencyclidine and analogues: Potential correlation with binding site identified with ^{3}H-phencyclidine. Biochem. Pharmacol. 33: 700-702, 1984.

Vincent, J.-P., Kartalovsky, B., Geneste, P., Kamenka, J.-M., and Lazdunski, M.: Interaction of phencyclidine ("angel dust") with a specific receptor in rat brain membranes. Proc. Natl. Acad. Sci. USA 76: 4678-4682, 1979.

Watkins, J.C. and Evans, R.H.: Excitatory amino acid transmitters. Ann. Rev. Pharmacol. Toxicol. 21: 165-204, 1981.

White, P.F., Way, W.L. and Trevor, A.J.: Ketamine—its pharmacology and therapeutic uses. Anesthesiol. 56: 119-136, 1982.

Wood, J.D. and Hertz, L.: Ketamine-induced changes in the GABA system of mouse brain. Neuropharmacol. 19: 805-808, 1980.

Yaksh, T.L. and Noueihed, R.: The physiology and pharmacology of spinal opiates. Ann. Rev. Pharmacol. Toxicol. 25: 433-462, 1985.

Zukin, S.R. and Zukin, R.S.: Specific [^{3}H]phencyclidine binding in rat central nervous system. Proc. Natl. Acad. Sci. USA 76: 5372-5379, 1979.

Status of Ketamine in Anesthesiology,
edited by E.F. Domino©1990, NPP Books
P.O. Box 1491, Ann Arbor, MI 48106

The Anticonvulsant Activity of Ketamine and Other Phencyclidine Receptor Ligands, with Particular Reference to N-Methyl-D-Aspartate Receptor Mediated Events

J. Church

Departments of Physiology and Anaesthesia
University of British Columbia
Vancouver, B.C., Canada

Introduction

Ever since the introduction of the anesthetic arylcyclohexylamines phencyclidine (PCP) and ketamine, controversy has existed over their complex profile of central effects. Despite useful properties such as analgesic activity, their widespread use has been precluded, not only because of their propensity to elicit psychotomimetic emergence reactions but also because of conflicting evidence concerning their possible epileptogenic properties. The purpose of this report is to outline briefly the background to the controversy surrounding the convulsant/anticonvulsant effects of the arylcyclohexylamines and then to place this in the modern context of the ability of these and related compounds to reduce neuronal excitations mediated by the N-methyl-D-aspartate (NMDA) subclass of excitatory amino acid (EAA) receptor. The latter effect will be discussed here only as it pertains to anticonvulsant activity. For a detailed review, the interested reader is referred to the chapter by Church and Lodge (this volume).

Early Background

In their original studies Chen *et al.* (1959) and Chen and Bohner (1961) reported that subanesthetic doses of PCP abolished maximal electroshock (MES), pentylenetetrazol (PTZ), and sound induced seizures in mice, although it was ineffective against those induced by strychnine and promoted seizures at supra-anesthetic doses. Ketamine had a similar profile of anticonvulsant activity, except that PTZ induced seizures could only be abolished by anesthetic doses of the drug and, importantly, even high doses failed to provoke seizures (McCarthy *et al.*, 1965; Chen *et al.*, 1966). Notably, even when PCP or ketamine failed to provide protection against strychnine induced seizures, they both significantly decreased the lethal effects of this convulsant (Chen *et al.*, 1959; McCarthy *et al.*, 1965).

The unusual spectrum of effects elicited by PCP and ketamine on overt behavior stimulated electroencephalographic (EEG) studies. Miyasaka and Domino (1968), for example, demonstrated in cats that ketamine anesthesia was associated with hypersynchronous *delta* wave activity in neocortical and thalamic areas and, paradoxically, *theta* "arousal" waves in the hippocampus, results which were interpreted as showing a functional dissociation between limbic and thalamo-neocortical systems (see also Corssen *et al.*, 1968). Similar cortical EEG findings were made in humans (Domino *et al.*, 1965). Ketamine, therefore, differed from more conventional anesthetic agents such as the barbiturates, which depressed all CNS areas, by depressing some regions of the neocortex and subcortical structures such as the thalamus, while at the same time activating parts of the limbic system such as the hippocampus.

The concept of differential actions of ketamine on various parts of the CNS was challenged by Mori *et al.* (1971) and Kayama and Iwama (1972) who reported that relatively high doses of ketamine affected cat neocortex and hippocampus in virtually identical ways, causing desynchronization of the EEG and inducing electrographic seizures without behavioral correlates in both areas. They concluded that, rather than being a dissociative anesthetic, ketamine interfered with consciousness by causing generalized CNS excitation and high frequency EEG changes akin to those seen in petit mal epilepsy. Winters (1972), in an editorial, labeled ketamine a CNS stimulant and speculated that the loss of consciousness produced by PCP and ketamine in humans was the result of "cataleptoid CNS excitation", sometimes associated with the development of electrographic limbic seizures (see also Winters *et al.*, 1972). He warned that a convulsing patient given ketamine might be pushed into status epilepticus and that the repeated use of ketamine in young patients might, by inducing epileptiform activity, produce brain damage.

On the basis of EEG data, a number of groups subsequently warned that ketamine, because it produced an anesthetic state characterized by a "preconvulsant state of catalepsy" (Manohar *et al.*, 1972), might precipitate seizures or accentuate EEG abnormalities in patients with pre-existing convulsive tendencies (*e.g.* Bennett *et al.*, 1973; Ferrer-Allado *et al.*, 1973). In addition, isolated reports began to appear describing the occurrence of seizures during ketamine anesthesia even in patients with no prior history of epilepsy, although in all such cases the doses of ketamine employed had been relatively high (*e.g.* Wyant, 1971; Thompson, 1972; Walker, 1972). Nevertheless, surveys of reported surgical series where ketamine was used as the sole anesthetic revealed an overall incidence of convulsions during ketamine anesthesia which was probably no higher than in patients anesthetized by other means (*e.g.* see Fisher, 1974). Little attention was paid at the time to the report by Corssen *et al.* (1968) that ketamine had proven to be an effective anticonvulsant in two patients undergoing pneumoencephalography who developed tonic-clonic convulsions.

The latter group of EEG studies were also criticized. Notably, Celesia and Chen (1974) argued that although ketamine could induce electrocorticographic spikes and synchronize EEG rhythms, these were not necessarily synonymous with epileptic activity. Further, they found that ketamine consistently suppressed focal seizures in cats induced by penicillin, suggesting that, rather than being a convulsant agent, ketamine in fact had a mild antiepileptic effect. In addition, the clinical reports of Bennett *et al.* (1973) and Ferrer-Allado *et al.* (1973) on the possible tendency of ketamine to precipitate seizures were challenged in controlled trials. Corssen *et al.* (1974) and Celesia *et al.* (1975) administered ketamine to healthy volunteers and patients with a history of active epilepsy and found no evidence that ketamine either aggravated or precipitated seizures. Indeed, Celesia *et al.* (1975) found ketamine to be less effective than natural sleep as an activator of epileptic discharges in patients with an unequivocal history of focal or generalized epilepsy.

The anticonvulsant activity of ketamine was further emphasized by clinical reports which appeared at this time. Low doses of ketamine were found to be an effective treatment for seizures in tetanus (Phillips *et al.*, 1970), eclamptic seizures (Rucci and Caroli, 1974), and febrile convulsions (Davis and Tolstoshev, 1976). Interestingly, in these reports ketamine had succeeded in aborting seizures after other, more generally accepted, therapies had failed (see also Corssen *et al.*, 1968; Fisher, 1974). This suggested that its anticonvulsant activity might reflect a mechanism of action somewhat different to that of conventional agents. It also became increasingly clear that convulsive activity was associated almost exclusively with high (near lethal, in the case of ketamine) doses of dissociative anesthetics, whereas anticonvulsant properties were evident at lower doses (*e.g.* see Chen *et al.*, 1959; McCarthy *et al.*, 1965; Corssen *et al.*, 1974; Leccese *et al.*, 1986). The severe behavioral disruption associated with such high doses of PCP and ketamine, in turn, suggested that their epileptogenic properties reflected a generalized toxic insult to the CNS rather than a selective action of these compounds.

Animal Studies

Since the early studies referred to above, many reports have verified the dose dependent anticonvulsant activity of PCP and ketamine against a wide variety of experimentally induced convulsions in a number of animal species. Both drugs are able to suppress PTZ, MES, NMDA, and sound induced seizures (Chen *et al.*, 1959, 1966; Taberner, 1976; Reder *et al.*, 1980; Bourn *et al.*, 1983; Sagratella *et al.*, 1983; Hayes and Balster, 1985; Leccese *et al.*, 1986; Leander *et al.*, 1988a,b). Similarly, both inhibit the generalization of epileptiform activity induced by penicillin (Celesia and Chen, 1974; Niglio *et al.*, 1985), and are active in the kindling model (Albertson *et al.*, 1980; Callaghan and Schwark, 1980; Bowyer and Winters, 1981; Bowyer, 1982; Freeman *et al.*, 1982; Gilbert, 1988). PCP also raises thresholds against flurothyl convulsions (Geller *et al.*, 1981), whereas ketamine ameliorates mercaptopropionic acid, high pressure, strychnine, bicuculline, and picrotoxin induced convulsions (Taberner, 1976; Myslobodsky *et al.*, 1981; Wardley-Smith *et al.*, 1988).

The anticonvulsant activity shown by PCP and ketamine is shared by other arylcyclohexylamines (*e.g.* tiletamine and the thienyl derivative of PCP; Chen *et al.*, 1969; Leccese *et al.*, 1986), as well as dissociative anesthetics from different chemical classes such as the 1,3-substituted dioxolanes, dexoxadrol and etoxadrol, and (-)-2-methyl-3,3-diphenyl-3-propanolamine ((-)-2-MDP; Hayes and Balster, 1985; Leander *et al.*, 1988b).

A variety of mechanisms have been proposed to account for this anticonvulsant activity, but in many cases the evidence is conflicting. Myslobodsky *et al.* (1981), for example, proposed modulation of noradrenergic and dopaminergic transmitter systems as the possible substrate for the anticonvulsant actions of ketamine and discounted *gamma*-aminobutyric acid (GABA) mediated effects (see also Taberner, 1976), whereas others (*e.g.* Wood and Hertz, 1980) specifically invoked an enhancement of GABA mediated inhibition as central to the anticonvulsant action of ketamine. In fact, a comparison of the relative anticonvulsant potency of dissociative anesthetics and related compounds (see below) with their actions on most neurotransmitter systems reveals only poor correlations (see Johnson and Snell, 1986; Johnson, 1987). Thus, although ketamine can inhibit the reuptake of central transmitter amines (such as dopamine and noradrenaline) and systems utilizing these transmitters have been implicated in the genesis or control of convulsive phenomena (Maynert *et al.*, 1975; see below), these effects are not consistently exhibited by other dissociative anesthetics or PCP like drugs which also possess anticonvulsant activity. Nor do naloxone, clonidine, physostigmine, or haloperidol affect the inhibitory influence of, for example, PCP on epileptiform activity, findings which suggest that the anticonvulsant action of dissociative anesthetics is not directly dependent upon neurotransmitter systems modulated by these drugs (see Geller *et al.*, 1981; Niglio *et al.*, 1985).

The PCP Receptor and NMDA Antagonism

An important advance in our understanding of the central actions of PCP and PCP like drugs came in the late 1970s with the description of a specific central binding site for these compounds. It is now recognized that there are in fact two distinct sites to which PCP like drugs bind, the PCP and the *sigma* receptor. In the present context, we are concerned only with the PCP receptor as selective *sigma* receptor ligands do not antagonize NMDA (see Church and Lodge, this volume). The only drugs which are able to displace [^{3}H]-PCP from the PCP receptor are other dissociative anesthetics and compounds which, from animal discrimination studies, are known to possess PCP like activity. Included in this latter group are benzomorphans (including cyclazocine and N-allylnormetazocine (NANM)), morphinans (*e.g.*, dextrorphan, dextromethorphan), and benz(f)isoquinolines (*e.g.*, LY154045). The apparent affinity of these compounds for the PCP site is highly correlated with their relative potency for eliciting PCP like discriminative stimuli, suggesting in turn that the PCP receptor might mediate at least some of the behavioral properties common to these groups of compounds (see Balster and Willetts, 1988). That these behavioral properties might include anticonvulsant activity was first suggested by Geller *et al.* (1981), who pointed out the similarity between the anticonvulsant effects of PCP, NANM and cyclazocine. Since then, a large number of compounds structurally unrelated to the arylcyclohexylamines, but having affinity for the PCP receptor, have been shown to exhibit anticonvulsant activity in a variety of *in vivo* models. Some of these are listed in Table 1. An extensive literature is also available

TABLE 1. PCP receptor ligands as anticonvulsants *in* vivo

Compound	*Species*	*Convulsant*	*Reference*
MK-801	Mouse/Rat	MES Bicuculline Kindling	Clineschmidt *et al.*, 1982; Gilbert, 1988; Leander *et al.*, 1988b; McNamara *et al.*, 1988
	Mouse	NMDA	Ferkany *et al.*, 1988
	Rat	Spontaneous	Peeters *et al.*, 1989
LY 154045	Mouse	MES	Leander *et al.*, 1988b
		NMDA	Leander *et al.*, 1988a
(±)-Cyclazocine	Mouse/Rat	PTZ	Harris & Pierson, 1964
		MES	Sagratella *et al.*, 1985; Berman & Adler, 1984
	Mouse	NMDA	Leander *et al.*, 1988a
	Rat	Flurothyl	Cowan *et al.*, 1979
		Kindling	Albertson *et al.*, 1984
	Rabbit	Penicillin	Massotti *et al.*, 1984
		Strychnine	Massotti *et al.*, 1984
(+)-and (−)-Cyclazocine	Rat	Flurothyl	Cowan *et al.*, 1979
		MES	Berman and Adler, 1984
(±)-NANM	Rat	MES	Leccese *et al.*, 1986
		Kindling	Albertson *et al.*, 1984
		Flurothyl	Cowan *et al.*, 1979
(+)-NANM	Mouse	PTZ	Hayes & Balster, 1985
		MES	Leander *et al.*, 1988b
		NMDA	Leander *et al.*, 1988a
Dextrorphan	Mouse/Rat	MES	Leander *et al.*, 1988b; Tortella *et al.*, 1988
	Mouse	NMDA	Ferkany *et al.*, 1988 Leander *et al.*, 1988a
Dextromethorphan	Mouse/Rat	MES	Tortella & Musacchio, 1986; Leander *et al.*, 1988b
	Mouse	NMDA	Ferkany *et al.*, 1988; Leander *et al.*, 1988a
	Rat	Kindling	Feeser *et al.*, 1988

on the ability of these drugs to suppress epileptiform discharges induced by a variety of means *in vitro* (*e.g.* Horne *et al.*, 1986; Thomson and West, 1986; Aram *et al.*, 1989; see Fig. 1).

The potency order exhibited for anticonvulsant activity by these structurally diverse compounds correlates well with their ability to displace [^{3}H]-PCP from its central binding site (*e.g.* Hayes and Balster, 1985), providing further evidence that the anticonvulsant properties of PCP like drugs might be mediated by their interaction with the PCP

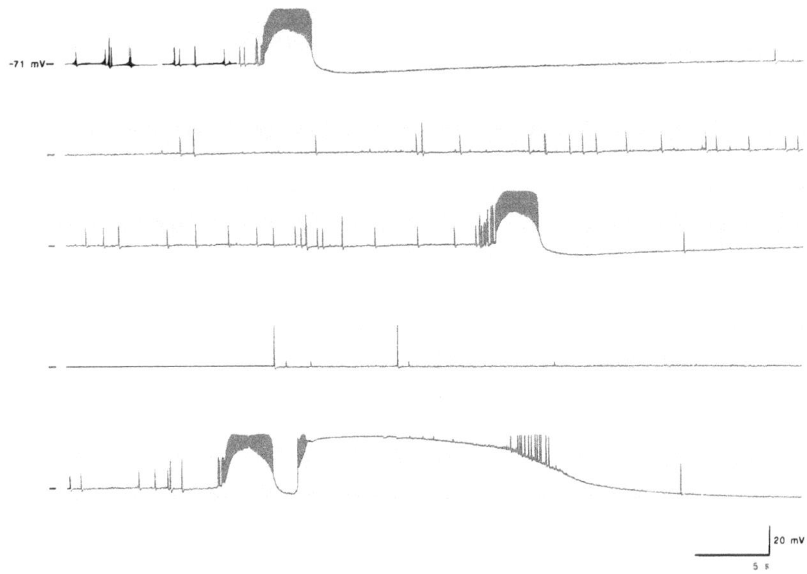

Fig. 1. Intracellular record of ictal activity in a rat CAl hippocampal pyramidal neuron *in vitro* obtained at resting membrane potential (-71 mV). Upper three traces are a continuous record of spontaneous activity, 170 min after the start of perfusion with a medium containing 72 mM bicarbonate (pH 7.9). Small upward deflections are brief (interictal) bursts. The fourth trace was obtained 10 min after addition of 20 μM of ketamine to the high bicarbonate medium. Lowermost trace shows recovery of epileptiform activity 30 min after washout of ketamine. (Church and McLennan, unpublished observations.).

receptor. Even so, the central question of the neurophysiological basis for the anticonvulsant efficacy of these drugs remained unclear until studies demonstrated that: a) the NMDA subclass of postsynaptic excitatory amino acid receptor plays an important role in the pathophysiology of convulsive phenomena, and b) that compounds with affinity for the PCP receptor selectively and noncompetitively reduce neuronal excitations mediated by the NMDA receptor.

A large body of evidence supports NMDA receptor involvement in both seizure initiation and the spread of seizure activity. First, their activation induces membrane potential shifts and burst discharges reminiscent of the depolarizing shifts which are the correlates of EEG interictal spikes (*e.g.* Dingledine *et al.*, 1986). Second, the NMDA receptor operated ionophore possesses a large Ca^{2+} conductance (see Mayer and Westbrook, 1987). NMDA receptor activation may, therefore, at least partly account for the dendritic Ca^{2+} spikes that may contribute to epileptiform discharge in many models of experimental epilepsy. Third, NMDA receptors have been shown to participate in synaptic transmission within the CNS, especially in circumstances of neuronal hyperactivity as may be found in an epileptic focus; they may, therefore, contribute to the propagation of epileptic activity through normal brain tissue (see Herron *et al.*, 1986). Fourth, seizure activity can be initiated experimentally by the systemic or focal intracerebral injection of excitatory amino acids, including NMDA (Patel *et al.*, 1988). Finally, competitive NMDA receptor antagonists such as 2-amino-7-phosphonoheptanoate are able not only to suppress a wide variety of experimentally induced seizures both *in vivo* (see Patel *et al.*, 1988) and *in vitro* (*e.g.* Dingledine *et al.*, 1986; Thomson and West, 1986; Aram *et al.*, 1989) but they also block epileptiform bursting in slices of human neocortex which exhibited interictal spiking prior to their excision (Avoli and Olivier, 1987).

The original finding that ketamine selectively reduced neuronal excitations evoked by NMDA (Anis *et al.*, 1983a) was followed by observations that this action was shared by other compounds which were also able to elicit PCP like interoceptive cues and which also had affinity for the PCP receptor (see above and Lodge *et al.*, 1988). Indeed, it now appears that the PCP receptor is part of a macromolecular complex which includes the NMDA recognition site and its associated ionophore and that PCP receptor ligands act as noncompetitive NMDA antagonists by blocking the NMDA receptor operated ionophore whilst the latter is in its activated configuration. These findings led to the suggestion (Church and Lodge, this volume) that reduced excitatory transmission at central synapses utilizing NMDA receptors underlies at least some of the behavioral properties common to PCP like compounds. In particular, because of the apparent importance of NMDA receptor mediated events in the genesis of convulsive phenomena, much recent interest has centered on the possibility that functional NMDA antagonism may underlie the anticonvulsant effects of PCP like drugs and, consequently, on the therapeutic potential of PCP like drugs as anticonvulsants.

Correlation Between NMDA Antagonist Potency and Anticonvulsant Efficacy for PCP Like Compounds

No selective antagonists are available for any of the behavioral effects elicited by the dissociative anesthetics or, with the exception of analgesia, *sigma* opioids such as cyclazocine. This means that, in order to invoke specific causative mechanisms for the behavioral effects of these drugs, one has to rely upon a comparison of relative potencies within a series of stereoisomers and analogues. Only if a strong correlation is observed between the relative potencies (in this case, NMDA antagonism) and the behavioral effect (in this case, anticonvulsant activity) in the system under study can one even indirectly imply the possibility of a causal relationship. Because ketamine is a NMDA antagonist and selective, competitive NMDA antagonists are known to possess anticonvulsant activity, this does not necessarily mean that the anticonvulsant efficacy of ketamine is due to its NMDA antagonist actions.

The relative anticonvulsant potency *in vivo* of a series of PCP receptor ligands has been examined in three published studies (Leander *et al.*, 1988a,b; Hayes and Balster, 1985) against NMDA, MES, and PTZ induced convulsions, respectively. A comparison of the rank order potency of a series of PCP like drugs as NMDA antagonists on rat spinal neurons *in vivo*, as tested by Lodge and colleagues, with their rank order as anticonvulsants in these studies (Table 2) reveals a good correlation, suggesting that the anticonvulsant properties of PCP like compounds may indeed be directly related to this effect. Although the rank order for NMDA antagonism in Table 2 has been estimated from *in vivo* experiments where compounds were applied by microelectrophoresis, a technique which is not well suited to providing quantitative measures of antagonism, a very similar rank order potency for many of the same drugs as NMDA antagonists has been obtained with known concentrations of the compounds *in vitro* (Lodge *et al.*, 1988; Aram *et al.*, 1989). In the study by Aram *et al.* (1989), where epileptiform activity was induced in rat neocortical slices by omission of Mg^{2+} from the bathing medium and, in the case of ketamine, by the addition of proconvulsant drugs (*e.g.* $GABA_A$ receptor antagonists and K^+ channel blockers), both competitive and noncompetitive (PCP like) NMDA antagonists reduced epileptiform bursts and afterpotentials with relative potencies which correlated well ($r>0.9$) with their NMDA antagonist potencies. Further, the absolute concentrations required for anticonvulsant activity were similar to those for block of NMDA evoked depolarizations. An example of the action of ketamine on epileptiform activity *in vitro* is shown in Fig. 1.

Reference to other studies which have examined the anticonvulsant activity of individual PCP like compounds extend the correlation between NMDA antagonist potency and anticonvulsant potency obtained in Table 2. Thus, the (+) isomer of ketamine is about 3 times as potent as the (-)

TABLE 2. Rank order of PCP like compounds as NMDA antagonists on rat spinal neurons *in vivo* following microelectrophoretic administration compared with rank order anticonvulsant potency as determined against NMDA induced convulsions in mice (Leander *et al.*, 1988a), against MES induced convulsions in mice (Leander *et al.*, 1988b), and against PTZ induced convulsions in mice (Hayes and Balster, 1985).

	Order as anticonvulsants:		
Order as NMDA antagonists:	***Leander* et al., *1988a***	***Leander* et al., *1988b***	***Hayes and Balster, 1985***
MK-801[a]	1[i]	1	n.t.
PCP[b]	2	2	1
LY 154045[c]	3	4	n.t.
Etoxadrol[d]	3	3	1
Dexoxadrol[d]	5	5	6
(±)-Cyclazocine[e]	5	n.t.	n.t.
(−)-2-MDP[f]	n.t.	n.t.	3
(+)-NANM[g]	7	6	4
Dextrorphan[h]	7	7	n.t.
Ketamine[b]	9	9	5
Dextromethorphan[h]	10	8	n.t.
(+)-2-MDP[f,j]	n.t.	n.t.	7
Levoxadrol[d,j,k]	n.t.	n.t.	7
LY 154005[c,j,k]	n.t.	10	n.t.

[a]Davies *et al.*, 1988; [b] Anis *et al.*, 1983a; [c]Berry and Lodge, 1984; [d]Berry *et al.*, 1984a; [e]Church and Lodge, unpublished; [f]Blake *et al.*, 1986; [g]Berry *et al.*, 1984b; [h]Church *et al.*, 1989; [i]taken from Leander *et al.*, 1988b; [j]compounds inactive as anticonvulsants; [k]compounds inactive as NMDA antagonists *in vivo* following microelectrophoretic application; n.t., not tested. Note that various compounds have been grouped as regards their potency as NMDA antagonists because absolute quantification cannot be achieved with the microelectrophoretic technique. Spearman rank order correlation coefficients of 0.86, 0.93 and 0.84, obtained by comparison of rank order potency for NMDA antagonism with rank order potency for anticonvulsant activity in the experiments by Leander and colleagues (1988a,b) and by Hayes and Balster (1985) respectively, are all significant at $P < 0.01$.

isomer in reducing NMDA-evoked neuronal excitations (Lodge *et al.*, 1982), a potency ratio similar to that obtained against sound induced convulsions in epilepsy prone rats (Bourn *et al.*, 1983). Similarly, (-)-cyclazocine is about twice as effective as its enantiomer against flurothyl induced seizures in rats (Cowan *et al.*, 1979), a ratio also seen for NMDA antagonism (Lodge *et al.*, 1984). In common with the dissociative anesthetics (*e.g.* Geller *et al.*, 1981; Bowyer, 1982), neither the anticonvulsant activity (Cowan *et al.*, 1979; Berman and Adler, 1984; Sagratella *et al.*, 1985; Tortella *et al.*, 1988) nor the NMDA antagonizing properties (Lodge *et al.*, 1988) of cyclazocine or other PCP like compounds are attenuated by naloxone.

Not only are the rank order potencies for PCP like drugs as NMDA antagonists and as anticonvulsants qualitatively similar, but also the systemic doses required for effective anticonvulsant activity are, in nearly every case, very like those which result in substantial NMDA antagonism (Table 3). Again, additional examples are available. Thus, 3 mg/kg cyclazocine protects against PTZ and flurothyl induced convulsions (*e.g.* Cowan *et al.*, 1979; Sagratella *et al.*, 1985) and inhibits the occurrence of the EEG and motor manifestations induced by the cortical application of penicillin or strychnine (Massotti *et al.*, 1984). The same dose substantially reduces NMDA evoked neuronal excitation (Anis *et al.*, 1983b).

Two points in particular regarding the correlations presented above require amplification. First, although dextrorphan is a more potent NMDA antagonist than ketamine when both drugs are applied by microelectrophoresis, the reverse is true after i.v. injection (Church *et al.*, 1989). This accounts for the apparent discrepancy between Tables 2 and 3 where the potency of dextrorphan relative to ketamine as a NMDA antagonist is reversed between the Tables. Second, in the study by Hayes and Balster (1985; Table 3), the relatively low potency of dexoxadrol as an anticonvulsant is surprising, given its good anticonvulsant activity in the study by Leander *et al.* (1988b) and its relatively high potency as a NMDA antagonist (Berry *et al.*, 1984a). Nevertheless, this finding is

TABLE 3. A comparison of the systemic doses of various PCP like drugs required for appreciable (70-90% reduction from control values) NMDA antagonism and for anticonvulsant activity. Doses listed under Leander *et al.*, 1988b are the ED_{50} values obtained against MES. Those listed under Hayes and Balster (1985) are P_{10} values, *i.e.* doses predicted to result in a 10-fold reduction in probability of tonic convulsions in response to PTZ.

I.V. doses (mg/kg) in rat for 70-90% reduction in NMDA evoked excitations		*Leander* et al. *1988b, ED_{50} (mg/kg s.c.)*	*Hayes and Balster 1985, P_{10} (mg/kg i.p.)*
MK-801	0.1- 0.3	0.15	n.t.
PCP	0.2- 0.5	1.5	3.7
Etoxadrol	1.8- 4.0	2.2	3.5
Dexoxadrol	1.9- 6.0	4.0	21.2
(+)-NANM	2.0- 5.0	7.1	6.9
Ketamine	2.0-10.0	15.1	12.5
(−)-2-MDP	4.0- 8.0	n.t.	5.9
Dextrorphan	8.0-16.0	9.6	n.t.
Dextromethorphan	> 50	11.8	n.t.
(+)-2-MDP	inactive	n.t.	inactive

Data for NMDA antagonism taken from studies cited in Table 2 except for (+)-2-MDP (unpublished); n.t., not tested.

consistent with the general observation that both competitive and non-competitive NMDA antagonists tend to be more efficacious against seizures induced by MES (or sound in genetically prone animals) than against those induced chemically. As an example, MK-801 (the most potent NMDA antagonist available) blocks clonic convulsions produced in mice by PTZ and tonic seizures caused by strychnine, but does so only at doses much higher than are required against MES or bicuculline (Clineschmidt *et al.*, 1982).

Modulating Influences

The rank order potency correlations presented here, together with those obtained from experiments *in vitro* (*e.g.* Aram *et al.*, 1989), not only imply a central role for NMDA receptors in many types of experimentally induced epileptiform activity but also strongly suggest that the shared anticonvulsant properties of structurally dissimilar compounds with PCP like activity may largely reflect their ability to reduce NMDA receptor mediated neuronal excitations. With regard to the dissociative anesthetics, it is important to emphasize that in experimental animals the doses required for effective anticonvulsant and NMDA blocking activity are less than those which produce surgical anesthesia. Ketamine 2 mg/kg i.v., for example, which produces a marked depression of NMDA evoked responses in the rat (Lodge *et al.*,1982), is at least 10 times less than the dose required for surgical anesthesia in that species (Flecknell, 1987). Similarly, *in vitro* 10-20 μM ketamine effectively blocks spontaneous and evoked epileptiform activity produced not only by perfusion with Mg^{2+}-free medium (a model of epileptiform activity which might be expected to be particularly sensitive to NMDA antagonists; see Mayer and Westbrook, 1987) but also by $GABA_A$ antagonists and by K^+ channel blockers (Aram *et al.*, 1989). These concentrations are also at least 10 times less than those seen after i.v. injection of 20 mg/kg ketamine in rats (Cohen *et al.*, 1974). Since there is little correlation between the NMDA antagonist/anticonvulsant and anesthetic potencies of dissociative anesthetics, it is evident that a comparison of the anticonvulsant effects of equianesthetic doses of dissociative anesthetics is not an adequate basis on which to examine the possible mechanism of the anticonvulsant actions of PCP like drugs. That anticonvulsant activity and NMDA antagonism are seen at subanesthetic doses is not to say, on the other hand, that effective anticonvulsant doses of PCP like drugs are devoid of adverse behavioral side effects in experimental animals. For example, Leander *et al.* (1988b) found that the anticonvulsant effects of a series of PCP like drugs occurred at only slightly lower doses than those which produced motor impairment (see also Ferkany *et al.*, 1988).

Other points regarding the anticonvulsant efficacy of PCP like drugs also require consideration. In particular, as outlined above, many PCP like drugs exhibit proconvulsant effects, although usually only when administered at doses which are somewhat higher than those which produce anticonvulsant activity (*e.g.* Chen *et al.*, 1959). PCP abusers, for example, may present with convulsions having ingested 0.5-1.0 mg/kg (Petersen and Stillman, 1978). Although little direct evidence is available, a number of mechanisms may plausibly be invoked to account for these proconvulsant actions. First, PCP like drugs are known to block neuronal K^+ channels (*e.g.* Lacey and Henderson, 1986). Blockade of presynaptic K^+ conductances would enhance Ca^{2+}-dependent transmitter release and might, in this way, provoke seizures. Importantly, this effect is seen only at high (*i.e.* convulsant) doses, whereas NMDA antagonism (and anticonvulsant activity) predominates at lower doses. Thus, whereas PCP, for example, depresses responses to NMDA in rat locus coeruleus neurons *in vitro* with an IC_{50} of 0.4 μM, K^+ channel mediated responses are reduced in the same tissue with IC_{50}s at least 10 times this value. Second, PCP like drugs have well documented effects on many central neurotransmitter systems apart from EAA mediated ones. Some of these actions may mask or limit the anticonvulsant activity afforded by the ability of PCP like drugs to reduce NMDA-evoked excitations and may, in themselves, promote seizure activity. Both PCP and ketamine, for example, can act as indirect dopamine agonists (see Johnson, 1987); raised levels of dopamine may facilitate seizure activity (see Maynert *et al.*, 1975). As was the case with K^+ channel blockade, higher concentrations of PCP are necessary to inhibit the uptake and enhance the release of [^{3}H]-dopamine than are required to inhibit NMDA stimulated dopamine release (see Johnson and Snell, 1986). Similarly, ketamine inhibits brain acetylcholinesterase and glutamate decarboxylase activities, although again it only does so if doses (or concentrations, *in vitro*) rather greater than those required for substantial NMDA antagonism are employed (*e.g.* 20 mg/kg i.v. in the rat; Cohen *et al.*, 1974). Both a reduction in GABA mediated inhibition and an enhancement of cholinergic transmission are potently convulsant (see Maynert *et al.*, 1975).

The net pharmacological effect of a PCP like drug *in vivo* would, of course, depend on the relative endogenous tone of each neurotransmitter system affected by the drug. Nevertheless, it is apparent that PCP like drugs, by and large, exhibit greater potency as antagonists of NMDA mediated responses, which would be expected to result in anticonvulsant activity, than they do on activities mediated by other neurotransmitter systems, some of which might be proconvulsant. Consequently, anticonvulsant activity might be expected to predominate at dose levels of PCP rather lower than those which might exhibit proconvulsant effects. In this regard, it is also important to note that PCP like compounds differ in their relative potencies for affecting each neurotransmitter system. MK-801, for example, is a more potent NMDA antagonist than PCP or ketamine but is less potent than either in inhibiting [^{3}H]-dopamine uptake (Snell *et al.*, 1988). This finding may, at least in part, account for the rather greater anticonvulsant potency of MK-801, relative to NMDA antagonist potency, than is seen with either PCP or ketamine (see Table 3).

Summary

At least one of the factors which deterred the widespread acceptance of ketamine was uncertainty about its profile of convulsant/anticonvulsant actions. Much recent work has demonstrated that, whereas high doses of ketamine and other PCP like compounds may be proconvulsant, at lower doses a dose related anticonvulsant effect is seen. Not only is there now excellent evidence that the anticonvulsant efficacy of these compounds is the result of their interaction with a specific central receptor (the PCP receptor), but also the reduction of NMDA receptor mediated events consequent upon the binding of these drugs to the PCP receptor provides a unifying neurophysiological explanation for their anticonvulsant effects.

It is nevertheless also clear that the possession by a PCP like drug of NMDA blocking activity will not alone determine its profile of convulsant/anticonvulsant activity in the whole animal. This will inevitably be determined by the relative strength of the interactions of a drug with numerous neurotransmitter systems as well as its nonspecific effects such as local anesthetic activity (see Cowan *et al.*, 1979). However, the strength of the various correlations between anticonvulsant activity and NMDA antagonist potency for PCP like drugs presented here and by others (Aram *et al.*, 1989) suggests that, despite their myriad other effects in the whole animal, functional NMDA antagonism is the major factor which determines the anticonvulsant efficacy of these compounds. It also appears as if the anticonvulsant effects of PCP like compounds are likely to be mediated quite independently from the mechanisms by which they induce seizures.

References

Albertson, T.E., Joy, R.M., and Stark, L.G.: Modification of kindled amygdaloid seizures by opiate agonists and antagonists. J. Pharmacol. Exp. Ther. 228: 620-627, 1984.

Albertson, T.E., Peterson, S.L., and Stark, L.G.: Anticonvulsant drugs and their antagonism of kindled amygdaloid seizures in rats. Neuropharmacol. 19: 643-652, 1980.

Anis, N.A., Berry, S.C., Burton, N.R., and Lodge, D.: The dissociative anesthetics, ketamine and phencyclidine, selectively reduce excitation of central mammalian neurones by N-methylaspartate. Br. J. Pharmacol. 79: 565-575, 1983a.

Anis, N.A., Berry, S.C., Burton, N.R., and Lodge, D.: Cyclazocine, like ketamine, blocks N-methylaspartate actions on spinal neurons in cat and rat. J. Physiol. 338: 37P, 1983b.

Aram, J.A., Martin, D., Tomczyk, M., Zeman, S., Millar, J., Pohler, G., and Lodge, D.: Neocortical epileptogenesis *in vitro*: Studies with N-methyl-D-aspartate, phencyclidine, *sigma* and dextromethorphan receptor ligands. J. Pharmacol. Exp. Ther. 248: 320-328, 1989.

Avoli, M. and Olivier, A.: Bursting in human epileptogenic neocortex is depressed by an N-methyl-D-aspartate antagonist. Neurosci. Lett. 76: 249-254, 1987.

Balster, R.L. and Willetts, J.: Receptor mediation of the discriminative stimulus properties of phencyclidine and *sigma* opioid agonists. In Transduction Mechanisms of Drug Stimuli, ed. by F.C. Colpaert and R.L. Balster, pp. 122-135, SpringerVerlag, Berlin, 1988.

Bennett, D.R., Madsen, J.A., Jordan, W.S., and Wiser, W.C.: Ketamine anesthesia in brain-damaged epileptics. Neurol. 23: 449-460, 1973.

Berman, E.F. and Adler, M.W.: The anticonvulsant effect of opioids and opioid peptides against maximal electroshock seizures in rats. Neuropharmacol. 23: 367-371, 1984.

Berry, S.C. and Lodge, D.: Benz(f)isoquinolines as excitatory amino acid antagonists: An indication of their mechanism of action? Biochem. Pharmacol. 33: 3829-3832, 1984.

Berry, S.C., Anis, N.A., and Lodge, D.: The effect of the dioxolanes on amino acid induced excitation in the mammalian spinal cord. Brain Res. 307: 85-90, 1984a.

Berry, S.C., Dawkins, S.L., and Lodge, D.: Comparison of *sigma* and *kappa* opiate receptor ligands as excitatory amino acid antagonists. Br. J. Pharmacol. 83: 179-185, 1984b.

Blake, J.C., Davies, S.N., Church, J., Martin, D., and Lodge, D.: 2-methyl-3,3-diphenyl-3-propanolamine (2-MDP) selectively antagonizes N-methylaspartate (NMA). Pharmacol. Biochem. Behav. 24: 23-25, 1986.

Bourn, W.M., Yang, D.J., and Davisson, J.N.: Effect of ketamine enantiomers on sound-induced convulsions in epilepsy prone rats. Pharmacol. Res. Comm. 15: 815-824, 1983.

Bowyer, J.F.: Phencyclidine inhibition of the rate of development of amygdaloid kindled seizures. Exp. Neurol. 75: 173-183, 1982.

Bowyer, J.F. and Winters, W.D.: The effects of various anesthetics on amygdaloid kindled seizures. Neuropharmacol. 20: 199-209, 1981.

Callaghan, D.A. and Schwark, W.S.: Pharmacological modification of amygdaloid-kindled seizures. Neuropharmacol. 19: 1131-1136, 1980.

Celesia, G.G. and Chen, R.-C.: Effects of ketamine on EEG activity in cats and monkeys. EEG Clin. Neurophysiol. 37: 345-353, 1974.

Celesia, G.G., Chen, R.-C., and Bamforth, B.J.: Effects of ketamine in epilepsy. Neurol. 25: 169-172, 1975.

Chen, G. and Bohner, B.: Anticonvulsant properties of 1-(1-phenylcyclohexyl)piperidine.HCl and certain other drugs. Proc. Soc. Exp. Biol. Med. 106: 632-635, 1961.

Chen, G., Ensor, C.R., and Bohner, B.: The pharmacology of 1-(1-phenylcyclohexyl)piperidine.HCl. J. Pharmacol. Exp. Ther. 127: 241-250, 1959.

Chen, G., Ensor, C.R., and Bohner, B.: The neuropharmacology of 2-(*o*-chlorophenyl)-2-(methylamino)cyclohexanone hydrochloride. J. Pharmacol. Exp. Ther. 152: 332-339, 1966.

Chen, G., Ensor, C.R., and Bohner, B.: The pharmacology of 2-(ethylamino)-2-(2-thienyl)-cyclohexanone.HCl (CI-634). J. Pharmacol. Exp Ther. 168: 171-179, 1969.

Church, J., Jones, M.G., Davies S.N., and Lodge, D.: Antitussive agents as N-methylaspartate antagonists: Further studies. Can. J. Physiol. Pharmacol. 67: 561-567, 1989.

Clineschmidt, B.V., Martin, G.E., and Bunting, P.R.: Anticonvulsant activity of (+)-5-methyl-10,11-dihydro-5H-dibenzo[a,d]-cyclohepten-5,10-imine (MK-801), a substance with potent anticonvulsant, central sympathomimetic, and apparent anxiolytic properties. Drug. Dev. Res. 2: 123-134, 1982.

Cohen, M.L., Chan, S.L., Bhargava, H.N., and Trevor, A.J.: Inhibition of mammalian brain acetylcholinesterase by ketamine. Biochem. Pharmacol. 23: 1647-1652, 1974.

Corssen, G., Little, S.C., and Tavakoli, M.: Ketamine and epilepsy. Anesth. Analg. 53: 319-335, 1974.

Corssen, G., Miyasaka, M., and Domino, E.F.: Changing concepts in pain control during surgery: Dissociative anesthesia with CI-581. Anesth. Analg. 47: 746-758, 1968.

Cowan, A., Geller, E.B., and Adler, M.W.: Classification of opioids on the basis of change in seizure threshold in rats. Science 206: 465-467, 1979.

Davies, S.N., Martin, D., Millar, J.D., Aram, J.A., Church, J., and Lodge, D.: Differences in results from *in vivo* and *in vitro* studies on the use-dependency of N-methylaspartate antagonism by MK-801 and other phencyclidine receptor ligands. Eur. J. Pharmacol. 145: 141-152, 1988.

Davis, R.W. and Tolstoshev, G.C.: Ketamine-use in severe febrile convulsions. Med. J. Austr. 1976ii: 465-466, 1976.

Dingledine, R., Hynes, M.A., and King, G.L.: Involvement of N-methyl-D-aspartate receptors in epileptiform bursting in the rat hippocampal slice. J. Physiol. 380: 175-189, 1986.

Domino, E.F., Chodoff, P. and Corssen, G.: Pharmacologic effects of CI-581, a new dissociative anesthetic, in man. Clin. Pharmacol. Ther. 6: 279-291, 1965.

Feeser, H.R., Kadis, J.L., and Prince, D.A.: Dextromethorphan, a common antitussive, reduces kindled amygdala seizures in the rat. Neurosci. Lett. 86: 340-345, 1988.

Ferkany, J.W., Borosky, S.A., Clissold, D.B., and Pontecorvo, M.J.: Dextromethorphan inhibits NMDA-induced convulsions. Eur. J. Pharmacol. 151: 151-154, 1988.

Ferrer-Allado, T., Brechner, V.L., Dymond, A., Cozen, H., and Crandall, P.: Ketamine-induced electroconvulsive phenomena in the human limbic and thalamic regions. Anesthesiol. 38: 333-344, 1973.

Fisher, M. McD.: Use of ketamine hydrochloride in the treatment of convulsions. Anaesth. Intens. Care 2: 266-268, 1974.

Flecknell, P.A.: Laboratory Animal Anaesthesia, Academic Press, London, 1987.

Freeman, F.G., Jarvis, M.F., and Duncan, P.M.: Phencyclidine raises kindled seizure thresholds. Pharmacol. Biochem. Behav. 16: 1009-1011, 1982.

Geller, E.B., Alder, L.H., Wojno, C., and Adler, M.W.: The anticonvulsant effect of phencyclidine in rats. Psychopharmacol. 74: 97-98, 1981.

Gilbert, M.E.: The NMDA-receptor antagonist, MK-801, suppresses limbic kindling and kindled seizures. Brain Res. 463: 90-99, 1988.

Harris, L.S. and Pierson, A.K.: Some narcotic antagonists in the benzomorphan series. J. Pharmacol. Exp. Ther. 143: 141-148, 1964.

Hayes, B.A. and Balster, R.L.: Anticonvulsant properties of phencyclidine-like drugs in mice. Eur. J. Pharmacol. 117: 121-125, 1985.

Herron, C.E., Lester, R.A.J., Coan, E.J., and Collingridge, G.L.: Frequency-dependent involvement of NMDA receptors in the hippocampus: A novel synaptic mechanism. Nature 322: 265-268, 1986.

Horne, A.L., Harrison, N.L., Turner, J.P., and Simmonds, M.A.: Spontaneous paroxysmal activity induced in zero magnesium and bicuculline: Suppression by NMDA antagonists and GABAmimetics. Eur. J. Pharmacol. 122: 231-238, 1986.

Johnson, K.M.: Neurochemistry and neurophysiology of phencyclidine. In Psychopharmacology: The Third Generation of Progress, ed. by H.Y. Meltzer, pp. 1581-1588, Raven Press, New York, 1987.

Johnson, K.M. and Snell, L.D.: Involvement of dopaminergic, cholinergic, and glutaminergic mechanisms in the actions of phencyclidine-like drugs. NIDA Res. Monogr. 64: 52-66, 1986.

Kayama, Y. and Iwama, K.: The EEG, evoked potentials, and single unit activity during ketamine anesthesia in cats. Anesthesiology 36: 316-328, 1972.

Lacey, M.G. and Henderson, G.: Actions of phencyclidine on rat locus coeruleus neurons *in vitro*. Neurosci. 17: 485-494, 1986.

Leander, J.D., Lawson, R.R., Ornstein, P.L., and Zimmerman, D. M.: N-methyl-D-aspartic acid-induced lethality in mice: Selective antagonism by phencyclidine-like drugs. Brain Res. 448: 115-120, 1988a.

Leander, J.D., Rathbun, R.C., and Zimmerman, D.M.: Anticonvulsant effects of phencyclidine-like drugs: Relation to N-methyl-D-aspartic acid antagonism. Brain Res. 454: 368-372, 1988b.

Leccese, A.P., Marquis, K.L., Mattia, A., and Moreton, J.E.: The convulsant and anticonvulsant effects of phencyclidine (PCP) and PCP analogues in the rat. Behav. Brain Res. 19: 163-169, 1986.

Lodge, D., Anis, N.A., and Burton, N.R.: Effects of optical isomers of ketamine on excitation of cat and rat spinal neurons by amino acids and acetylcholine. Neurosci. Lett. 29: 281-286, 1982.

Lodge, D., Aram, J.A., Church, J., Davies, S.N., Martin, D., Millar, J., and Zeman, S.: *Sigma* opiates and excitatory amino acids. In Excitatory Amino Acids in Health and Disease, ed. by D. Lodge, pp. 237-259, John Wiley and Sons, Chichester, 1988.

Lodge, D., Berry, S.C., Church, J., Martin, D., McGhee, A., Lai, H.-M., and Thomson, A.M.: Isomers of cyclazocine as excitatory amino acid antagonists. Neuropeptides 5: 245-248, 1984.

Manohar, S., Maxwell, D., and Winters, W.D.: Development of EEG seizure activity during and after chronic ketamine administration in the rat. Neuropharmacol. 11: 819-826, 1972.

Massotti, M., Sagratella, S., Argiolas, L., and Mele, L.: Influence of morphine and cyclazocine on the cortical epileptic foci in rabbits. Brain Res. 310: 201-212, 1984.

Mayer, M.L. and Westbrook, G.L.: The physiology of excitatory amino acids in the vertebrate central nervous system. Prog. Neurobiol. 28: 197-276, 1987.

Maynert, E.W., Marczynski, T.J., and Browning, R.A.: The role of the neurotransmitters in the epilepsies. In Advances in Neurology, Vol. 7, ed. by W.J. Friedlander, pp. 79-147, Raven Press, New York, 1975.

McCarthy, D.A., Chen, G., Kaump, D.H., and Ensor, C.: General anesthetic and other pharmacological properties of 2-(o-chlorophenyl)-2-(methylamino)cyclohexanone HCl (CI-581). J. New Drugs 5: 21-33, 1965.

McNamara, J.O., Russell, R.D., Rigsbee, L., and Bonhaus, D.W.: Anticonvulsant and antiepileptogenic actions of MK-801 in the kindling and electroshock models. Neuropharmacol. 27: 563-568, 1988.

Miyasaka, M. and Domino, E.F.: Neuronal mechanisms of ketamine-induced anesthsia. Int. J. Neuropharmacol. 7: 557-573, 1968.

Mori, K., Kawamata, M., Mitani, H., Yamazaki, Y., and Fujita, M.: A neurophysiologic study of ketamine anesthesia in the cat. Anesthesiol. 35: 373-383, 1971.

Myslobodsky, M.S., Golovchinsky, V., and Mintz, M.: Ketamine: Convulsant or anticonvulsant? Pharmacol. Biochem. Behav. 14: 27-33, 1981.

Niglio, T., Sagratella, S., and Scotti de Carolis, A.: An investigation on the anticonvulsant activity of phencyclidine and ketamine in rabbits. Br. J. Pharmacol. 86: 694P, 1985.

Patel, S., Chapman, A.G., Millan, M.H., and Meldrum, B.S.: Epilepsy and excitatory amino acid antagonists. In Excitatory Amino Acids in Health and

Disease, ed. by D. Lodge, pp. 353-378, John Wiley and Sons Ltd., Chichester, 1988.

Peeters, B.W.M.M., Van Rijn, C.M., Van Luijtelaar, E.L.J.M., and Coenen, A.M.L.: Antiepileptic and behavioral actions of MK-801 in an animal model of spontaneous absence epilepsy. Epilepsy Res. 3: 178-181, 1989.

Petersen, R.C. and Stillman, R.C.: Phencyclidine: An overview. NIDA Res. Monogr. 21: 1-17, 1978.

Phillips, L.A., Seruvatu, S.G., Rika, P.N., and Tirikula, U.: Anaesthesia for the surgeon-anaesthetist in difficult situations. Anaesthesia 25: 36-45, 1970.

Reder, B.S., Trapp, L.D., and Troutman, K.C.: Ketamine suppression of chemically induced convulsions in the two day old white leghorn cockerel. Anesth. Analg. 59: 406-409, 1980.

Rucci, F.S. and Caroli, G.: Ketamine and eclampsia (letter). Br. J. Anaesth. 46: 546, 1974.

Sagratella, S., Niglio, T., Ortolani, E., Scotti de Carolis, A., and Pezzola, A.: Phencyclidine-like effect of cyclazocine on pentylentetrazol-induced seizures in laboratory animals. Pharmacol. Biochem. Behav. 22: 515-519, 1985.

Sagratella, S., Passarelli, F., and Scotti de Carolis, A.: An EEG investigation on the effects of phencyclidine on pentylenetetrazol convulsions in rats and rabbits. Arch. Int. Pharmacodyn. 266: 294-307, 1983.

Snell, L.D., Yi, S.-J., and Johnson, K.M.: Comparison of the effects of MK-801 and phencyclidine on catecholamine uptake and NMDA-induced norepinephrine release. Eur. J. Pharmacol. 145: 223-226, 1988.

Taberner, P.V.: The anticonvulsant activity of ketamine against seizures induced by pentylenetetrazol and mercaptopropionic acid. Eur. J. Pharmacol. 39: 305-311, 1976.

Thompson, G.E.: Ketamine-induced convulsions (letter). Anesthesiol. 37: 662-663, 1972.

Thomson, A.M. and West, D.C.: N-methylaspartate receptors mediate epileptiform activity evoked in some, but not all, conditions in rat neocortical slices. Neurosci. 19: 1161-1177, 1986.

Tortella, F.C. and Musacchio, J.M.: Dextromethorphan and carbetapentane: Centrally acting non-opioid antitussive agents with novel anticonvulsant properties. Brain Res. 383: 314-318, 1986.

Tortella, F.C., Ferkany, J.W., and Pontecorvo, M.J.: Anticonvulsant effects of dextrorphan in rats: Possible involvement in dextromethorphan-induced seizure protection. Life Sci. 42: 2509-2514, 1988.

Walker, A.K.Y.: Intramuscular ketamine in a developing country. Anaesthesia 27: 408-414, 1972.

Wardley-Smith, B., Little, H.J.,and Halsey, M.J.: Lack of correlation between the anaesthetic and anticonvulsant potencies of Althesin, ketamine and methohexitone. Br. J. Anaesth. 60: 140-145, 1988.

Winters, W.D.: Epilepsy or anesthesia with ketamine (Editorial view). Anesthesiol. 36: 309-312, 1972.

Winters, W.D., Ferrer-Allado, T., Guzman-Flores, C., and Alcaraz, M.: The cataleptic state induced by ketamine: A review of the neuropharmacology of anesthesia. Neuropharmacol. 11: 303-315, 1972.

Wood, J.D. and Hertz, L.: Ketamine-induced changes in the GABA system of mouse brain. Neuropharmacol. 19: 805-808, 1980.

Wyant, G.M.: Intramuscular Ketalar (CI-581) in paediatric anesthesia. Canad. Anaesth. Soc. J. 18: 72-83, 1971.

Status of Ketamine in Anesthesiology,
edited by E.F. Domino©1990, NPP Books
P.O. Box 1491, Ann Arbor, MI 48106

Anticonvulsant Action of Ketamine in Laboratory Animals

L. Velíšek and P. Mareš

Institute of Physiology
Czechoslovak Academy of Sciences
Prague, Czechoslovakia

Introduction

Ketamine is a drug commonly used as a dissociative anesthetic predominantly for limited surgery in the young and elderly (Winters, 1976). Its anticonvulsant properties have often been described (Taberner, 1976; Myslobodsky *et al.*, 1981; Bourn *et al.*, 1983; Sagratella *et al.*, 1983; Hayes and Balster, 1985; Leccese *et al.*, 1986). On the other hand, proconvulsant and/or convulsant effects of ketamine also have been found (DeVore *et al.*, 1976; Myslobodsky *et al.*, 1981; Gourie *et al.*, 1983; Kayama, 1983). These contradictory results might be due either to the dose of ketamine, as suggested by Myslobodsky *et al.* (1981), or to a specific action of ketamine only against certain types of seizures with a possible proconvulsant action in other types. Such a dual action is known in human epilepsy. For example, phenytoin is effective against partial and generalized tonic-clonic seizures, but aggravates absences (Meinardi and Magnus, 1974).

Results and Discussion

We studied the possible anticonvulsant action of ketamine in adult and immature experimental animals. The results from developing animals are of clinical significance because ketamine is frequently used in children (Winters, 1976). Because ketamine is a noncompetitive NMDA antagonist, such data may also increase knowledge about the significance of N-methyl-D-aspartate (NMDA) receptors in epileptic seizures and their development. Ketamine blocks the associated NMDA ionic channel (Anis *et al.*, 1983; Leander *et al.*, 1987). As the first step, we examined the effects of i.p. ketamine on sleeping times in immature rats (Marešová *et al.*, 1989). The duration of ketamine induced sleeping time decreased with age, whereas the latency to the loss of the righting reflex increased during maturation. A dose of 80 mg/kg, which led to the loss of the righting reflex in only 5 out of 20 adult rats, occasionally resulted in respiratory disturbances and death in 7 and 12 day old rat pups. In addition, jerks and movements resembling clonic seizures appeared in 12 and 18 day old rat pups. EEG recordings demonstrated the presence of sharp elements which were mostly complexes of spikes and waves or sharp and slow waves, especially in the 12 day old animals. The possible anticonvulsant action of ketamine was studied in various animal models of generalized and partial seizures.

Models of generalized seizures

Ketamine has been tested in various generalized seizure models elicited by maximal electroshock (Leccese *et al.*, 1986; Ornstein *et al.*, 1987), systemic pentylenetetrazol, picrotoxin, and 3-mercaptopropionic acid (Myslobodsky *et al.*, 1981; Taberner, 1976; Hayes and Balster, 1985), systemic aminophylline (Czuczwar *et al.*, 1987), and by loud sound in epilepsy prone animals (Bourn *et al.*, 1983). All of these researchers found ketamine to be anticonvulsant in adult animals. However, different seizure patterns were found during ontogenesis after treatment with the aforementioned drugs (*e.g.*, Mareš and Velíšek, 1983).

In our study, performed in 7, 12, 18, 25, and 90 day old rats, we tried to show the anticonvulsant profile of ketamine (1-40 mg/kg i.p.) against pentylenetetrazol (100 mg/kg s.c.) induced seizures. We found that ketamine in doses of 10 and 20 mg/kg efficiently suppressed generalized tonic-clonic seizures without influencing minimal (pure clonic) seizures. A 40 mg/kg dose of ketamine was not as effective as the 10 and 20 mg/kg doses in 25 and 90 day old animals (Table 1, Velíšek *et al.*, 1989).

TABLE 1. Incidence of major generalized tonic-clonic seizures induced by pentylenetetrazol in rats*

Age in days	*Control*	*Dose of ketamine (mg/kg)*				
		1	*5*	*10*	*20*	*40*
7	16/16	7/8	0/8	0/9	x	x
12	12/13	7/8	2/8	0/8	0/7	x
18	8/8	8/8	0/7	0/10	0/8	x
25	10/11	7/7	1/8	0/8	0/9	2/8
90	9/12	5/8	2/8	0/8	0/8	0/8

* The first number indicates the number of animals showing a major seizure within the subgroup; the second number indicates the total number of rats in the subgroup.
x–Dose was not tested.

To determine if the efficacy of ketamine against pentylenetetrazol induced generalized tonic-clonic seizures might represent a general phenomenon, the effects of ketamine in the same dose range were studied against bicuculline and picrotoxin induced seizures in groups of rats of identical age (doses indicated in Fig. 1). The results demonstrated that ketamine was active in suppression of major (generalized tonic-clonic) seizures, whereas the effects against minimal (pure clonic) seizures

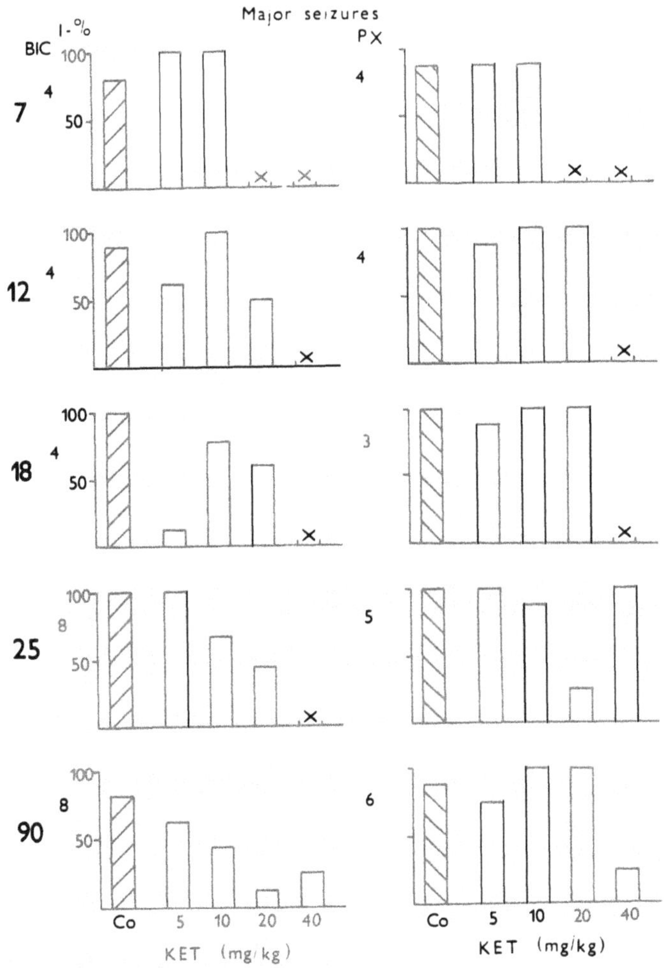

Fig. 1. Incidence of major (tonic-clonic) seizures induced by bicuculline (left) and picrotoxin (right). From top to bottom—rats 7, 12, 18, 25, and 90 days old; Abscissa—doses of ketamine; CO = controls without ketamine; ordinate incidence of seizures; x = dose was not tested.

seemed to be negligible. This effect was more pronounced in the case of bicuculline induced seizures. Picrotoxin induced generalized tonic-clonic seizures were only delayed by ketamine. Ketamine also delayed the time to death induced by picrotoxin.

Our studies also demonstrated the greater effectiveness of ketamine in rat pups, which is in accordance with findings regarding NMDA receptor supersensitivity in young animals (Tsumoto *et al.*, 1987). The action of ketamine against the generalized tonic-clonic pattern was clearly demonstrated, suggesting that NMDA receptors may play a prominent role in this type of seizure. The generator of this seizure pattern is hypothetically in the brainstem which is where one may look for the site of action of ketamine on a macrolevel (Browning, 1985).

Models of partial seizures

There are only a few reports of the action of ketamine in models of partial seizures with complex symptomatology, *i.e.*, limbic and temporal lobe seizures. Ketamine was found to suppress afterdischarges elicited by amygdaloid kindling in adult rats with an inverted U shaped dose response. Its behavioral effects were also dose dependent (Bowyer and Winters, 1981). In an *in vitro* study (Brady and Swann, 1986), ketamine was shown to eliminate the afterdischarges evoked by orthodromic stimulation of CA3 neurons in immature hippocampal slices, suggesting that the hippocampus also contains a number of ketamine binding sites.

We decided to study the action of ketamine (5-40 mg/kg i.p.) in a model of complex partial seizures evoked by the rhythmic stimulation of the dorsal hippocampus of unrestrained animals aged 12, 18, 25, and 90 days. The drug was given immediately after the first of 4 stimulations (intervals 15 min in 90 day old rats; 10 min in pups). Ketamine (20 or 40 mg/kg i.p.) depressed the duration of afterdischarge in adult rats but its effect on a behavioral correlate ("wet dog shakes") was transient and was observed only following the largest dose. On the other hand, no effect of ketamine was noted on the duration of afterdischarge in 12 day old rats. However, the dose dependent attenuation of "wet dog shakes" was observed in this age group. Eighteen and 25 day old animals showed a continuous transition from the results found in 12 day old rats to those observed in adults (Table 2). Our results suggest two different effects of ketamine. One is associated with a reduction of afterdischarge and develops later, whereas the other is associated with behavior and prevails in young animals. These conclusions are in agreement with much of the published data describing various mechanisms of action of ketamine (see Myslobodsky *et al.*, 1981

TABLE. 2 Effects of ketamine on hippocampal afterdischarges and their behavioral sequelae in rats

Stimulation	***Mean ± S.E. Afterdischarge Duration (sec)***										
	12 day old			18 day old			25 day old		90 day old		
1st	26 ±3	30 ±2	23 ±3	32 ±5	15 ±2	18 ±1	16 ±2	16 ±2	20 ±2	21 ±2	22 ±3
	Dose of ketamine mg/kg i.p.*										
	5	10	20	10	20	40	10	20	10	20	40
2nd	25 ±2	24 ±6	22 ±10	12 ±3	9 ±2	12 ±4	9 ±4	5 ±2	6 ±2	5 ±2	2 ±1
3rd	28 ±2	29 ±2	27 ±4	24 ±6	24 ±4	41 ±7	12 ±4	13 ±3	15 ±2	9 ±2	6 ±2
4th	33 ±3	29 ±2	32 ±4	32 ±5	19 ±2	35 ±8	18 ±4	14 ±5	10 ±2	22 ±1	12 ±1
	Mean ± S.E. Number of Wet Dog Shakes										
1st	8 ±.4	9 ±1	10 ±1	10 ±2	9 ±1	11 ±1	10 ±2	14 ±3	4 ±2	3 ±1	3 ±1
	Dose of ketamine mg/kg i.p.*										
	5	10	20	10	20	40	10	20	10	20	40
2nd	5 ±1	2 ±.3	.2 ±.1	2 ±1	.1 ±.1	0 ±0	8 ±5	1 ±.6	2 ±1	1 ±1	.4 ±.2
3rd	8 ±1	4 ±1	1 ±.4	4 ±2	3 ±1	1 ±.4	15 ±7	8 ±3	9 ±2	4 ±2	.4 ±.2
4th	10 ±1	6 ±1	2 ±1	8 ±2	5 ±1	3 ±1	20 ±8	10 ±6	6 ±2	5 ±2	1 ±.5

*Ketamine was administered following the first stimulation.

for a review of this subject). However, suppression of the afterdischarge seen in adults was not as marked as the action of ketamine against the generalized tonic-clonic seizure pattern. The role of ketamine in suppressing hippocampal afterdischarge seems to be moderate.

The action of ketamine in neocortical foci, *i.e.*, in the model of simple partial seizures, was described by DeVore *et al.* (1976). These authors found that ketamine activates and promotes epileptic foci induced by cobalt-gelatine in the neocortex of adult rats. They described the spike-wave frequency of the focus to be increased by 600% following ketamine treatment. However, another study (Aram and Lodge, 1987) performed *in vitro* revealed that the ketamine block of epileptiform activity induced by alkalosis in neocortical slices is in concentrations which are relevant to NMDA receptor blockade. The role of ketamine in simple partial seizure models deserves further extensive study.

Summary

One can conclude that ketamine exhibits a potent anticonvulsant action against generalized tonic-clonic seizures. Its efficacy in other models is either moderate or negligible. Its proconvulsant effect might be due to another mechanism which is set into an action by larger doses of ketamine. The sensitivity to ketamine is greatest in very young animals and decreases with age.

References

Anis, N.A., Berry, S.C., Burton, N.R., and Lodge, D.: The dissociative anesthetics, ketamine and phencyclidine, selectively reduce excitation of central mammalian neurones by N-methyl-D-aspartate. Br. J. Pharmacol. 79: 565-575, 1983.

Aram, J.A. and Lodge, D.: Epileptiform activity induced by alkalosis in rat neocortical slices: Block by antagonists of N-methyl-D-aspartate. Neurosci. Lett. 83: 345-350, 1987.

Black, J.A., Golden, G.T., and Fariello, R.G.: Ketamine activation of corticoreticular epilepsy. Neurol. 30: 315-318, 1980.

Bourn, W.M., Yang, D.J., and Davisson, J.N.: Effect of ketamine enantiomers on sound induced epilepsy in prone rats. Pharmacol. Res. Commun. 15: 815-824, 1983.

Bowyer, J.F. and Winters, W.D.: The effects of various anesthetics on amygdaloid kindled seizures. Neuropharmacol. 20: 199-209, 1981.

Brady, R.J. and Swann, J.W.: Ketamine selectively suppresses synchronized afterdischarge in immature hippocampus. Neurosci. Lett. 69: 143-149, 1986.

Browning, R.A.: Role of the brainstem reticular formation in tonic-clonic seizures: Lesion and pharmacological studies. Fed. Proc. 44: 2425-2431, 1985.

Czuczwar, S.J., Janusz, W., Wamil, A., and Kleinrok, Z.: Inhibition of aminophylline-induced convulsions in mice by antiepileptic drugs and other agents. Eur. J. Pharmacol. 144: 309-315, 1987.

DeVore, G.R., McQueen, J.K., and Woodbury, D.M.: Ketamine hydrochloride and its effect on a chronic cobalt epileptic cortical focus. Epilepsia 17: 111-117, 1976.

Gourie, D.M., Cherian, L., and Shankar, S.K.: Seizures in cats induced by ketamine hydrochloride anesthesia. Indian J. Med. Res. 77: 525-528, 1983.

Hayes, B.A. and Balster, R.L.: Anticonvulsant properties of phencyclidine-like drugs in mice. Eur. J. Pharmacol. 117: 121-125, 1985.

Kayama, Y.: Stimulant and depressant effects of ketamine on neocortical activity in cats. Brit. J. Anaesth. 55: 655-660, 1983.

Leander, J.D., Ornstein, P.L., and Zimmerman, D.M.: Antagonism of NMDA-induced lethality and behavioral effects by phencyclidine-like drugs. In Excitatory Amino Acid Transmission, Hicks, T.P., Lodge, D., and McLennan, H., eds., pp. 197-204, Alan R. Liss, Inc., New York, 1987.

Leccese, A.P., Marquis, K.L., Mattia, A., and Moreton, J.E.: The convulsant and anticonvulsant effects of phencyclidine (PCP) and PCP analogues in the rat. Behav. Brain Res. 19: 163-169, 1986.

Mareš, P. and Velíšek, L.: Influence of ethosuximide on metrazol induced seizures during ontogenesis in rats. Activ. Nerv. Super. 25: 295-298, 1983.

Marešová, D., Mareš, P., Zouhar, A., Trojan, S., and Vidner, P.: Ontogenetic development of ketamine-induced sleeping time and electrocenticographic changes in rats. Dev. Pharmacol. Ther. 12:179-187, 1989.

Meinardi, H. and Magnus, O.: Drug therapy. Clinical application. In Handbook of Clinical Neurology, Vol. 15, Magnus, O. and deHaas, A.M.L., eds., pp. 664-672, North-Holland Publishing Co., Amsterdam, 1974.

Myslobodsky, M.S., Golovchinsky, V., and Mintz, M.: Ketamine: Convulsant or anticonvulsant? Pharmacol. Biochem. Behav. 14: 27-33, 1981.

Ornstein, P., Zimmerman, D.M., Hynes, M.D., III, and Leander, J.D.: Anticonvulsant, motor impairment and stimulatory effects of NMDA antagonists and phencyclidine-like compounds in mice. In Excitatory Amino Acid Transmission, Hicks, T.P., Lodge, D., and McLennan, H., eds., pp. 123-136, Alan R. Liss, Inc., New York, 1987.

Sagratella, S., Passarelli, F., and Scotti de Carolis, A.: An EEG investigation on the effects of phencyclidine on pentylenetetrazol convulsions in rats and rabbits. Arch. Int. Pharmacodyn. Ther. 266: 294-307, 1983.

Taberner, P.V.: The anticonvulsant activity of ketamine against seizures induced by pentylenetetrazol and mercaptoproionic acid. Eur. J. Pharmacol. 39: 305-311, 1976.

Tsumoto, T., Hagihara, K., Sato, H., and Hata, Y.: NMDA receptors in the visual cortex of young kittens are more effective than those of adult cats. Nature 327: 513-514, 1987.

Velíšek, L., Mikolášová, R., Blanková-Vaňková, S., and Mareš, P.: Effects of ketamine on metrazol-induced seizures during ontogenesis in rats. Pharmacol. Biochem. Behav. 32: 405-410, 1989.

Winters, W.D.: Effects of drugs on the electrical activity of the brain: Anesthetics. Ann. Rev. Pharmacol. Toxicol. 16: 413-426, 1976.

Status of Ketamine in Anesthesiology,
edited by E.F. Domino©1990, NPP Books
P.O. Box 1491, Ann Arbor, MI 48106

Ketamine Reduces NMDA Receptor Mediated Neurotoxicity in Cortical Cultures

D.W. Choi

Department of Neurology
Stanford University Medical Center
Stanford, CA

INTRODUCTION

The anesthetic, ketamine, interacts with the phencyclidine (PCP) binding site in the NDMA receptor activated channel, interfering with the influx of cations through the channel and thus noncompetitively antagonizing the actions of NMDA agonists (Zukin and Zukin, 1979; Lodge *et al.*, 1987). The relationship between this defined action of ketamine and its anesthetic effects has not yet been fully clarified. However, its ability to act as an NMDA antagonist raises the possibility that it could have beneficial effects in several disease settings, including stroke, cardiac arrest, prolonged seizures, and trauma, where overactivation of NMDA receptors may contribute importantly to the pathogenesis of neuronal cell loss (Simon *et al.*, 1984; Wieloch, 1985; Rothman and Olney, 1987; Choi, 1988). This possibility is supported by experimental evidence suggesting that ketamine can reduce hypoxic neuronal injury both *in vitro* (Weiss *et al.*, 1986) and *in vivo* (Natale *et al.*, 1988; Marcoux *et al.*, this volume).

We have previously used murine neocortical cell cultures to quantitatively characterize the ability of several other PCP or *sigma* ligands to block NMDA receptor mediated neurotoxicity (Goldberg *et al.*, 1988). We report here an extension of this study to include ketamine.

MATERIALS AND METHODS

Mixed cultures of neurons and glia were prepared from fetal mice (embryonic days 14-18), generally as previously described (Choi *et al.*, 1987). Dissociated neocortices were plated on modified polystyrene (Falcon Primaria) 16 mm culture wells (0.28-0.34 $x10^6$ cells/well), in

Eagle's minimal essential medium (MEM), and supplemented with 10% horse serum, 10% fetal bovine serum, glutamine (2 mM), and glucose (total 21 mM). Cultures were maintained at 37° C in a humidified 5% CO_2 atmosphere. Non neuronal cell division was inhibited after 5-10 days *in vitro* by a 1-3 day exposure to 10 μM cytosine arabinoside. Subsequently, cells were fed twice a week by exchange with a similar medium lacking fetal serum. Cultures were selected for study between 15-21 days *in vitro*, at which time phase bright neurons could be readily distinguished from the underlying glial monolayer.

Cultures were exposed to NMDA or glutamate dissolved in a tris buffered physiological salt solution at room temperature (Choi *et al.*, 1987). After 5 min, the solution was removed by washing with serum free culture medium (supplemented with extra glucose, total 25 mM), and cultures were returned to the incubator for 20-24 hr. Kainate and quinolinate were comparatively weak neurotoxins with 5 min exposure. In order to produce widespread neuronal loss, cultures were exposed to these compounds for 24 hr (in the 37° C incubator, using serum free culture medium supplemented with glucose).

Morphologic features of cell injury were assessed by phase contrast microscopy, augmented in some cases by examination of trypan blue exclusion. Quantitation of neuronal loss was obtained by measurement of extracellular lactate dehydrogenase (LDH), released by damaged neurons into the culture medium 24 hr after the onset of excitotoxic exposure. The background LDH released by sister cultures exposed to sham wash alone was always subtracted from experimental values to yield the signal specifically associated with excitotoxicity. Control studies demonstrated that this LDH signal correlated closely with the number of neurons damaged by glutamate (Koh and Choi, 1987). As described here, glia were not visibly injured by these experimental manipulations, and there was minimal LDH release from pure glial cultures exposed to excitotoxins.

Results

A 5 min exposure to 500 μM NMDA invariably produced widespread acute neuronal swelling within 30 min, followed over the ensuing day by extensive destruction of neurons and processes, and substantial release of LDH into the culture medium. Addition to the exposure medium of 100 μM ketamine blocked both the morphological and biochemical (LDH) evidence of neuronal injury (Fig. 1). Ketamine also blocked the neurotoxicity of the NMDA receptor agonist quinolinate, but

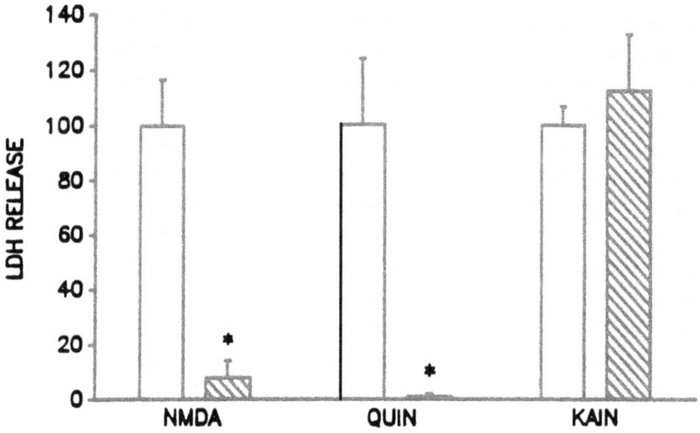

Fig. 1. Ketamine is a selective antagonist of NMDA mediated neurotoxicity. Cultures were exposed to NMDA (500 μM), kainate (KAIN, 100 μM), or quinolinate (QUIN, 1 mM), either alone (control, open bars) or in the presence of 100 μM ketamine (shaded bars). A matched set of sister cultures were used for each, with or without antagonist comparison. Bars depict mean ± S.E. (N = 3-4 cultures) LDH efflux to the bathing medium, scaled to mean LDH present in the appropriate antagonist free control (= 100), and following subtraction of the background efflux present in cultures exposed to sham wash only. * Significantly different from control ($P < 0.01$), two tailed "t" test.

had no effect on neuronal injury produced by exposure to the non NMDA agonist kainate (Fig. 1).

Ketamine antagonism of NMDA induced neuronal injury was concentration dependent, with little protective effect at 1 μM, and intermediate protective effect at 10 μM (Fig. 2).

We have previously shown that selective blockade of NMDA receptor mediated neurotoxicity suffices to largely attenuate the neurotoxicity produced by brief exposure to the endogenous broad spectrum agonist, glutamate (Choi *et al.*, 1988). As predicted by this precedent, ketamine produced a concentration dependent reduction in glutamate neurotoxicity with potency and efficacy similar to its ability to reduce NMDA neurotoxicity (Fig. 3).

The table below summarizes the relative potencies of ketamine and other PCP ligands (Goldberg *et al.*, 1988) against NMDA induced neuronal injury in our cortical culture system. EC_{50} values represent the concentration of antagonist required to reduce neuronal injury produced by exposure to 500 μM NMDA for 5 min, rounded to the nearest 1/2 log unit.

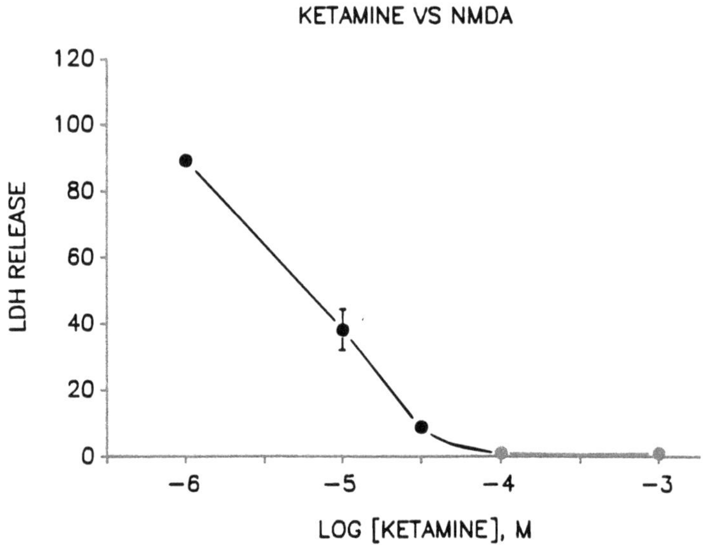

Fig. 2. Concentration dependence of ketamine antagonism of NMDA induced neuronal injury. Sister cultures were exposed to 500 μM NMDA for 5 min in the presence of the indicated concentration of ketamine. Each point depicts LDH release (mean ± S.E., N = 3-4 at each concentration), scaled to mean value seen in unprotected controls (= 100).

EC_{50} for neuroprotective action *vs* NMDA

Drug	*EC_{50} (μM)*
MK-801	0.3
Phencyclidine	1
(+)-Cyclazocine	10
(+)-SKF 10,047	10
Ketamine	10
Pentazocine	30

Discussion

Ketamine, in common with other PCP or *sigma* ligands, blocked NMDA receptor mediated late neuronal loss in cortical cell cultures. This protective action was concentration dependent between 1 and 100 M with an EC_{50} of about 10 μM. It was also selective. Ketamine blocked the neurotoxicity of NMDA or the endogenous NMDA agonist, quinolinate, but did not block the neurotoxicity of the non-NMDA agonist, kainate. These findings are compatible with the reported ability of ketamine to block selectively NMDA induced acute excitotoxic neuronal swelling in

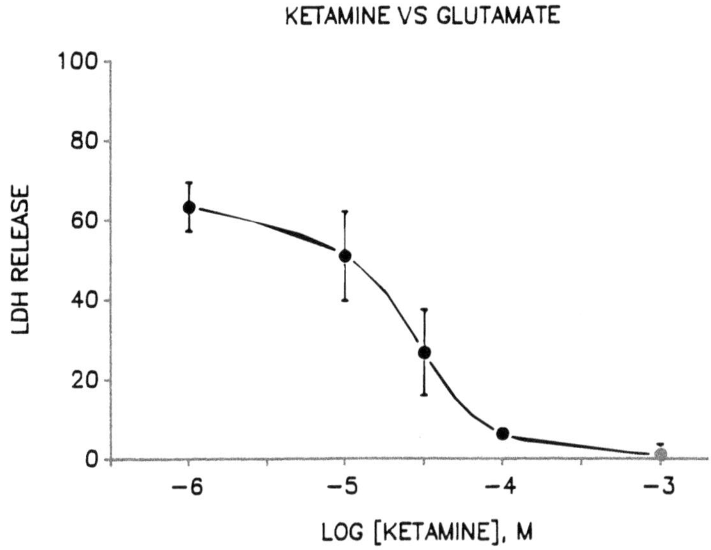

Fig. 3. Concentration dependence of ketamine antagonism of glutamate induced neuronal injury. Sister cultures were exposed to 500 μM glutamate for 5 min in the presence of the indicated concentration of ketamine. Bars depict LDH release (mean ± S.E., N = 3-4 at each concentration), scaled to mean values seen in unprotected controls (= 100).

the chick retina (Olney *et al.*, 1986). The neuroprotection to other tested PCP or *sigma* ligands is more consistent with rank affinity for the PCP site than for the *sigma* site (Zukin and Zukin, 1979; Mendelsohn *et al.*, 1985; Largent *et al.*, 1986), supporting the widely accepted idea that it is the PCP site which is directly involved in antagonism of NMDA receptor induced neurotoxicity.

The ability of ketamine to reduce the late neuronal loss induced by brief glutamate exposure suggests that it could have neuroprotective value in certain types of acute brain injury. However, present results only provide a specific cellular basis for neuroprotection. Whether or not ketamine will actually reduce neuronal loss *in vivo* will depend on additional factors not studied in these cell culture experiments. As discussed elsewhere in this volume, ketamine has several effects outside the glutamate system that could be relevant to brain injury. In particular, the ability of ketamine to increase brain metabolism and cerebral blood flow could be deleterious in the setting of ischemia or raised intercranial pressure. The net effect of ketamine on neuronal survival in these settings thus might reflect an interplay between a beneficial parenchymal neuroprotective action and a deleterious prometabolic action. In addition, at least in small animals, the results of Marcoux and colleagues (reported elsewhere in this volume) underscore the possible importance of temperature effects in influencing ketamine neuroprotection, as originally emphasized by Pulsinelli and colleagues.

Still, the availability of ketamine as a clinical anesthetic makes it an attractive candidate for cautious exploration of possible neuroprotective actions (Albers *et al.*, 1989). The best settings for initial exploration would probably be those in which a need for a general anesthetic, and a risk for brain ischemia, coincide. Substantial safety issues would need to be considered in study design, but ultimately only clinical trial can test the utility of the NMDA antagonist strategy in man. Neuroprotection could represent an important new indication for ketamine or structurally related compounds.

Acknowledgements

I thank V. Viseskul and K. Rose for technical assistance. This work was supported by NIH grant NS12151. Ketamine was kindly suppplied by Dr. F. Marcoux at Parke-Davis.

References

Albers, G.W., Goldberg, M.P. and Choi, D.W.: N-methyl-D-aspartate antagonists: Ready for clinical trial in brain ischemia? Ann. Neurol. 25: 398-403, 1989.

Choi, D.W.: Glutamate neurotoxicity and diseases of the nervous system. Neuron 1: 623-634, 1988.

Choi, D.W., Maulucci-Gedde, M.A. and Kriegstein, A.R.: Glutamate neurotoxicity in cortical cell culture. J. Neurosci. 7: 357-368, 1987.

Goldberg, M.P., Viseskul, V. and Choi, D.W.: Phencyclidine receptor ligands attenuate cortical neuronal injury after N-methyl-D-aspartate exposure hypoxia. J. Pharmacol. Exp. Ther. 245: 1081-1087, 1988.

Koh, J.Y. and Choi, D.W.: Quantitative determination of glutamate mediated cortical neuronal injury in cell culture by lactate dehydrogenase efflux assay. J. Neurosci. Meth. 20: 83-90, 1987.

Largent, B.L., Gundlach, A.L. and Snyder, S.H.: Pharmacological and autoradiographic discrimination of *sigma* and phencyclidine receptor binding sites in brain with (+)-[^{3}H] SKF 10,047, (+)-[^{3}H]-3-[3-hydroxyphenyl]-N-(1-propyl)piperidine and [^{3}H]-1-[1-(2-thienyl)cyclohexyl]piperidine. J. Pharmacol. Exp. Ther. 238: 739-748, 1986.

Lodge, D., Aram, J.W., Church, J., Davies, S.N., Martin, D., O'Shaughnessy, C.T. and Zeman, S.: Excitatory amino acids and phencyclidine-like drugs.

In Excitatory Amino Acid Transmission, ed. by T.P. Hicks, D. Lodge and H. McLennan, Liss, New York, NY, pp 83-89, 1987.

Mendelsohn, L.G., Kalra, V., Johnson, B.G. and Kirchner, G.A.: *Sigma* opiate receptor: Characterization and co-identity with the phencyclidine receptor. J. Pharmacol. Exp. Ther. 233: 597-602, 1985.

Natale, J.E., Schott, R.J. and D'Alecy, L.G.: Ketamine reduces neurologic deficit following 10 minutes of cardiac arrest and resuscitation in canines. In *Sigma* and Phencyclidine Compounds as Molecular Probes in Biology, ed. by E.F. Domino and J.-M. Kamenka, NPP Books, Ann Arbor, MI, pp 717-726, 1988.

Olney, J.W., Price, M.T., Fuller, T.A., Labruyere, J., Samson, L., Carpenter, M. and Mahan, K.: The anti-excitotoxic effects of certain anesthetics, analgesics and sedative-hypnotics. Neurosci. Lett. 68: 29-34, 1986.

Rothman, S.M. and Olney, J.W.: Glutamate and pathophysiology of hypoxic-ischemic brain damage. Ann. Neurol. 19: 105-111, 1987.

Simon, R.P., Swan, J.H., Griffiths, T. and Meldrum, B.S.: Blockade of N-methyl-D-aspartate receptors may protect against ischemic damage in the brain. Science 226: 850-852, 1984.

Wieloch, T.: Hypoglycemia-induced neuronal damage prevented by an N-methyl-D-aspartate antagonist. Science 230: 681-683, 1985.

Weiss, J., Goldberg, M.P., and Choi, D.W.: Ketamine protects cultured neocortical neurons from hypoxic injury. Brain Res. 380: 186-190, 1986.

Zukin, R.S. and Zukin, S.R.: Specific [^{3}H]phencyclidine binding in the rat central nervous system. Proc. Natl. Acad. Sci. USA 76: 5372-5376, 1979.

Status of Ketamine in Anesthesiology,
edited by E.F. Domino©1990, NPP Books
P.O. Box 1491, Ann Arbor, MI 48106

Ketamine Anesthesia Reduces Ischemic Hippocampal Neuronal Injury

F. W. Marcoux, J. E. Goodrich, and M. A. Dominick

Departments of Pharmacology and Pathology
and Experimental Toxicology
Parke-Davis Pharmaceutical Research Division
Warner-Lambert Company
Ann Arbor, MI

INTRODUCTION

Ketamine hydrochloride is an established dissociative anesthetic (Domino *et al.*, 1965; White *et al.*, 1982). Unlike barbiturate anesthetics, which are CNS depressants, ketamine is reported to increase cerebral metabolism (Dawson *et al.*, 1971). Since some barbiturates have shown beneficial activity in experimental models of cerebral ischemia (Hoff *et al.*, 1975), and such activity has been explained as the result of decreased metabolic requirements in the compromised brain (Steen and Michenfelder, 1978), an increased cerebral metabolic demand with ketamine anesthesia might be expected to exacerbate ischemic neuronal injury. However, ketamine antagonizes the action of excitatory amino acids in the CNS (Anis *et al.*, 1983; Lodge and Anis, 1984), a pharmacological action proposed to be of therapeutic benefit in the treatment of stroke (Rothman and Olney, 1986) and reported to be effective in reducing experimentally induced cerebral infarction (Simon *et al.*, 1984). Indeed, ketamine is neuroprotective *in vitro* in conditions which are proposed to mimic hypoxic/ischemic brain injury *in vivo* (Choi, this volume).

The present study extends observations made previously (Marcoux *et al.*, 1988a and Marcoux *et al.*, 1988b), where ketamine was shown to prevent hypoxia induced neuronal calcium accumulation and injury in cell culture and ischemic hippocampal injury in gerbils. Here the *in vivo* findings are reexamined with core body temperature measurements presented for ketamine treated gerbils. At the anesthetic dose of 150 mg/kg ketamine reduced ischemic hippocampal injury significantly and caused an insignificant 1°C fall in core body temperature. The combined effects of hypothermia and anesthesia produced by the higher 200 mg/kg dose conferred substantial neuroprotection.

Materials and Methods

Mongolian gerbils were anesthetized with ether-air or ketamine hydrochloride (Ketalar) and subjected to temporary bilateral carotid artery occlusion. The vulnerability of the brain to this procedure is unique in the gerbil species because the confluence of cerebral blood supply at the circle of Willis is incomplete (Levy and Brierley, 1974), rendering the cerebral hemispheres specifically dependent on carotid blood flow (Osburne and Halsey, 1975). Thus, even relatively short periods of ischemia in gerbils can lead to neuronal necrosis (Kirino, 1982).

A midline incision was made under anesthesia ventrally in the neck and both common carotid arteries were dissected free. Aneurysm clips were positioned across each carotid artery within 3 min of the initial incision. Skin clips were used to reappose the neck tissues, leaving the aneurysm clips in place. Gerbils were returned to the upright prone position and the aneurysm clips were removed 10 min postocclusion.

Eighty gerbils were used in 6 treatment groups, of which 61 survived treatment and bilateral carotid occlusion. Seven gerbils in the unoperated vehicle control group (VCL CNTL) were treated with 0.9% NaCl (10 ml/kg b. wt., i.p.) and were given no anesthesia. Eight gerbils in the ketamine control group (KET CNTL) were given the high dose of ketamine (200 mg/kg, i.p.), but did not undergo surgery. Eleven gerbils in the bilateral carotid occlusion control group (BCO CNTL) were subjected to 10 min of bilateral carotid occlusion under brief ether anesthesia. The 3 ketamine treatment groups were 100, 150 and 200 mg/kg (KET 100, KET 150 and KET 200), with 11, 11 and 12 gerbils per group, respectively. The 100 mg/kg treatment group represented a borderline anesthetic dose, and ether was used to supplement anesthesia during placement of the aneurysm clips. The 150 mg/kg treatment group represented an anesthetic dose, requiring no supplemental ether. The 200 mg/kg treatment group showed deep anesthesia. All ketamine treated groups were given a single i.p. injection 30 min prior to placement of the aneurysm clips. Core body temperature was determined by rectal probe 30 minutes after i.p. injection of either vehicle (BCO CNTL group) or ketamine.

Fifteen to 17 days after bilateral carotid occlusion, the brains of the gerbils were fixed *in situ* by transcardiac perfusion with buffered formalin. A 5 mm coronal section through the dorsal hippocampus was processed for histopathologic examination by routine paraffin technique. Beginning approximately 1.8 mm caudal to the bregma and proceeding rostrally, 3 serial sections 300 mm apart were stained with hematoxylin and eosin, examined in a blinded fashion, and graded on the severity of ischemic neuronal injury of pyramidal cells of the CA1 region. Pyramidal cell injury in the CA1 region of the hippocampus was graded on the basis of a pilot study as follows: grade 0, no decrease in density of neuronal perikarya; grade 1, degenerate or necrotic neurons distributed in clusters or individually in a segmental pattern; grade 2, unilateral partial depletion of neurons (incomplete, multifocal or segmental loss of neurons in the CA1 region); grade 3, bilateral partial depletion of neurons; grade 4, unilateral marked depletion of neurons (diffuse loss of neurons in the CA1 region) or marked depletion unilaterally with contralateral partial depletion of neurons; grade 5, bilateral marked depletion of neurons. A weighted least squares analysis of variance with X^2 statistics was used to compare mean histopathological grades between groups. A Bonferroni approximation ($P < 0.008$ for tests between 6 groups) was used to correct for multiple comparisons.

Results

Mean histopathological grades and body temperatures by treatment group are shown in Fig. 1.

Core body temperature in the BCO CNTL group was 38.3 ± 0.3°C and not different from gerbils caged at ambient room temperature (38.1 ± 0.2°C). Body temperature in the KET 100 and KET 150 groups was 38.4 ± 0.2°C and 37.4 ± 0.7°C, respectively, and not different from that in the BCO CNTL group. Body temperature in the KET 200 group was significantly depressed to 34.4 ± 0.4°C.

Minor neuronal injury was seen infrequently in the VCL and KET CNTL groups. In contrast, the average grade was 4.7 ± 0.13 for the BCO CNTL group. The ketamine treated groups showed a dose related amelioration in the severity of ischemic injury to pyramidal cells in dorsal hippocampus. The KET 100, 150 and 200 groups showed mean ± SE histopathological grades of 4 ± 0.41, 3.2 ± 0.53 and 1.5 ± 0.47, respectively. In the KET 200 group, 9 of 12 brains were scored as 0 or 1.

Discussion

Ketamine anesthesia, which did not produce significant core hypothermia (150 mg/kg), ameliorated the histopathological consequences of temporary global cerebral ischemia observed in ether anesthetized con-

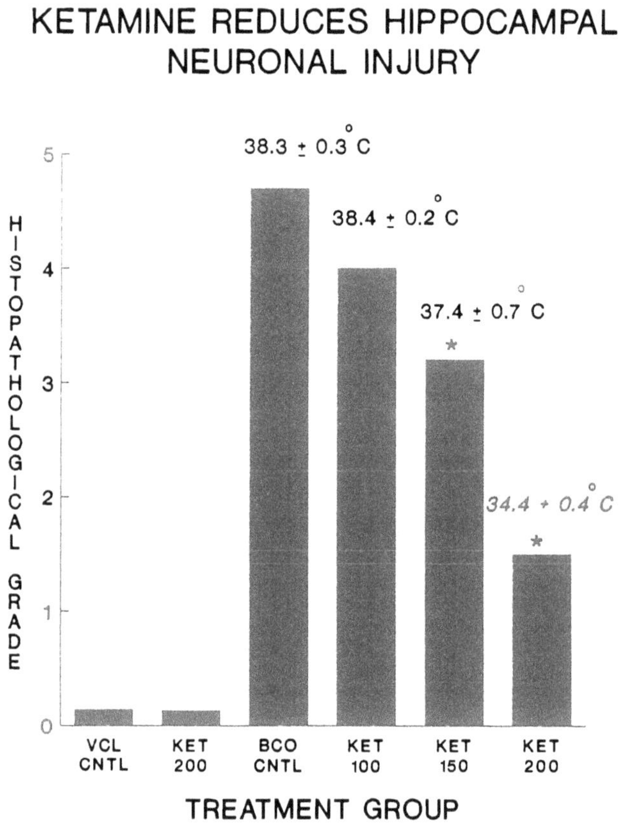

Fig. 1: Mean histopathoiogical grades and body temperatures by treatment group. Core body tempertures were not different for the BCO CNTL, KET 100 and KET 150 groups. Core body temperature in the KET 200 group (italics) was significantly depressed from BCO CNTL. Mean histopathological grades for KET 150 and KET 200 groups (*) were significantly less than for BCO CNTL.

trols. A higher dose of ketamine (200 mg/kg), which produced hypothermia, was associated with a pronounced protective effect, with 3/4 of the treated animals showing only segmental or no hippocampal cell injury. Hypothermia alone can protect the brain from temporary global cerebral ischemia (Busto *et al.*, 1987). Although body temperature in the KET 150 group was not statistically different from that in the BCO CNTL group, it was lower, and this was the lowest dose at which neuroprotection was observed. In experiments to be described in detail elsewhere, we examined the neuroprotective effects of other agents which produced body temperature falls equivalent to and greater than that observed in the KET

150 group. For example, in this same gerbil model, the adenosine agonist, cyclohexyladenosine (CHA) produced hypothermia at doses of 0.1 and 0.3 mg/kg, i.p. (36.5 ± 0.3°C and 33.7 ± 0.4°C, respectively), but neuroprotection only at the higher dose. Thus, the 0.1 mg/kg CHA treatment produced a greater fall in core body temperature than did the 150 mg/kg ketamine treatment. However, the ketamine treatment (histopathological grade = 3.2 ± 0.53 vs 4.7 ± 0.13 BCO CNTL) was neuroprotective and the CHA treatment was not (histopathological grade = 4.8 ± 0.1 vs 4.7 ± 0.1 BCO CNTL). Thus, ketamine's neuroprotective effect at 150 mg/kg in this model is not due to a statistically insignificant fall in core body temperature. The pronounced neuroprotection afforded by the high anesthetic dose of ketamine (200 mg/kg) was likely contributed to by marked hypothermia (Ikonomidou *et al.*, 1989).

In conclusion, ketamine reduces ischemic hippocampal neuronal injury in this gerbil model by a mechanism which is independent of core body hypothermia. This is consistent with similar reports of neuroprotection in other models of brain ischemia using anesthetized, normothermically maintained rodents (*i.e.*, Church *et al.*, 1988). Although ketamine's neuroprotective effects against ischemic brain injury fit with reports of other NMDA antagonists (Albers *et al.*, 1989), other pharmacological mechanisms may be involved. Finally, although our findings dissociate ketamine's neuroprotective actions from core body hypothermia, measurements of intra ischemic brain temperature (Busto *et al.*, 1987) will be required to resolve this issue completely.

References

Albers, G.W., Goldberg, M.P., and Choi, D.W.: N-methyl-D-aspartate antagonists: Ready for clinical trial in brain ischemia? Ann. Neurol. 25: 398-403, 1989.

Anis, N.A., Berry, S.C., Burton, N.R., and Lodge, D.: The dissociative anaesthetics, ketamine and phencyclidine, selectively reduce excitation of central mammalian neurones by N-methyl-D-aspartate. Br. J. Pharmacol. 79: 565-575, 1983.

Busto, R., Dietrich, W.D., Globus, M.Y-T, Valedes, Scheinberg, P., and Ginsberg, M.D.: Small differences in intraischemic brain temperature critically determine the extent of ischemic neuronal injury. J. Cerebral Blood Flow & Metab. 7: 729-738, 1987.

Church, J., Zeman, S., and Lodge, D.: The neuroprotective action of ketamine and MK-801 after transient cerebral ischemia in rats. Anesthesiol. 69: 702-709, 1988.

Dawson, B., Michenfelder, J.D., and Theye, R.A.: Effects of ketamine on canine cerebral blood flow and metabolism: Modification by prior administration of thiopental. Anesth. Analg. 50: 443-447, 1971.

Domino, E.F., Chodoff, P., and Corssen, G.: Pharmacologic effects of CI-581, a new dissociative anesthetic, in man. Clin. Pharm. Ther. 6: 279-291, 1965.

Hoff, J.I., Smith, A.L., Hankinson, H.L., and Nielson, S.L.: Barbiturate protection from cerebral ischemia in primates. Stroke 6: 28-33, 1975.

Ikonomidou, C., Mosinger, J.L. and Olney, J.N., Hypothermia enhances protective effect of MK-801 against hypoxic/ischemic brain damage in infant rats. Brain Research, 487: 184-187, 1989.

Kirino, T.: Delayed neuronal death in the gerbil hippocampus following ischemia. Brain Res. 239: 57-69, 1982.

Levy, D.E. and Brierley, J.B.: Communications between vertebro-basilar and carotid arterial circulations in the gerbil. Exp. Neurol. 45: 503-508, 1974.

Lodge, D. and Anis, N.A.: Effects of ketamine and three other anaesthetics on spinal reflexes and inhibitions in the cat. Br. J. Anaesth. 56: 1143-1151, 1984.

Marcoux, F.W., Goodrich, J.E., Probert, Jr., A.W., and Dominick, M.A.: Ketamine prevents glutamate-induced calcium influx and ischemic nerve cell injury. In *Sigma* and Phencyclidine-Like Compounds as Molecular Probes in Biology, E.F. Domino and J.-M. Kamenka, Eds., pp. 735-746, NPP Books, Ann Arbor, 1988a.

Marcoux, F.W., Goodrich, J.E., and Dominick, M.A.: Ketamine prevents ischemic neuronal injury. Brain Res. 452: 329-335, 1988b.

Osburne, R.C. and Halsey, Jr., J.H.: Cerebral blood flow. A predictor of recovery from ischemia in the gerbil. Arch. Neurol. 32: 457-461, 1975.

Rothman, S. and Olney, J.W.: Glutamate and the pathophysiology of hypoxic-ischemic brain damage. Ann. Neurol. 19: 105-111, 1986.

Simon, R.P., Swan, J.H., Griffith, T., and Meldrum, B.S.: Blockade of N-methyl-D-aspartate receptors may protect against ischemic damage in the brain. Science 226: 850-852, 1984.

Steen, P.A. and Michenfelder, J.D.: Cerebral protection with barbiturates. Stroke 9: 140-142, 1978.

White, P.F., Way, W.L., and Trevor, A.J.: Ketamine-its pharmacology and therapeutic uses. Anesthesiol. 56: 119-136, 1982.

Status of Ketamine in Anesthesiology,
edited by E.F. Domino©1990, NPP Books
P.O. Box 1491, Ann Arbor, MI 48106

Neuroprotective Effects of Ketamine in a Rodent Model of Peptide Induced Spinal Cord Injury: Anatomical and Physiological Correlates

D.D. Rigamonti, A. Martinez-Arizala, and J.B. Long

Walter Reed Institute of Research
Washington, D.C.

INTRODUCTION

The dissociative anesthetic, ketamine, first described in a clinical setting by Corssen and Domino (1966), also increases blood flow to the brain following hypovolemic shock in rodents (Idvall *et al.*, 1980; Idvall, 1981) and protects limbic structures during carotid occlusion in gerbils (Marcoux *et al.*, 1988). During spinal cord ischemia produced by aortic occlusion, ketamine increases the duration of ischemia needed to produce hindlimb paralysis in the rabbit (Robertson *et al.*, 1986). A standardized model of spinal cord ischemia in the rat is rather challenging since the collateral circulation is profuse and segmental radicular arteries are interconnected. A novel approach to produce spinal cord ischemia in this species is through intrathecal injection of the endogenous opiate peptides both called dynorphin A (1-13 and 1-17; dyn means powerful). These peptides cause permanent hindlimb paralysis (Przewlocki *et al.*, 1983), decreased spinal cord blood flow and ischemia (Long *et al.*, 1987), and neuropathological changes (Petras and Long, 1989). We have observed that increased doses of dynorphin A (1-13) were needed to produce paralysis and affect the somatosensory evoked responses when injected into animals anesthetized with ketamine for several hours (Rigamonti *et al.*, 1987). Therefore, we began a series of anatomical and physiological experiments to correlate the protective effects of ketamine on the neuropathological and neurophysiological changes induced by intrathecal injection of these peptides.

METHODS

Anatomical experiments

Adult male Sprague Dawley rats were anesthetized with halothane and suspended in a stereotaxic unit. A parasagittal skin and paraspinous muscle incision exposed the lower lumbar lamina and the fourth lumbar vertebral interspace. Injections were delivered through a 30 gauge needle that was passed between the L4 and L5 vertebra into the underlying spinal subarachnoid space. Animals were divided into 4 experimental groups: Group I, 0.9% NaCl (saline) injected controls; Group II, dynorphin plus ketamine (2 μmol); Group III, dynorphin plus ketamine (4 μmol); Group IV, dynorphin plus saline. The dynorphin A (1-17) dose was kept constant at 20 nmol, an amount previously determined to produce total hindlimb paralysis in halothane anesthetized animals. The rats were reanesthetized at 72 hr postinjection and perfused transcardially with physiological saline followed by a 10% formalin solution for fixation. Perfusion pressure was maintained between 60-80 mm Hg. The spinal cords were dissected from the spinal canal, and a cord segment extending 35 mm rostral from the tip of the conus medullaris was removed. The cord was divided into 6 segments and sectioned either transversely or horizontally. Cross sections were prepared at 3 levels: the sacral cord (10 mm from the termination of the cord), the 6th lumbar segment, and the lumbar enlargement 35 mm from the tip of the coccygeal segments. The intervening cord segments were sectioned horizontally. The tissue was stained according to the methods of Nissl, with hematoxylin and eosin, and with luxol fast blue. Tissue was subsequently evaluated independently by 3 observers blinded to the experimental treatment. Histological scores were assigned using the following criteria, and the lesion rating mean was calculated and plotted using a SAS statistical package:

1. Normal
2. Mild necrosis of the gray matter (less than 30%) with ischemic cell changes and edema
3. Moderate necrosis of the gray matter (less than 60%) with edematous white matter
4. Severe necrosis involving both gray (greater than 90%) and adjacent white matter, edema, cellular infiltration, and glial proliferation

Neurophysiological experiments

Preliminary experiments were designed to record somatosensory evoked potentials (SSEP) following dynorphin A (1-13, i.t. 50 nmol) exposure. This dose routinely produced hindlimb paralysis in halothane anesthetized animals. Adult male Sprague Dawley rats (N = 20), anesthetized with ketamine and xylazine (70 and 6 mg/kg, respectively) and maintained under anesthesia with the same drugs throughout the 3-4 hr experiment, were mounted in a stereotaxic frame and the skull overlying the somatosensory (SSI) receiving area for the hindlimb exposed. A low impedance silver chloride electrode pair was placed 10 mm rostral to bregma and at the site of maximum cortical response to monitor the somatosensory evoked response following stimulation of the medial and lateral plantar nerves in the contralateral hindlimb. Square wave pulses of 0.1 msec duration were used at a current strength 10 times the threshold for muscle twitch at a frequency of 1 Hz. The cortical response was averaged (N = 300) using standard amplification procedures with a Nicolet Pathfinder. Peak amplitude and latency were measured, either on line or from a plot of the generated analog signal (SSEP). Dynorphin A (1-13) was injected after a baseline SSEP was established and recordings were conducted for 1 hr. Animals were then allowed to recover and the motor activity monitored and recorded at 24 hr.

A second series of experiments was designed to test increased doses (50-200 nmol, dynorphin A 1-13, i.t.) in adult Sprague Dawley rats (N = 22). The same stimulation and recording procedures were used throughout. The motor scores of the animals were recorded at 24 hr. Motor scores were assigned using the following criteria in both experiments:

Score	Function
3	Normal motor function
2	Paraparesis, with ability to support weight and walk with impairment, or make walking movements without supporting weight
1	Severe paraparesis, in which animals could make voluntary hindlimb movements but not walking movements
0	Total paralysis, with complete absence of any hindlimb movement

Results

Neuroanatomical evaluation consistently revealed extensive neural injury throughout the sacral cord and lumbar enlargement following injection of 20 nmol of dynorphin A (1-17). The neuropathological changes, found throughout the gray matter, were characterized by wide-

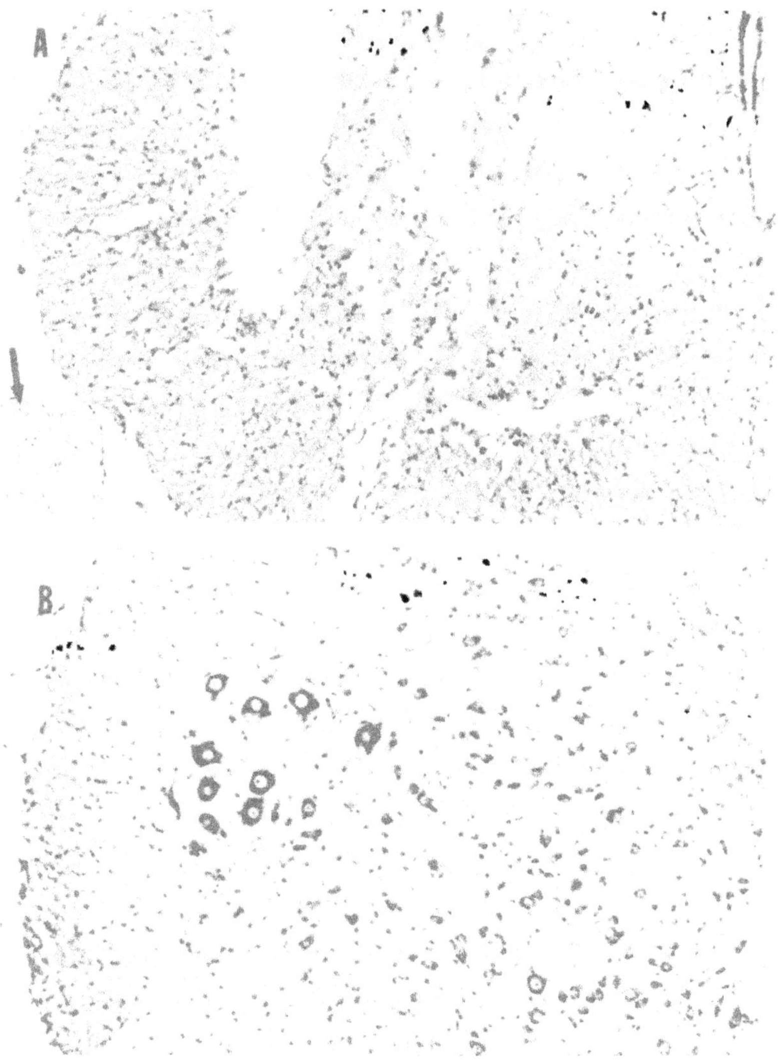

Fig. 1. Light photomicrographs of the lower lumbar (L6) spinal cord perfused 72 hr after injection (i.t.) of either dynorphin (A) or dynorphin with ketamine (2 μmol, B). Note extensive tissue necrosis following peptide exposure. (A) These paralyzed animals show extensive neuropathological changes in the gray and white matter with both neurons and glia being involved. Segmental ventral roots (arrow) are also affected. This is typical of the injury seen throughout the lumbosacral cord. However, dynorphin injected rats cotreated with ketamine (B) maintain neurons in the ventral horn with glial proliferation and only slight changes in the white matter of the sixth lumbar spinal cord segment. Nissl stain. X25.

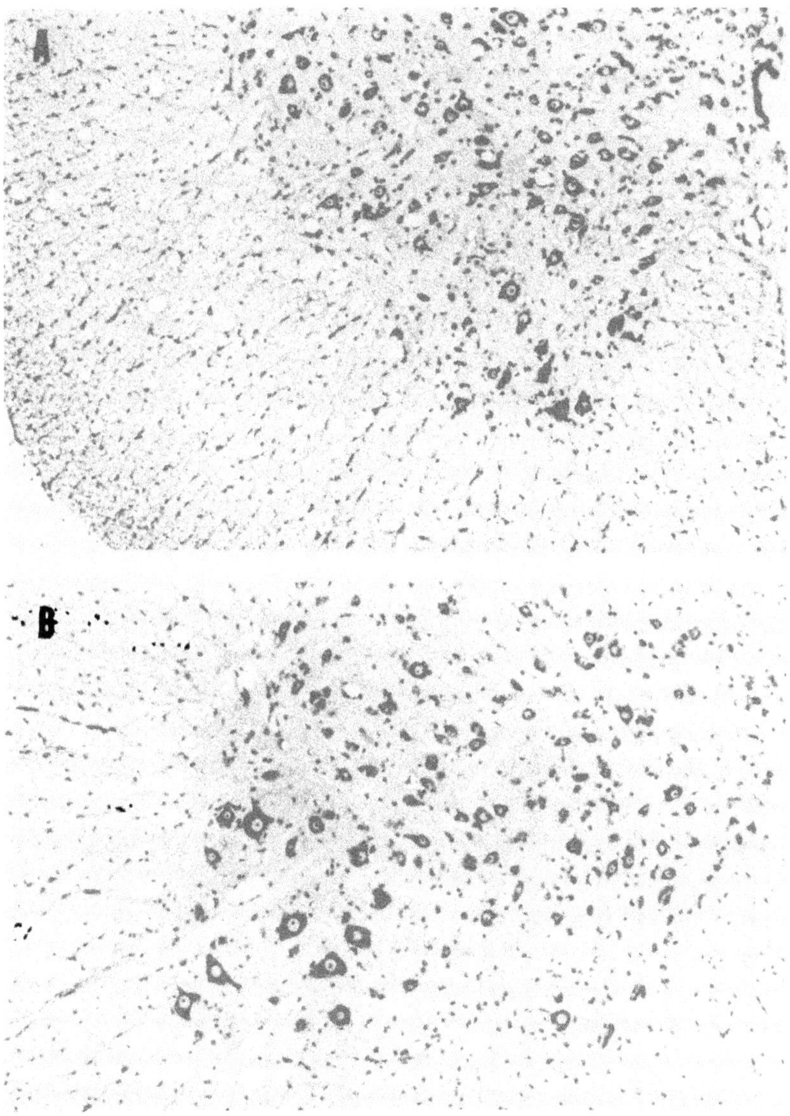

Fig. 2. Light photomicrographs of the lumbar enlargement from a dynorphin plus ketamine (4 μmol, A) and a saline injected control (B). The ketamine treated animals show some loss of motoneurons and slight glial proliferation when compared to control animals at 72 hr postinjection. Nissl stain. A, X25; B, X50.

spread ischemic and necrotic cell changes, diffuse gliosis, and cellular infiltration in these paralyzed animals (Fig. 1A). In contrast, after coinjection of dynorphin and ketamine, animals showed sparing of dorsal and ventral horn neurons in the lower lumbar segment (L6) and lumbar enlargement (Figs. 1B, 2). Mean histopathological grades for each treatment group are shown in Figs. 3, 4, and 5. Dynorphin treated animals were uniformly paralyzed and exhibited extensive neuropathology throughout the lumbosacral cord. Rats injected with dynorphin plus ketamine (2 mol) exhibited protection of the lumbar enlargement and lower lumbar (L6) segment. Rats treated with dynorphin plus ketamine (4 μmol) exhibited a greater degree of protection at the same levels of the spinal cord (lumbar enlargement and L6). All animals treated with either dose of ketamine plus dynorphin were weight bearing.

The neurophysiological responses (SSEP) in preliminary experi-

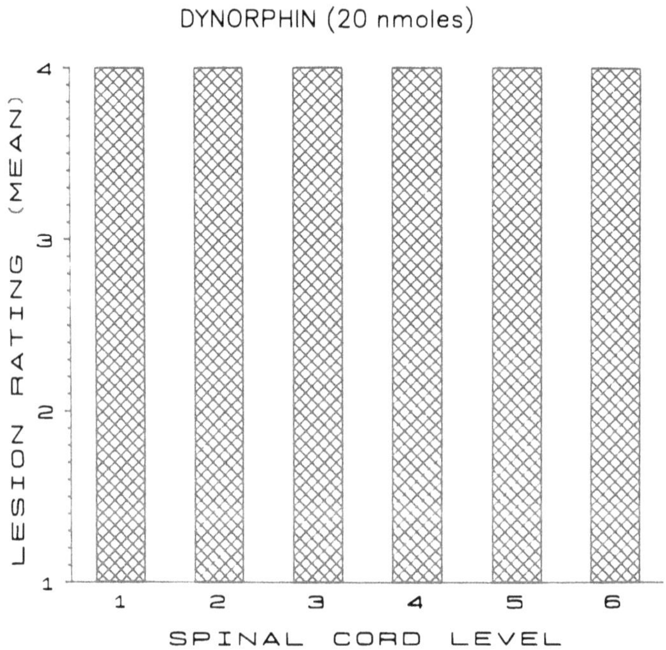

Fig. 3. Summary of histopathological results following dynorphin plus saline intrathecal coinjection to the lumbosacral cord in halothane anesthetized animals (N=4). Transverse (1,3,5) and horizontal (2,4,6) sections were evaluated by 3 observers and graded on a scale of 1-4. Dynorphin (20 nmol) produced extensive neuropathological changes (grade 4) in all spinal cord segments examined in these paralyzed animals 72 hr postinjection.

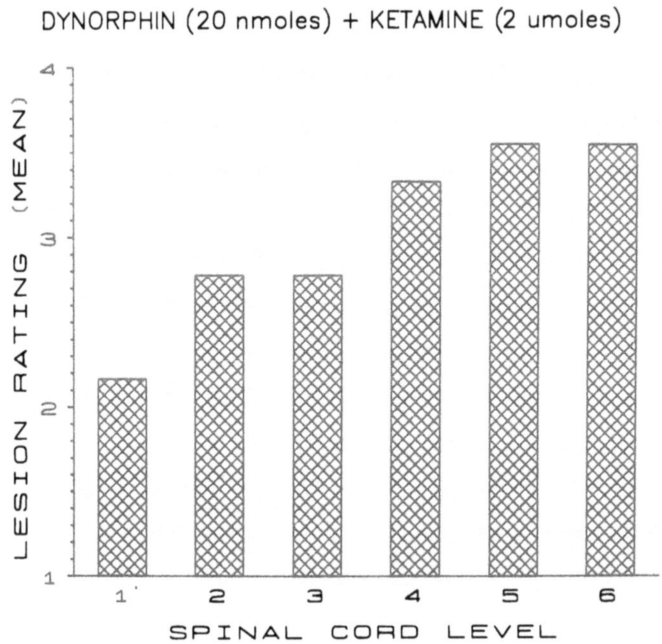

Fig. 4. Summary of histopathological results following dynorphin and ketamine (2 μmol, N = 4) intrathecal coinjection. Maximum protection was observed in the lumbar enlargement (level 1,2) and the sixth lumbar spinal cord segment (level 3). The sacral cord exhibited minimal protection in all of these animals which could support their own weight but walked with impairment.

ments with animals receiving 50 nmol of dynorphin while anesthetized with ketamine for several hours (2-4) showed little change in either latency or amplitude of the cortical response (Fig. 6). The subsequent motor scores were rarely abnormal. However, increased doses of dynorphin (100-200 nmol) in ketamine anesthetized rats produced a reduction of the SSEP beginning shortly after the injection of dynorphin (Fig. 7). In these animals, there was a correlation between the length of time of SSEP reduction with the resultant motor score (Fig. 8). Specifically, all animals showing a 50% reduction in the maximum amplitude of the SSEP of <30 min were walking and weight bearing at 24 hr and all but one of the remaining animals were either paralyzed or expired.

Discussion

When injected intrathecally, dynorphin produces a significant dose related reduction in blood flow in the rodent lumbosacral cord (37-75%)

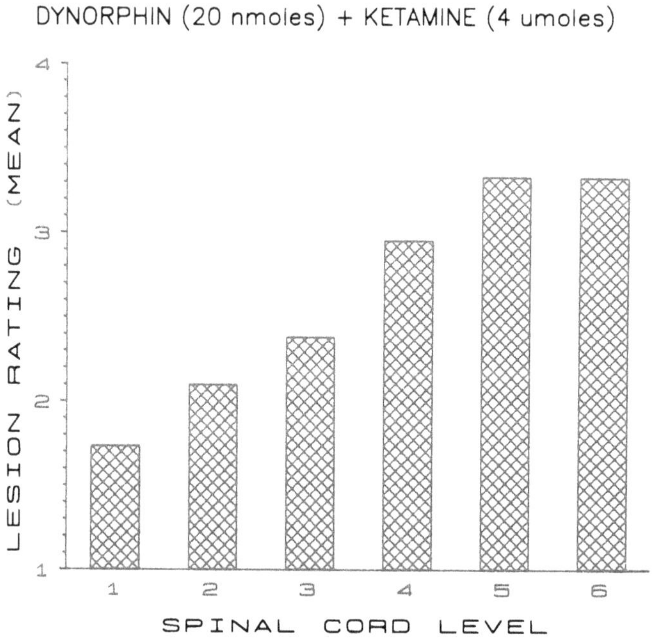

Fig. 5. Summary of histopathological results following dynorphin and ketamine (4 μmol, N = 7) intrathecal coinjection. Maximum protection was observed in the lumbar enlargement and was dose dependent. All animals could walk and were weight bearing.

without altering cardiac output or blood flow to the brain or cervical spinal cord (Long *et al.*, 1987). The resultant secondary changes in nociceptive responses, loss of EMG activity, and paralysis are thought to be caused, at least in part, by this ischemic insult. Neuropathological changes found after dynorphin exposure parallel the ischemic spinal cord changes reported to occur in a variety of animals following aortic occlusion (DeGirolami and Zivin, 1982). This injury primarily produces central gray matter necrosis and glial proliferation. It secondarily causes edema in the surrounding white matter. Interestingly, both ketamine and MK-801 (Rigamonti *et al.*, 1989), two NMDA receptor antagonists, attenuate these neuropathological changes. Both intra- and extracranial blood vessels of the rat are innervated by neural fibers containing dynorphin, and presumably receptors located on the underlying blood vessels respond to their input (Moskowitz *et al.*, 1987). We have observed that the vasoconstriction of pial vessels of the parietal cortex by topical

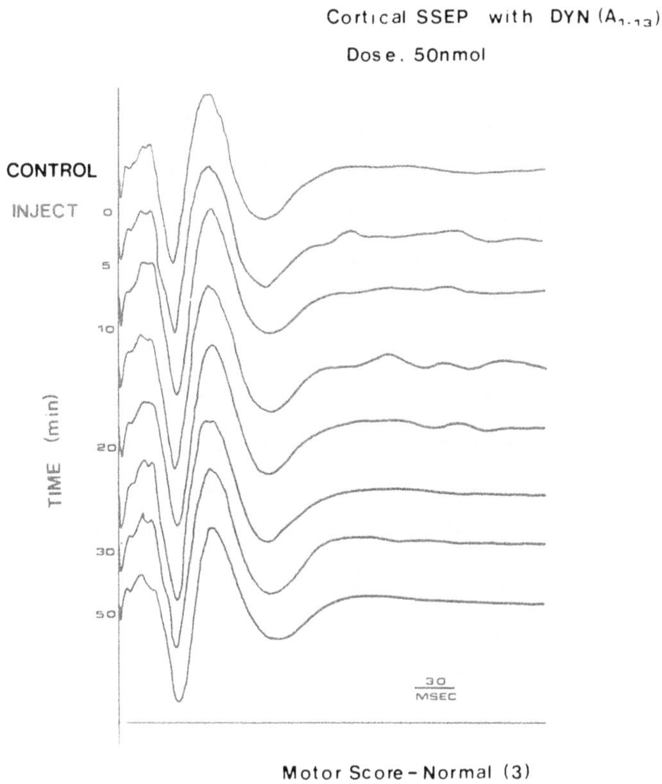

Fig. 6. Somatosensory evoked potential (SSEP) recorded from the cerebral cortex in the ketamine anesthetized animal following stimulation of the contralateral sciatic nerve. Following injection of 50 nmol of dynorphin, a dose which always produced a loss of the SSEP in halothane anesthetized animals, the SSEP amplitude and latency were unaffected for 50 min. The motor score at 24 hr was normal.

dynorphin application appears to be attenuated by simultaneous exposure to ketamine (unpublished observations). Thus: 1) vascular receptors for dynorphin associated with similar innervations in the spinal cord may account for the blood flow reductions and the resultant ischemic response to dynorphin exposure, and 2) ketamine may blunt dynorphin induced vasoconstriction and thereby improve recovery.

The cortical somatosensory response (SSEP) decreases following a reduction of spinal cord blood flow (Berenstein *et al.*, 1983; Schramm and Jones, 1985), and changes in the SSEP 5-10 min after dynorphin

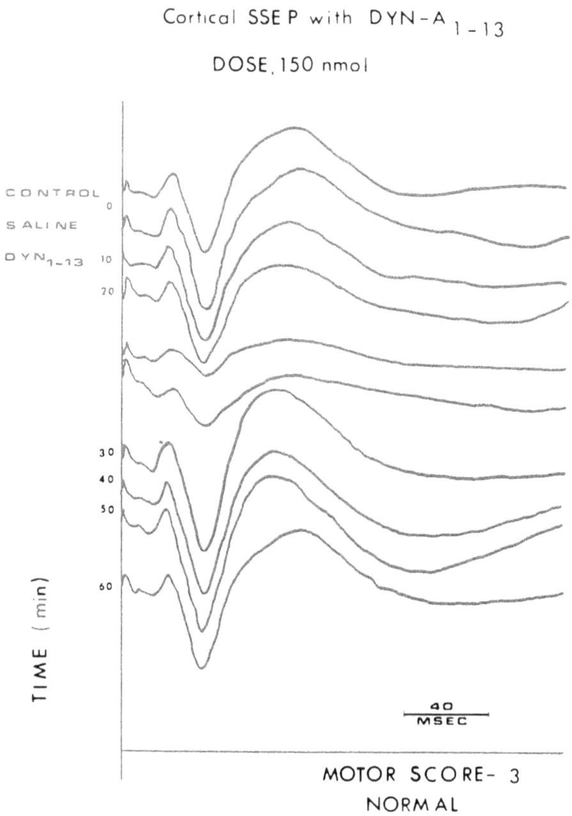

Fig. 7. Cortical SSEP recorded in ketamine anesthetized rats following contralateral sciatic nerve stimulation. There was a decreased amplitude for only 10 min following injection of 150 nmol of dynorphin and normal motor function 24 hr postinjection. This dose always produced permanent paralysis in halothane anesthetized animals and persistent loss of the SSEP.

exposure correlate well with other reported effects of ischemia on long tract neural conduction in the spinal cord (Kobrine *et al.*, 1979). The loss of the cortical response for greater than 30 min has also been used to predict paralysis in the clinical setting following spinal cord surgical procedures. The loss of the SSEP for greater than 30 min was a reliable indicator to predict paralysis in this model. Of current interest are changes not only in the dorsal column, the location of fibers which transmit the SSEP to the cerebral cortex, but also in segmental reflex activity in the spinal cord following dynorphin exposure. Spinal cord reflexes are altered when exposed to dynorphin (Caudle and Isaac, 1988) and ketamine

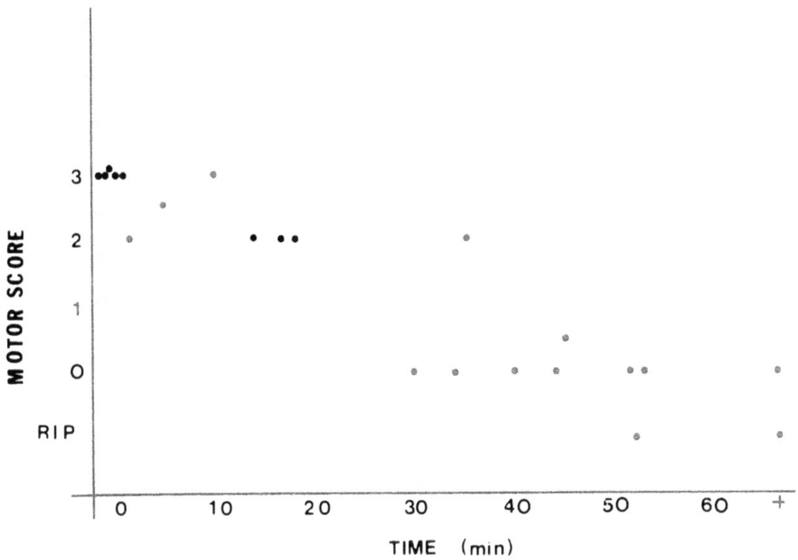

Fig. 8. Comparison of change in the somatosensory evoked response (SSEP) and subsequent motor score of animals (N = 22) receiving dynorphin (i.t. 50-200 nmol) while anesthetized with ketamine. After recording a baseline cortical SSEP (control) the lumbosacral cord was exposed to dynorphin and the change in maximum peak amplitude over time was measured. All animals with a 50% reduction of the maximum peak amplitude of the SSEP for <30 min were weight bearing the following day (Motor score 3 is normal and 0 is paralyzed). Animals (88%) with a 50% reduction of the maximum peak response for greater than 30 min were subsequently paralyzed or expired (RIP). All animals receiving 50-200 nmol of dynorphin with halothane anesthesia were consistently paralyzed.

(Lodge and Anis, 1984). We are currently examining the interaction of ketamine and dynorphin when simultaneously applied to the spinal cord.

Acknowledgements

The authors would like to thank Ms. Rhoda King for expert histological support during this study, Ms. Karen Daniel and Mrs. Jean Paige for preparation of the manuscript, and Dr. Ray Genovese for assistance in preparing the histopathology charts. "The views of the author do not purport to reflect the positions of the Department of the Army of the Department of Defense. (Para. 4-3, AR 360-365). Research was conducted in compliance with the Animal Welfare Act, and other Federal statutes and regulations relating to animals and experiments involving animals and adheres to principles stated in the Guide for the Care and Use of Laboratory Animals, NIH Publication 86-23, 1985 edition."

References

Berenstein, A., Young, W., Ranshoff, J., Benjamin, V., and Merkin, H.: Somatosensory evoked potentials (SEP) during spinal angiography and therapeutic transvascular embolization. J. Neurosurg. 60: 777-785, 1983.

Caudle, R.M. and Isaac, L.: Influence of Dynorphin (1-13) on spinal reflexes in the rat. J. Pharmacol. Exp. Ther. 246: 508-513, 1988.

Corssen, G. and Domino, E.F.: Dissociative anesthesia: Further pharmacologic studies and first clinical experiences with the phencyclidine derivative CI-581. Anesth. Analg. 45: 29-40, 1966.

DeGirolami, U. and Zivin, J.A.: Neuropathology of experimental spinal cord ischemia in the rabbit. J. Neuropathol. Exp. Neurol. 41: 129-149, 1982.

Idvall, J.: Influence of ketamine anesthesia on cardiac output and tissue perfusion in rats subjected to hemorrhage. Anesthesiol. 55: 297-304, 1981.

Idvall, J., Aronsen, K.F., and Stenberg, P.: Tissue perfusion and distribution of cardiac output during ketamine anesthesia in normovolemic rats. Acta Anesth. Scand. 24: 257-263, 1980.

Kobrine, A.J., Evans, D.E., and Rizzoli, H.V.: Experimental acute balloon compression of the spinal cord: Factors affecting disappearance and return of the spinal evoked response. J. Neurosurg. 51: 841-845, 1979.

Lodge, D. and Anis, N.A.: Effects of ketamine and three other anesthetics on spinal reflexes and inhibitions in the cat. Br. J. Anesth. 56: 1143-1151, 1984.

Long, J.B., Kinney, R.C., Malcolm, D.S., Graeber, G.M., and Holaday, J.W.: Intrathecal dynorphin A 1-13 and dynorphin A 3-13 reduce rat spinal cord blood flow by non-opioid mechanisms. Brain Res. 436: 374-379, 1987.

Marcoux, F.W., Goodrich, J.E., and Dominick, M.A.: Ketamine prevents ischemic neuronal injury. Brain Res. 452: 329-335, 1988.

Moskowitz, M.A., Saito, K., Brezina, L., and Dickson, J.: Nerve fibers surrounding intracranial and extracranial vessels from human and other species contain dynorphin-like immunoreactivity. Neurosci. 23: 731-737, 1987.

Petras, J.M. and Long, J.B.: Dynorphin and somatostatin induce spinal cord injury: Neuroanatomical findings in the rat. Neurol. 39: 388, 1989.

Przewlocki, R., Shearman, G.T., and Herz, A.: Mixed opioid/ nonopioid effects of dynorphin and dynorphin related peptides after their intrathecal injection in rats. Neuropeptides 3: 233-240, 1983.

Rigamonti, D.D., Long, J.B., Tortella, F.C., Gussio, R.P., Martinez-Arizala, A., and Holaday, J.W.: Somatosensory evoked potentials following intrathecal Dynorphin A 1-13 injection in the rat. Soc. Neurosci. Abstr. 13: 474, 1987.

Rigamonti, D.D., Martinez-Arizala, A., Genovese, R.F., Holaday, J.W., and

Long, J.B.: MK-801 neuroprotective effects in a rodent model of peptide induced spinal cord injury: A histological study. Soc. Neurosci. Abstr. 14: 1113, 1989.

Robertson, C.S., Foltz, R., Grossman, R.G., and Goodman, J.C.: Protection against experimental spinal cord injury. J. Neurosurg. 64: 633-642, 1986.

Schramm, J. and Jones, S.J., Eds.: Spinal Cord Monitoring. 1st Edition, Springer-Verlag, Berlin, 1985.

KEY WORD INDEX

This index is based upon key words and therefore is incomplete. The reader should refer to the Table of Contents for individual chapters that summarize in detail various topics related to ketamine.

www.ingramcontent.com/pod-product-compliance
Ingram Content Group UK Ltd.
Pitfield, Milton Keynes, MK11 3LW, UK
UKHW052229270726
14060UKWH00004B/682

9 780916 1823